D0931416

TEXTBOOK OF VETERINARY HISTOLOGY

TEXTBOOK OF VETERINARY HISTOLOGY

H.-DIETER DELLMANN

Professor of Veterinary Anatomy
Iowa State University
Ames, Iowa

ESTHER M. BROWN

Professor of Veterinary Anatomy
University of Missouri
Columbia, Missouri

Third Edition

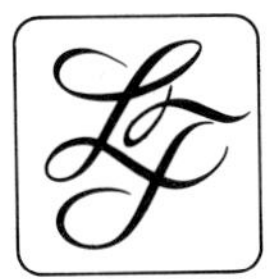

LEA & FEBIGER *Philadelphia* *1987*

Lea & Febiger
600 Washington Square
Philadelphia, PA 19106-4198
U.S.A.
(215) 922-1330

First Edition, 1976
Reprinted, 1978
Spanish Edition by Editorial Acribia, Zargoza, Spain
Japanese Edition by Gakusosha Company, Tokyo, Japan
Italian Edition by Grasso, Bologna, Italy
Portuguese Edition by Editora Guanabara Koogan, Rio de Janeiro, Brazil

Second Edition, 1981
Reprinted, 1983

Library of Congress Cataloging-in-Publication Data

Dellmann, H.-Dieter.
Textbook of veterinary histology.

Bibliography: p.
Includes index.
1. Veterinary histology. I. Brown, Esther Marie, 1923- . II. Title.
SF757.3.D438 1986 636.089'1018 85-23801
ISBN 0-8121-1010-2

Copyright © 1987 by Lea & Febiger. Copyright under the International Copyright Union. All Rights Reserved. This book is protected by copyright. No part of it may be reproduced in any manner or by any means without written permission from the publisher.

PRINTED IN THE UNITED STATES OF AMERICA

Print number: 3 2 1

Preface

The wide distribution and use of the second edition of this textbook has been rewarding to all the authors and has provided great incentive and encouragement during the preparation of the third edition. As with the previous editions, this edition is intended primarily for courses in veterinary histology. We have not deviated from our original concept of limiting the text to those facts considered essential for veterinary medical students. We are convinced that this book provides a solid basis for the understanding of microscopic structure and related functions and prepares the student well for other areas such as Physiology, Pharmacology, Pathology, Theriogenology, and Immunology.

Extensive rewriting and updating, often incorporating comments and suggestions from histologists all over the world, together with the expert contributions of several new authors, have produced a textbook that we are proud to present to our readers.

We wish to thank Barbara Bremer and Glenda Burkheimer for typing the manuscript. A special thanks goes to Gary Brimer for numerous histologic preparations and help in the darkroom. We also wish to express our gratitude to Amy S. Norwitz and Samuel A. Rondinelli, from Lea & Febiger, for their suggestions, their attention to detail, and their patience in the successful completion of this third edition.

We hope that this textbook will continue to support veterinary students in their pursuit of knowledge and to aid veterinary histologists in their teaching endeavors.

Ames, Iowa H.-Dieter Dellmann
Columbia, Missouri Esther M. Brown

Contributors

Adams, D.R.
Dept. of Veterinary Anatomy
College of Veterinary Medicine
Iowa State University
Ames, Iowa

Björkman, Nils
Professor
Dept. of Anatomy
Veterinary and Agricultural University
Copenhagen, Denmark

Brown, Esther M.
Professor
Department of Veterinary Biomedical Sciences
College of Veterinary Medicine
University of Missouri
Columbia, Missouri

Calhoun, M. Louis
Distinguished Emeritus Professor
Anatomy Department
College of Veterinary Medicine
Michigan State University
East Lansing, Michigan

Cardinet, G.H., III
Department of Anatomy
Davis School of Veterinary Medicine
University of California
Davis, California

Collier, Linda
Department of Veterinary Pathology
College of Veterinary Medicine
University of Missouri
Columbia, Missouri

Dantzer, Vibeke
Associate Professor
Department of Anatomy
Veterinary and Agricultural University
Copenhagen, Denmark

Dellmann, H.-Dieter
Professor
Department of Veterinary Anatomy, Physiology, and Pharmacology
College of Veterinary Medicine
Iowa State University
Ames, Iowa

Fletcher, Thomas F.
Professor of Veterinary Anatomy
Department of Veterinary Biology
College of Veterinary Medicine
University of Minnesota
St. Paul, Minnesota

Nicander, Lennart
The Veterinary College of Norway
Department of Anatomy
Norway

Plopper, C.G.
Department of Anatomy
Davis School of Veterinary Medicine
University of California
Davis, California

Priedkalns, Jānis
Elder Professor
Department of Anatomy and Histology
Faculty of Medicine
University of Adelaide
Adelaide, South Australia

Stinson, Al W.
Professor
Anatomy Department
College of Veterinary Medicine
Michigan State University
East Lansing, Michigan

Venable, John H.
Professor
Department of Anatomy
Colorado State University
Fort Collins, Colorado

Wrobel, Karl-Heinz
Professor
Lehrstuhl für Morphologie und Anatomie
Universität Regensburg
Regensburg, Germany

Contents

1

Cytology

H.-DIETER DELLMANN

The cell is the smallest structural unit of living material of a multicellular organism. Surrounded by the cell membrane, the cell is composed of a membrane-bounded nucleus and cytoplasm that contains specialized organelles and inclusions.

STRUCTURAL ORGANIZATION OF THE CELL

Cellular shape, size, and structure vary widely and express adaptations for the specific functions of each cell in specialized tissues and organs. However, despite varying degrees of functional differentiation and thus variation in cell structure, most cells share general structural characteristics (Fig. 1–1).

Cytoplasmic Organelles

Organelles are small structures whose particular organization gives them a specific function in the metabolism of the cell. Organelles lie within the ground substance, or hyaloplasm, an aqueous gel composed of proteins (including various enzymes), lipids, and carbohydrates, either alone or forming combinations such as lipoproteins, glycoproteins, proteoglycans, or mucoproteins. It also contains various inorganic materials such as Ca^{++}, Na^{+}, and K^{+}. All these constituents play a role in cell function and in the maintenance of the intracellular environment.

Most cytoplasmic organelles, in addition to the nucleus, are bounded by similarly structured membranes that participate in numerous cell functions, such as protein synthesis, secretion, phagocytosis, respiration, and transmembrane transport.

CELL MEMBRANE. Also known as the plasma membrane, plasmalemma, or cytolemma, the membrane surrounding the cell measures 8 to 10 nm in width and thus is too thin to be resolved with the light microscope (LM), unless the membrane is sectioned obliquely and enough of the cell coat is exposed to stain, or the membrane-coat complex is thick enough to absorb stain.

With the electron microscope (EM), the cell membrane can be visualized as a trilaminar membrane consisting of an outer and inner lamina, each lamina electron-dense and about 2.5 nm thick, and an electron-lucent intermediate lamina about 3 nm thick (Fig. 1–2). Models of the plasmalemma have been determined using a variety of special physical and chemical techniques. The most widely accepted one is the fluid mosaic model of Singer and Nicholson. According to this model, the

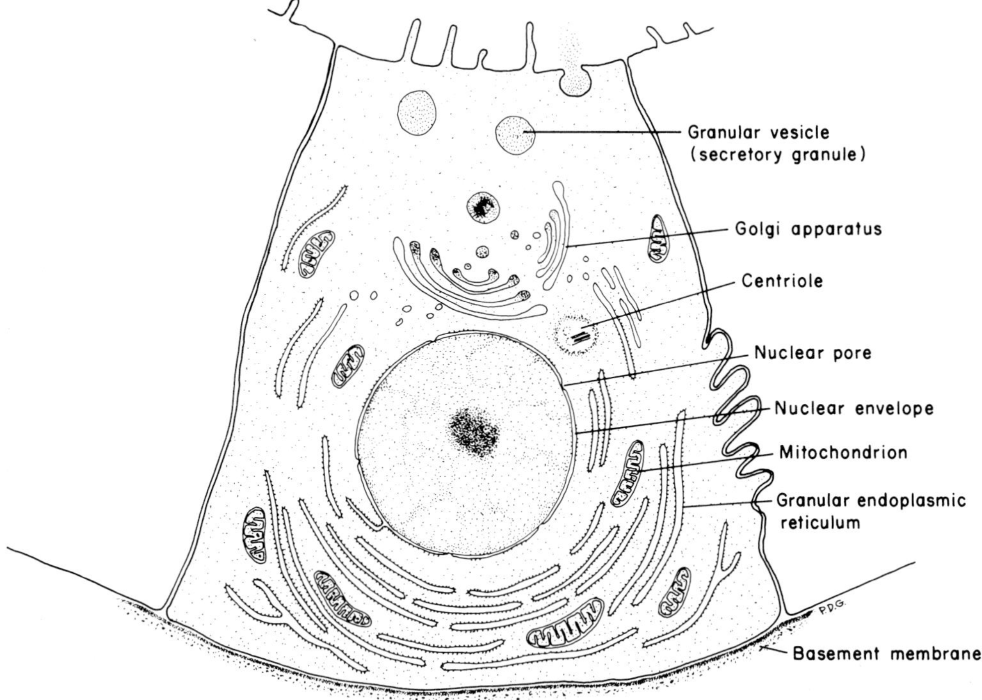

Fig. 1–1. *Schematic drawing of the general organization of a cell.*

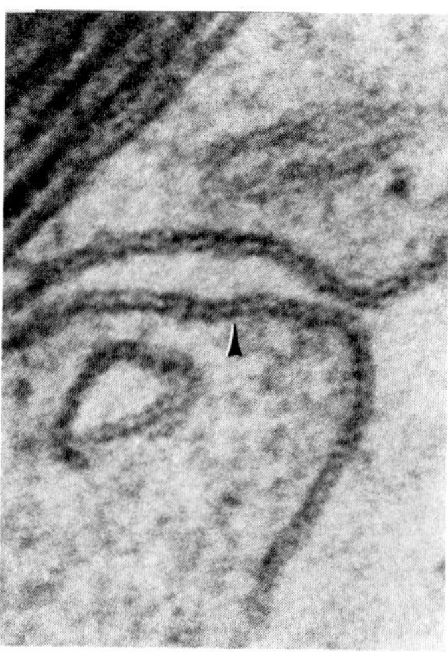

Fig. 1–2. *Electron micrograph of the infolded trilaminar plasma membrane (arrow) of a neurolemmocyte. ×327,680.*

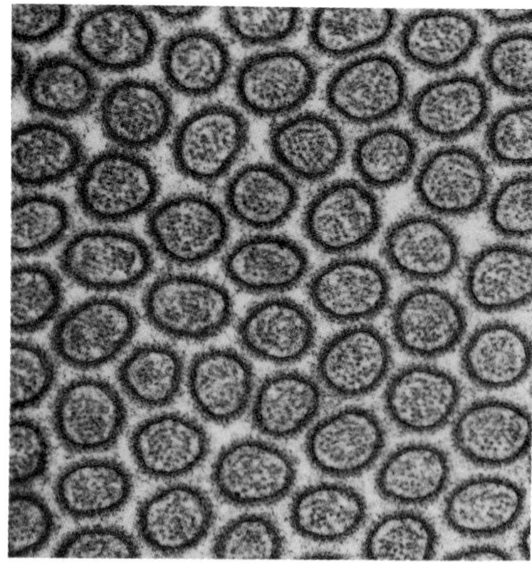

Fig. 1–3. *Cross section through microvilli of an intestinal absorptive cell, small intestine, rat. Notice the distinct glycocalyx and the cross sections of numerous actin filaments. ×66,000.*

cell membrane consists of two leaflets composed primarily of phospholipid molecules that are arranged perpendicularly to the cell surface. The polar, hydrophilic ends of these molecules face both the cytoplasmic and extracellular surfaces; their nonpolar, hydrophobic ends oppose each other in the center of the membrane, which is likewise the preferential site of cholesterol molecules. Within this lipid bilayer lie the proteins, most of which are intrinsic and amphipathetic, with their hydrophilic ends protruding from the outer or inner membrane surface and with their hydrophobic ends embedded among the hydrophobic fatty acids in the center of the membrane. Some proteins (transmembrane proteins) may cross the membrane and protrude at both surfaces. Extrinsic proteins are present at the cytoplasmic surface in contact with either intrinsic proteins or the polar ends of the phospholipid molecules. Membrane lipids and proteins are not necessarily in a fixed position but may change their location within the plane of the membrane; however, the lipids appear to be confined largely to their own monolayer.

Carbohydrates that are attached to the membrane lipids or proteins protrude from the external surface of the membrane. This extrinsic cell coat, referred to as glycocalyx, is present on all cells; on some cells, as for example on the microvilli of the intestinal absorptive cells, it is particularly dense (Fig. 1–3) (see Chapter 2).

The cell membrane plays an essential role in cell function. It is selectively permeable, depending on the lipid content of the membrane, and it contains "pumps" that regulate ion concentrations within the cell and in its immediate vicinity. The cell membrane also contains a variety of enzymes. Body cells, especially in aggregates such as epithelia, are held together by their cell coats. Specific receptor sites within the cell coat mediate important cell functions, such as endocytosis and phagocytosis, antigen recognition, and antibody production; hormone-triggered cellular events likewise depend upon specific surface receptors.

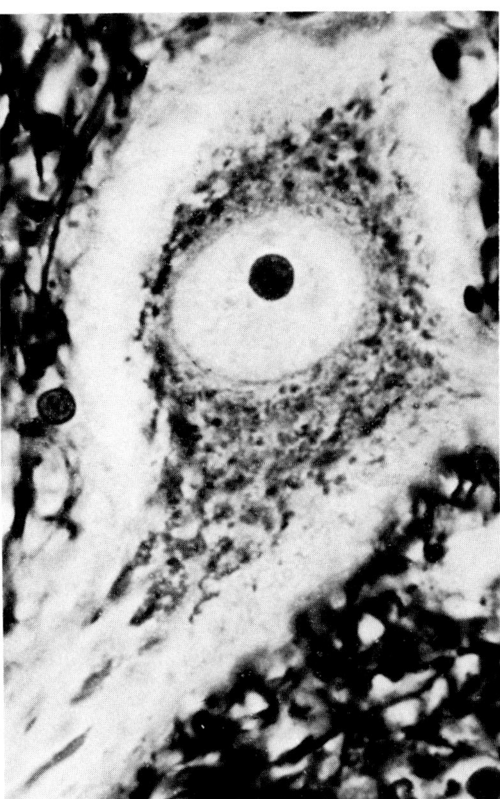

Fig. 1–4. *Motor nerve cell from the spinal cord, dog. The ergastoplasm or chromatophilic substance is visible as dark, pleomorphic masses throughout the cytoplasm. The nucleus contains a distinct nucleolus. Cresyl violet–Luxol fast blue. ×1100.*

ENDOPLASMIC RETICULUM. The endoplasmic reticulum occurs in two functionally and structurally distinct varieties, the rough-surfaced endoplasmic reticulum (rER) and the smooth endoplasmic reticulum (sER).

The *rough endoplasmic reticulum* consists of a continuous network of flat and wide sacs, referred to as cisternae (see Fig. 1–5). The cytoplasmic surface of the limiting membrane is studded with ribosomes (thus the designation "rough"). Aggregates of rER appear as basophilic regions within many cells, such as nerve cells (Fig. 1–4) and pancreatic acinar cells. These regions are referred to as the ergastoplasm or chromidial substance. The rER functions primarily in the biosynthesis of a large variety of proteins destined for either extracellular or intracellular use (e.g., secretory proteins, lysosomal proteins, membrane proteins) and is thus abundant in protein-secreting cells, such as pancreatic acinar cells and plasma cells, but it occurs likewise in virtually all nucleated cells. Another important function of the rER is the glycosylation of proteins to form glycoproteins, which takes place at the luminal site of the rER membranes.

Ribosomes are small particles (15 × 25 nm in diameter) composed of a large and a small subunit. Prior to protein synthesis, these two subunits exist as separate entities. The large subunit consists of three molecules of rRNA and approximately 45 different proteins; the small subunit consists of one molecule of rRNA and about 33 different proteins. The ribosome has two grooves, one for the mRNA and one for the growing polypeptide chain. Protein synthesis at the ribosomes begins with the binding of the small ribosomal subunit, which initially is still a separate entity, to the initiation site of a mRNA, with the aid of an initiator tRNA inserted at a P site (see below) and the subsequent attachment of the large subunit. Thus a functional ribosome is formed, which will now begin the synthesis of a protein chain with the insertion of a tRNA at an A site.

Each ribosome contains two binding sites for tRNAs. One site holds the tRNA attached to the growing end of the polypeptide chain (P site); the other site holds the tRNA that carries the amino acid to be added to the polypeptide chain (A site). Following the binding of tRNA to the A site, the tRNA at the P site uncouples from the last amino acid of the growing polypeptide chain, which at the same time is joined by a peptide bond to the new amino acid at the A site. Finally the ribosome moves one codon (three nucleotides) along the mRNA, releasing the uncoupled tRNA from the P site and moving the tRNA from the A site to the P site, thus freeing the A site for the attachment of a new mRNA. The elongating polypeptide chain slides along its groove on the ribosome. If the protein to be synthesized is destined to be segregated into the cisternal lumen, a special signal peptide at the beginning of the growing polypeptide chain is thought to interact with a receptor protein on the ER membrane to which the ribosome attaches. This signal peptide is absent when the synthesized proteins are to be used by the cell. The polypeptide chain is then transferred across the membrane into the lumen of the cisterna, where it is released following completion of the translation process. At this time the ribosome detaches from the membrane and dissociates into its two subunits. If the proteins are synthesized within the cytosol, a new ribosome attaches to the mRNA as soon as the preceding one has moved far enough along the mRNA to make space for the new one. In this manner, polyribosomes or polysomes are formed (Fig. 1–5), indicating actively translating mRNA.

The *smooth endoplasmic reticulum* consists of a network of tubules that, in most cells, are the ribosome-free terminal portions of rER (referred to as transitional ER). These tubules give rise to transfer vesicles that carry substances synthesized within the rER to other locations, especially to the Golgi complex. In steroid hormone synthesizing cells and striated muscle cells, however, the sER carries out major cell functions and is more abundantly developed, consisting of single vesicles and an anastomosing network of tubules of rather uniform size, often in an irregular, tortuous, and entangled arrangement (Fig., 1–6). In these cells it may be visualized at the light-microscopic level with silver impregnation methods.

The sER participates in a wide variety of functions: steroid hormone synthesis in the testicular interstitial cells, the cells of the corpus luteum, and those of the adrenal cortex; synthesis of complex lipids and

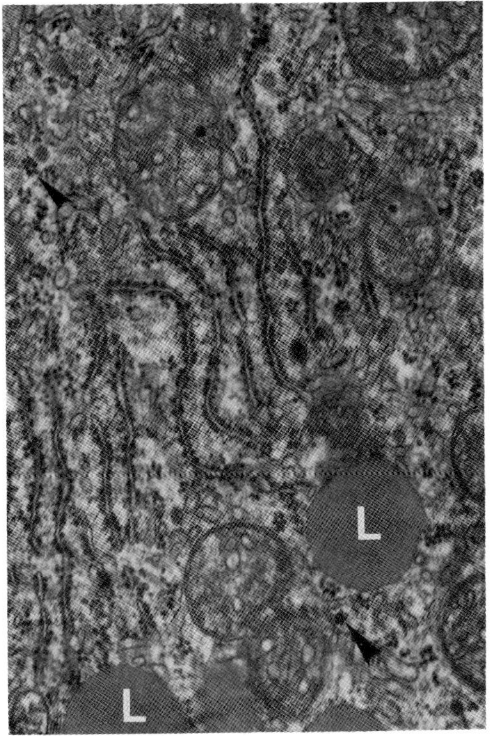

Fig. 1–5. *Cisternae of rough endoplasmic reticulum with their characteristic ribosomes; also notice the presence of polyribosomes (arrowheads) and lipid droplets (L). Luteal cell, rat. ×30,000.*

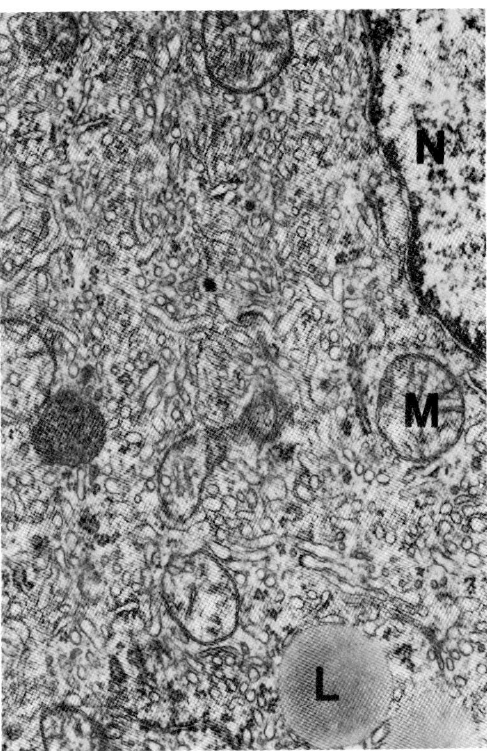

Fig. 1–6. *This cell contains an abundant smooth endoplasmic reticulum, mitochondria (M) and lipid droplets (L) in the vicinity of the nucleus (N). Adrenal cortex, rat. ×19,500.*

drug detoxification in hepatocytes; lipid resynthesis in the intestinal absorptive cells; release and capture of Ca^{++} ions in striated muscle cells; and concentration of Cl^{-} ions in gastric parietal cells.

ANNULATE LAMELLAE. Stacks of membrane-bounded cisternae with numerous pore complexes, identical to isolated nuclear envelopes, are present in germ cells and cells with high protein synthesis. Their functional significance is unknown.

GOLGI COMPLEX. The Golgi complex, or internal reticular apparatus, when stained with silver salts or osmium appears as a black network of cisternae. In routine light-microscopic preparations, it may be visible as a lighter-stained region called the negative Golgi image.

At the fine-structural level, the Golgi complex consists of one or several stacks of parallel membrane-bounded cisternae and associated vesicles and tubules at the lateral surfaces and at either face of the stacks (Fig. 1–7). Thus, one recognizes a *cis-face, stacks,* and a *trans-face.* The cis-face, also referred to as the forming face, consists of a network of tubules. These are adjacent to and continuous with the parallel saccules of the stack. A network of anastomosing tubules connects the saccules within each layer of the stack and also connects adjacent layers. The trans- or maturing face of the Golgi complex is composed of a tubular and cisternal network connected to the stack. The transmost cisternal element of the Golgi complex, frequently referred to as GERL (Golgi-associated ER involved in lysosome formation), should be considered an integral component of the Golgi complex that apparently shares many, and probably all, of its functions.

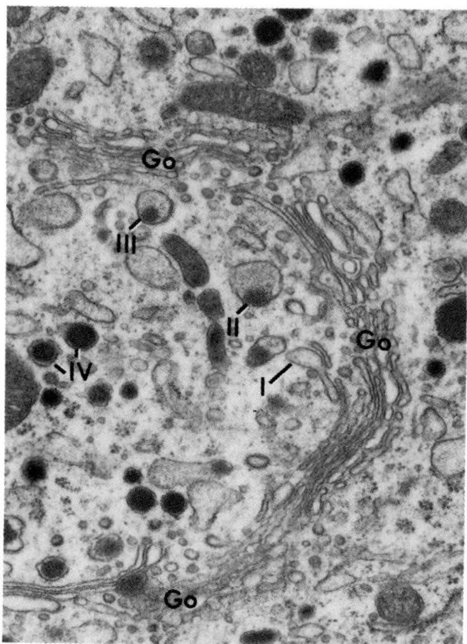

Fig. 1–7. *Electron micrograph of the Golgi complex (Go) and surrounding cytoplasm of a cell of the pars intermedia, adenohypophysis, rat. Notice the difference in the electron density of the content of the secretory vesicles in the concave (trans) side of the Golgi cisternae, Sequence of the maturation process of the secretory vesicles (I, II, III, IV).* ×*22,680.*

Proteins and membranes from the rER are transferred to the Golgi complex at the cis-face by means of transport vesicles (including coated vesicles). Within the cisternal lumen occurs covalent modification of the oligosaccharides that were coupled to proteins in the rER, terminal glycosylation, sulfation, and phosphorylation. The process of proteolytic conversion of protein prohormones is initiated in the Golgi complex. Proteins are concentrated and sorted into vesicles (condensing vacuoles or vesicles), which eventually separate from the Golgi complex at its trans-face.

Concentrated secretory proteins are contained within secretory vesicles that migrate toward the cell surface, where they are discharged from the cell by exocytosis. This process involves fusion of the vesicular membrane, formation of an opening, and delivery of the vesicular content into the extracellular space. Since this process involves integration of the vesicular membrane into the cell membrane, the surface area of the latter would increase in secretory cells if the vesicular membrane were not removed. After exocytosis, the vesicular membrane is indeed retrieved intact, a process called endocytosis, and it moves in vesicular form toward the dilated rims of the trans-Golgi cisternae and fuses with them to be reutilized in the secretory process. Endocytosis refers also to the uptake of substrates and their selective transport across (transcytosis) or within the cell. The uptake of fluid from the extracellular environment is called pinocytosis and gives rise to pinocytotic vesicles (Figs. 1–8 and 1–9). These are either macropinocytotic vesicles, visible at the LM level, or micropinocytotic vesicles, visible only with the EM.

LYSOSOMES. Most commonly, two general types of lysosomes are distinguished: primary lysosomes and secondary lysosomes. *Primary lysosomes* contain nothing but hydrolytic enzymes, while *secondary lysosomes* are the result of the fusion of primary lysosomes with a variety of membrane-bound substrates. *Primary lysosomes* originate as coated vesicles from the trans-most cisterna (GERL) of the Golgi complex (Fig. 1–8). As they move away from the Golgi complex, the primary lysosomes shed their clathrin coat and become smooth vesicles, which enables them to fuse with heterophagosomes, autophagosomes, secretory vesicles, and endocytotic vesicles to form secondary lysosomes of diverse structure. *Heterophagosomes* are formed by invagination of the plasma membrane around large particulate matter, such as bacteria.

When elements of the granular ER, mitochondria, and other cytoplasmic organelles lose their ability to function, they become segregated within segments of the sER and form *autophagosomes,* which subsequently fuse with primary lysosomes to form autophagic vacuoles (Fig. 1–8). *Crinophagic vacuoles* result from the fusion of

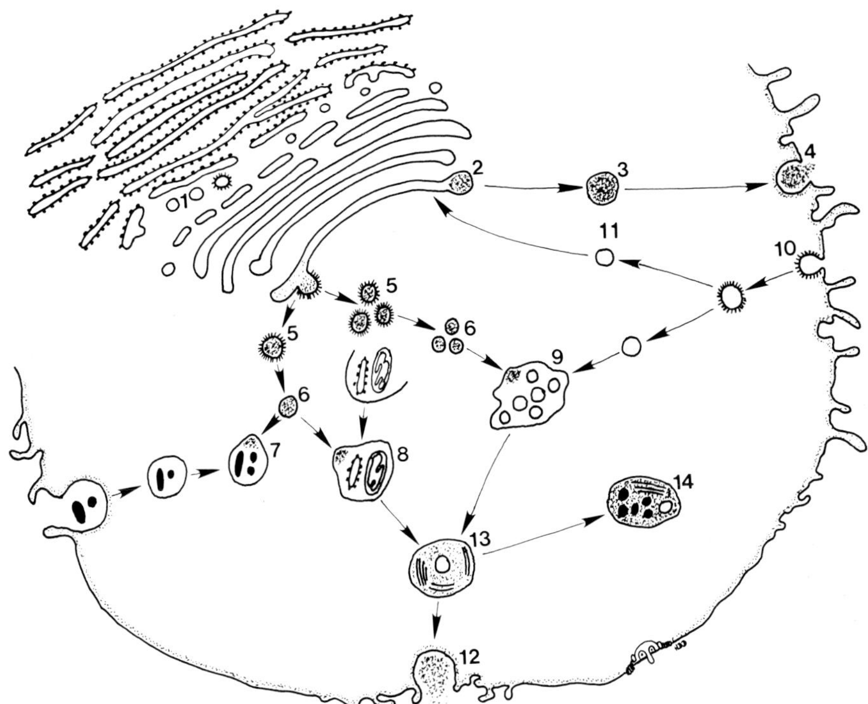

Fig. 1–8. *From the rER, transport vesicles (1) join the cis-face of the Golgi complex. Condensing vesicles (2) separate from the trans-face of the Golgi complex to form secretory vesicles (3) whose contents are released by exocytosis (4). In addition, primary lysosomes originate from the Golgi complex as coated vesicles (5), become smooth vesicles (6), and merge with heterophagosomes (7) of phagocytotic origin, autophagosomes (8), or multivesicular bodies (9) whose vesicles are of pinocytotic origin (10), to form secondary lysosomes. Pinocytotic vesicles may also be reincorporated into the Golgi complex (11). Secondary lysosomes may release the end product of lysosomal digestion from the cell (12). Indigestible residues within residual bodies (13) may be permanently stored as lipofuscin (14).*

aged, damaged, or excess secretory vesicles with primary lysosomes. *Multivesicular bodies* are a special form of heterolysosomes. They are large, membrane-bounded sacs containing varying numbers of small vesicles (50 to 75 nm in diameter), probably of pinocytotic origin, surrounded by lysosomal enzymes (Fig. 1–10).

Lysosomal enzymes are optimally active at pH 5. The lysosomal membrane is impermeable to these enzymes but not to terminal products of heterophagy, autophagy, and crinophagy (i.e., enzymatic digestion of the contents of secondary lysosomes), which diffuse through the membrane to be excreted or reutilized. However, the permeability of the bounding membrane may change under certain circumstances, such as lack of oxygen, regression of the mammary gland, or involution during embryonic development. The enzymes are then liberated into the cytoplasm and the cells are destroyed.

In advanced stages of degradation, laminated concentric membrane-bounded structures represent the indigestible residues of lysosomal activity and are variably referred to as *dense lamellar bodies, myelinated bodies,* or *residual bodies* (Fig. 1–11); they may also occur as *vacuolated dense bodies* (Fig. 1–12). The contents of these secondary lysosomes may either be released from the cell or remain permanently within the cell as lipofuscin pigment (Figs. 1–8 and 1–12).

PEROXISOMES. Peroxisomes are membrane-bounded spherical organelles with finely granular material and frequently

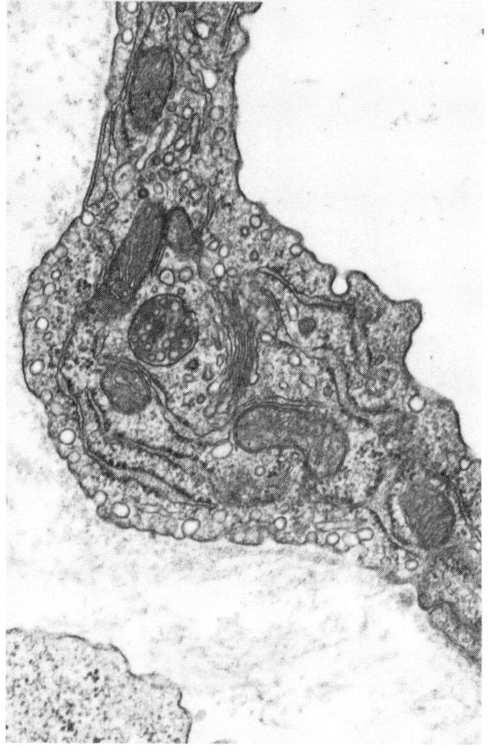

Fig. 1–9. *Numerous pinocytotic vesicles are forming at the surface and are present within the cytoplasm of this capillary endothelial cell. ×26,000.*

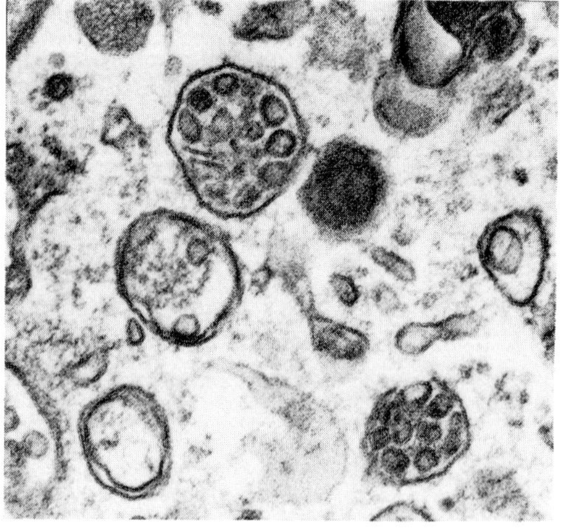

Fig. 1–10. *Multivesicular bodies, neurohypophysis, rat. ×66,000.*

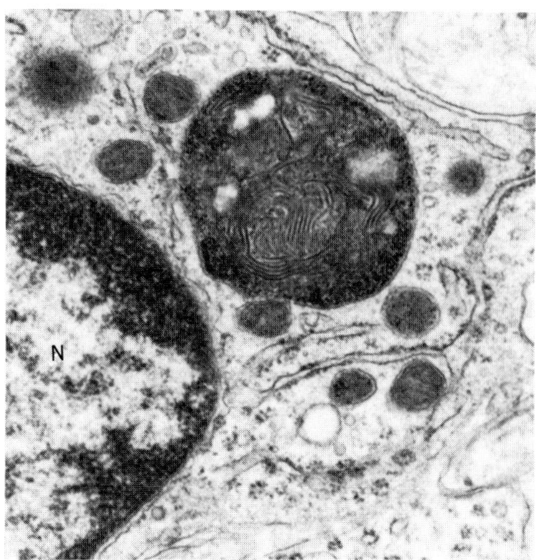

Fig. 1–11. *Large dense lamellar body in a corticotropic cell, adenohypophysis, rat. Nucleus (N) with peripheral heterochromatin. ×10,150.*

crystalline electron-dense inclusions, which are particularly abundant in hepatocytes and the epithelial cells of the proximal convoluted tubule of the kidney. They are a major site of oxygen utilization within the cell and are particularly rich in catalase and hydrogen peroxide. Peroxisomes are involved in various detoxifying reactions and in the breakdown of fatty acids to acetyl CoA.

MITOCHONDRIA. When living cells are stained with supravital dyes such as Janus Green B, mitochondria become visible as small rods or spheres approximately 0.2 μm in diameter and up to 12 μm long. Mitochondria are the chief source of ATP (energy) for the cell and are thus particularly numerous in cells with high metabolic activity. In many cells, mitochondria appear to be distributed randomly and change their location continually, while in others they are stationary at sites of high ATP consumption, such as in the basal processes of the epithelial cells of the convoluted tubules of the kidney (Fig. 1–13).

With the electron microscope, mitochondria are seen to be bounded by two membranes (Figs. 1–13 and 1–14). The outer

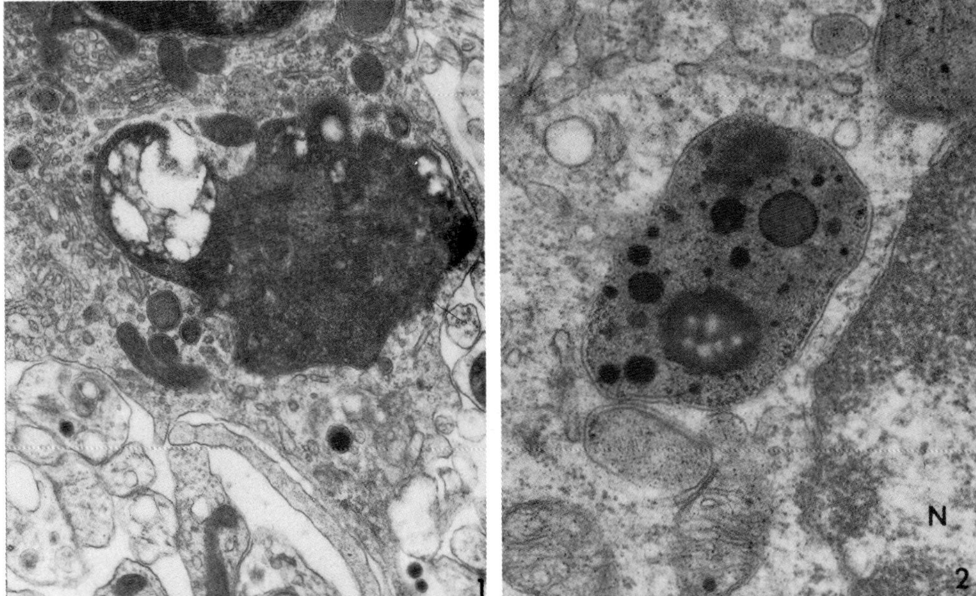

Fig. 1–12. *1, Vacuolated dense body in a glial cell, subfornical organ, rat.* ×*7900. 2, Lipofuscin granule in a corticotropic cell, adenohypophysis, rat. Nucleus (N).* ×*29,850.*

membrane is a smooth, saclike structure. The inner membrane is thrown into folds (cristae mitochondriales) (Fig. 1–13) or cylindric or prismatic tubules (tubuli) (Fig. 1–14) that project into the interior of the mitochondrion. On the inner surface of the inner membrane are located elementary particles that are part of a transmembrane protein (ATP synthetase) complex. Fatty acids and pyruvate, the end products of glycolysis in the cytoplasm, are transported into the mitochondrial matrix, where they are metabolized by matrix enzymes to produce acetyl CoA. This is enzymatically oxidized in the citric acid cycle, which yields mainly CO_2 and NADH (nicotinamide adenine dinucleotide hydride). NADH is the main source of electrons that are transported along the respiratory chain; its three major respiratory enzyme complexes are proteins embedded in the inner mitochondrial membrane. The energy generated during this transport is used to pump protons from the mitochondrial matrix into the intermembranous space, where they create an electrochemical proton gradient across the inner mitochondrial membrane. This drives protons back through the ATP synthetase, which synthesizes ATP from ADP and P_i in the mitochondrial matrix.

The inner membrane encloses a space occupied by the matrix, which contains occasional granules that are binding sites of calcium and other divalent cations. In addition, the mitochondrial matrix contains DNA of the circular (viral) type and ribosomal, transfer, and messenger RNAs. Mitochondria do not replicate by de novo synthesis, but grow and divide. This process involves two protein synthesis machineries, that of the mitochondrion and that of the cell (cytosol), from which proteins are transported into the mitochondrial matrix through the mitochondrial membranes.

Cytoskeleton

Microfilaments, myosin, intermediate filaments, and microtubules, together with a variety of proteins that interconnect these structures or link them to other structures

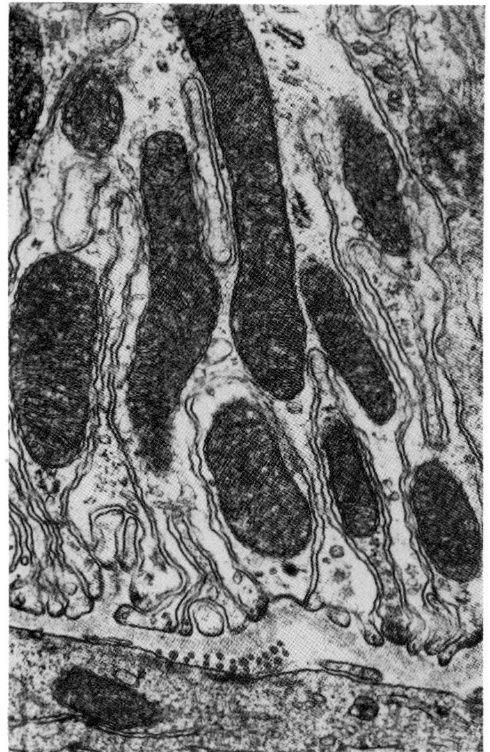

Fig. 1–13. *Mitochondria in the interdigitating processes of the cell base of adjacent cells of the proximal convoluted tubules of the kidney, rat.* ×*22,000.*

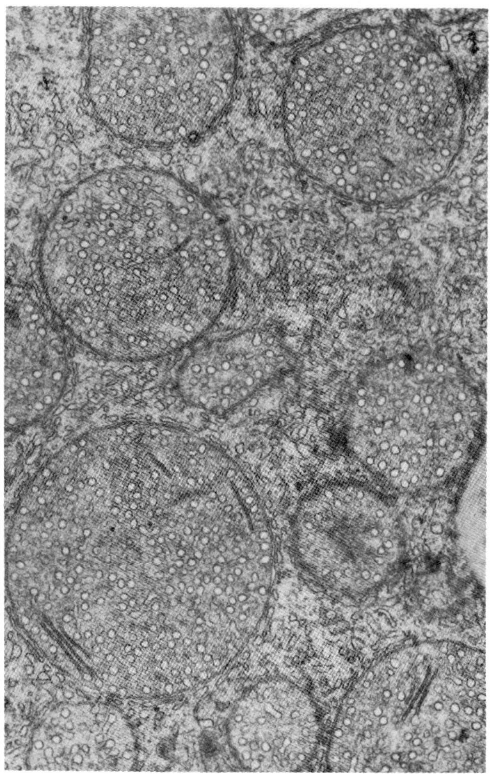

Fig. 1–14. *Mitochondria in the adrenal cortex, rat. The cylindric tubules of the inner membrane that project into the mitochondrial matrix are mostly cross sectioned.* ×*22,100.*

such as the plasma membrane or secretory granules, make up the *cytoskeleton.* They often form complex meshworks that maintain cell shape and stability and are responsible for cell movements.

Microfilaments are about 1.0 μm long and 5 to 8 nm in diameter. They are composed of the protein actin, which is associated with two accessory proteins, troponin and tropomyosin. Actin is one of the major components of muscle cells (for a more detailed description, see Chapter 5); it is present in a wide variety of other cells as well. For example, actin filaments are abundant in microvilli (Figs. 1–3 and 1–15) and stereocilia, in which they play a primarily supportive role. In migrating and growing cells such as macrophages and developing nerve cells, they are responsible for cell movements. Furthermore, actin filaments occur throughout the cytoplasm of virtually every cell and are in particularly high concentration in the subplasmalemmal cytoplasm, where they are attached to the proteins in the plasma membrane.

Myosin in its thick filamentous form (about 1.5 μm long and 15 nm in diameter) occurs only in muscle cells (see Chapter 5). Almost all mammalian cells, however, contain myosin in the small filamentous form, usually not detectable with the electron microscope. The interaction of this myosin with cytoplasmic actin filaments is responsible for changes in cell shape and movements of the cell surface and of the entire cell, as well as for the separation of dividing cells.

Intermediate filaments measure 8 to 10 nm in diameter and are of varying chemical composition. They include *neurofilaments* of

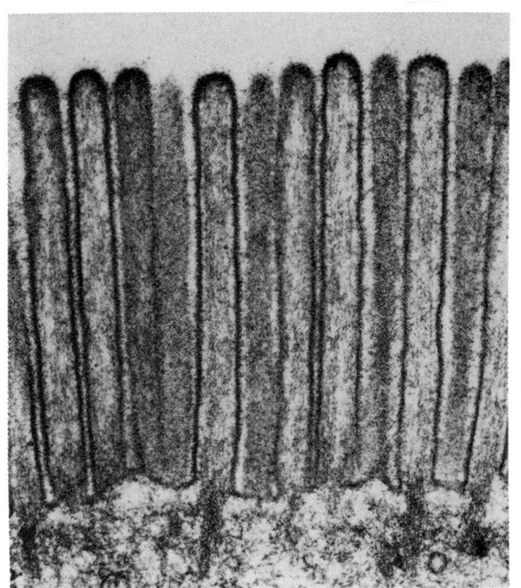

Fig. 1–15. *The microvilli at the apical surface of an intestinal absorptive cell contain numerous microfilaments that project into the terminal web. ×39,000.*

neurons (Fig. 1–16), *glial filaments* in astrocytes, and *keratin filaments,* also referred to as tonofilaments, of epithelial cells. *Vimentin* filaments are present in most other cells (for example, fibroblasts) and coexist with other intermediate fibrillary proteins such as desmin in muscle (see Chapter 5) and glial fibrillary acid protein in glial cells (see Chapter 6). The primary function of these filaments appears to be a structural one, i.e., they maintain cell shape, and since they are an integral part of spot desmosomes, they also play an important role in epithelial cell adhesion.

Microtubules vary in length and measure 25 nm in diameter. Protofilaments of globular tubulin polypeptides are assembled in the cytoplasm from tubulin dimers to form the microtubule wall. Usually 13 of these protofilaments are arranged side by side in a cross section of that wall. Microtubules are stable, permanent structures in cilia, flagella, centrioles, and basal bodies. Cytoskeletal microtubules and those of the mitotic spindle are highly labile structures and are in a continuous state of assembly and disassembly. Antimitotic drugs such as colchicine and vincristine inhibit microtubule assembly and thus cell division by preventing the addition of tubulin dimers and by inducing microtubule depolymerization.

In addition to their essential role in cell division, microtubules have the distinct cytoskeletal function of determining the distribution of microfilaments and intermediate filaments within the cell and thus specifying their polarity. Microtubules are, for example, essential for the growth of processes in developing nerve cells as well as for the transport of various organelles (see page 121) from the perikaryon to the

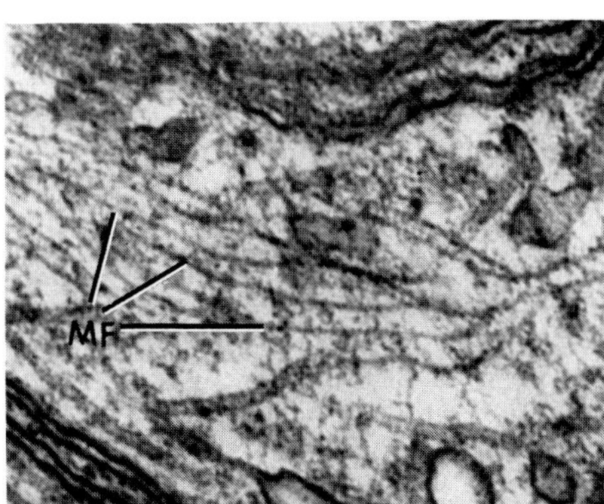

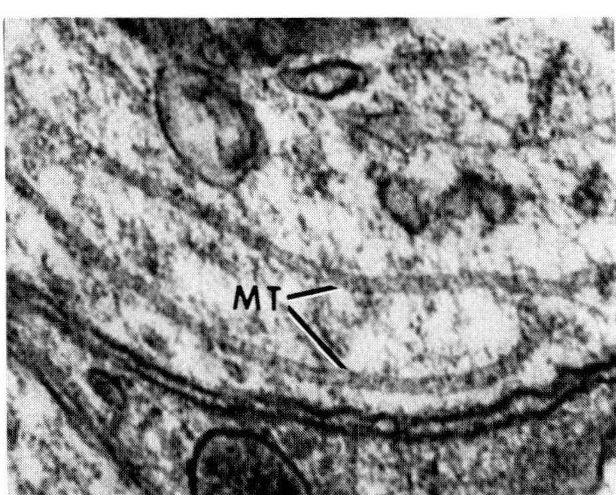

Fig. 1–16. *Electron micrographs of microfilaments (MF) and microtubules (MT) in neurosecretory nerve fibers, neurohypophysis, rat. ×55,060.*

periphery (Fig. 1–16). Exactly how these movements take place is still unknown.

In interphase cells, microtubules terminate in a special region of the cell, the *cell center* or centrosome, that contains a pair of *centrioles.* At the fine structural level, a centriole is composed of nine groups of three microtubules in longitudinal and parallel arrangement. They form a cylinder 0.1 to 0.2 μm in diameter and 0.2 to 0.3 mm long and are thus barely visible with the light microscope. Each centriole is surrounded by finely granular, pericentriolar material that appears to be the organizing center for cytoplasmic microtubules.

The orderly arranged microtubules of cilia (see p. 17) terminate in *basal bodies* whose structure is essentially identical to that of centrioles.

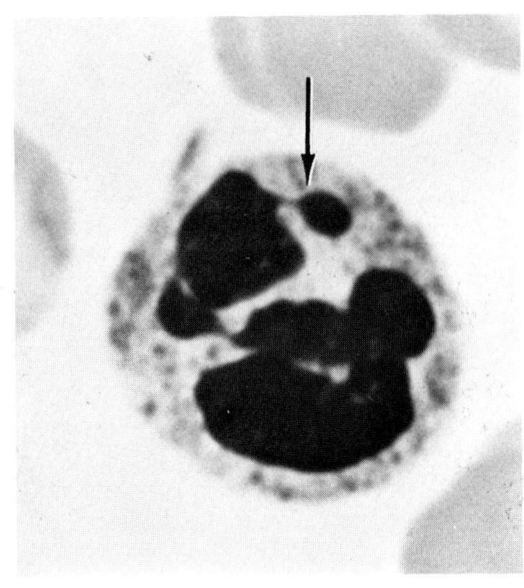

Fig. 1–17. *Sex chromatin (arrow), polymorphonuclear leukocyte, large ruminant. ×3300.*

Cytoplasmic Inclusions

GLYCOGEN. Glycogen, the major storage form of carbohydrate, is particularly abundant in liver cells. In routine histologic sections, glycogen remains unstained, but it can be demonstrated selectively by the PAS reaction or Best's carmine stain. At the fine-structural level, glycogen occurs either as single, electron-dense granules 10 to 40 nm in diameter (β particles) or as larger assemblies of these granules, forming rosette configurations called α particles.

LIPID. Fat is stored primarily in adipose cells, but is also present in a variety of other cells. Since most routine histologic techniques involve the use of fat solvents, lipids, are demonstrated only with special techniques, such as osmic acid fixation, which renders fat resistant to extraction, or Sudan III-stained frozen sections. With the electron microscope, lipid is seen in the form of droplets devoid of a bounding membrane and of varying size, shape, and electron density (Figs. 1–5 and 1–6).

MELANIN. This dark-brown to black pigment occurs primarily in the eye and in the common integument where it is synthesized by melanocytes and secreted as melanin granules, which are incorporated by the keratinocytes.

HEMOSIDERIN. This pigment is the result of hemoglobin degradation following phagocytosis of erythrocytes by the macrophages of the spleen, liver, bone marrow, and hemal lymph nodes. This golden-brown pigment contains iron, which permits its distinction from other pigments of similar color. With the electron microscope, dense particles of ferritin, an iron-containing protein, are visible within hemosiderin.

LIPOFUSCIN. Golden-brownish aggregates of lipofuscin, stainable with certain fat dyes, are commonly found in cardiac muscle, liver, and some nerve cells. Lipofuscin is composed of the indigestible residues of phagocytosis, autophagy, and crinophagy and is thus the morphologically heterogeneous end product of lysosomal activity (Fig. 1–12). Since the amount of pigment increases with the age of the animal, lipofuscin inclusions are often referred to as "wear-and-tear" pigment.

Nucleus

The nucleus carries information about the multiple functions of cells and the organism in deoxyribonucleic acid (DNA), which when combined with basic proteins forms deoxyribonucleoprotein (DNP). Although all the cells of a given organism contain the same genetic information in their DNA, repression and derepression of genes varies among different cell types and thus accounts for differences in structure and function. DNA serves as a template for messenger, transfer, and ribosomal ribonucleic acids (RNA), which are transferred to the cytoplasm where they are involved in the translation of the encoded message into the synthesis of proteins. Cells are most commonly observed during interphase of the cell cycle, when they perform their various specialized functions. Most commonly, nuclei are spherical to ovoid, but they may also be spindle-shaped (smooth muscle), bean- or kidney-shaped (monocytes), or multilobulated (neutrophilic leukocytes) (Fig. 1–17). The interphase nucleus contains chromatin and one nucleolus or several nucleoli within its nucleoplasm and is surrounded by the nuclear envelope.

NUCLEAR ENVELOPE. The nuclear envelope consists of two concentric membranes separated by a perinuclear space 25 nm wide. The outer nuclear membrane may be studded with ribosomes, and it is continuous with the membranes of both the rER and the sER (Fig. 1–18). It is thus part of the secretory machinery of the cell and as such may contain secretory products in secretory cells. At the inner surface of the inner membrane, polypeptides that bind to membrane proteins and to which specific sites of (hetero-) chromatin are attached form a granular lamina. The nuclear envelope, granular lamina, and attached heterochromatin account for the staining affinity of the nuclear envelope as seen with the LM. The nuclear envelope is interrupted by numerous pores where the outer and inner nuclear membranes fuse. Together with large protein granules in octagonal arrangement and a central granule within the pore, they form nuclear pore complexes, through which the nucleus communicates with the cytoplasm (Fig. 1–18).

CHROMATIN. Chromatin represents the DNP of chromosomes and occurs in two forms, heterochromatin and euchromatin. With the light microscope *heterochromatin* is visible as irregular clumps or threads of basophilic material, often preferentially located at the nuclear periphery (Fig. 1–11) or scattered throughout the nucleus, or found in association with the nucleolus (nucleolus-associated chromatin). Heterochromatin consists of the tightly coiled portions of chromosomes that lie entangled within the nucleus. Here genes are repressed and transcription does not take place. Heterochromatin is thus the predominant form of chromatin in relatively inactive cells. Uncoiled portions of chromatin, known as *euchromatin,* in which information is transcribed from DNA responsible for directing protein synthesis in the cytoplasm, remain essentially unstained and are thus indistinguishable from nucleoplasm. Euchromatin is particularly abundant in relatively active cells. The fine-structural correlates of hetero- and euchromatin are readily identified with the EM as regions of granular material of varying electron density (Fig. 1–11). Because of the high degree of coiling, tangling, and folding, details of chromatin fine structure that can be demonstrated with special in vivo techniques are not apparent.

Most mammalian nuclei are sexually dimorphic, since one of the paired chromosomes remains heterochromatic during interphase in the female. This sex chromatin (Barr body) appears either as an almost spherical chromatin condensation underneath the nuclear envelope of most cells of females or as a prominent nuclear appendage in neutrophilic leukocytes (Fig. 1–17).

NUCLEOLUS. The nucleolus is a conspicuous, spherical, basophilic organelle (Fig. 1–4) within which the subunits of ribosomes (ribosomal RNA) are synthesized be-

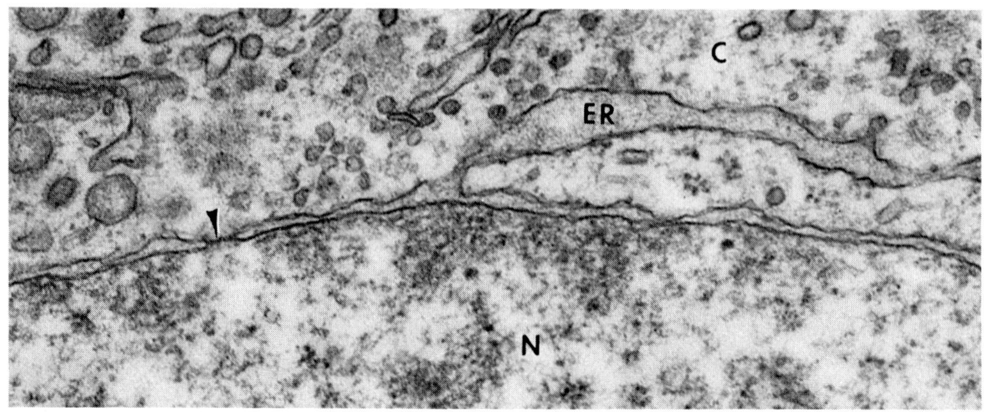

Fig. 1–18. *Electron micrograph of part of the nucleus (N) and the cytoplasm (C) of a glial cell, neurohypophysis, large ruminant. The nuclear envelope contains pores (arrow) closed by a diaphragm. Notice the continuity between the outer nuclear membrane and the endoplasmic reticulum (ER).* ×60,000.

fore their release into the cytoplasm, where they undergo changes before their assembly into ribosomes. Nucleoli are permanently located at specific constrictions of certain chromosomes, the nucleolar organizing sites, where that portion of DNA that is transcribed to ribosomal RNA is located.

With the electron microscope the nucleolus is seen to be composed of granular RNP (pars granulosa) and fibrillar RNP (pars fibrosa), which is supposedly an immature form of the RNP granules.

CELL DIVISION

Maintenance of most cell populations of the mature organism and proliferation of cells during growth occur through cell division. The life cycle of a somatic cell (as opposed to the reproductive or germ cell) is divided into two phases. The phase between divisions is called the *interphase,* during which the exact replication of the genetic material takes place. In the dividing phase, referred to as *mitosis,* the DNA is equally distributed to the daughter cells, enabling them to perform the same functions as the mother cell.

Interphase

Interphase is subdivided into three phases. The G_1 (gap 1) or *preduplication phase* is the period between the previous mitosis and the beginning of DNA duplication. Most cells are in this stage while they perform their particular functions. For example, adult nerve cells never divide, but remain in the G_1 phase during the lifetime of the organism. During the following S or *synthesis phase,* DNA replication occurs, resulting in two daughter chromosomes, each of which consists of 50% original (parental) and 50% replicated (new) DNA. The daughter chromosomes are referred to as *chromatids* as long as they remain attached to the centromere, where the spindle microtubules are later attached. Following completion of the S phase and before mitosis begins, the cell passes through a rather short G_2 (gap 2) or *postduplication phase.* During this phase the duplication of the centrioles, which began during S phase, is completed.

Mitosis

Mitosis lasts between 30 and 90 minutes. Although a continuous event, it is divided into four consecutive phases: (1) prophase, (2) metaphase, (3) anaphase, and (4) telophase.

Upon entering *prophase,* the cell hypertrophies and assumes a spherical shape by

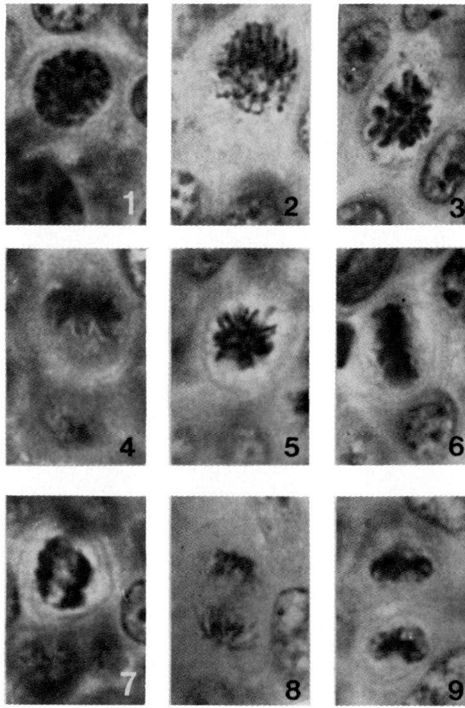

Fig. 1–19. *Mitotic divisions in the epithelial cells of the epiglottis, sheep. 1–3: Prophase, 4–6: metaphase; 7,8: anaphase; 9: telophase. H & E. ×1250. (Courtesy of A. Hansen.)*

retracting its processes and losing surface differentiations (Fig. 1–19). The chromosomes become visible, and as prophase proceeds they shorten, thicken, and coil and are seen to consist of two chromatids. The pairs of centrioles move to the opposite poles of the cell; microtubules begin to develop and eventually form the interpolar microtubules. In more advanced prophase, the nuclear envelope distintegrates and the nucleolus disappears. The cell becomes elongated.

When the chromosomes are arranged with their centromeres all in the same plane, the equatorial plane, the cell is in *metaphase* (Fig. 1–19). The arms of the bent chromosomes are directed toward the poles of the cell. On each side of the centromere is a small disklike structure, the kinetochore. After the nuclear envelope disintegrates, the kinetochore initiates the formation of chromosomal microtubules, so that the mitotic spindle now consists of two sets of microtubules.

The addition of colchicine to rapidly dividing cells in culture inhibits spindle formation and causes arrest of mitosis. The chromosomes also become more condensed, and because of their characteristic shapes, they can be used to establish the karyotype of an individual.

During *anaphase,* the centromere of each chromosome splits, and the separated chromatids of each chromosome, now called the daughter chromosomes, move to the opposite poles of the cell, while the mitotic spindle continues to elongate (Fig. 1–19).

Telophase is characterized by an elongation and unwinding of the chromosomes, with an ultimate return to the interphase condition (Fig. 1–19). At the same time the nuclear envelope begins to reassemble, and the nucleolus is reconstituted in association with the nucleolar organizer region of the chromosomes. The cleavage furrow, a constriction that began to develop late in anaphase, deepens in the middle of the elongated cell. The slender cytoplasmic bridge contains microtubules embedded in an electron-dense material, referred to as the midbody. The bridge eventually breaks and the two halves, one containing the midbody, retract to their respective daughter cells, thus completing cytokinesis.

Meiosis

In contrast to the somatic cells, which have a diploid set of chromosomes, the male and female reproductive cells (spermatozoon and oocyte) possess a haploid number of chromosomes. Since they derive from diploid precursors, these germ cells undergo a special type of division, during which the number of chromosomes is reduced by one half. This process is referred to as *meiosis* and will be discussed in detail in Chapter 12.

FUNCTIONAL MORPHOLOGY OF THE CELL

In the following paragraphs, cell structures will be discussed as they relate to specific cell functions. This will eliminate repetitious descriptions in the histology and organology chapters, where only those differences that reflect specialized functions of certain cells will be discussed.

Specializations for Cell Attachment and Communication

Intercellular attachments are visible with the light microscope. Examples are intercellular bridges with desmosomes in stratified squamous epithelium, and terminal bars between simple columnar epithelial cells. Detailed information, however, is obtained only with the electron microscope, which has led to the classification of intercellular attachments as adhering, impermeable, and communicating junctions.

ADHERING JUNCTIONS. Three types of junctions are classified as adhering junctions: belt desmosomes, spot desmosomes, and hemidesmosomes. The *belt desmosome,* or *zonula adherens,* surrounds epithelial cells in a belt-like fashion. The two plasma membranes are separated by a space 20 nm wide filled with filamentous intercellular material. On their cytoplasmic surface, the membranes are coated with electron-dense material closely associated with microfilaments coursing parallel to the plasma membrane and with those of the terminal web.

A *spot desmosome* or *macula adherens* is a disklike structure approximately 200 to 400 nm in diameter. It is characterized by an intercellular space that is about 20 nm wide and contains electron-dense fine filamentous material that often forms an intermediate dense line (Fig. 1–20). This material probably consists of filaments that connect the adjacent plasma membranes. Beneath the plasma membrane of each interacting cell is an attachment plaque of electron-dense amorphous material. Intermediate filaments either terminate within these plaques or form hairpin loops. Since these filaments cross the entire cell, a virtually continuous filamentous network permeates many cellular aggregates, such as epithelia, and enables them to resist mechanical stress and maintain their integrity.

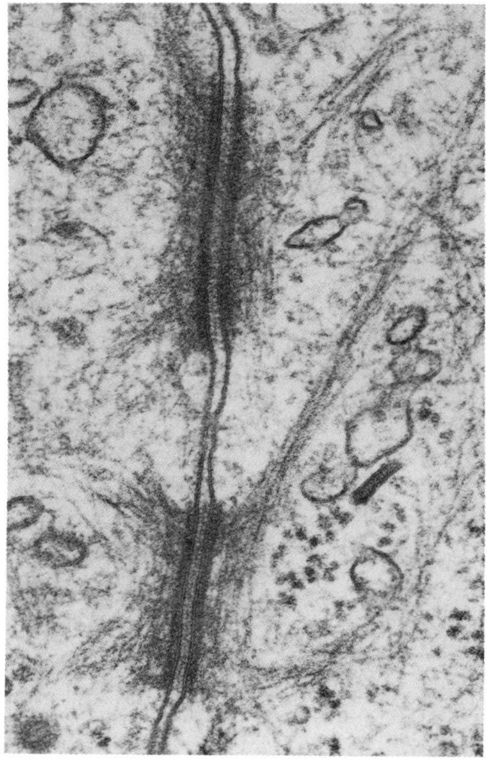

Fig. 1–20. *Desmosomes between two neurohypophysial glial cells, frog. Notice the distinct intermediate dense lines and the filaments that form hairpin loops.* ×70,000.

Hemidesmosomes consist of only one half of a desmosome; they are a means of attaching epithelial cells to the basal lamina.

IMPERMEABLE JUNCTIONS. The only impermeable junction in the mammalian organism is the *tight junction,* or *zonula occludens.* It seals neighboring cells together in a beltlike fashion and constitutes a barrier preventing the passage of substances from the lumen to the intercellular space and thus to the internal environment of the organism. Tight junctions, however, may be

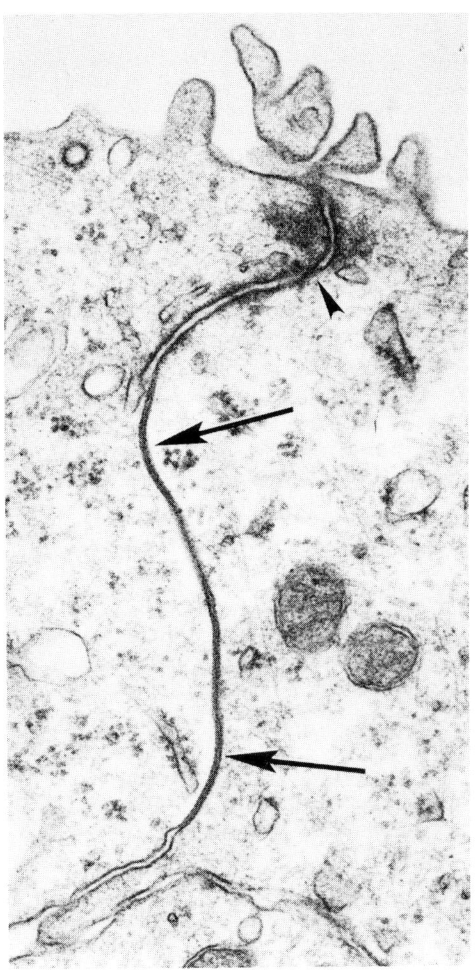

Fig. 1–21. *Zonula adherens (arrowhead) and extensive gap junctions (arrows) between two ependymal cells. ×42,000.*

selectively permeable to certain substances. As yet, no structural differences have been detected between impermeable and selectively permeable tight junctions. They are also thought to maintain cell polarity by preventing the movement of membranes and their associated specific functional complexes (e.g., enzymes). At tight junctions, integral proteins of the outer laminae of adjacent cell membranes are fused in irregular anastomosing rows or ridges across the intercellular space over a distance of 0.1 to 0.5 μm.

The intercellular connections between apices of intestinal epithelial cells are composed of three fine structural components, a zonula occludens, a zonula adherens, and a macula adherens. These are collectively referred to as the *junctional complex.*

COMMUNICATING JUNCTIONS. *Gap junctions* are classified as communicating junctions where the intercellular space is narrowed to approximately 2 nm (Fig. 1–21). This gap is bridged by connexons formed by six integral membrane proteins of the apposed membranes, which are complementary and interlock. These proteins constitute the hexagonal wall of a hydrophilic channel, 1.5 nm in diameter. Gap junctions allow the direct passage of ions and small molecules from cell to cell, thus permitting the conduction of electrical impulses and possibly functional synchronization and metabolic cooperation of cells. Gap junctions are thus of considerable functional importance, and it is not surprising that they are present in virtually all tissues of the organism, with the exception of skeletal muscle, spermatozoa, and circulating blood cells.

Specializations of the Free Surface

CILIA AND FLAGELLA. Ciliated cells are commonly found in the respiratory system, where they function in the movement of a mucous film. They also occur in the male and female reproductive systems, where they promote the propulsion of spermatozoa and oocytes. Several hundred cilia may be found on a single cell. Cilia are about 0.2 μm in diameter and between 5 and 15 μm long and thus are visible with the light microscope. At the fine-structural level, cilia consist of an axoneme surrounded by the plasma membrane. The axoneme is composed of nine doublet microtubules around two central single microtubules. The two central microtubules are complete. However, one microtubule of each doublet is complete while the other is a partial microtubule, whose wall is made of 10 rather than 13 subunits and is fused to the wall of the complete microtubule. At regular intervals, pairs of sidearms (dynein) project from the microtubules; furthermore, adjacent doublets are linked by an elastic protein, nexin. From each of the nine doublets, radial spokes extend toward the central pair around which slender protein arms form the inner sheath. The tubules extend throughout the entire length of the cilium, from the apex to the *basal body* located at the base of the cilium. The two central tubules terminate at the base plate, an electron-dense disk; the peripheral doublets are continuous with the inner pair of microtubules of the triplets of the basal body.

Cilia are rigid during their effective stroke, e.g., when propelling mucus, and become flexible during their return, or recovery, stroke. They function in a metachronal rhythm, in which each row of cilia beats in sequence. During ciliary movement, doublets of microtubules slide in relation to one another, using energy provided by the splitting of ATP through ATPase located within the dynein arms.

A single long cilium is referred to as a *flagellum.* The most prominent example of a flagellated cell is the mammalian spermatozoon, whose flagellum may be several hundred micrometers long; it uses undulatory movements for its propulsion.

MICROVILLI. In cells whose principal function is absorption, the free surface has a varying number of cytoplasmic evaginations called microvilli (Fig. 1–15). These are observable with the light microscope when they are particularly numerous and densely packed, as in the small intestine (striated border) and the proximal convoluted tubule of the kidney (brush border). With the electron microscope, the microvilli are seen to be slender cylindrical processes, approximately 0.1 μm in diameter and of variable length. They contain a core of actin filaments, which extend from their attachment to a region of amorphous material at the tips of the microvilli into the terminal web, which is also mainly composed of actin filaments. Whether the myosin, which it also contains, is of any functional significance for the microvilli is an open question.

Another variety of microvilli are those present at the luminal surface of the epithelial lining of the epididymis. They are slender and often branching cytoplasmic processes of varying length with a microfilamentous core that extends into the apical cytoplasm.

STEREOCILIA. The hair cells of the spiral organ, or organ of hearing, and the receptor cells in the vestibular sensory receptors have long, rigid microvilli that are commonly referred to as stereocilia. They also contain a core of actin filaments that apparently confers rigidity to these structures and enables them to detect minute movements of their fluid environment.

REFERENCES

Alberts, B., Bray, D., Lewis, F., Raff, M., Roberts, K., and Watson, J.D.: Molecular Biology of the Cell. New York and London, Garland Publishing, Inc., 1983.

Brinkley, B.R., and Porter, K.R. (eds.): International Cell Biology, 1976–1977. New York Rockefeller University Press, 1977.

Cantin, M. (ed.): Cell Biology of the Secretory Process. Basel, Karger, 1984.

Dingle, J.T., and Dean, R.T. (eds.): Lysosomes in Biology and Pathology. Vol. 5. Amsterdam, North-Holland, 1976.

Dustin, P.: Microtubules. Berlin, Springer-Verlag, 1978.

Farquhar, M.G.: Multiple pathways of exocytosis, endocytosis, and membrane recycling: validation of a Golgi route. Fed Proc *42*:2407, 1983.

Goldfischer, S.: The internal reticular apparatus of Camillo Golgi: A complex heterogeneous organelle enriched in acid, neutral and alkaline phosphatases, and involved in glycolisation, secretion, membrane flow, lysosome formation and intracellular digestion. J Histochem Cytochem *30*:717, 1982.

Larsen, W.J.: Biological implications of gap junction structure, distribution and composition. A review. Tissue Cell *15*:645, 1983.

Lentz, T.L.: Cell Fine Structure. Philadelphia, W.B. Saunders, 1971.

Novikoff, A.B.: The endoplasmic reticulum: a cytochemist's view (a review). Proc Natl Acad Sci USA *73*:2781, 1976.

Porter, K.R., and Bonneville, M.A.: An Introduction to the Fine Structure of Cells and Tissues. 4th Ed. Philadelphia, Lea & Febiger, 1973.

Revel, J.P., Henning, U., and Fox, C.F. (eds.): Cell shape and surface architecture. Prog Clin Biol Res Vol. 17. New York, Liss, 1977.

Singer, S.J., and Nicolson, G.L.: The fluid mosaic model of the structure of cell membranes. Science. *175*:720, 1972.

2

Epithelium

AL W. STINSON
ESTHER M. BROWN
M. LOIS CALHOUN

Epithelium consists of a sheet of aggregated cells of similar type and constitutes the external and internal surface of the body. In addition to forming the surface covering, growths of epithelial cells proliferate into the underlying tissue to form glands and hair follicles.

All three embryonic germ layers take part in the formation of epithelium. Ectoderm is the origin of the epithelium of the external body surfaces. Most of the epithelium of the digestive and respiratory systems originates from entoderm, and mesoderm gives rise to the lining of the vascular system, the closed body cavities, and parts of the urogenital system.

Epithelium is separated from the underlying connective tissue by a thin membrane, which may be a *basement membrane* composed of two layers, a *basal lamina* and a *reticular lamina,* or the basal lamina alone. The basal lamina, common to all epithelia, is an amorphous sheet containing type IV collagen, which does not form typical collagen fibrils, proteoglycans, laminin, and fibronectin. The latter two components are both glycoproteins. The composition of the reticular lamina is not well characterized; however, it is visible by light microscopy when treated with either PAS reagent or silver stains. In addition to underlying all epithelia, a basal lamina is found around muscle cells and neurolemmocytes and between epithelia in the renal corpuscle, where it has a special filtration role. The constituents of the basal lamina derive from both the epithelium and the adjacent connective tissue.

Because blood and lymph vessels do not penetrate the basement membrane, the epithelial cells must receive their nutritional support by diffusion of tissue fluids from the underlying connective tissue.

Epithelial cells are specialized for a variety of different functions, among which are protection, absorption, secretion, excretion, and formation of barriers for selective permeability.

The classification of the various epithelial types is based on the shape of the epithelial cells and the number of layers present. *Simple epithelium* is any single layer of epithelial cells resting on the basement membrane. *Stratified epithelium* is composed of two or more layers of cells with only the basal cell layer resting on the basement membrane. The names given to the various types of stratified epithelia are based on the shape of the surface cells without regard to the shape of those within the deeper layers.

CLASSIFICATION AND MICROSCOPIC STRUCTURE

Simple Squamous Epithelium

Simple squamous epithelium consists of a single layer of thin, flat, scalelike cells. On surface view (Fig. 2–1), the cells have an irregular shape with a slightly serrated border. They fit together to form a continuous sheet. A spherical or oval nucleus, near the center of the cell, gives a slightly elevated appearance to this area. On cross section, the cell appears thicker in the area of the nucleus and has thin attenuated strands of cytoplasm on either side (Fig. 2–1). Simple squamous epithelium lines moist, internal surfaces, such as the closed body cavities, the heart and the blood and lymph vessels.

The simple squamous epithelium lining the closed body cavities (pleural, pericardial, and peritoneal) is called *mesothelium;* that lining the heart, blood, and lymph vessels is referred to as *endothelium. Mesenchymal epithelium* is a special type of simple squamous epithelium that lines the subarachnoid and subdural spaces, the anterior chamber of the eye, and the perilymphatic spaces of the ear. It is variously referred to as mesothelium and endothelium.

Simple Cuboidal Epithelium

Simple cuboidal epithelium is a single layer of cells whose width and height are approximately equal. These cells appear as squares in cross sections but are more hexagonal when seen from the surface (Fig. 2–2). When the height is slightly less than the width of a cell, it is known as low cuboidal epithelium, and when the height is slightly greater than the width, the epithelium is called tall cuboidal epithelium. It should be emphasized that the classification of epithelia is not always clear-cut, and many times intermediate forms are present that require some subjective judgment regarding classification. Cuboidal epithelium lines the ducts of glands and covers the choroid plexus and ciliary body. Depend-

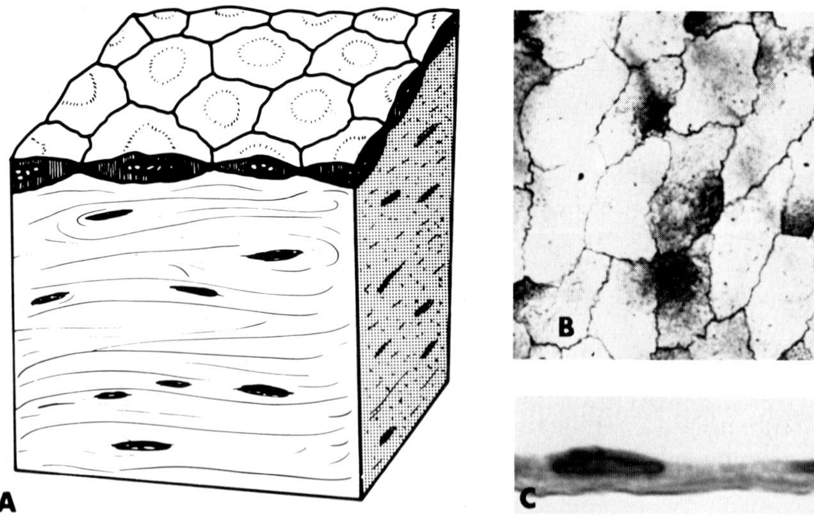

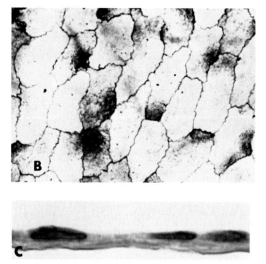

Fig. 2–1. *Simple squamous epithelium, A, Schematic drawing. B, Surface view of silvered mesothelium, mensentery. Silver stain. ×500. C, Cross section of mesothelium, peritoneum on the surface of the urinary bladder. H & E. ×1200. (A and C, from Stinson, A.W., and Brown, E.M.: Veterinary Histology Slide Sets. East Lansing, Mich., Michigan State University, Instructional Media Center, 1970.)*

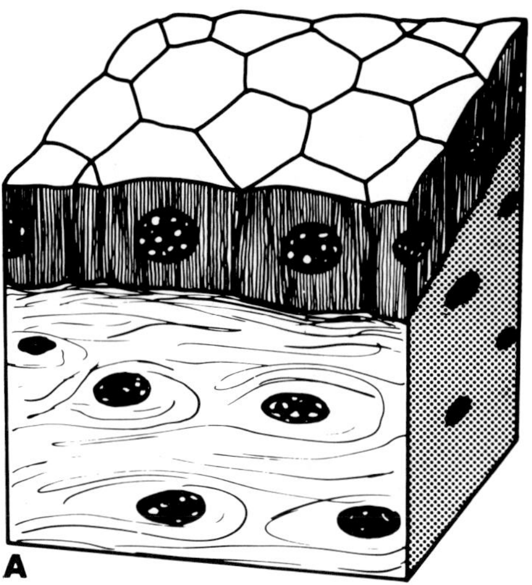

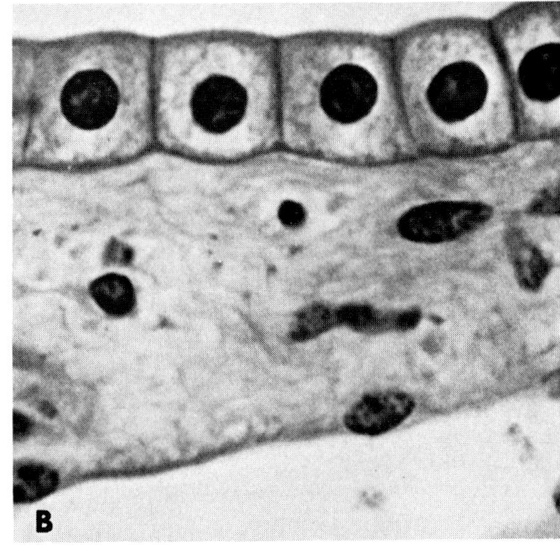

Fig. 2–2. *Simple cuboidal epithelium. A, Schematic drawing. B, Collecting duct, kidney, horse. H & E. ×900. (A, from Stinson, A.W., and Brown, E.M.: Veterinary Histology Slide Sets. East Lansing, Mich., Michigan State University, Instructional Media Center, 1970).*

ing on location, these cells may have an absorptive or secretory function. When they form small, spherical glandular secretory units (acini), they must assume a pyramidal shape. Thus, they are called *pyramidal* or *glandular epithelia* (see Fig. 2–18).

Simple Columnar Epithelium

Simple columnar epithelium consists of tall, narrow cells having considerably greater height than width (Fig. 2–3). Usually, the nuclei are oval and are located near the base of each cell. Generally, simple columnar epithelium lines organs that perform secretory and absorptive functions.

Pseudostratified Columnar Epithelium

Pseudostratified columnar epithelium is composed of a single layer of cells, but because the cells are irregular in shape and size, their nuclei are located at various levels; therefore, the epithelium appears to have several layers (Fig. 2–4). In this type of epithelium, all cells rest on the basement membrane but not all reach the surface. Those reaching the surface are either ciliated or goblet cells (unicellular mucous glands), and the short, peg-shaped cells lie between the taller cells. It is believed that the short cells serve as progenitors of the columnar cells. The goblet cells produce a mucous film that traps dust particles, and the ciliated cells move the dust-laden mucus to the body opening. Pseudostratified epithelium is found in the respiratory and reproductive systems.

Stratified Squamous Epithelium

Stratified squamous epithelium consists of several layers of cells, with only the superficial cells having a squamous shape. Two types of stratified squamous epithelium are recognized (Fig. 2–5). The *keratinized form* has cells on the surface layer that have lost their nuclei and are filled with keratin, a water-resistant protein that forms a protective barrier against the destructive forces of the environment. In the *nonkeratinized form,* the flattened superficial cells retain their nuclei.

Three to five distinct cell layers are present in stratified squamous epithelium. The deepest layer of cells next to the basal lam-

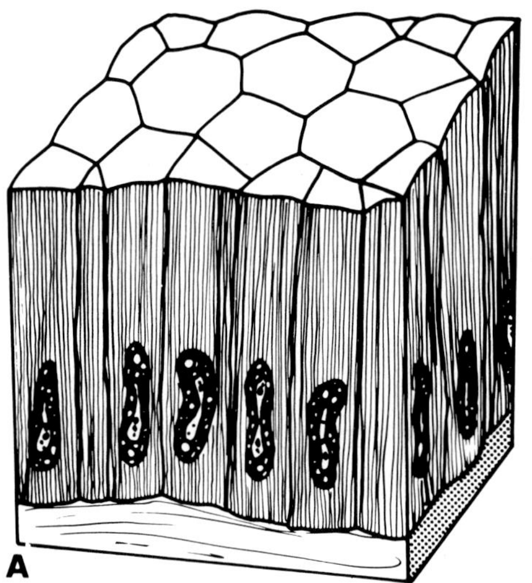

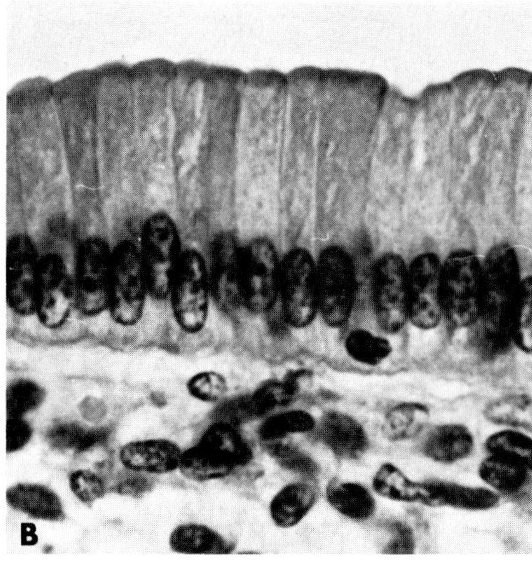

Fig. 2–3. *Simple columnar epithelium. A, Schematic drawing. B, Lining of gallbladder, pig H & E. ×900. (A, from Stinson, A.W., and Brown, E.M.: Veterinary Histology Slide Sets. East Lansing, Mich., Michigan State University. Instructional Media Center, 1970.)*

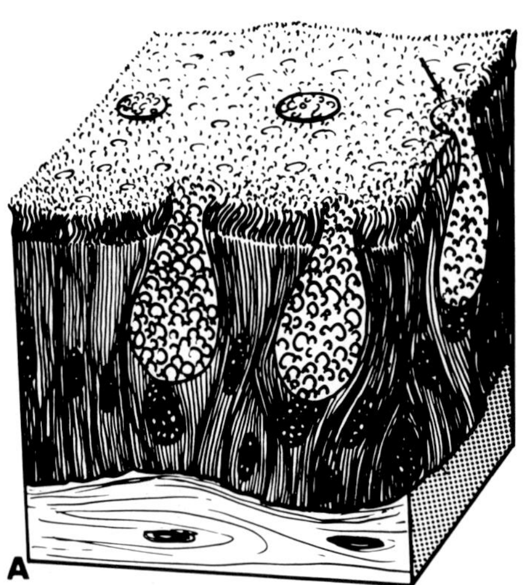

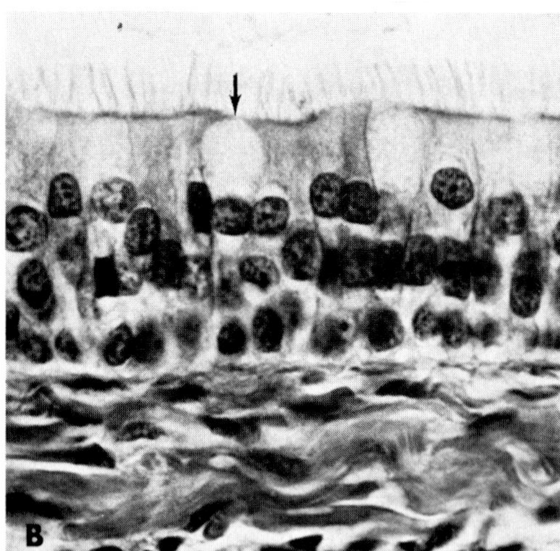

Fig. 2–4. *Pseudostratified columnar epithelium with goblet cells. A, Schematic drawing. B, Trachea, dog. Arrow points to goblet cell. H & E. ×1200. (A, from Stinson, A.W., and Brown, E.M.: Veterinary Histology Slide Sets. East Lansing, Mich., Michigan State University, Instructional Media Center, 1970.)*

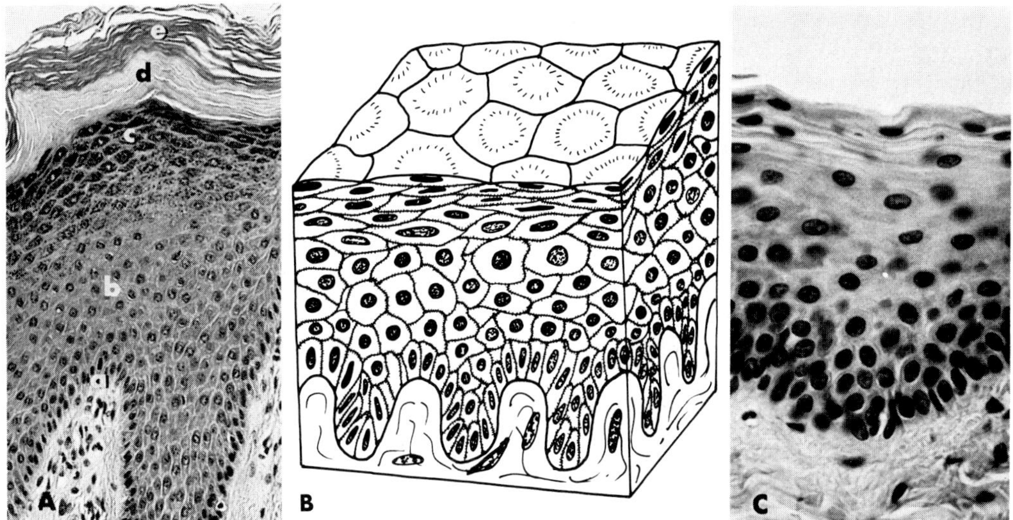

Fig. 2–5. *Keratinized stratified squamous epithelium. A, Teat, cow. Stratum basale (a), stratum spinosum (b), stratum granulosum (c), stratum lucidum (d), stratum corneum (e). H & E. ×150. B, Schematic drawing. C, Nonkeratinized squamous epithelium, lip, cat. H & E. ×380. (A, from Stinson, A.W., and Brown, E.M.: Veterinary Histology Slide Sets. East Lansing, Mich., Michigan State University, Instructional Media Center, 1970.)*

ina is the *stratum basale* (Fig. 2–5), which is a single layer of cuboidal to columnar cells. The next layer is the *stratum spinosum* (Fig. 2–5), composed of a varying number of layers of polyhedral cells tightly adhered to each other by numerous desmosomes. In ordinary histologic preparations, the cytoplasm between the desmosomal attachment shrinks, and wherever the cells remain attached, small spiny processes radiate from the surface of the cells. This appearance gives rise to the name of the layer, stratum spinosum, or "spiny layer." Actually, these spiny processes contain tonofibrils condensed at the site of the desmosomes (Fig. 2–6). Numerous mitotic figures occur in the lower layer of the stratum spinosum as well as in the stratum basale. Therefore, this region is referred to as the *stratum germinativum* because it gives rise to the cells that move into the upper layers of the epithelium.

As the cells from the stratum spinosum move toward the surface, they become more flattened and accumulate keratohyaline granules in their cytoplasm. The nature of these granules will be discussed later. This layer of granulated cells is the

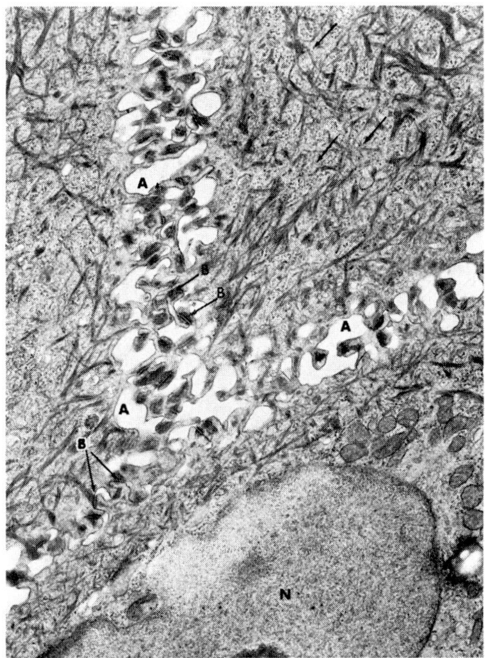

Fig. 2–6. *Electron micrograph of stratum spinosum, rumen epithelium, at junction of three cells, with nucleus (N) of one visible at lower left. Intercellular canaliculi (A) are located between desmosomal attachments (B). Polyribosomes (arrows) are present throughout the cytoplasm. Osmium. ×6700.*

stratum granulosum and is not present in all stratified squamous epithelia. It is absent in nonkeratinized epithelium as well as in the keratinized forms that produce hard keratin, such as that found in the wall of the hoof and in the horn of ruminants.

The *stratum lucidum* occurs only in nonhairy skin regions (Fig. 2–5). It is a layer of flattened keratinized cells between the stratum granulosum and the stratum corneum and has a translucent appearance because it contains *eleidin,* a protein similar to keratin but with a somewhat different staining affinity.

The outermost layer of stratified squamous epithelium is the *stratum corneum.* It consists of dead, keratinized cells that are fairly resistant to environmental irritants. During keratinization, the nuclei become pyknotic and subsequently disappear. A true stratum corneum is not present in non-keratinized stratified squamous epithelium found on moist surfaces. In these locations the cells are flat but retain their nuclei and keratins. Groups of cells in the outermost layer of the stratum corneum become loose and separate. This process gives rise to the descriptive term *stratum disjunctum.*

In areas where stratified squamous epithelium is keratinized, the cells undergo a series of transformations as they move from the stratum basale to the surface layer. The process of keratinization involves the gradual disappearance of Golgi complexes, mitochondria, and nuclei, and a decreased lysosomal activity with a concurrent accumulation of tonofilaments.

Stratum basale cells are rich in polyribosomes that are concerned with the synthesis of tonofilaments. As these germinative cells move up into the stratum spinosum, the tonofilaments condense into bundles (tonofibrils) and become attached to desmosomes (Fig. 2–6). The cells in the granular layer are flat and contain numerous keratohyaline granules, which are readily visible with the light microscope. With the EM, the tonofilaments are seen to

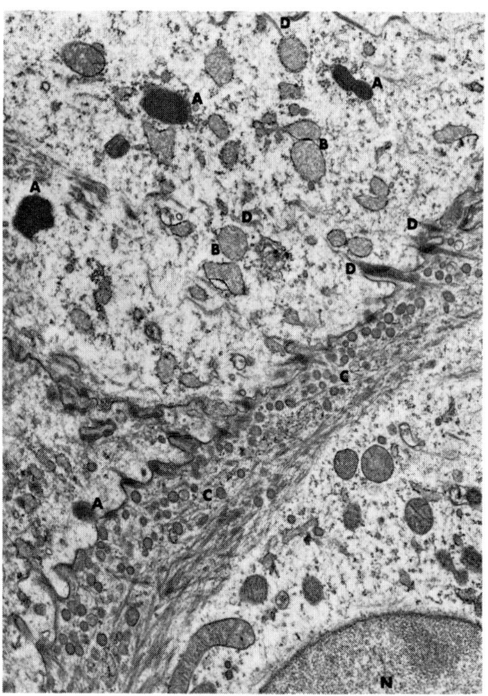

Fig. 2–7. *Electron micrograph of stratum granulosum, rumen epithelium. The dark granules (A) are the keratohyaline granules. The lighter granules (B) are keratohyaline granules in various states of development. The numerous small granules (C) near the cell surface of the lower cell are membrane-coating granules. Tonofilaments (D) extend into the upper cell and near developing keratohyaline granules. Nucleus (N). Osmium.* ×6720.

extend into the periphery of the cell, intermingling with the granules (Fig. 2–7). In addition to the keratinohyaline granules, the cells in the uppermost layer of the stratum granulosum contain oval granules (100 to 500 nm) composed of alternating light and dark lamellae. These *membrane coating granules* are produced by the Golgi complex (Fig. 2–7). The granules are located at the cell periphery, and eventually the granule contents is secreted by exocytosis. This material may be the primary water barrier. By the time the cells reach the stratum lucidum, they are more elongated and flattened, and all the cell organelles are gone. With the light microscope, only the cell outlines are visible, and the cytoplasm appears homogeneous. Ultrastructural examination reveals densely

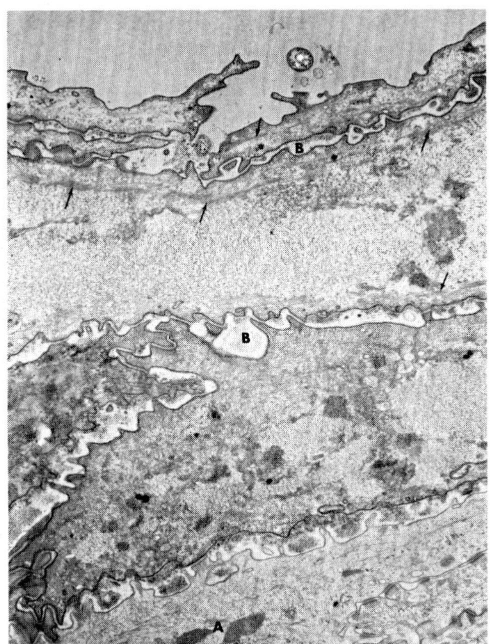

Fig. 2–8. *Electron micrograph of stratum corneum, rumen epithelium. Keratohyaline granules (A) are in the lower cell with the three upper cells in various stages of keratinization. Tonofilaments (arrows) appear at cell periphery. Notice the extensive intercellular spaces (B) indicating ease of desquamation. Because this was from a moist surface, its appearance is somewhat different from that of a dry surface. Osmium. ×6720.*

packed filaments embedded in a dense matrix, and it is possible that this extensive fibrillar matrix is derived from the keratohyaline granules. Cells in the stratum corneum appear lifeless, and as those on the surface dry they flake off (Fig. 2–8). This desquamation process is probably the result of weakened desmosomal junctions between the surface cells.

Stratified Cuboidal Epithelium

Stratified cuboidal epithelium consists of two or more layers of cells, with a surface layer of typical cuboidal cells. Frequently, it occurs as a distinct two-layered epithelium (Fig. 2–9) lining the excretory ducts of glands.

Stratified Columnar Epithelium

Stratified columnar epithelium is made up of several layers of cells. The superficial layer of tall, prismatic cells does not extend to the basement membrane (Fig. 2–10). The deeper layers are composed of smaller polyhedral cells that do not reach the surface. This type of epithelium may be found in the distal portion of the urethra, as circumscribed areas in the transitional epithelium, in the parotid and mandibular ducts, and in the lacrimal sac and duct.

Transitional Epithelium

Transitional epithelium is a pseudostratified type with a wide variety of appearances and is restricted to the urinary system. It lines hollow organs capable of considerable distention, such as the urinary bladder. Therefore, the shape of the epithelial cells depends on the degree of the organ distention at the time of fixation. When the epithelium is under little tension, the surface cells are large and "pillow-shaped," whereas the deeper cells are smaller and irregularly shaped (Fig. 2–11). The cells increase in size from the basal layers to the superficial layers. When the epithelium is stretched, the cells become flattened and elongated, and the total height of the epithelium decreases.

The luminal surface of transitional epithelial cells appears relatively smooth with the light microscope. However, in electron micrographs areas of thickened plasma membrane or plaques anchored by numerous cytoplasmic filaments are seen on the luminal cell membrane. These thick areas develop from Golgi vesicles. The region between the membrane plaques has a normal plasmalemma, and when the bladder contracts the plaques fold together much like a hinge, producing typical transitional epithelial surface ridges. Upon distention they unfold, allowing expansion of the luminal surface.

Because urine is hypertonic, the surface

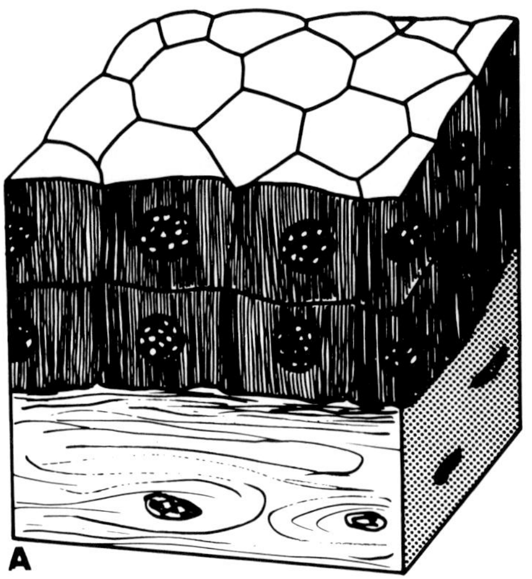

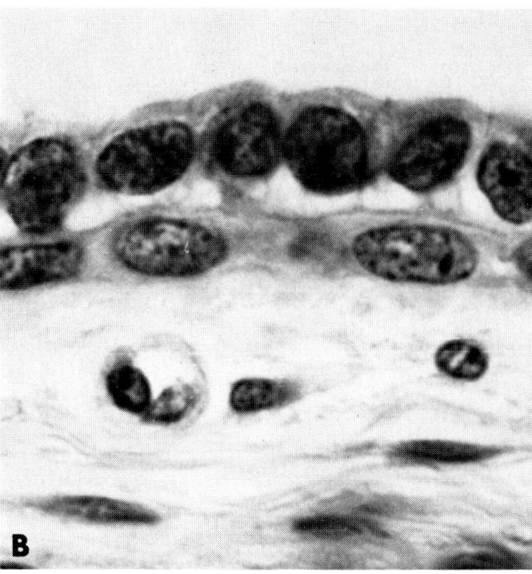

Fig. 2–9. *Two-layered cuboidal epithelium. A, Schematic drawing. B, Duct of carpal gland, pig. H & E. ×1400. (A, from Stinson, A.W., and Brown, E.M.: Veterinary Histology Slide Sets. East Lansing, Mich., Michigan State University, Instructional Media Center, 1970.)*

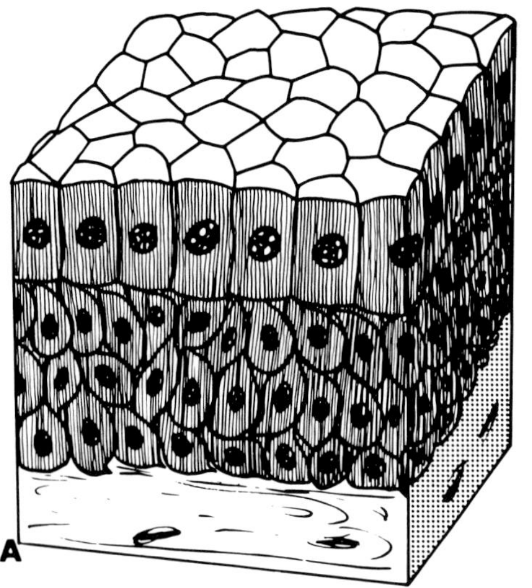

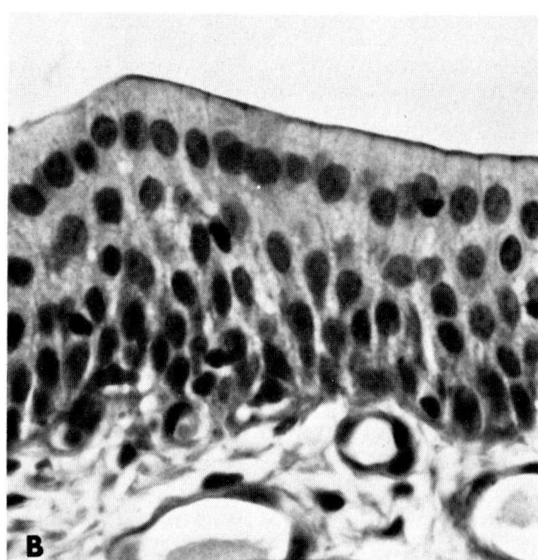

Fig. 2–10. *Stratified columnar epithelium. A, Schematic drawing. B, Penile urethra, horse. H & E. ×620. (A, from Stinson, A.W., and Brown, E.M.: Veterinary Histology Slide Sets, East Lansing, Mich., Michigan State University, Instructional Media Center, 1970.)*

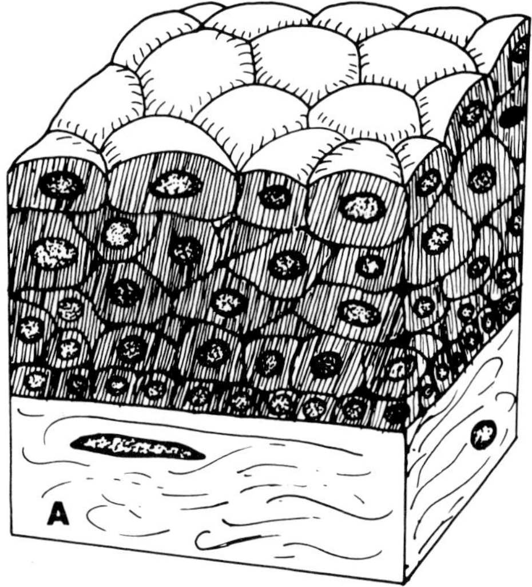

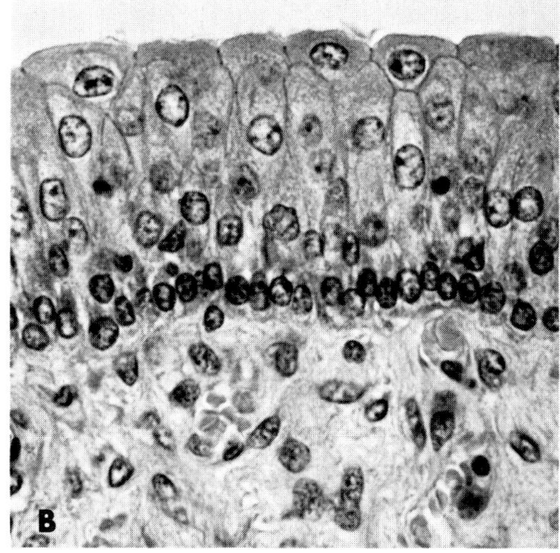

Fig. 2–11. *Transitional epithelium. A, Schematic drawing. B, Urinary bladder, pig. H & E. ×480 (A, from Stinson, A.W., and Brown, E.M.: Veterinary Histology Slide Sets. East Lansing, Mich., Michigan State University, Instructional Media Center, 1970.)*

epithelium of the bladder is a barrier to the diffusion of water from the subepithelial tissue. Morphologic evidence of this diffusion barrier is the increased thickness of the outer layer of the plasmalemma as compared to the thickness of the innermost layer. In addition, there is a concentration of tonofilaments immediately beneath the luminal surface, which probably aids in preventing diffusion. Moreover, intercellular diffusion is prevented by junctional complexes located between the surface cells.

Recent fine-structural studies of developing transitional epithelium indicate that when the epithelium becomes multilayered and the cells elongate and overlap each other, all remain attached to the basement membrane by slender cytoplasmic processes, much like the attachment in pseudostratified epithelium. This type of attachment allows the cells to form a parallel alignment when the urinary bladder is distended; thus, fewer layers of cells are seen.

SPECIAL CHARACTERISTICS

The location of cellular organelles and variations in luminal, basal, and lateral cell membranes characterize a definite polarized organization of epithelial cells. While some of these special morphologic and functional features are discussed in detail in other chapters, it seems worthwhile to emphasize those associated with epithelial cells here.

Surface Modifications

APICAL MEMBRANE. The luminal surface membrane proteins in most epithelial cells are different from those associated with lateral or basal membranes. For example, the kidney tubular epithelial membranes contain alkaline phosphatase, whereas those in the intestinal cells contain enzymes to hydrolyze sugars.

MICROVILLI. Cells whose chief function is absorption have long cytoplasmic extensions on their free surface called *microvilli.* Because microvilli are so numerous and regularly arranged, under the light microscope the cell surface appears striated. This observation led to the term *striated border.* In electron micrographs, each microvillus is seen to be composed of cytoplasm with a central core of fine filaments (Fig. 2–10).

In addition to having absorptive function, microvilli contain enzymes for splitting disaccharides. Although microvilli are particularly well developed on the cells of the small intestine and the proximal tubules in the kidney, they are also present on practically all cells involved in absorption.

STEREOCILIA. Extremely long microvilli, prevalent in the epithelium lining the tubules in the epididymis, are called *stereocilia.* This is an unfortunate name, because they are not cilia but long cytoplasmic extensions, which increase the surface area for absorption. Their ultrastructure is described in Chapter 12.

CILIA. The epithelia lining the respiratory system and portions of the male and female reproductive systems have motile processes on their surfaces called *cilia.* They are much longer than microvilli and are easily visualized with the light microscope. They serve a protective function in the respiratory system, and in all likelihood aid in the movement of ova and spermatozoa through various portions of the respective reproductive organs. For a description of ultrastructural details, refer to Chapter 1.

GLYCOCALYX. A carbohydrate-rich surface coat, the glycocalyx is present on the surfaces of all cells, and it is particularly well developed on microvilli of epithelial cells. This PAS-positive layer contains various enzyme systems that enhance absorption.

BASAL CELL MEMBRANE. The basal portion of many epithelial cell types contains Na-K ATPase, an important hydrolytic enzyme system responsible for the outward and inward transport of Na and K, respectively. Transcytotic vesicles, seen at or near the basal cell membrane of the intestinal epithelium of neonatal animals, transport immunoglobulins from colostrum. The basal surface of epithelial cells in endocrine organs have hormone receptors, and in epithelial cells whose chief function is resorption (e.g., kidney tubules), the basal cell membrane displays complex infoldings closely associated with numerous mitochondria (see Chapter 11).

Internal Support Structures and Cellular Attachments

TONOFILAMENTS. An internal support for the various types of epithelial cells is related to the structure, location, and function of intercellular attachments. This meshwork of cytoplasmic filaments, referred to as the *cytoplasmic network* or *cell web,* is composed of individual ultrastructural units, called *tonofilaments,* which are too small to be resolved with the light microscope. However, bundles of tonofilaments, called *tonofibrils,* are visible with the light microscope in stratified squamous epithelial cells. Although these filaments are distributed throughout the cell, they are concentrated at sites of cell-to-cell attachments. In columnar epithelial cells, tonofilaments concentrated at the apex of the cells are called the *terminal web.* Filaments from the web continue into the microvilli for internal support, and they are condensed near the intercellular attachment sites.

JUNCTIONAL COMPLEX. As discussed in Chapter 1, the junctional complex, which holds epithelial cells together, is composed of three different types of junctions: (1) zonula occludens, (2) zonula adherens, and (3) macula adherens. With the light microscope, the junctional complex appears as a dense bar or dot near the juxtaluminal surface.

DESMOSOMES. Cellular attachments between stratified squamous epithelial cells are particularly prominent in the stratum spinosum. These cellular attachments are desmosomes (see Chapter 1), which are similar to spot-welds because they occur only at certain sites around the cell membrane; thus the term *macula adherens.* Shrinkage caused by histologic processing separates the cells, except where desmosomes hold adjacent cells together (Fig. 2–6). This widens the intracellular spaces, and the cytoplasm at the desmosomal junctions appears as dark-stained, spiny processes with the light microscope. The cells in the stratum basale contain hemidesmosomes that anchor the cells to the extracellular matrix below. Desmosomes are not confined to stratified squamous epithelium; indeed, they are common in many other types of epithelial cells.

GAP JUNCTIONS. As discussed in Chapter 1, gap junctions are found between epithelial cells in many locations. They function primarily as a passageway for ions and small molecules, and cells connected by gap junctions are ionically and metabolically coupled.

Table 2–1.
Classifications of Glands

Classifications of Glands
Morphologic characteristics
Unicellular glands
Multicellular glands
Intraepithelial
Extraepithelial
Endocrine
Exocrine
Simple
Tubular—straight, coiled, branched
Acinar (alveolar)—single, branched
Tubuloacinar (tubuloalveolar)
Compound
Tubular
Acinar (alveolar)
Tubuloacinar (tubuloalveolar)
Type of secretory product
Serous
Mucous
Mixed (seromucous)
Mode of secretion
Merocrine
Apocrine
Holocrine
Cytocrine

GLANDS

Epithelial cells may be modified into secretory structures, or *glands,* of varying complexities. Most internal organs of the body contain glands in one form or another, and their secretory products may be widely distributed.

General Classification

Glands are classified according to several different structural and functional characteristics to facilitate discussion (Table 2–1).

Morphologic Characteristics

Unicellular glands consist of a single secretory cell in a nonsecretory epithelium. The goblet cell is an example of this type of gland. It is a specialized epithelial cell that produces mucinogen, which is released onto the epithelial surface. As this secretory material is synthesized, it fills and expands the apical portion of the cell and forces the nucleus into the slender basal portion, giving the cell a distinct goblet shape (Fig. 2–4).

Multicellular glands are composed of more than one cell, and most of the glands belong in this classification. They may occur as a cluster of only a few secretory cells within a surface epithelium, forming *intraepithelial glands,* or as large accumulations of cells that have proliferated into the underlying connective tissue, forming *extraepithelial glands.*

Endocrine glands are multicellular glands that do not have a system of ducts to convey their secretory product to sites of utilization. Instead, the secretory product (hormone) is released directly into the intercellular fluid, from which it is transported to a site of action by the blood and lymph.

Exocrine glands are multicellular glands with a system of ducts through which their secretory products are transported to the sites of utilization. Exocrine glands are either *simple glands,* consisting of a single or several secretory units connected to the surface through an unbranched duct, or *compound glands* with a large number of secretory units emptying into a branched duct system.

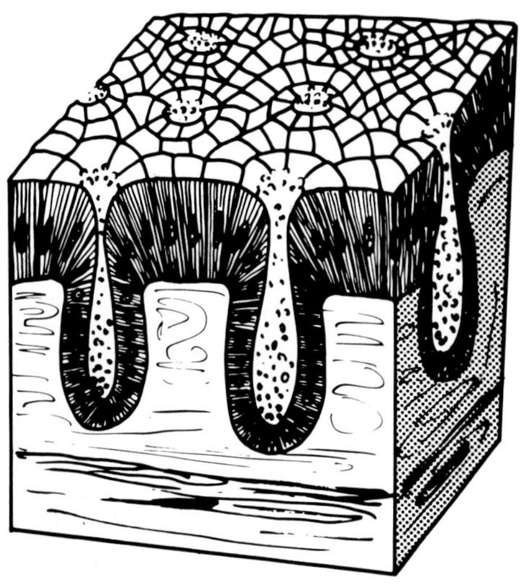
A

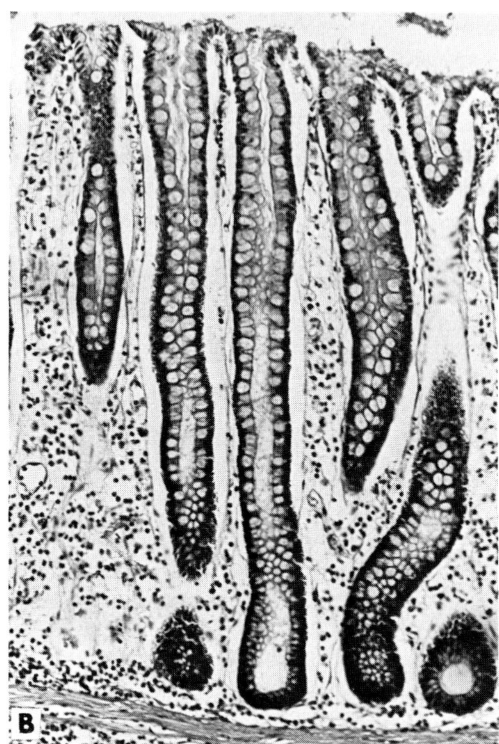

Fig. 2–12. *Simple tubular glands. A, Schematic drawing. B, Large intestine, dog. H & E. ×120. (A, from Stinson, A.W., and Brown, E.M.: Veterinary Histology Slide Sets. East Lansing, Mich., Michigan State University, Instructional Media Center, 1970.)*

Simple Glands

Simple exocrine glands have secretory units of various shapes and dispositions. These morphologic characteristics form the basis for the following types. *Simple straight tubular glands,* such as those in the large intestine, pursue a straight, unbranched course in the underlying tissue and open directly onto the surface (Fig. 2–12). *Simple coiled tubular glands* have their terminal portion disposed in coils or convolutions. In histologic sections, the secretory unit appears as a cluster of cross-sectional profiles (Fig. 2–13). Sweat glands of the skin are good examples of this type. *Simple branched tubular glands* have a branched terminal portion (Fig. 2–14). The branches converge into a single tube near the opening onto the surface, and both portions are lined with secretory cells. The glands of the stomach are typical simple branched tubular glands.

Simple acinar and *simple alveolar glands* are similar because they have an enlarged, spherical secretory unit connected to the surface by a constricted portion (Fig. 2–15). The lumen of the acinus is small and narrow, but that of the alveolus is large and distended (Fig. 21–16). The simple forms of this type are relatively rare. Some of the sebaceous glands are the simple acinar type, whereas the simple alveolar type is found in the skin of amphibians. *Simple branched acinar* and *simple branched alveolar glands* are more common than unbranched glands. In these types, two or more acini or alveoli occur together, and their secretory product empties through a common opening. Many of the larger sebaceous glands of the skin are of the branched acinar type.

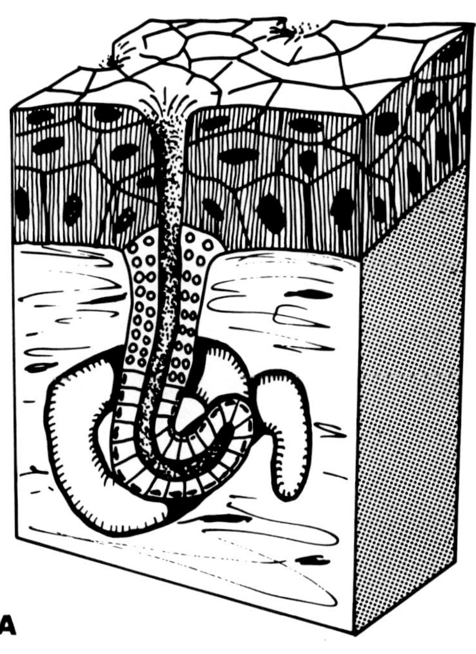

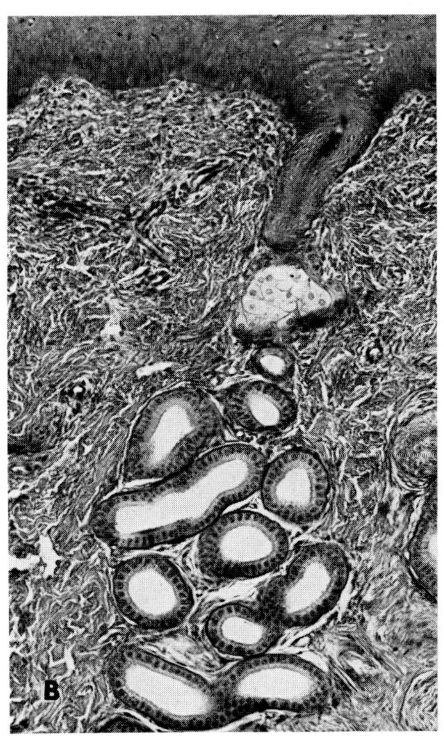

Fig. 2–13. *Simple coiled tubular gland. A, Schematic drawing. B, Ceruminous gland, cow. H & E. ×120. (A and B, from Stinson, A.W., and Brown, E.M.: Veterinary Histology Slide Sets. East Lansing, Mich., Michigan State University. Instructional Media Center, 1970.)*

Simple tubuloacinar and *tubuloalveolar glands* have secretory units composed of both a tubular portion and an enlarged terminal acinus or alveolus and occur only in the branched form. The minor salivary glands that empty into the oral cavity are classified as this type.

Compound Glands

Compound glands are composed of the same types of secretory units as the simple glands but have elaborate duct systems that branch repeatedly. Compound glands are classified into tubular, acinar, alveolar, tubuloacinar, and tubuloalveolar types. Figure 2–17 illustrates the various types of secretory units and ducts found in compound glands.

PARENCHYMA. Compound glands are composed of secretory units and ducts, collectively termed *parenchyma;* the supportive or connective tissue elements make up the *stroma.* Large glands are partly or completely divided into *lobes,* which are large, easily recognized structural units. The lobes are further subdivided by connective tissue into *lobules,* which in turn are composed of a number of *secretory units* (Fig. 2–18). Some of the smaller compound glands have only lobules and secretory units. The various segments of the duct system of compound glands are identified by their location within a gland.

The duct that drains the entire gland is the *main duct* and is formed by the convergence of the *lobar ducts,* the large ducts that drain the lobes. Ducts located within the lobes are called *intralobar ducts,* and those located in the connective tissue between the lobes are *interlobar ducts* (Fig. 2–17–H). The smaller ducts associated with the lob-

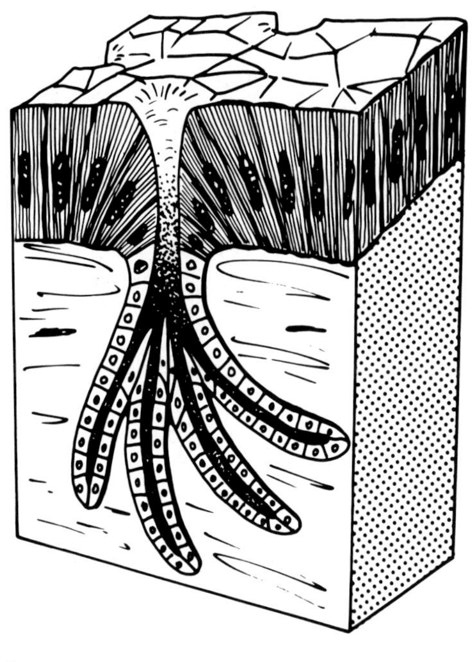

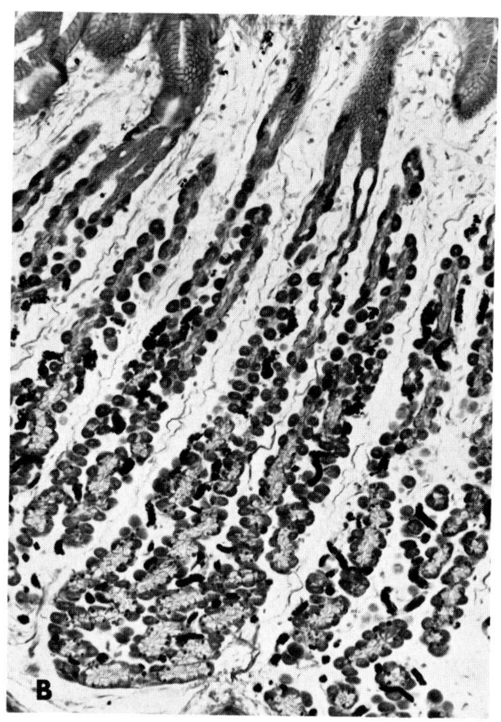

Fig. 2–14. *Branched tubular gland. A, Schematic drawing. B, Fundic stomach, dog. H & E. ×120. (A, from Stinson, A.W., and Brown, E.M.: Veterinary Histology Slide Sets. East Lansing, Mich., Michigan State University, Instructional Media Center, 1970.)*

ules are either *interlobular* (located in the connective tissue between the lobules) or *intralobular* (located within the lobule) (Fig. 2–18).

In some glands, such as the parotid salivary gland, portions of the intralobular ducts also contribute to the secretory product and thus are called *secretory ducts.* These ducts are also called *striated ducts,* because their cells have large numbers of mitochondria oriented perpendicularly to the long axis of the cell and located between the infoldings of the basal plasmalemma, giving the cells a striated appearance (Fig. 2–17–G). *Intercalated ducts* are small nonsecretory ducts that connect the secretory units with the secretory duct (Fig. 2–17–E).

The general term *excretory duct* describes any of the above-mentioned ducts that function only to transport the secretory product to the site of utilization. They do not contribute to the secretory product as do the secretory ducts.

STROMA. The *stroma* of compound glands includes the capsule and the internal supportive framework (Fig. 2–18). The capsule, composed of collagen, elastic, and reticular fibers, completely surrounds the gland and gives rise to connective tissue sheets (septa) or strands (trabeculae) that extend well into the parenchyma. These septa clearly define the lobes and lobules and provide support for the various interlobar and interlobular ducts. Fine reticular fibers encircle the individual secretory units.

Types of Secretory Units

Both simple and compound glands may be classified as mucous, serous, or seromucous, based on the type of secretory product. In *serous glands,* which produce a thin, watery product, the cells of the secretory units usually have spherical nuclei

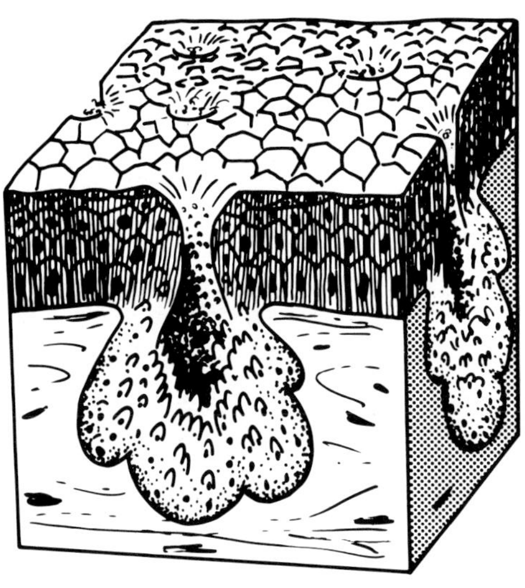

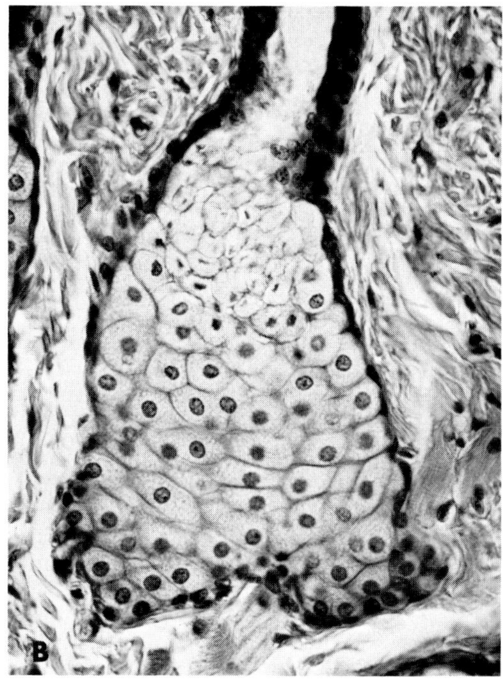

Fig. 2–15. *Simple acinar gland. A, Schematic drawing. B, Sebaceous gland, nostril, horse. H & E. ×300. (A, from Stinson, A.W., and Brown, E.M.: Veterinary Histology Slide Sets. East Lansing, Mich., Michigan State University, Instructional Media Center, 1970.)*

near the center of the cells, and the apical cytoplasm is filled with small secretory granules (Fig. 2–17–F). These granules are precursors of enzymes produced by many of the serous glands and are called *zymogen granules.* The parotid salivary gland and the exocrine portion of the pancreas are typical serous glands.

Mucous glands produce a thick, viscous secretion (mucus), forming a protective coating over the lining of hollow organs that communicate with the outside of the body (Fig. 2–17–B). The cells of the mucus-secreting units are filled with mucinogen, the precursor of mucus, which stains light with hematoxylin and eosin.

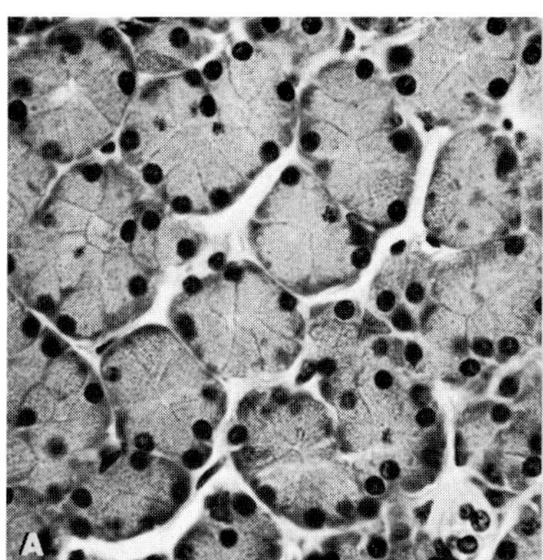

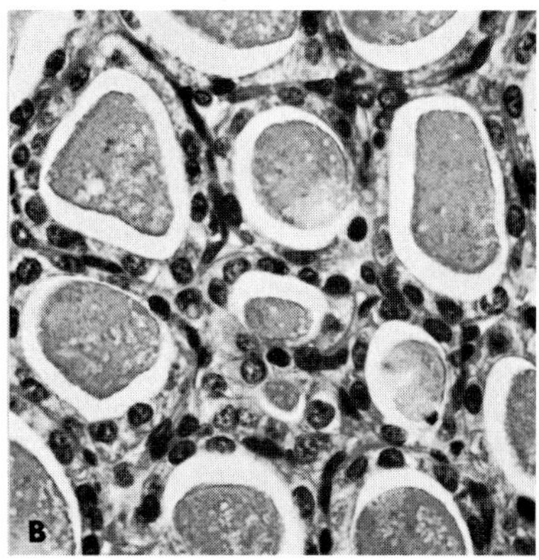

Fig. 2–16. *A, Acinar-type secretory unit characterized by small lumen, parotid gland, horse. H & E. ×480. B, Alveolar-type secretory unit with a large lumen, mammary gland, sow. H & E. ×480.*

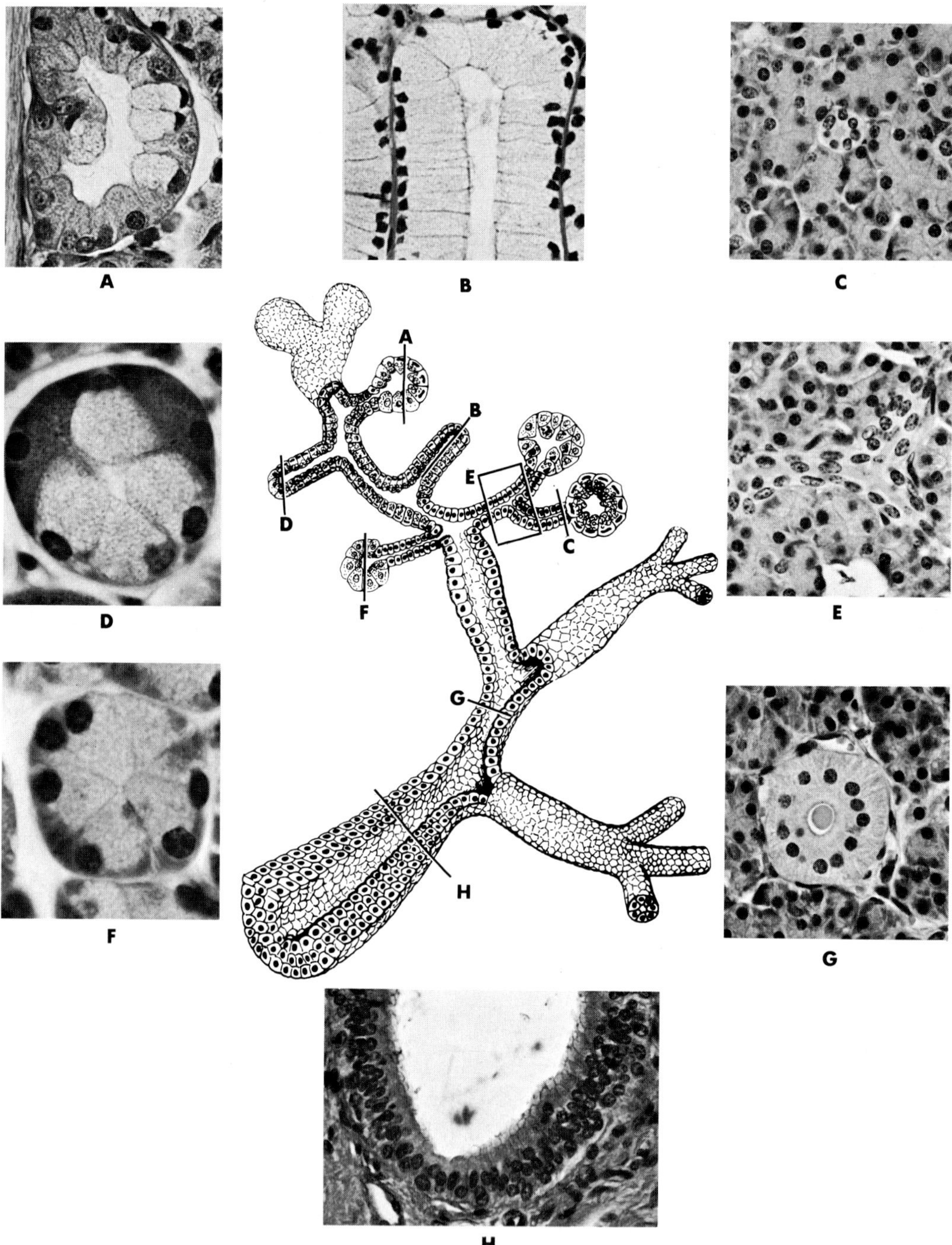

Fig. 2–17. *Schematic composite drawings and photomicrographs of the duct system and secretory units of a multilobular gland. The photomicrographs correspond to the areas labeled A through H. A, Seromucous gland, trachea, pig. Trichrome, ×600. B, Mucous tubular gland, bulbourethral gland, bull. H & E. ×480. C, Cross section of intercalated duct, parotid gland, horse. H & E. ×480. D, Secretory unit from seromucous salivary gland with serous demilunes, horse, H & E. ×1000. E, Longitudinal section through intercalated duct, parotid gland, horse. H & E. × 480. F, Serous acinus, parotid salivary gland, horse. H & E. ×1200. G, Striated salivary duct, parotid gland, horse. H & E. ×480. H, Interlobular salivary duct, mandibular salivary gland, dog. H & E. ×300. (Drawing, from Stinson, A.W., and Brown, E.M.: Veterinary Histology Slide Sets. East Lansing, Mich., Michigan State University, Instructional Media Center, 1970.)*

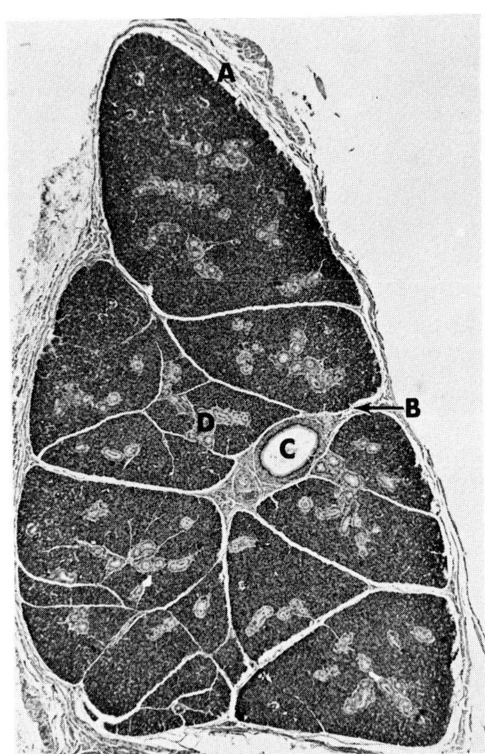

Fig. 2–18. *Parotid salivary gland, horse. Capsule (A); interlobular connective tissue (B); interlobular collecting duct (C); intralobular collecting ducts (D). H & E. ×30.*

The nuclei are displaced toward the basal part of the cell and are usually flattened against the cell membrane.

Seromucous glands contain both mucous and serous cells. The combinations of these two types of cells vary considerably from one gland to another. Some secretory units contain both serous and mucous cells intermixed (Fig. 2–17–A). Frequently, the serous cells are located at the periphery of the mucus-secretory unit and are half-moon- or crescent-shaped clusters of cells called *serous demilunes* (Fig. 2–17–D). They empty their serous secretory product into the lumen by way of intercellular canaliculi. Some seromucous tubuloacinar glands have a mucous tubular unit with a terminal serous acinus. Other seromucous glands are composed of a mixture of all mucous acini and all serous acini, rather than each acinus having some serous and some mucous cells.

Modes of Secretion

The mode by which the secretory product is released from the cell forms the basis for a third classification of glands. The *merocrine* (sometimes called *eccrine*) mode of secretion is one in which the product is released as small secretory granules (Fig. 2–19–A). Because the intracellular secretory granules are usually enclosed within a membrane, they are referred to as *granulated vesicles.* When the granulated vesicle touches the plasmalemma, the two membranes fuse, and the bounding membrane becomes incorporated into the plasmalemma. The secretory product is thus discharged from the cell without any disruption of the plasmalemma. This is an example of exocytosis.

In the *apocrine* secretory mode, the intracellular secretory droplet is surrounded by the unit membrane. As it migrates into the cell apex, the cell plasmalemma invaginates beneath the droplet, forming a constriction so that the droplet bulges into the gland lumen (Fig. 2–19–B). Actual scission of the apical cap occurs at the constriction, and the membrane-bounded droplet, together with a rim of cytoplasm and plasmalemma, is released from the cell, leaving the cell membrane intact. Apocrine glands (e.g., mammary gland) in the secretory state are easily recognized; however, when they are in a resting phase with no secretory droplets, it is difficult to differentiate them from merocrine glands.

In the *holocrine* mode of secretion, the entire cell is extruded and constitutes the secretory product (Fig. 2–19–C). The sebaceous glands of the skin are typical holocrine glands. The cell becomes filled with lipid secretion granules and moves toward the duct; the entire cell then disintegrates and its content is extruded into the duct.

The *cytocrine* mode of secretion is an unusual transfer of secretory material from

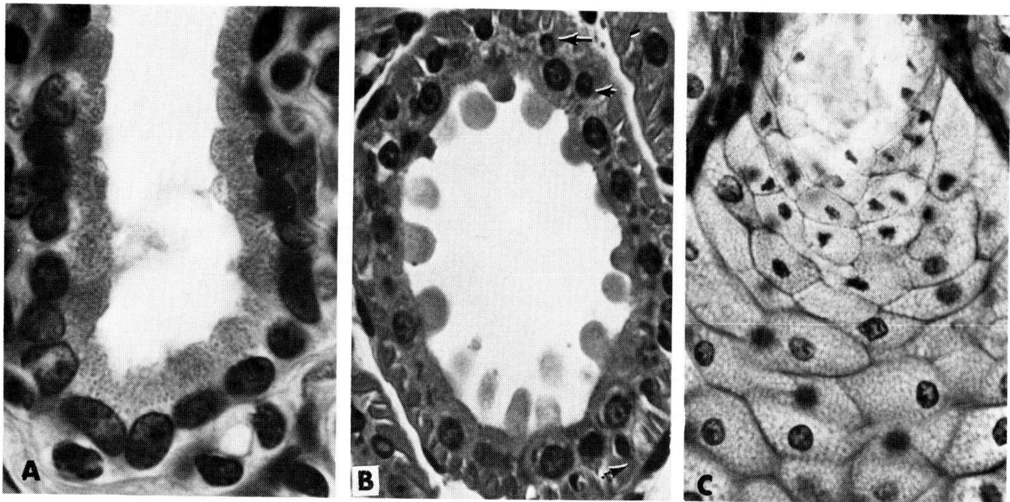

Fig. 2–19. *Secretory units illustrating the various modes of secretion. A, Merocrine gland, prostate, dog. H & E, ×1200. B, Apocrine gland, skin, pig, with myoepithelial cells at arrows. H & E. ×610. C, Holocrine sebaceous gland, horse. H & E. ×480.*

one cell to the cytoplasm of another cell. This occurs when the melanocyte of the epidermis transfers the brown melanin pigment into the cytoplasm of the keratinocyte.

Myoepithelial Cells

In addition to the secretory cells, some simple and compound glands have modified epithelial cells with contractile properties, the *myoepithelial cells,* which contain attenuated cytoplasmic processes interposed between the secretory cells and the basement membrane. The processes form a basketlike network around the secretory unit, and contraction of them forces the secretory product into the duct system. Myoepithelial cells are especially well developed in sweat and mammary glands (Fig. 2–19–B).

REFERENCES

Bharadwaj, M.B., and Calhoun, M.L.: Histology of the urethral epithelium of domestic animals. Am J Vet Res *20*:841, 1959.

Bretscher, A., and Weber, K.: Fimbrin, a new microfilament-associated protein present in microvilli and other cell surface structures. J Cell Biol *86*:335, 1980.

Hashimoto, K.: The eccrine and apocrine glands and their function. *In* The Physiology and Pathophysiology of the Skin. Vol. 5. Edited by A. Jarret. New York, Academic Press, 1978.

Martin, B.F., and Wong, Y.C.: Development and maturation of the bladder epithelium of the guinea pig. Acta Anat *110*:359, 1981.

Phillips, S.J., and Griffin, T.: Scanning electron microscope evidence that human urothelium is a pseudostratified epithelium. Anat Rec *211*:153A, 1985.

Severs, J.J., and Hicks, R.M.: Analysis of membrane structure in transitional epithelium of rat urinary bladder. 2. The discoidal vesicles and golgi apparatus: Their role in luminal membrane biogenesis. J Ultrastruct Res *69*:279, 1979.

Steinert, P.M., Cantieri, J.S., Teller, D.C., Lonsdale-Eccles, J.D., and Dale, B.A.: Characterization of a class of cationic proteins that specifically interact with intermediate filaments. Proc Natl Acad Sci USA *78*:4097, 1981.

Thaslaff, I., Barrach, H.J., Foidart, J.M., Vaheri, A., Pratt, R.H., and Martin, G.R.: Changes in the distribution of laminin, Type IV collagen, B.M./1 proteoglycan and fibronectin during mouse tooth development. Dev Biol *81*:182, 1981.

Yancey, S.B., Nicholoson, B.J., and Revel, J.P.: The dynamic state of liver gap junctions. J Supramolec Struct Cell Biochem *16*:221, 1981.

3

Connective and Supportive Tissues

H.-DIETER DELLMANN
ESTHER M. BROWN

Connective and supportive tissues have great morphologic, topographic, and structural diversities. Their primary functions are to connect other tissues, to provide a framework, and to support the entire body by means of cartilage and bones. These tissues also play an important role in heat regulation and defense and repair mechanisms.

A common characteristic of all connective and supportive tissues is their mesodermal origin. However, it should be noted that the ectoderm of the head region also participates in the formation of connective and supportive tissues. Embryonic connective tissue, or mesenchyme, arises from the mesodermal somites and lateral layers of the somatic and splanchnic mesoderm. Subsequently, all other connective and supportive tissues are derived from mesenchyme.

CLASSIFICATION

Based on occurrence, connective and supportive tissues are classified into two large groups with several subgroups (Table 3–1).

Table 3–1.
Classification of Connective and Supportive Tissues

I. Embryonic connective tissue
   A. Mesenchyme
   B. Gelatinous connective tissue
II. Adult connective and supportive tissues
   A. Adult connective tissues
      1. Loose connective tissue
      2. Dense irregular connective tissue
      3. Dense regular connective tissue
         a. Collagen
         b. Elastic
      4. Reticular connective tissue
      5. Adipose tissue
         a. White adipose tissue
         b. Brown adipose tissue
   B. Adult supportive tissues
      1. Cartilage
         a. Hyaline cartilage
         b. Elastic cartilage
         c. Fibrocartilage
      2. Bone
      3. Notochord (chorda dorsalis)
      4. Cementum and dentin (teeth)

All connective and supportive tissues are composed of cells, fibers, and amorphous ground substance in varying proportions. Mesenchyme, however, lacks fibers during early development.

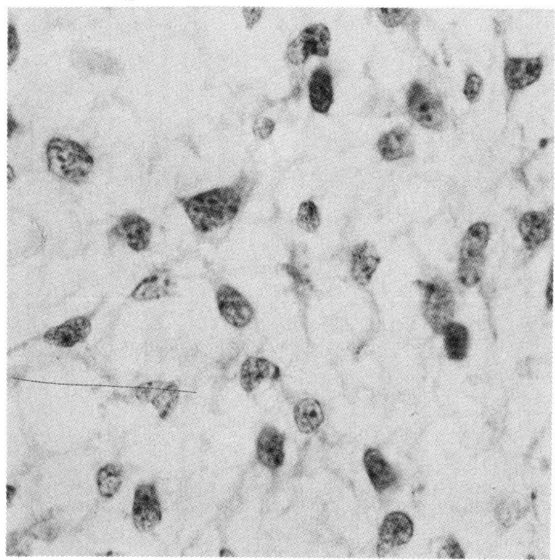

Fig. 3–1. *Mesenchymal cells, rat embryo. ×800.*

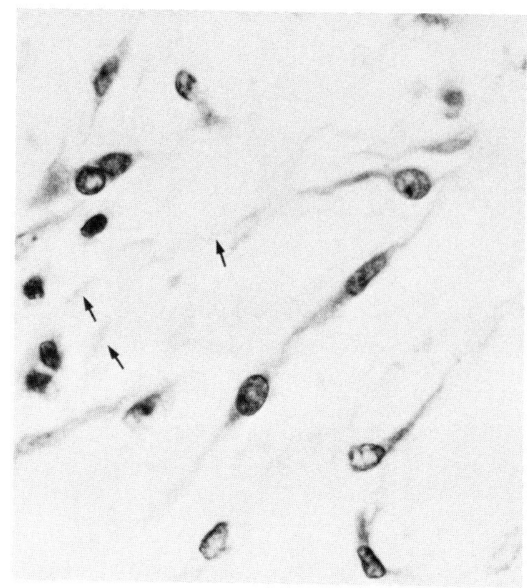

Fig. 3–2. *Gelatinous connective tissue, umbilical cord, pig. A few collagen fibers (arrows) are present. H & E. ×800.*

EMBRYONIC CONNECTIVE TISSUES

Mesenchyme

Mesenchyme is composed of irregularly shaped mesenchymal cells with many and often long processes (Fig. 3–1). The processes may be in contact with those of adjacent cells and thus form a three-dimensional network. Mesenchyme cells undergo numerous mitotic cell divisions and continuously change their shape and location to adapt to the transformations that occur during embryonic growth. During early development, mesenchyme does not contain fibers, and the abundant amorphous ground substance fills the wide intercellular spaces.

Mesenchyme gives rise to the various types of adult connective tissues, as well as blood and blood vessels. As mesenchyme differentiates into other connective tissue types, some of the transitional forms are not easily distinguished.

Gelatinous Connective Tissue

Gelatinous or mucous connective tissue is found primarily in the embryonic hypodermis and umbilical cord. It is characterized by stellate fibroblasts; these form a network whose meshes are occupied by a viscous, gel-like amorphous ground substance that has a positive reaction for mucin and contains collagen fibrils (Fig. 3–2). In the adult organism, gelatinous connective tissue occurs in the core of the papillae on the reticular folds and the omasal laminae, and in the bovine glans penis.

ADULT CONNECTIVE AND SUPPORTIVE TISSUES

Connective tissues consist of cells, intercellular fibers, and amorphous ground substance. The cells of the different types of connective tissue possess varying structural characteristics; the fibers, however, vary only in quantity and arrangement. The amorphous ground substance, likewise, has certain common properties. Therefore, the description of fibers and ground substance will precede that of the various types of adult connective and supportive tissues.

Connective Tissue Fibers

Three types of connective tissue fibers can be distinguished: collagen, reticular, and elastic.

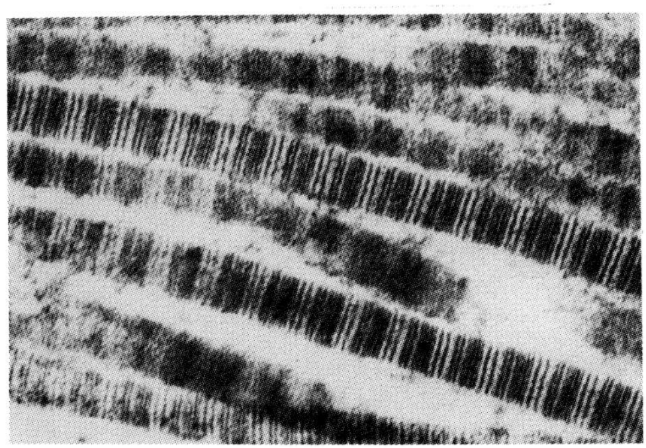

Fig. 3–3. *Electron micrograph of collagen fibrils with characteristic cross striations.* ×*88,000.*

COLLAGEN FIBERS

Collagen polypeptide chains are synthesized in the rER as pro-α-chains that contain extension peptides at both ends. Within the rER cisternae, these pro-α-chains assemble into triple helices to form procollagen molecules. These are transferred to the Golgi complex, packaged into secretory vesicles, and released by exocytosis. The extracellular enzymatic cleavage of the extension peptides yields collagen (or tropocollagen) molecules. These in turn assemble in the extracellular matrix to form collagen fibrils. Collagen fibrils are only visible with the EM and are long (up to several micrometers) structures of varying diameter (10 to 300 μm) with characteristic cross-striations repeated at 67-nm intervals (Fig. 3–3). Bundles of these fibrils form collagen fibers of indefinite length and several micrometers in diameter that are visible in the light microscope (see Fig. 3–15).

Inter- and intramolecular covalent cross-links are formed extracellularly, and their extent and type differs from tissue to tissue. For example, a particularly prominent cross-linkage is present in tendons and ligaments that are characterized by high tensile strength. Likewise, the number, thickness, length, and three-dimensional orientation of the collagen fibers are subject to great variations and depend on the functional properties of a given type of connective tissue.

Collagen fibrils are composed of collagen molecules consisting of three polypeptide helices, referred to as alpha chains, which are coiled around each other in a superhelix. Collagen alpha chains are rich in glycine and lysine and also contain large amounts of hydroxylysine (type I, IV, and V collagen) or hydroxyproline (type III collagen). The repeating cross-striational pattern is very likely due to rows of collagen molecules arranged in an end-to-end fashion with each molecule overlapping the adjacent one by approximately one quarter of its length and stabilized by covalent intermolecular cross-links.

Five genetically distinct types of collagen have been identified, each having alpha chains with a different amino acid sequence, called α1 (I) through α1 (V), α2 (V), and α3 (V). Type I is the most commonly occurring collagen (bone, skin, tendon, ligaments) and consists of two α1 (I) and one α2 (I) chain. Type II collagen predominates in cartilage, with three identical α1 (II) chains. Type III collagen, with three identical α1 (III) chains, is found in embryonic connective tissues and skin. The alpha chain composition of type IV and type V collagen is still controversial. Type IV collagen occurs in the basal laminae of the adult organism; type V occurs mainly in the embryo and a variety of locations of the adult. Neither of these collagens form fibrils.

Fresh collagen fibers are white, and in histologic preparations they stain with acid dyes. Thus, they are red to pink in H & E–stained sections, red with van Gieson's method, and blue in Mallory's and Masson's triple stain (green when light green is used).

Collagen fibers are digested by collagenase, trypsin, and pepsin in an acid environment and are dissolved by strong acids. In weak acids, they swell from uptake of water. When boiled, collagen fibers become hydrated and yield gelatin.

Because collagen fibers have a wavy arrangement (Fig. 3–4), they are flexible and

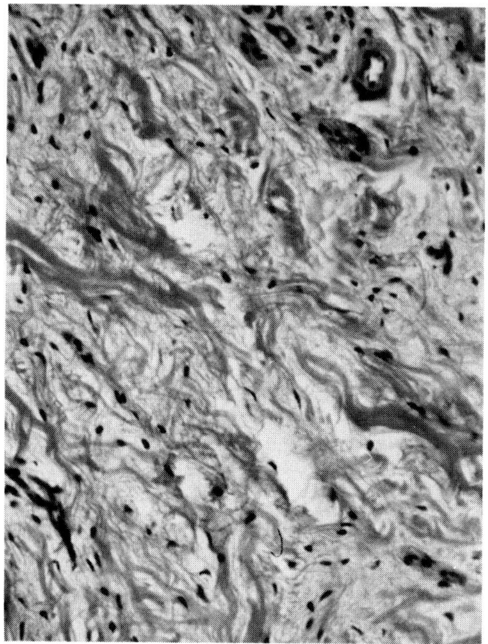

Fig. 3–4. *Dense irregular connective tissue, hard palate, dog. Notice the interlacing bundles of collagen fibers and associated fibroblasts. H & E. ×200.*

can adapt to the movements and changes in size of the organs with which they are associated. Collagen fibers themselves are characterized by a high tensile strength and can be stretched only to approximately 5% of their initial length. Consequently, they are found wherever high tensile strength is required, such as in tendons, ligaments, and organ capsules.

RETICULAR FIBERS

In routine histologic preparations, reticular fibers are not visible. It is only with certain silver impregnations (thus the term argyrophilic or argentaffin fibers) or with the periodic acid-Schiff (PAS) reagent that these fibers can be seen. They form delicate, flexible networks around capillaries, muscle fibers, nerves, adipose cells, and hepatocytes, and serve as a scaffolding to support cells or cell groups of endocrine, lymphatic, and blood-forming organs (Fig. 3–5). They are an integral part of basement membranes.

The fine-structural and biochemical analysis of reticular fibers has revealed that they are actually individual collagen fibrils (type III collagen) coated by proteoglycans and glycoproteins. It is that coating that processes the affinity for silver salts (Fig. 3–5). When individual fibers are bundled to form collagen fibers, the coating is supposedly displaced and the argyrophilia disappears.

ELASTIC FIBERS

Elastic fibers or sheets (laminae) are present in organs whose normal function requires elasticity, in addition to tensile strength.

Elastic fibers can be stretched as much as 2½ times their original length, to which they return when released. Elastic fibers are found in organs whose normal functions require great elasticity, such as the external ear, vocal cords, trachea, lungs, ligamentum nuchae, skin, and arteries (Fig. 3–6).

Elastic fibers usually occur as individual, branching and anastomosing fibers. Their diameter varies within a wide range, from 0.2 to 5.0 μm in loose connective tissue to as large as 12 μm in elastic ligaments, such as the ligamentum nuchae (Fig. 3–7). In H & E–stained histologic sections, the larger elastic fibers in elastic ligaments are readily distinguished as highly refractile, light pink strands; they are stainable by certain selective dyes such as orcein and resorcin-fuchsin.

The main component of elastic fibers is *elastin,* an amorphous protein of low electron density. The elastin molecules are randomly coiled and joined by stable, covalent cross-links, the two major ones of which are desmosine and isodesmosine, the two derivatives of lysine. The secondary component of elastic fibers is microfibrils, approximately 11 nm in diameter, which are embedded in the periphery of elastic fibers.

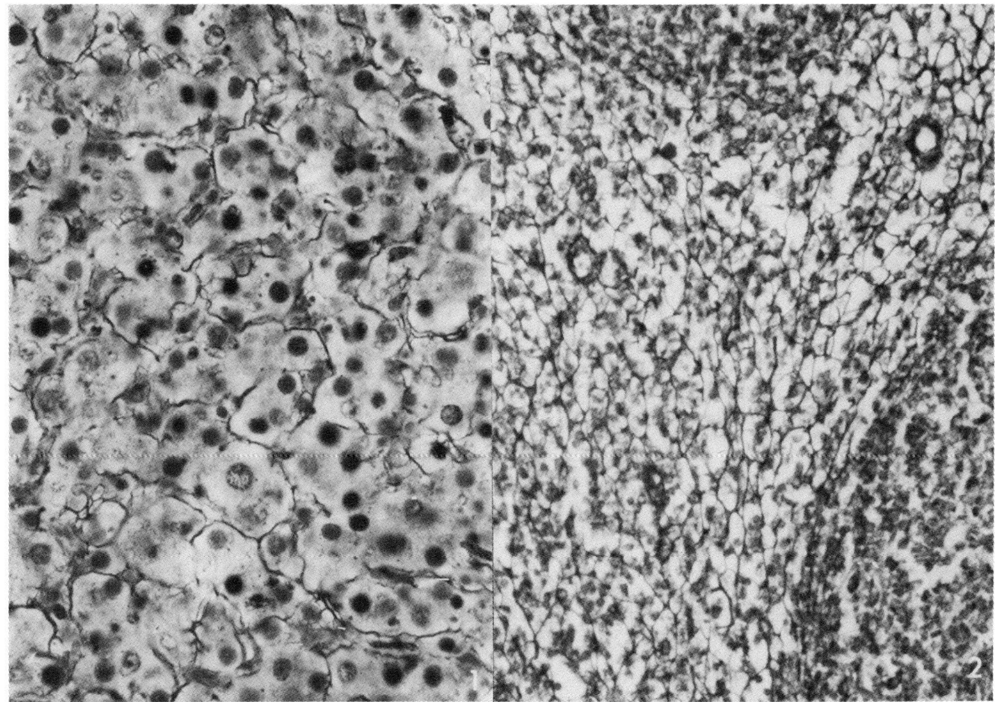

Fig. 3–5. *Reticular fibers. 1, Liver, pig. Achucarro silver impregnation. ×435. 2, Lymph node, dog. Palmgren silver impregnation. ×230.*

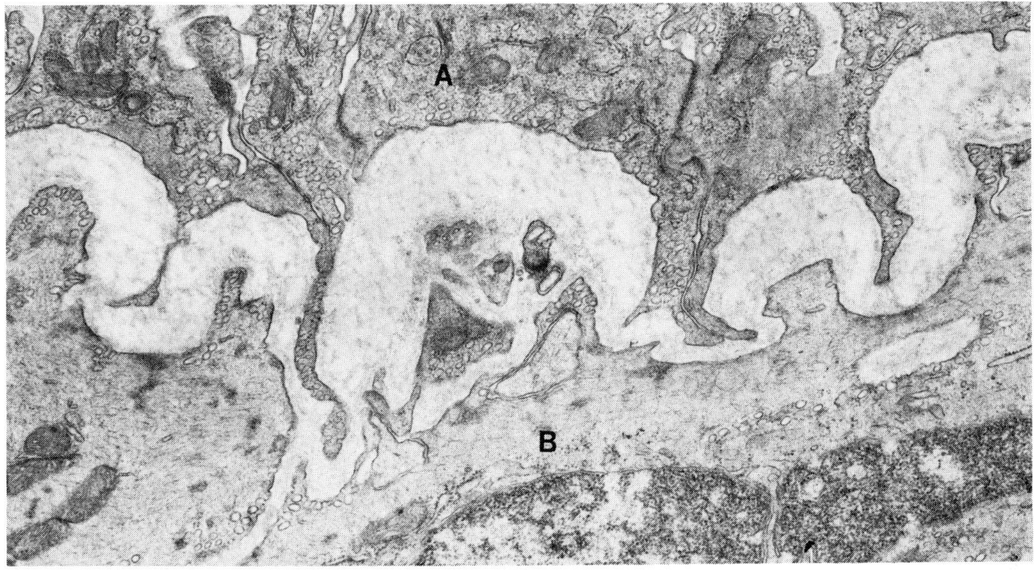

Fig. 3–6. *Electron micrograph of a portion of an arteriole wall with the internal elastic lamina between endothelium (A) and smooth muscle (B). ×14,500.*

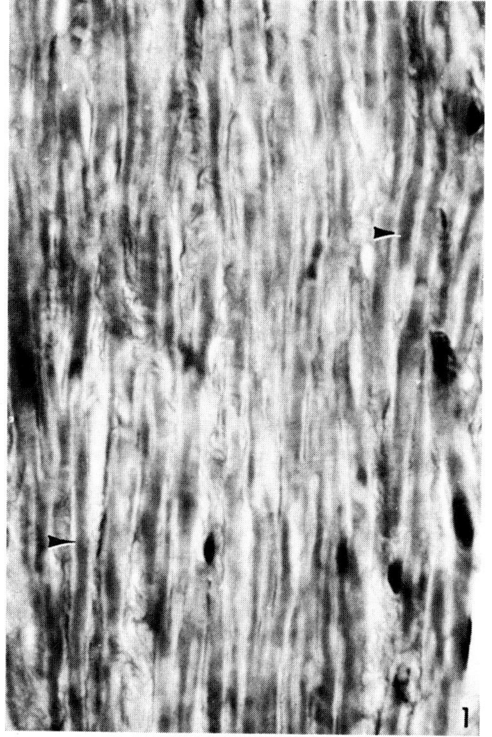

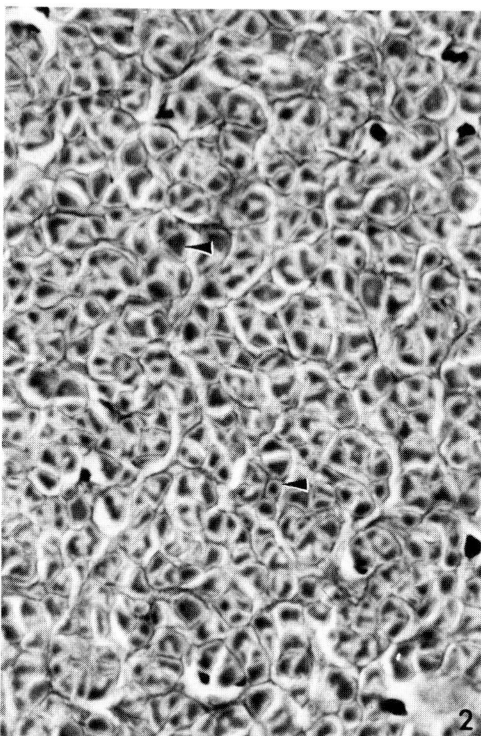

Fig. 3–7. *Ligamentum nuchae, large ruminant. 1, Longitudinal section; 2, cross section. Notice that the large elastic fibers (arrows) are surrounded by networks of collagen fibers. Crossmon's trichrome.* ×600.

The microfibrillar material is a glycoprotein rich in cystine.

Elastin is synthesized by fibroblasts and smooth muscle cells as tropoelastin, i.e., single polypeptide chains that are transformed into elastin, cross-linked, and assembled in the extracellular space. The microfibrils are secreted prior to elastin and provide a scaffolding on which elastin forms fibers and sheets.

Ground Substance

The fibers and cells of connective tissue are embedded in an amorphous ground substance composed predominantly of various *proteoglycans*. Proteoglycans in low concentrations are not detected by H & E–stained sections, but when present in higher concentrations, as in hyaline cartilage, they stain with basophilic dyes. When stained with toluidine blue or crystal violet, a metachromatic reaction occurs, i.e., the amorphous ground substance stains a different color from that of the dye solution.

Proteoglycans consist of multiple polysaccharide side chains (glycosaminoglycans) bound to a protein core. Seven major types of proteoglycans can be distinguished. *Hyaluronic acid* is a nonsulfated glycosaminoglycan that is not linked to a protein. It is a large, long molecule that forms networks whose spaces are filled with tissue fluid; the resulting gel is particularly abundant in vitreous humor and synovial fluid and is also found in the umbilical cord, loose connective tissue, skin, and cartilage. *Chondroitin-4-sulfate* and *chondroitin-6-sulfate* are abundant in cartilage, bone, skin, and cornea. *Dermatan sulfate* is found in skin, tendon, ligamentum nuchae, sclera, and lung. *Keratan sulfate* is present in cartilage, bone, and cornea. *Heparan sulfate* is found in arteries and the lung, and *heparin,* in mast cells, the lung, liver, and skin. The latter six proteoglycans are all of the sulfated variety.

The glycosaminoglycans of proteoglycans are highly hydrophilic; they form hydrated gels that by virtue of their high water content are highly resistant to pressure. The intercellular fluid in the proteoglycan meshwork permits diffusion of nutrients and metabolites and is thus essential in the maintenance of a proper environment for connective tissue fibers and cells. The proportions of the various proteoglycans in a given type of connective tissue determine to a large degree the morphologic and functional properties of that tissue.

Fibronectin, a major product of mesenchymal cells, is a fiber-forming protein that binds to various structures including the cell membrane, collagen, elastin, and proteoglycans and very likely mediates the connection between cytoskeleton and the extracellular matrix. Fibronectin plays a role in a variety of processes such as cell adhesion, cell differentiation, cell growth, homeostasis, and phagocytosis. *Laminin* is a large glycoprotein. It is the major constituent of basal laminae and is synthesized by the cells that are in contact with it (e.g., epithelial cells, smooth muscle cells, neurolemmocytes). It is present in the lamina rara (lucida) of basal laminae and specifically attaches the cell to the lamina densa, in which type IV collagen forms a nonfibrous network of considerable strength and elasticity.

Adult Connective Tissues

LOOSE CONNECTIVE TISSUE

Loose, irregularly arranged, or areolar connective tissue is the most widely distributed type of connective tissue in the adult animal (Fig. 3–8).

Loose connective tissue is present around blood vessels and nerves and between muscle bundles and the layers of smooth musculature of hollow organs. It is found beneath many epithelia, where it provides support and a vascular supply. It makes up the interstitial tissue in most organs, allowing easy movements and shifting of organs.

Loose connective tissue predominates in the pia mater and arachnoid. Adipose cells in varying numbers regularly occur in loose connective tissue and are particularly abundant in that of the hypodermis.

Many important functions are carried out by loose connective tissue. They range from the purely mechanical, such as support and dampening effects in various locations, to more sophisticated functions, such as participation in tissue repair, defense activities (inflammation), and water metabolism (edema).

Cells are relatively more abundant than fibers in loose connective tissue. The various cell types are divided into two groups: one population of fixed cells, which includes fibroblasts, pericytes, and adipose cells, and another population of wandering or free cells whose presence depends largely upon the functional state of the tissue.

Fixed Cells of Loose Connective Tissue

FIBROBLASTS. The most common fixed cell of loose connective tissues is the fibroblast. When lying between connective tissue fibers, fibroblasts are generally elongated and spindle-shaped, and their nuclei are surrounded by a small amount of pale cytoplasm. Active fibroblasts are found in the developing organism and in the connective tissue involved in wound repair.

In adult connective tissue, the fiber-forming cells are relatively inactive and are commonly referred to as *fibrocytes* (see Fig. 3–15). The fine structure of fibrocytes reflects their relative inactivity. The rER, free ribosomes, transfer and secretory vesicles, mitochondria, and lysosomes are all sparse, and the Golgi complex is small. In the more active *fibroblasts,* these organelles are more

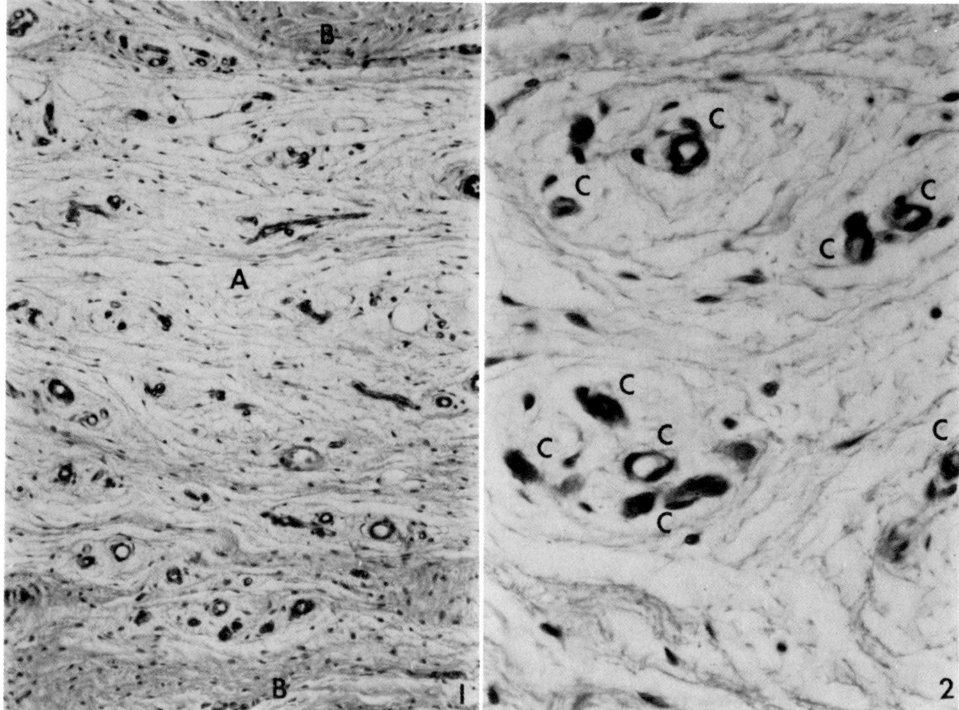

Fig. 3–8. *Loose connective tissue, digital cushion, cat. 1, Notice the loose texture of the loose connective tissue (A) in comparison with the dense irregular connective tissue (B), and the rich blood supply. H & E. ×130. 2, Capillaries (C) within a loosely arranged collagen fiber network associated with a few fibroblasts. H & E. ×435.*

numerous and/or extensive, and granulated secretory vesicles are seen to discharge their contents (procollagen, proteoglycans, proelastin, etc.) into the intercellular space. Fibroblasts also possess a larger nucleus with a prominent nucleolus, more abundant and basophilic cytoplasm, and long processes contacting adjacent cells.

PERICYTES. Pericytes are elongated pericapillary cells (Fig. 3–9) surrounded by a basal lamina that is continuous with the capillary basal lamina. These cells have a fusiform nucleus, and the relatively sparse cytoplasm that extends into slender processes contains many mitochondria, rER, free ribosomes, and a small Golgi complex (see Fig. 7–8).

Pericytes are considered undifferentiated cells that may give up their fixed pericapillary position and move into the surrounding connective tissue; they may serve

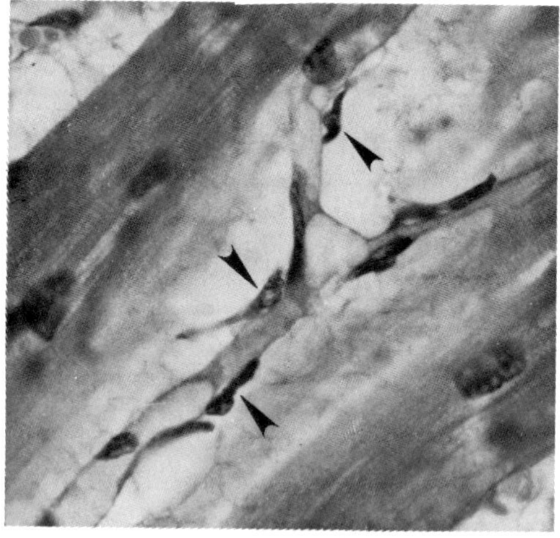

Fig. 3–9. *Myocardial capillary, pig, surrounded by pericytes (arrow). H & E. ×650.*

as progenitor cells for fibroblasts, chondroblasts, osteoblasts, and smooth muscle cells whenever the need arises.

ADIPOSE CELLS. Adipose cells are also referred to as *fat cells* or *adipocytes*. Fat cells, single or in groups, are normal components of loose connective tissue, but whenever they outnumber all other cell types, the tissue is called *adipose tissue* (see p. 50). Mature adipocytes are spherical or polyhedral cells, measuring up to 120 μm in diameter. Most of the cell is occupied by a single large lipid droplet that reduces the cytoplasm to a thin peripheral layer containing the flattened nucleus, small Golgi complex, ER, free ribosomes, and mitochondria.

Free Cells of Loose Connective Tissue

MACROPHAGES. Macrophages in nonreactive loose connective tissue are usually fixed, but they become motile in response to stimulation. They are derived from blood monocytes that migrate into the loose connective tissue (see page 82). In routine light-microscopic sections, fixed macrophages or histiocytes are difficult or even impossible to distinguish from fibroblasts. When histochemically stained for lysosomal enzymes, such as acid phosphatase, they have a strong, positive reaction. Stimulated macrophages, however, are large, ovoid, or spherical cells with foamy cytoplasm readily distinguishable with the light microscope. At the fine-structural level, they are characterized by numerous filopodia (fine, threadlike processes), abundant ribosomes, short cisternae of rER, mitochondria, a Golgi complex, and especially numerous lysosomes and phagosomes, or phagolysosomes (Fig. 3–10). Multinucleated giant cells or foreign-body giant cells (Fig. 3–11) are the result of a fusion of several mononuclear phagocytes in response to the presence of foreign material too large to be phagocytized by a single macrophage.

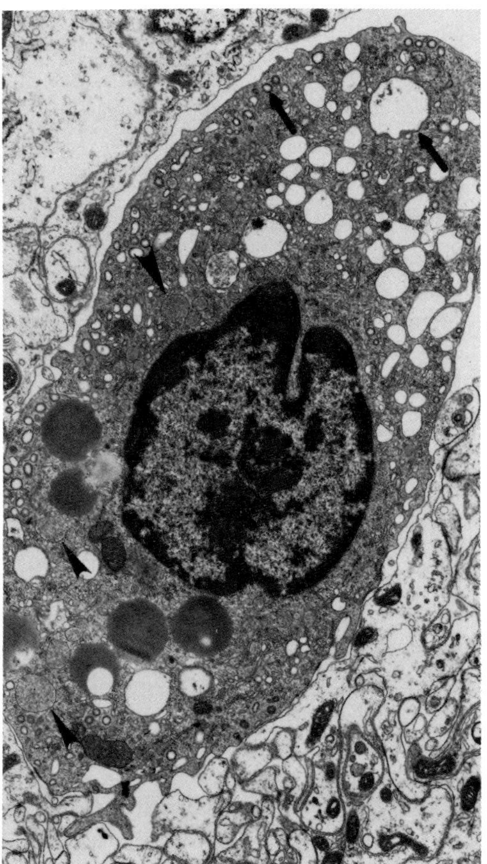

Fig. 3–10. *Macrophage containing abundant pinocytotic vacuoles (arrows) and phagolysosomes (arrowheads).* ×*7800.*

A variety of stimuli (e.g., infectious agents, lymphokines) cause macrophages to move to those parts of the organism (by chemotaxis) where they are needed, to accumulate there and to become phagocytic. Macrophages engulf material by pinocytosis and phagocytosis; these processes may be nonspecific, in which particles are engulfed indiscriminately (e.g., dust particles in the lung), or they may be highy specific, in which particle-bound recognition factors (IgG, IgM, and the third component of complement C3) interact with specific receptors on the macrophage surface, called Fc receptors, and initiate particle attachment and phagocytosis.

Macrophages synthesize and secrete many substances that are a reflection of

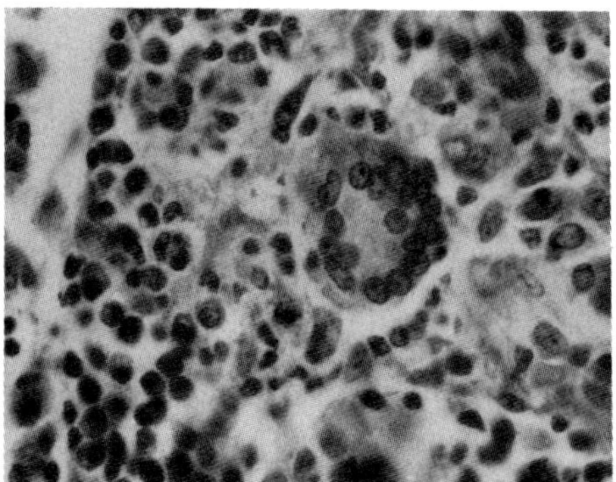

Fig. 3–11. *Multinucleated giant cell, lymph node, sheep. Crossmon's trichrome. ×435.*

their multiple and varied functions. These substances include lysozyme that lyses the wall of many bacteria; interferon, an antiviral factor; protein involved in complement activation; prostaglandin; mitogenic protein (interleukin) essential for the proliferation and survival of B- and T-lymphocytes; and superoxide (O_3), hydroxyradicals (OH), and hydrogen peroxide (H_2O_2), important components of the bactericidal and cytocidal (tumor cells) activities of macrophages.

MAST CELLS. Mast cells are common in loose connective tissue, especially that of the skin and intestine, and are often particularly abundant around blood vessels. They are large, polymorphic, spherical, or ovoid cells that contain numerous large metachromatic granules (Fig. 3–12). At the fine-structural level, the granules are seen to be membrane-bounded and to have either crystalline, lamellar, or fine granular characteristics. The remaining cytoplasm is occupied by an extensive Golgi complex, cisternae of rER, free ribosomes, and mitochondria.

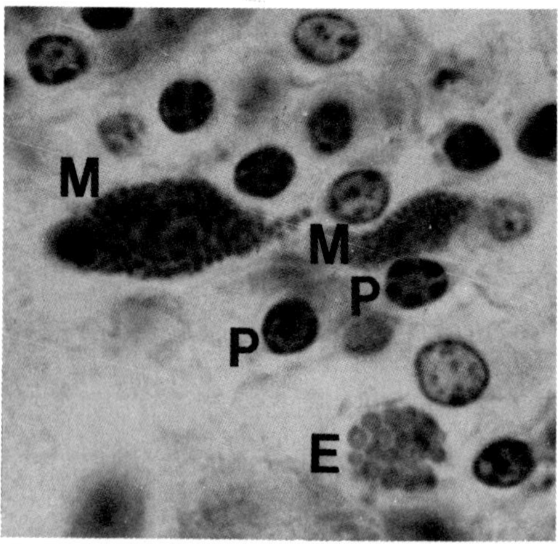

Fig. 3–12. *Mast cells (M) in the propria of the colon of the horse are readily distinguished from eosinophilic leukocytes (E) by the size and staining affinity of their granules. The nuclei of plasma cells (P) have a characteristic chromatin pattern. Crossmon's trichrome. ×1470.*

In allergic and anaphylactic reactions, interaction of antigens with antibodies bound to the surface of sensitized mast cells induces granule release by exocytosis. These granules contain histamine, heparin, and, in the mouse and rat, serotonin and a variety of other so-called mediators. The liberated serotonin is a vasoconstrictor, as is histamine, which also causes increased permeability of small venules which permits leakage of plasma resulting in edema. This is a localized inflammatory reaction designed to dispose of foreign antigens rapidly. Heparin is an anticoagulant whose role in connective tissue is not clear. Eosinophil chemotactic factors attract eosinophils commonly observed in parasitic infestations of the intestinal mucosa.

PLASMA CELLS. Plasma cells are spherical, ovoid, or pear-shaped cells with a spherical, eccentric nucleus. The chromatin is often arranged in peripherally located clumps or in centrally converging strands that give it a "cartwheel" appearance (Fig. 3–12). The cytoplasm is intensely basophilic, and often a negative Golgi image can be observed readily. At the fine-structural level, in addition to an extensive Golgi complex, the cytoplasm contains an abundant rER, whose often dilated cisternae contain slightly granular and moderately electron-dense material (Fig. 3–13), free ribosomes, and mitochondria. Plasma cells may also contain spherical inclusions, referred to as *Russell bodies,* located within dilated portions of the ER (Fig. 3–13). Russell bodies

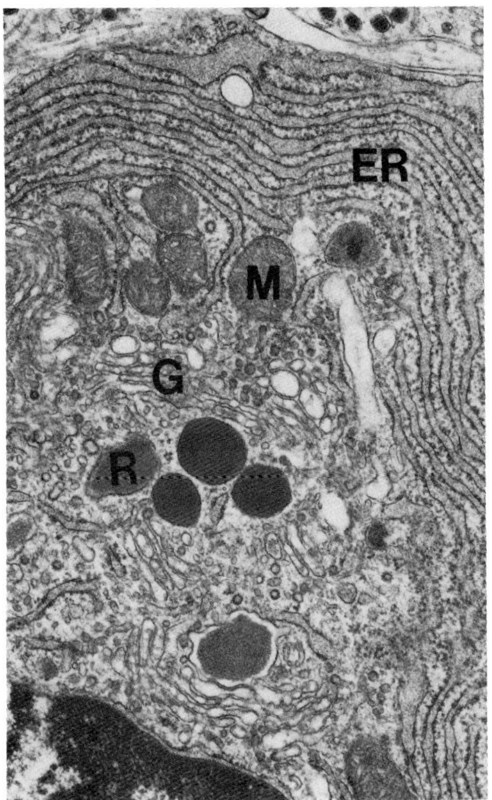

Fig. 3–13. *Part of a plasma cell with abundant rough ER (ER), mitochondria (M), extensive Golgi complex (G), and Russell bodies (R).* ×*19,500.*

give a positive reaction for immunoglobulin.

Plasma cells are particularly abundant in the loose connective tissue of the propria of the gastrointestinal tract, the respiratory system, and the female reproductive system, but they are relatively scarce in the loose connective tissue of other body areas. They are most numerous in lymphatic tissue.

Plasma cells do not originate in loose connective tissue but develop from B-lymphocytes that migrate from the blood; they produce circulating or humoral antibodies (see Chapter 8).

MELANOCYTES. Large pigmented cells of neural crest origin with numerous long, branching processes are referred to as *melanocytes* (Fig. 3–14). They occur in various

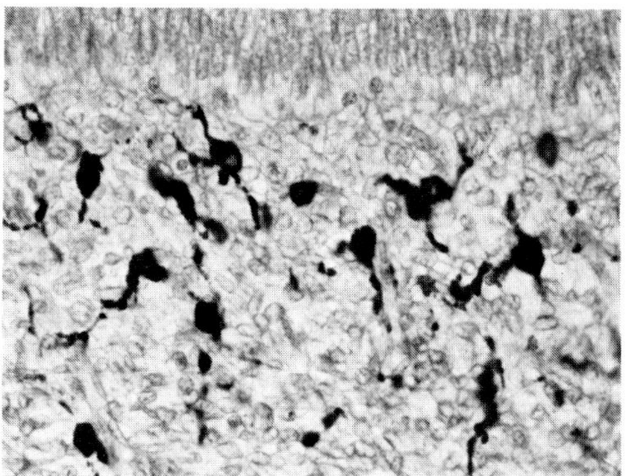

Fig. 3–14. *Melanocytes in the propria of a uterine caruncle, sheep. H & E.* ×*325.*

locations such as the dermis, uterine caruncles of sheep, meninges, choroid, and iris. Their significance will be discussed in connection with these organs.

OTHER FREE CELLS OF LOOSE CONNECTIVE TISSUE. Depending on its location and various other factors (infestation by parasites, presence of bacteria, and the like), loose connective tissue may contain a varying number of lymphocytes, monocytes, and granulocytes (especially eosinophils [Fig. 3–12] and neutrophils). The structure and function of these free cells will be discussed in the section on blood (Chapter 4).

Fibers of Loose Connective Tissue

The connective tissue fibers are loosely arranged and include all three fiber types: recticular, collagen, and elastic. Their relative abundance and orientation are subject to wide variations and depend largely upon the location and specific function of the tissue.

Amorphous Ground Substance of Loose Connective Tissue

The amorphous ground substance of loose connective tissue is composed of proteoglycans that form a three-dimensional network filled with tissue or intercellular fluid. In the larger interstices, this fluid has the ability of limited circulation. Substances dissolved in it (e.g., metabolites) can either circulate together with the intercellular fluid or diffuse through the amorphous ground substance and thus have ready access to connective tissue cells. Tissue fluid is formed at the arterial end of capillaries and absorbed by either venous or lymph capillaries.

DENSE CONNECTIVE TISSUE

The fibers in dense connective tissue are more abundant than cells and amorphous ground substance. Dense connective tissue is commonly classified as either *dense irregular connective tissue,* with a seemingly random orientation of the fiber bundles, or *dense regular connective tissue,* in which fibers are oriented in a regular pattern.

Dense Irregular Connective Tissue

Dense irregular connective tissue has essentially the same cell population as loose connective tissue, although fibrocytes usually predominate (Fig. 3–4). The other cell types are difficult to identify.

Collagen fibers predominate in dense irregular connective tissue. They are generally arranged in bundles that cross each other at varying angles. In thin aponeuroses or muscle fasciae, for example, these bundles are located in a single plane and withstand stretching parallel to fiber orientation. In thick aponeuroses, muscular fascia, organ capsules, dermis, and the like, the bundles are superimposed in several planes and interlace with one another in three planes: longitudinal, vertical, and horizontal. This allows for adaptation to changes in the size of an organ or the diameter of a muscle. Such stretching forces can be withstood in any direction. The fact that organ capsules and muscle fasciae are continuous with the trabeculae or the connective tissue between muscle bundles (perimysium) adds to the strength of these structures and makes overstretching rather difficult. The presence of elastic networks facilitates a fast return to resting conditions.

Dense irregular connective tissue is found in a variety of locations, such as the propria of the initial portions of the digestive system, the capsule of the lung (visceral pleura), the capsules of various organs (spleen, liver, kidney, testis), fasciae, aponeuroses, joint capsules, pericardium, and dermis. Special functional and morphologic features will be discussed with the various organ systems.

Dense Regular Connective Tissue

Dense regular connective tissue occurs in two varieties, as collagen tendons and ligaments and as elastic ligaments. In both types, the fibers are arranged in the same plane and direction, according to specific functional requirements.

COLLAGEN TENDONS AND LIGAMENTS. The great tensile strength of collagen tendons and ligaments is reflected in their structure. They consist of fascicles of parallel collagen fibers (Fig. 3–15). These fascicles are bound together by sparse, loose connective tissue that forms a protective sheath around the blood vessels and nerves of the tendon and that is continuous with the *peritendineum,* the loose connective tissue around the tendon. Repair of a severed tendon is effected by the fibroblasts of this loose connective tissue; those of the fiber bundles are believed to remain essentially inactive.

The fibrocytes between the collagen fibers are long, flat cells (Fig. 3–15) of varying shape, with winglike cytoplasmic processes extending between adjacent collagen fibers, giving them a stellate appearance in cross section.

The typical tendon structure may be altered at points of insertion to bone or cartilage or where tendons course around bones. Wherever tendons insert on bones or cartilage, the dense regular collagenous tissue becomes fibrocartilage at the point

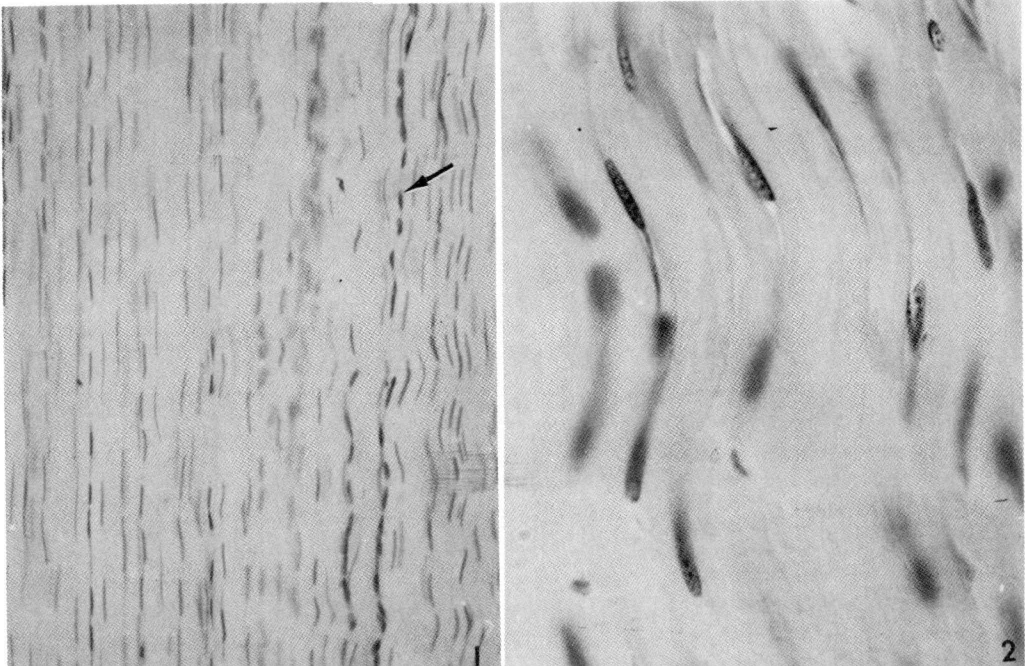

Fig. 3–15. *Longitudinal section through a tendon. 1, Notice the line of nuclei (arrow), indicative of loose connective tissue, surrounding blood vessels and nerves. H & E. ×226. 2, Spindle-shaped fibrocytes among collagen fibers. H & E. ×660.*

of attachment. In areas where tendons course around bones, they are subjected not only to pulling forces but also to pressure, which causes the cells to enlarge and to become encapsulated, so that the tissue appears very similar to fibrocartilage.

The motility of the tendon is assured either by the surrounding peritendineum or by a tendon sheath. The latter consists of a visceral and a parietal portion. The visceral portion is tightly anchored to the tendon and separated from the parietal portion by a fluid-filled synovial cavity. The two portions are connected by a mesotendineum. Both the parietal and the visceral portions comprise a fibrous layer of dense irregular connective tissue and a synovial layer whose structure is similar to that of synovial membranes.

ELASTIC LIGAMENTS. Branching and interconnected parallel elastic fibers surrounded by loose connective tissue make up elastic ligaments (Fig. 3–7). The ligamentum nuchae and the elastic fasciae of the abdominal musculature of herbivores are examples of elastic ligaments.

RETICULAR CONNECTIVE TISSUE

The stroma of all lymphatic organs (spleen, lymph node, hemal lymph node, hemal node, tonsils), diffuse lymphatic tissue, solitary lymphatic nodules, and bone marrow is made up of reticular connective tissue. This tissue is composed of stellate reticular cells and a complex three-dimensional network of reticular fibers (Fig. 3–16) (see Chapter 8).

ADIPOSE TISSUE

Adipose tissue, or fat, is a specialized type of connective tissue that, in addition to performing insulating and mechanical functions, plays an important role in the metabolism of the organism. Two types of

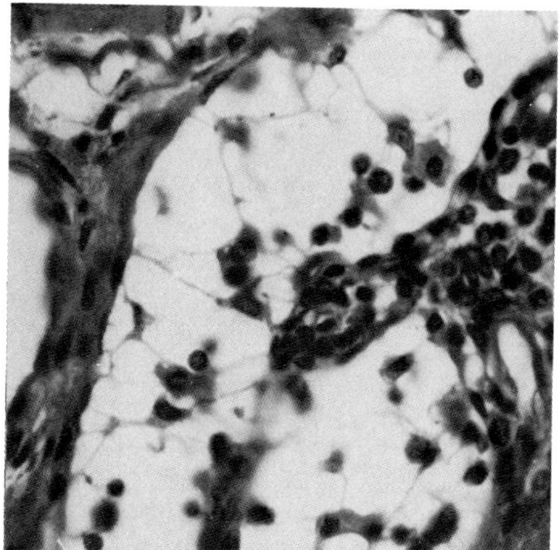

Fig. 3–16. *Reticular connective tissue, lymph node, sheep. Notice the numerous interconnected reticular cells which form a three-dimensional network. H & E. ×600.*

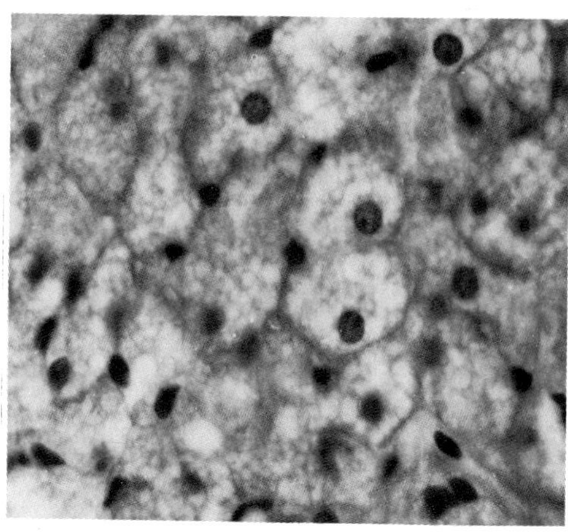

Fig. 3–18. *Brown adipose tissue. Notice the numerous, small lipid inclusions. H & E. ×600.*

adipose tissue, white and brown, are distinguished in most mammals by differences in color, vascularity, structure and function.

White Adipose Tissue

White fat is partitioned by septa of loose connective tissue into clusters of adipose cells referred to as lobules. Each adipose cell is surrounded by a delicate network of collagen and reticular fibers that supports

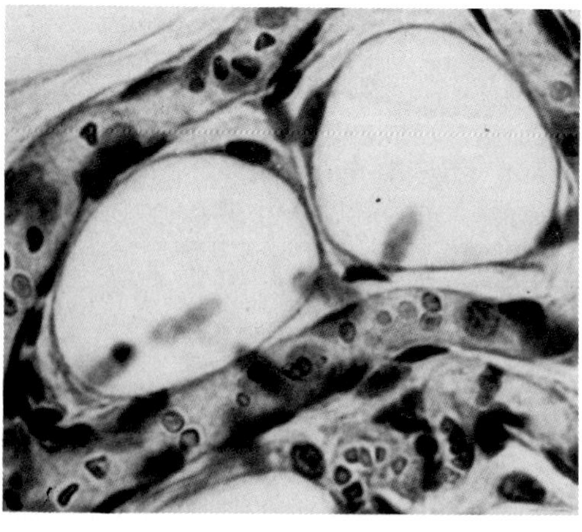

Fig. 3–17. *Two white adipocytes surrounded by capillaries. H & E. ×630. (Courtesy of Dr. A. Hansen.)*

a dense capillary plexus and nerve fibers. In addition, the narrow intercellular spaces contain a few fibrocytes, mast cells, and sparse amorphous ground substance.

The polygonal adipose cells measure up to 200 μm in diameter and contain a single large lipid droplet, and therefore are also called *unilocular adipocytes* (Fig. 3–17). The lipid droplet is surrounded by a thin layer of cytoplasm that contains a flattened nucleus, a small Golgi complex, ER, and mitochondria. The lipid inclusion is not membrane-bounded, but the cytoplasm adjacent to its surface often contains microfilaments.

Because fat is rapidly dissolved by most of the dehydration and/or clearing agents commonly used for the preparation of histologic sections, adipose cells appear as large clear spaces surrounded by a thin layer of cytoplasm (Fig. 3–17). When properly treated, the lipid can be preserved and stained with certain dyes such as osmium tetroxide or Sudan III.

Brown Adipose Tissue

Brown fat cells are usually considerably smaller than white ones. Their outstanding characteristic is the presence of multiple small individual lipid droplets scattered throughout the cytoplasm (*multilocular adipocyte* (Fig. 3–18). Both the Golgi complex and ER are rather inconspicuous, but a large number of mitochondria are present, whose high concentration of cytochromes is primarily responsible for the brown color of the tissue. The intercellular connective tissue has the same characteristics as that of white adipose tissue; capillaries form a dense plexus and the adipocytes are directly innervated by adrenergic axons.

Brown adipose tissue is particularly common and abundant in rodents and hibernating mammals, where it is located primarily in the axillary and neck regions (interscapular fat body), along the thoracic aorta and in the mediastinum, in the mesenteries, and around the aorta and vena cava dorsal to the kidney; however, it may also be found in the same locations in domestic mammals.

Function of Adipose Tissue

One of the most important functions of adipose tissue is its participation in fat metabolism. Regardless of whether the organism has to draw on its fat reserves to supplement food intake, there is an extremely rapid turnover of intracellular fat, with a continuous withdrawal and deposit.

Intracellular lipids are synthesized mainly from fatty acids, but also from carbohydrates and proteins. The fatty acids necessary for lipid synthesis are derived from the enzymatic breakdown by lipoprotein lipase of the triglycerides contained in blood chylomicrons or lipoproteins (see Chapter 10); following their uptake by the adipocytes, the fatty acids are resynthesized to triglycerides.

Under hormonal (insulin) or nervous (norepinephrine) control, intracellular enzymatic hydrolysis of triglycerides takes place, and fatty acids and glycerol are released into the blood and catabolized in energy-yielding reactions. In brown adipocytes, mitochondrial respiration is uncoupled from ATP synthesis; thus the oxidation of stored fat generates heat rather than ATP, causing a rise in body temperature in arousing hibernating mammals.

In mammalian subcutaneous connective tissue, the adipose tissue component serves as a thermal and mechanical insulator. In the foot pads and digital cushions, adipose tissue is associated with bundles of collagen and elastic fibers. This combination of fibers and fat cells allows the adipose tissue to act as a dampening cushion, and at the same time the cells are protected by the great tensile strength of the collagen fibers. Following deformation, the elastic fibers allow the adipose cells to return to normal shape.

Adult Supportive Tissues

CARTILAGE

Cartilage is the connective tissue specialized for a supportive role. It is composed of cells, the *chondrocytes,* fibers, and a gel-like ground substance. It possesses considerable tensile strength, because the intercellular substance is laced with collagen and elastic fibers, and the firm but pliable ground substance enhances its weight-bearing ability.

On the basis of different structural characteristics of the fibers and amorphous ground substance, three types of cartilage are distinguishable: hyaline cartilage, elastic cartilage, and fibrocartilage.

Hyaline Cartilage

Hyaline cartilage is found on the articulating surfaces of bones and provides support in the nose, larynx, trachea, and bronchi. It forms most of the entire appendicular and axial skeleton in the embryo.

Knowledge of cartilage formation is important in understanding the development of embryonic bone models, epiphyseal

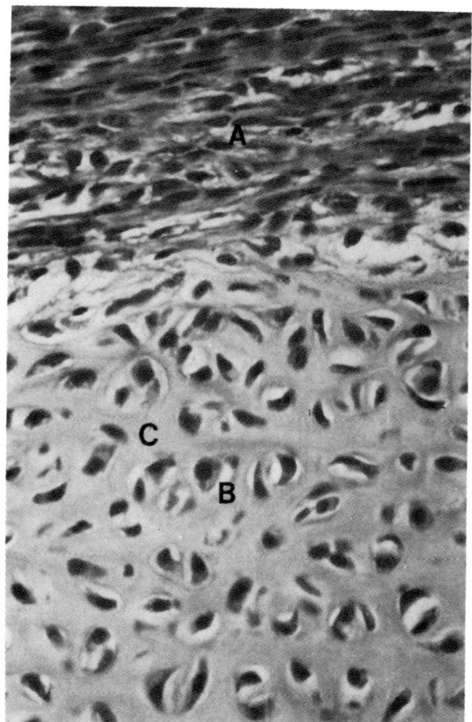

Fig. 3–19. *Immature hyaline cartilage, dog. The perichondrium (A) borders the cartilage composed of chondrocytes in lacunae (B) and intercellular ground substance (C). H & E. ×400.*

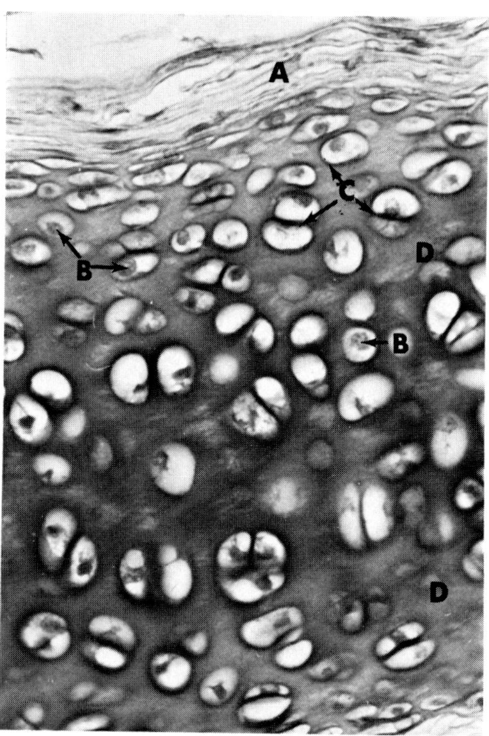

Fig. 3–20. *Mature hyaline cartilage, dog. The fibrous perichondrium (A) surrounds the cartilage mass. The chondrocytes (B) lie in lacunae. The territorial matrix (C) is darker than the interterritorial matrix (D). H & E. ×425.*

plates, and bone formation. For these reasons, it will be considered first.

DEVELOPMENT. The first indication of cartilage formation within the embryo is a clustering of mesenchyme cells. These cells enlarge, withdraw their processes, and synthesize and secrete amorphous ground substance and procollagen. They are then referred to as *chondroblasts,* and the cell clusters are called *centers of chondrification.* As the intercellular substances increase, the cells become spherical and isolated from each other in compartments called *lacunae* (Fig. 3–19); at this point they are called *chondrocytes.*

Chondroblasts undergo several mitotic divisions, and after each division, new intercellular ground substance separates the two daughter cells. This process leads to substantial expansion of the cartilage from within and is referred to as *interstitial growth.* Concurrently, the mesenchyme surrounding the cartilage primordium differentiates into the *perichondrium,* made up of two distinct layers. The layer immediately adjacent to the cartilage, composed of chondroblasts, is called the *cellular* or *chondrogenic layer.* These chondroblasts secrete some components of the ground substance and the fibers and become chondrocytes. In this way, new cells are added to the periphery of the cartilage, and the process is called *appositional growth.* The ability of the chondrogenic layer to produce cartilage persists into adult life, but it is dormant until there is a need for new cartilage. The outer *fibrous layer* of the perichondrium is made up of irregularly arranged collagen fibers and fibroblasts.

MICROSCOPIC STRUCTURE. The chondrocytes in mature hyaline cartilage vary in size. As a result of appositional growth, those immediately beneath the perichondrium are small, and their lacunae are elliptical with their long axes parallel to the surface. Deep within the cartilage, where interstitial growth occurs, the cells are larger and more polyhedral in shape (Fig. 3–20). Some lacunae contain only one cell; others contain two, four, or sometimes six cells. These multicellular lacunae are called *cell nests* or *isogenous cell groups,* because each cluster is the progeny of one cell from repeated mitotic divisions. Chondrocytes have a spherical nucleus with one or more nucleoli, and in living cartilage the cell fills the lacunae. However, in stained sections the cell surface is seen to be separated from the lacunar walls because of shrinkage. Active chondrocytes have an abundant rER and Golgi complex. The uneven cellular borders have short cytoplasmic processes extending into the intercellular substance. Glycogen and lipid accumulate in old chondrocytes, and in routine preparation the cells appear vacuolated.

The amorphous ground substance is a firm gel laced with collagen fibers. Because the fibers have the same index of refraction as the amorphous ground substance, they cannot be seen in the usual preparations. The ground substance contains the proteoglycans chondroitin sulfate, keratan sulfate, and hyaluronic acid, all of which play an important role in the transport of water and electrolytes. The proteoglycans are bound to the collagen fibrils, thereby forming a loose network that functions as a molecular sieve limiting movement of larger molecules. The matrix is intensely basophilic, reacts positively with PAS, and exhibits a marked metachromasia when stained with toluidine blue. Surrounding each lacuna is the *territorial matrix,* which has a functionally special region immediately adjacent to the chondrocyte, the *pericellular matrix.* The chondrocyte plasmalemma and the pericellular matrix may function together in the polymerization of collagen and proteoglycans. The area farther away from the lacunae, the *interterritorial matrix,* stains lighter than the territorial matrix because of increased numbers of collagen fibers (Fig. 3–20).

NUTRITION. Unlike other connective tissues cartilage is nonvascular. Therefore, the chondrocytes must depend on diffusion of nutrients through the gelled intercellular substance from capillaries outside the perichondrium. When, for some reason, the intercellular matrix becomes calcified, diffusion is no longer possible, and the cartilage cells die. This occurs in aging and is a natural phenomenon in endochondral bone development.

Elastic Cartilage

Elastic cartilage is found wherever there is need for elasticity as well as some rigidity, such as in the external ear, epiglottis, and external auditory canal. It is also part of the corniculate and cuneiform cartilages of the larynx.

In addition to all the structural components of hyaline cartilage, elastic cartilage possesses a dense network of elastic fibers that are visible in ordinary H & E preparations. During development, the fibroblasts produce undifferentiated fibrils that later become elastic fibers. The elastic fibers are few in number near the perichondrium but form a dense network within the cartilaginous mass (Fig. 3–21).

Fibrocartilage

Of the three cartilage types, fibrocartilage occurs least frequently. It is a transitional form merging with hyaline cartilage, tendons, and ligaments. It is found in the intervertebral disks and makes up the menisci of the stifle joint. In the dog, the atrial and ventricular heart muscles are joined together by fibrocartilage.

The most striking characteristic of fibrocartilage is the presence of numerous collagen fibers in the intercellular substance. The microscopic appearance of fibrocartilage may vary with location. Fibrocarti-

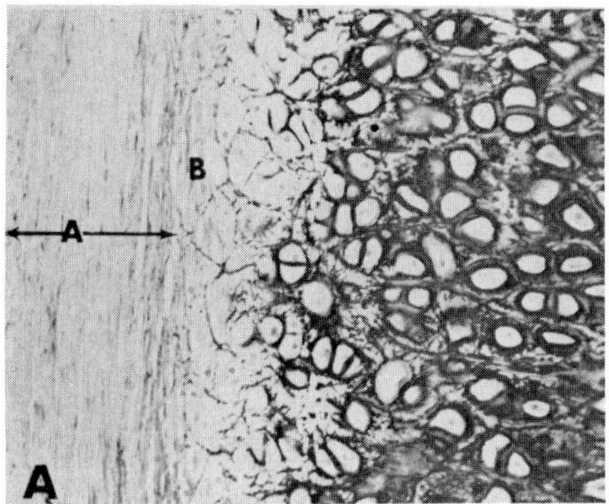

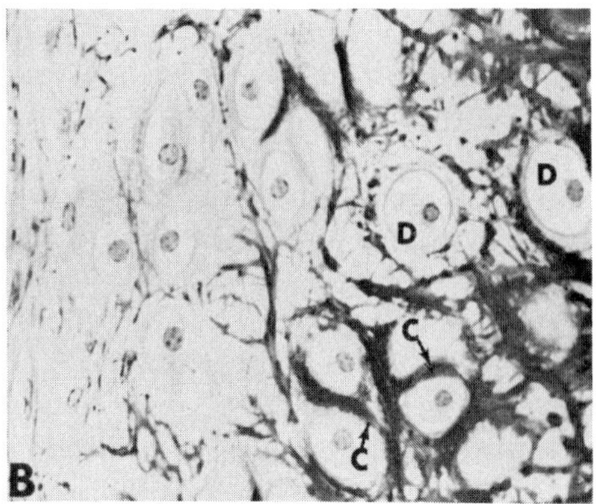

Fig. 3–21. *Elastic cartilage, external ear, dog. A, Perichondrium (A) with elastic fibers (black) penetrating the cellular layer (B). ×80. B, High power magnification illustrates elastic fibers (C) coursing through the matrix. The chondrocytes (D) nearly fill the lacunae. Verhoeff's stain. ×425.*

lage that attaches ligaments and tendons to bone has large collagen fiber bundles dispersed in a plane parallel to the direction of the pulling forces, with rows of small lacunae containing chondrocytes between collagen bundles (Fig. 3–22A). In the fibrocartilaginous cardiac skeleton of the dog, the chondrocytes and collagen fibers are distributed more randomly (Fig. 3–22B). The amorphous ground substance is most abundant in the vicinity of the cells so that the collagen fiber bundles do not become infiltrated with matrix. Fibrocartilage lacks a distinct perichondrium, al-

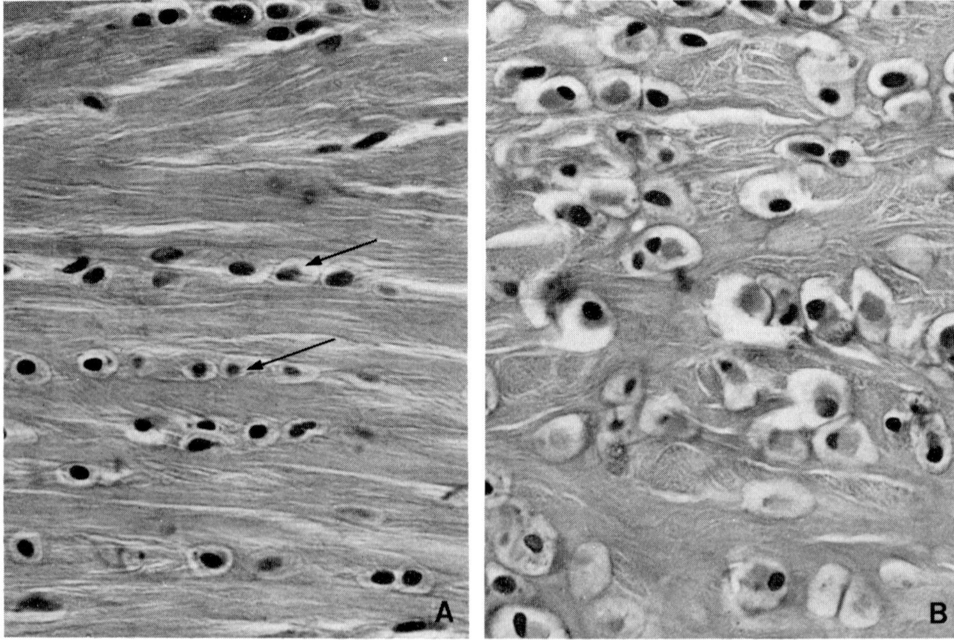

Fig. 3–22. *Fibrocartilage at ligament insertion on bone, dog. A, The lacunae (arrows) are oriented in the plane of pulling forces. H & E. ×300. B, Cardiac skeleton, dog. The lacunae and collagenous fibers are randomly arranged. H & E. ×570.*

though in some locations it is surrounded by collagen fibers. However, a cellular chondrogenic layer is absent.

BONE

Bone is a connective tissue with cells and fibers embedded in a hard, unbending substance well suited for the supportive and protective functions it performs. Bone gives internal support to the entire body and provides for attachment of the muscles and tendons necessary for movement. It protects the brain and organs in the thoracic cavity and houses the bone marrow. Bone also functions metabolically by providing a source of calcium to maintain proper blood calcium levels.

Bone is a dynamic tissue that is renewed and remodeled throughout the life of all mammals. Its construction is unique because it provides the greatest tensile strength with the least amount of weight of any tissue.

Structural and Functional Characteristics

Before the structure of adult bone is described, it is helpful to consider three fundamental morphologic and functional characteristics of bone that differentiate it from cartilage: a canalicular system, a direct vascular supply, and its growth process.

Cartilage is entirely dependent upon diffusion for nourishment; bone, however, has a unique canal system for supplying the cells with metabolites. When the bony matrix (osteoid) is secreted by the bone-producing cells, the *osteoblasts,* the cell body is trapped in a lacuna, and it becomes an *osteocyte.* The long cytoplasmic extensions of the osteocyte become encased in tiny canals. These passageways, called *canaliculi,* extend from one lacuna to another and to the bone surface, where they lie in close association with capillaries. Therefore, canaliculi permeate the bony matrix, providing a conduit system for the nourishment of the mature bone cells, the osteocytes.

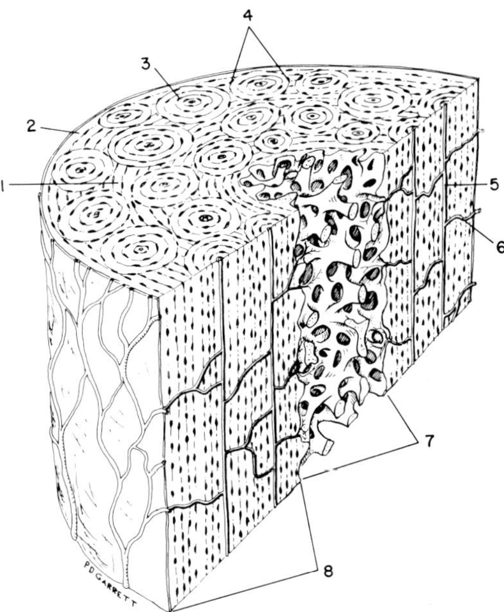

Fig. 3–23. *Schematic drawing of adult bone, illustrating bony lamellae and cortical and cancellous bone. (1) Interstitial lamellae; (2) outer circumferential lamellae; (3) osteon lamellae; (4) osteon; (5) central canal; (6) perforating canal; (7) cancellous or spongy bone; (8) cortical bone.*

The extensive capillary supply of bone further enhances the efficiency of the canalicular system. In fact, osteocytes are not more than one tenth of a millimeter away from a capillary.

Unlike cartilage, bone grows by apposition only. Because the intercellular substance calcifies so rapidly, interstitial growth of bone is not possible. Therefore, bone increases in size and changes shape by adding layers to one or more of its surfaces.

Macroscopic Structure

In a longitudinal section a typical long bone is seen to be composed of an outer solid mass called *compact* or *cortical bone* and inner *spongy* or *trabecular* bone that has a honeycomb appearance because of the lattice arrangement of the bony spicules. There is no sharp demarcation between these two types; they merge together gradually (Fig. 3–23).

In the mid-shaft or *diaphysis,* the compact bone makes up the wall of a hollow cylinder enclosing the *medullary* or *marrow cavity.* The ends of long bones, the *epiphyses,* are composed primarily of spongy or trabecular bone, and the communicating spaces, which are filled with marrow, are continuous with the marrow cavity of the diaphysis. In an immature animal, the diaphysis and epiphysis are separated by a cartilaginous *epiphyseal disk* located adjacent to the *metaphysis.* The epiphyseal surfaces are covered with hyaline cartilage, the *articular cartilage.*

Types of Histologic Preparations

The heavy mineral deposits in bone make ordinary sectioning difficult. However, when these minerals are removed by a process referred to as decalcification, the bone sample can be embedded in paraffin and cut like any soft tissue. Decalcifying agents such as formic acid, nitric acid, or commercial chelating agents remove the inorganic ions while not affecting the cells and organic intercellular substances.

Undecalcified preparations are made either by grinding slices of dried bone until they are thin enough to see through, or by embedding bone in one of the hard synthetic resins and cutting it with a special steel knife or a cutting disc embedded with diamond dust. Such preparations are often devoid of cells, but because the mineral content is still present it is possible to study bone growth, mineralization, and density. Different information is obtained from each type of bone preparation.

Microscopic Structure

A cross section of ground, undecalcified compact bone is composed of bony matrix deposited in layers or *lamellae* (2 to 8 μm thick) with lacunae between each layer (Figs. 3–23 and 3–24). Radiating from the lacunae are the branching canaliculi that penetrate and join canaliculi of adjacent lamellae (Figs. 3–24 and 3–25). Thus the lacunae and canaliculi form an extensive system of interconnecting passageways for the transport of nutrients.

Bony lamellae are seen in three distinct patterns: concentric, interstitial, and circumferential. *Concentric lamellae* are layers of bone surrounding longitudinally oriented channels forming definitive cylindric structures called *osteons* or *haversian systems.* Between the osteons are many irregularly shaped groups of lamellae, *interstitial lamellae.* Definite lines, called *cement lines,* delimit each haversian and interstitial system. They stain differently because the area is collagen-poor and devoid of canaliculi. Cement lines that appear scalloped or irregular occur when bone formation follows a phase of bone removal or resorption and are called *reversal lines.* Those that have a smooth contour are called *arrest lines* and are the result of bone formation occurring after a period of interruption. The external and internal surfaces of compact bone from adult animals are composed of continuous concentric bony lamellae extending around the shaft. These are the *inner* and *outer circumferential lamellae.* In a longitudinal section of bone, the lamellae appear as bands coursing parallel to the long axis of the bone.

Osteons are arranged around longitudinal channels, called *central canals,* that contain capillaries, lymphatic vessels, and nonmyelinated nerve fibers, all supported by connective tissue. Central canals are connected with each other and with the free surface by transverse or horizontal channels, *perforating canals* (Fig. 3–24). Classically, central canals were described as the vertical or longitudinal canals, and perforating canals as the horizontal channels. However, osteons are known to branch and anastomose, producing a complicated tridimensional configuration, with the result that some central canals may course obliquely and appear at first glance to be

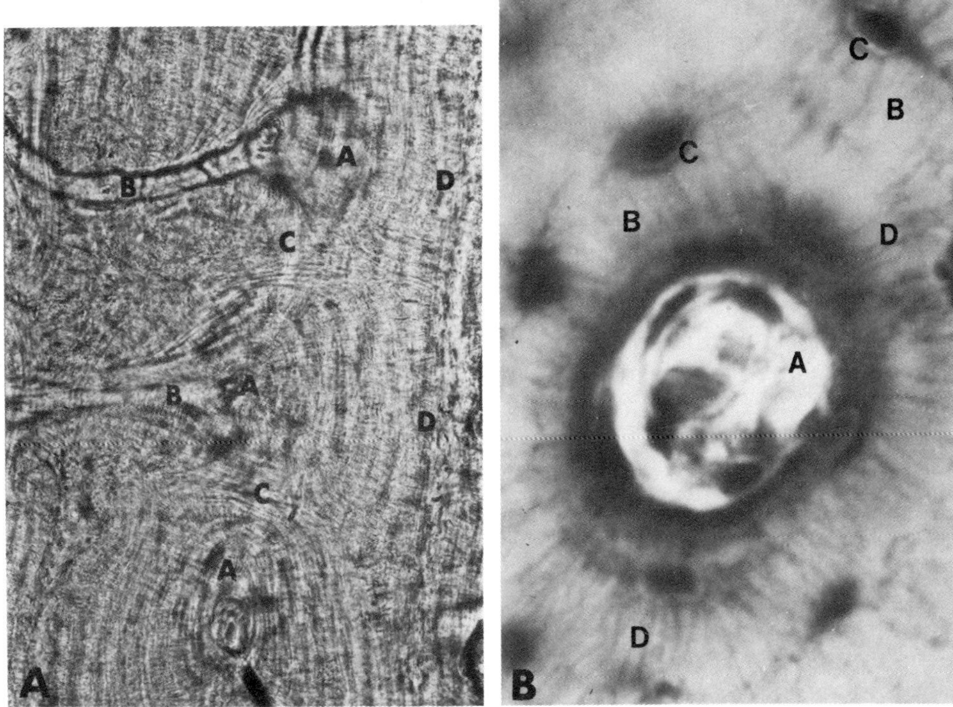

Fig. 3–24. *Ground bone, dog. A, Three osteons (A); two perforating canals (B); interstitial lamellae (C); and circumferential lamellae (D). ×80. B, Decalcified bone, dog. Central canal (A) surrounded by bony lamellae (B). Osteocytes (C) in lacunae with canaliculi (D) coursing from one lamella to another. H & E. ×1400. (Courtesy of A. Hansen.)*

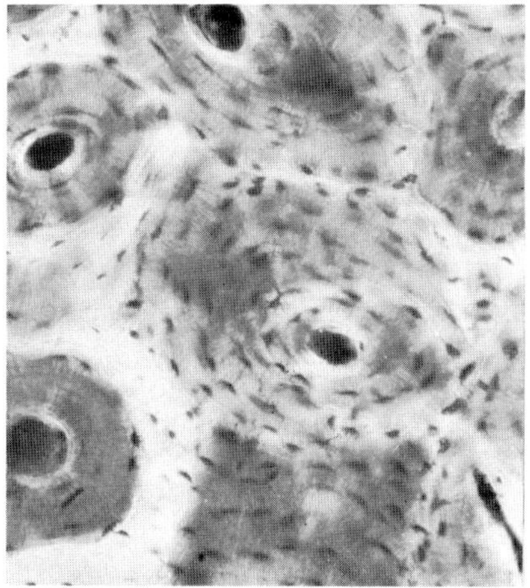

Fig. 3–25. *Ground bone, dog. Several lacunae with connecting canaliculi from adjacent lamellae. (From Dellmann, H.-D.: Veterinary Histology: An Outline Text-Atlas. Philadelphia, Lea & Febiger, 1971.)*

perforating canals. This need not cause any confusion, because central canals are always surrounded by concentric lamellae and perforating canals are not. The mechanisms involved in producing this lamellar arrangement of bone will be discussed in the section on osteogenesis.

In decalcified bone, the cells, fibers, and organic intracellular matrix are all well preserved, whereas the three distinct lamellar patterns are not as well defined.

The osteocyte is the principal cell of mature bone and resides in a lacuna surrounded by the calcified interstitial substance. Numerous long, slender processes extend from the cell body into the canaliculi, where they contact processes of adjacent osteocytes. These cell processes contain microfilaments, and gap junctions are present where they join those of other osteocytes. Young osteocytes are much like osteoblasts, but as they mature, the Golgi complex and rER are reduced and lysosomes increase in number.

The exact way in which osteocytes preserve the integrity of bone matrix is not completely understood. The long cellular processes have the intracellular machinery that allows them to shorten and lengthen. This activity may serve as a "pump" to move fluid through lacunae and canaliculi to transfer metabolites from the bone surface. The lysosomal enzymes in osteocytes may help to maintain the mineral content of the matrix, but their function in calcium release is probably minimal, since it is the osteoclast (to be described later) that plays the major role in bone resorption. Osteocytes may remove and replace perilacunar bone, a 1-μm layer immediately adjacent to the osteocyte. Because perilacunar bone has a lower mineral content, it is more soluble and thus can exchange minerals with the surrounding extracellular fluid. Therefore, perilacunar bone may be a mineral reservoir, with little contribution to the structural integrity of bone. Perilacunar bone removal is called osteocytic osteolysis; the extent to which this removal occurs is unclear. Nonetheless, osteocytes are necessary in preserving bone structure because when they die, osteoclasts immediately move to the area to resorb the bone.

The organic intercellular substance of bone contains sulfated glycosaminoglycans, glycoproteins, some blood-derived albumin and collagen. The collagen fibers in each osteonal lamellae course in a spiral direction with respect to the long axis of the central canal. In addition to their spiral orientation, the collagen fibers course at right angles to those in each adjacent lamella. This arrangement imparts considerable strength to each osteon.

The inorganic matter of bone is made up of submicroscopic hydroxyapatite crystals deposited as slender needles within the collagen fibers. Such an efficient arrangement enhances the tensile strength so characteristic of bone. The principal ions in bone salt are Ca, CO_3, PO_4, and OH, and there are substantial amounts of Na, Mg, and Fe. Bone, then, is a major storehouse for calcium and phosphorus, which are mobilized whenever they are needed.

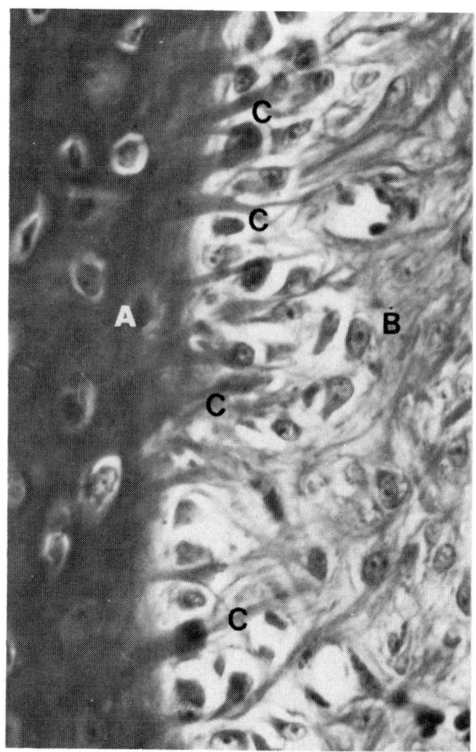

Fig. 3–26. *Decalcified bone, cat. Bone (A) with periosteum (B) attached by perforating fibers (C). H & E. ×500. (Courtesy of A. Hansen.)*

Most bones are invested with a tough layer of connective tissue, *the periosteum.* It has two layers: an inner or cellular *osteogenic* layer that provides cells to form bone, and an outer *fibrous* layer made up of irregularly arranged collagen fibers and blood vessels. The vessels branch and enter the perforating canals and ultimately reach the osteons. The cellular layer is more evident in young animals than in adults. The periosteum is attached firmly to the bone by bundles of coarse collagen fibers that extend into the outer circumferential and interstitial lamellae of the bone. These fibers are called *perforating fibers,* and they become incorporated into the bony matrix as surface lamellae are formed (Fig. 3–26). A periosteum is absent on the articulating surfaces covered with hyaline cartilage and at sites where tendons and ligaments insert on bones. The marrow cavity and osteonal canals are lined with a delicate layer of bone-lining cells, the *endosteum.* These bone-lining cells are probably quiescent osteoblasts and are joined to each other by gap junctions between the long cell processes. Some cells send processes into canaliculi to join those of nearby osteocytes. Bone-lining cells possess the potential to become active bone-secreting cells, particularly during fracture healing (see p. 66). Recently, it has been suggested that these cells form an ion barrier so that the fluid flowing through the lacunae and canaliculi is separated from the interstitial fluid. In addition, endosteal cells may play a role in mineral homeostasis by regulating the flow of calcium and phosphate in and out of bone fluids and thus maintaining an optimum microenvironment for the growth of bone crystals.

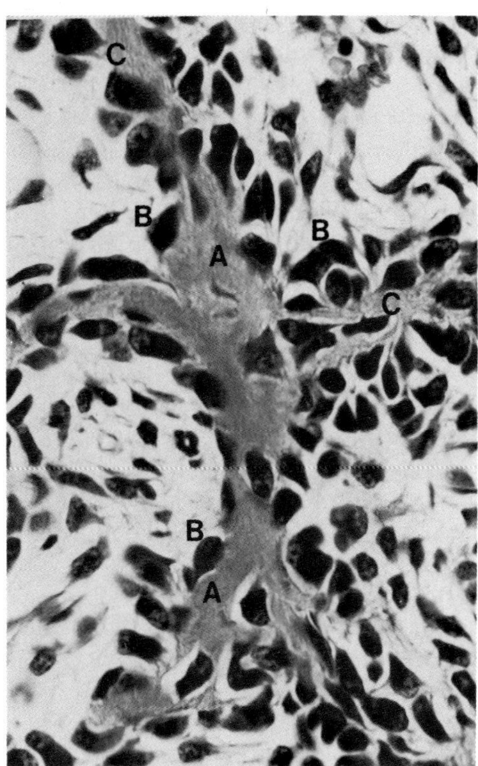

Fig. 3–27. *Developing bone. Bone spicule (A) is formed by osteoblasts (B) surrounding the immature bone. Collagen fibers (C) are visible in bony matrix, thus it is called woven bone. H & E. ×540. (Courtesy of A. Hansen.)*

OSTEOGENESIS

Regardless of where bone develops, it does so by a process of transformation from an existing connective tissue. There are two different types of bone development, both of which depend on specific cells differentiating within two different environments.

When bone forms directly from mesenchyme, the process is termed *intramembranous ossification.* This term arose because the mesenchyme that fills the sites where bone will form is in a layer, and hence membranous.

The process of bone formation in preexisting cartilage models is termed *endochondral* or *intracartilaginous ossification.* During this process, calcified cartilage is replaced by bone.

The terms intramembranous and endochondral indicate the type of environment in which the bone forms and do not refer to any given type of bone. Essentially there are only two kinds of bone, immature and mature. Immature bone is the first bone formed and has more cells and collagen and less mineral substance than mature bone. It is called *woven bone* because the thick bundles of collagen fibrils arranged in an irregular, interanastomosing fashion are readily visible within the matrix (Fig. 3–27). This immature bone, or *primary spongiosa,* is eventually replaced by mature bone, the *secondary spongiosa.*

Intramembranous Ossification

The bones of the vault of the skull develop by intramembranous ossification. Such sites in the embryo are occupied by stellate-shaped mesenchymal cells whose processes connect with one another. As capillaries invade these areas, the cells become spherical, and their processes thicken as they differentiate into *osteoblasts,* the bone-forming cells. These cells begin to synthesize and secrete the organic matrix and contribute to the mineralization process as well. Osteoblasts first secrete the organic matrix, the chief component of which is collagen, and the remaining constituents of the ground substance are produced somewhat later. During early intramembranous osteogenesis, osteoblasts become surrounded by an incompletely mineralized matrix, called *osteoid,* within which collagen fibers are visible (Fig. 3–27). Gradually, more osteoid is produced, followed by complete mineralization. As a result, some osteoblasts become trapped within their lacunae and become osteocytes, while others move away and secrete more matrix. These small, isolated pieces of bone within the mesenchyme are called the *centers of ossification,* which ultimately radiate in several directions to join other bony *spicules,* forming beams or *trabeculae* (Fig. 3–28). Such bone is called *trabecular, spongy,* or *cancellous* bone.

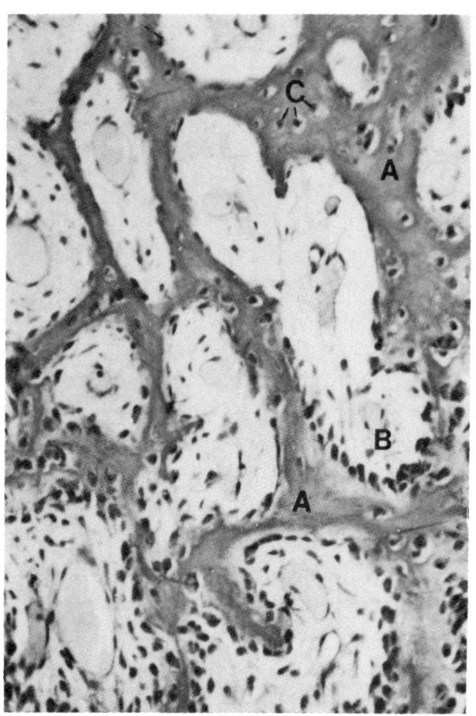

Fig. 3–28. *Trabecular bone (A) of intramembranous osteogenesis has osteoblasts (B) and osteocytes (C) within lacunae. Notice the prominent blood vessels in the mesenchyme. H & E. ×175.*

Osteoblasts are spherical cells with abundant basophilic cytoplasm owing to the well-developed rER. They have a prominent Golgi complex, and their long cytoplasmic processes have actin filaments. As the osteoblasts synthesize and secrete the organic matrix, plasmalemma buds, called *matrix vesicles,* form along the cell margin and pinch off. Matrix vesicles contain lipid, accumulate calcium ions, and have alkaline phosphatase activity, all of which are required to initiate and maintain the process of mineralization.

COMPACT BONE. As the bony trabeculae increase in width and length by the addition of new lamellae, all of the mesenchyme is replaced by bone. When this occurs, cancellous bone becomes compact bone. (For details of lamellar formation, see p. 65.)

The efficiency of the canalicular system in the transport of nutrients to the osteocytes is enhanced by the adjacent channels for blood vessels. In cancellous bone, the spaces between the trabeculae have an intensive vascular supply. Therefore, when cancellous bone is transformed into compact bone, the blood vessels and associated mesenchyme eventually are surrounded by concentric bony lamellae. These central vessels supply nutrients to the osteocytes via the canaliculi.

RESORPTION. Bone resorption accompanies bone formation, so that newly formed trabecular bone is often seen with large multinucleated cells called *osteoclasts,* closely apposed on one surface (Fig. 3–29). Bone resorption occurs when these cells are stimulated by the parathyroid hormone.

Osteoclasts originate from blood monocytes and enter the site of future bone by way of the capillaries and, after osteogenesis begins, are attracted by minerals in the extracellular tissue fluid to calcified bone

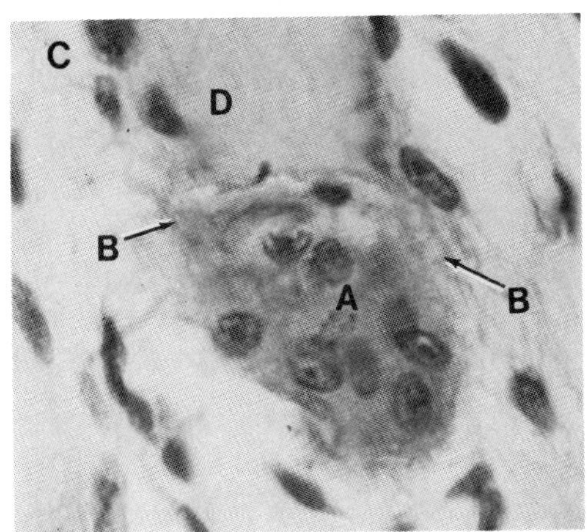

Fig. 3–29. *Osteoclast (A) in an erosion lacuna, resorbing bone. The ruffled border (B) is visible at the cell–bone junction. Osteoblasts (C) are forming bone (D). H & E. ×960.*

surfaces not occupied by osteoblasts. Several monocytes fuse to form the large, multinucleated cells. Osteoclasts, 40 to 70 μm in size with 15 to 30 nuclei, are usually seen on bony spicules in small depressions called *erosion lacunae* (Fig. 3–29).

Four major cytoplasmic areas are involved in bone resorption. The outermost portion of the cell is called the *ruffled border* because the plasmalemma is thrown into numerous long microvilli that penetrate the bone surface (Fig. 3–29). Adjacent to the ruffled border is a clear zone that has many actin-containing filaments. A third zone is filled with membrane-bounded vesicles that originate from the base of the microvilli. The basal zone is the innermost area, containing the nuclei, mitochondria, rER, and an extensive Golgi complex. Hydrolytic enzymes released from the osteoclast microvilli digest the noncollagenous organic matrix, allowing the collagen fibrils of the bone to persist long enough to be seen as a fuzzy border. Further proteolytic enzymatic activity dissolves the remaining collagen.

The manner in which the inorganic matrix is resorbed and released into the blood is still somewhat obscure. The most plausible explanation is that the osteoclasts secrete a substance that lowers the pH of the tissue fluid in the area of the ruffled border. The resulting acidic environment causes the relatively insoluble calcium phosphate crystals of bone to act as a buffer, and their continued buffering activity gradually converts them to the more soluble acid salts. In other words, bone mineral is dissolved through the effect of its own buffering action on the local acidity.

Endochondral Ossification

Bones of the extremities, vertebral column, pelvis, and base of the skull are formed initially of hyaline cartilage models that are replaced by bone in the developing embryo.

PRIMARY CENTER OF OSSIFICATION. As the cartilage model grows both in width and in length, it reaches a stage when most of the growth occurs at the ends of the model, while the chondrocytes in the midsection mature and enlarge, so that the intercellular substance between the hypertrophied cells becomes extremely thin (Fig. 3–30). With cellular hypertrophy and thinning of the matrix, the chondrocytes release matrix vesicles, similar to those of osteoblasts, that promote mineralization. This prevents the hypertrophied chondrocytes from receiving adequate nutrition and results in their degeneration and death. The intercellular matrix breaks up, leaving large cavities laced with calcified cartilage spicules.

Concomitantly the perichondrium is invaded by numerous capillaries, which change the environment of the chondrogenic layer. These pluripotential or progenitor cells differentiate into osteoblasts and form a thin shell of bone around the midsection of the cartilage, providing strength to the degenerating model. This *periosteal band* or *bony collar* forms by intramembranous ossification, and the perichondrium becomes the periosteum. Blood vessels are essential in activating the osteogenic potencies of the inner layer of the perichondrium, whose cells retain the abil-

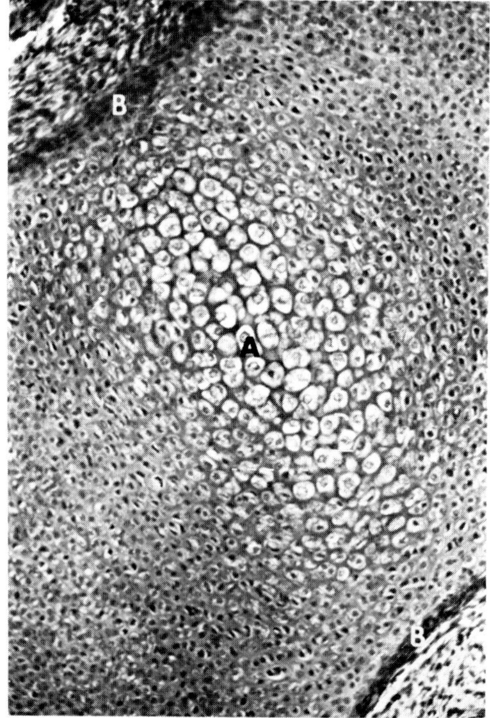

Fig. 3–30. *Cartilage model of a long bone, dog. Hypertrophied cartilage cells (A) are in center of the model. Notice the thin partitions between the enlarged lacunae; perichondrium (B). H & E. ×80.*

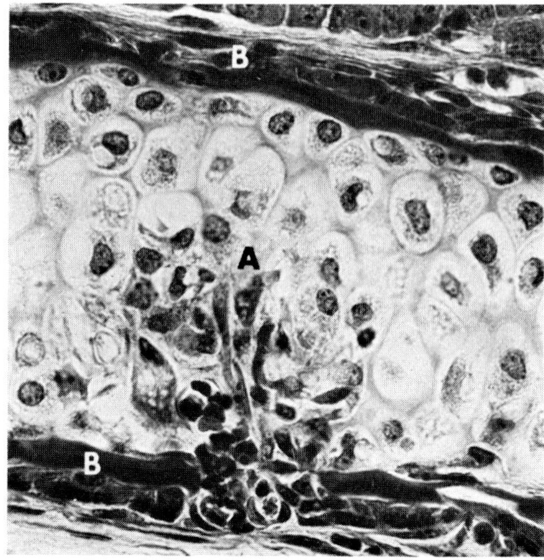

Fig. 3–31. *Primary center of ossification, cat. Periosteal bud (A) entering hypertrophied cartilage. Perichondrium (B). Crossmon's trichrome. ×570.*

ity to differentiate into either chondroblasts or osteoblasts throughout their life. This is especially significant in fracture healing, during which cartilage forms in areas relatively devoid of capillaries and is eventually replaced by bone as soon as capillaries grow into the area (see p. 66).

After the bony collar forms around the midsection of the model, blood vessels from the periosteum invade the area of the degenerating cartilage cells, thereby raising the oxygen level. Pericytes, osteogenic cells from the periosteum, and undifferentiated mesenchyme cells all accompany the invading capillaries. These blood vessels and their associated cells constitute the *periosteal bud.* When the periosteal bud reaches the interior of the midsection of the cartilage model, the *primary center of ossification* is established (Fig. 3–31). Under the influence of inductive bone-forming factors in the blood plasma, the pericytes and the osteogenic cells that accompany the capillaries differentiate into osteoblasts. These cells cluster around fragments of the calcified cartilage, begin to synthesize and secrete osteoid, and somewhat later contribute to the mineralization process. Such osteoblastic activity continues until bony trabeculae form that have cores of calcified cartilage. This is primary spongiosa, much of which will be entirely resorbed. In H & E preparations, the blue-stained cartilage core is surrounded by pink-stained immature bone.

While the primary center of ossification is forming, the cartilage at each end of the model continues to proliferate by interstitial growth, resulting in an increase in the length of the model. The capillaries from the primary center of ossification continue to invade the model toward both epiphyses, which extends bone formation throughout the cartilage model. The chondrocytes undergo the same sequence of events as described previously. Because the periosteum continues to add bone to the periphery, the primary spongiosa in the center is no longer needed for support. Therefore,

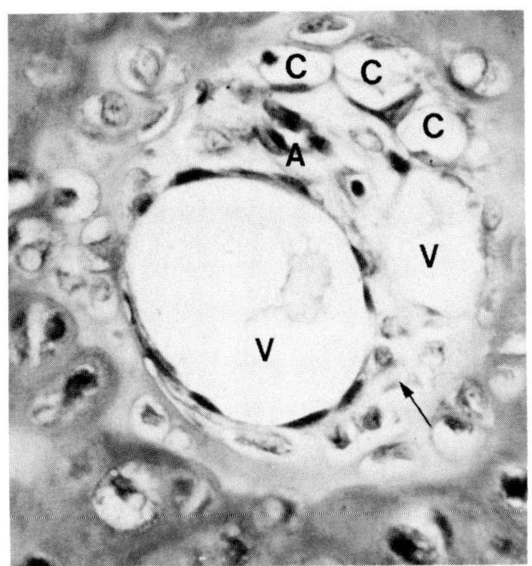

Fig. 3–32. *Cartilage canal in epiphysis of day-old puppy containing an arteriole (A), venules (V), and glomerular capillaries (C) degenerating cartilage at arrow.*

most of it is resorbed by osteoclasts, thus forming the marrow cavity, which becomes filled with hemopoietic tissue brought in with the periosteal bud.

SECONDARY CENTERS OF OSSIFICATION. The epiphyses of the larger long bones have centers of ossification, referred to as *secondary centers.* While it is generally accepted that hyaline cartilage is avascular, the epiphyseal cartilage of newborn animals is well supplied with cartilage canals containing arterioles, venules, and nonmyelinated nerve fibers, all surrounded by connective tissue (Fig. 3–32). These canals arise from the perichondrium and are evenly spaced throughout the epiphysis, providing nutrients to a given area. They do not enter the epiphyseal disk or penetrate the future articular cartilage. The arterioles of these canals end in a capillary glomerulus, and the initial sites of ossification occur as multiple foci adjacent to the glomeruli. When ossification begins, the chondrocytes next to the glomerulus of the cartilage canal degenerate and the matrix calcifies. This process is followed by circularly oriented layers of hypertrophic and dividing chondrocytes. Thus, this cellular arrangement resembles that of the growth zones in the epiphyseal disk, or *physis.* Since the connective tissue in the cartilage canals is continuous with the perichondrium, these cells have the same osteogenic potential for bone formation. Ultimately these foci fuse into a single secondary center of ossification, forming spongy bone in the epiphysis.

Ossification does not replace all the epiphyseal cartilage. Enough remains to serve as the articular cartilage, and a transverse disk of cartilage is left between the diaphysis and the epiphysis. In domestic animals, this physis persists until puberty and then it too is replaced by bone.

GROWTH OF BONES IN LENGTH. The epiphyseal disk, sometimes referred to as the epiphyseal-metaphyseal complex, functions to lengthen bone and to provide a scaffolding for constructing metaphyseal cancellous bone. Continued interstitial growth of the cartilage cells in the epiphyseal disk, involving chondrocytic hyperplasia and the active secretion of proteoglycans, serves to lengthen the long bones.

A longitudinal section through the epiphyseal disk of a growing bone has four zones or regions (Fig. 3–33). From the epiphysis to the diaphysis, the following zones are present:

1. The zone of resting cartilage is adjacent to the bone and marrow cavity of the epiphysis. Here the small chondrocytes are dispersed in an irregular pattern.

2. In the zone of cell proliferation, the cartilage cells are somewhat larger and tend to form rows or columns at right angles to the epiphysis (Fig. 3–34). Because this is the area where new cells are produced, numerous mitotic figures are present.

3. In the zone of cell maturation, the cells are arranged in columns (Fig. 3–35). As maturation progresses, the cells increase in size, accumulate glycogen, and begin to produce phosphatase, which initiates calcification.

4. The zone of calcification and ossifi-

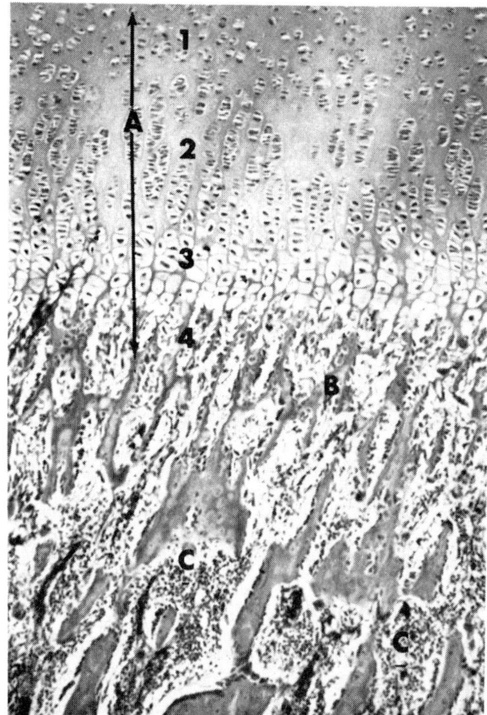

Fig. 3–33. *Growing bone, ulna, dog. Epiphyseal plate (A) has four zones (1, 2, 3, 4; see text). Trabecular bone (B) with bone marrow cells (C) between bony spicules. H & E. ×65.*

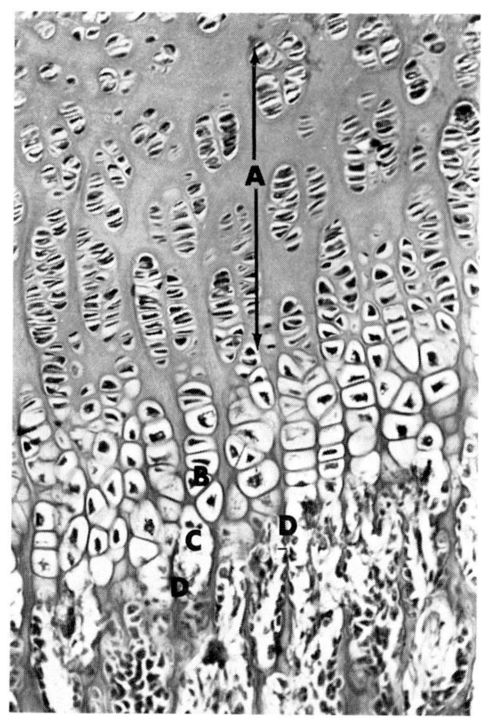

Fig. 3–34. *Growing bone, ulna, dog. Zones of cartilage cell alignment (A), hypertrophy (B), degeneration (C) and calcification (D). H & E. ×80.*

cation is thin and composed of one or two cell layers (Fig. 3–35). Most cells are degenerating, and the calcified cartilage partitions between the lacunae in a given column disintegrate rapidly. *Chondroclasts,* large multinucleated cells, remove much of the calcified cartilage by lytic action similar to that of osteoclasts. The thicker calcified partitions between the cell columns are the main sites for early bone deposition. Osteoblasts lining up along the sides of these cartilaginous spicules result in the formation of longitudinally oriented bony trabeculae with calcified cartilage cores (Fig. 3–35). Because the cartilage cores are continuous with the cartilaginous intercellular substance of the disk, the new bony trabeculae are anchored firmly to the epiphyseal disk. As fast as bone is added to the trabeculae, osteoclasts begin to resorb it from the free diaphyseal ends projecting toward the marrow cavity. This continuous process serves not only to lengthen the entire bone but also to increase the length of the metaphysis.

In longitudinal sections through the growth plate, the bony trabeculae and their cartilage cores resemble separate stalks attached to the growth plate. However, in a cross section taken through the diaphyseal side of the epiphyseal disk, each trabecula is actually a wall between adjacent tubes filled with osteogenic cells and capillaries. The osteogenic cells differentiate into osteoblasts and produce a layer of osteoid inside the tubes so that the immature bone, seen as a covering of the cartilaginous cores in longitudinal sections, actually lines the cartilage tubes (Figs. 3–36 and 3–37). In the central part of the epiphyseal disk the cartilaginous tubes usually have but a single layer of immature bone, the primary spongiosa, which eventually will be resorbed

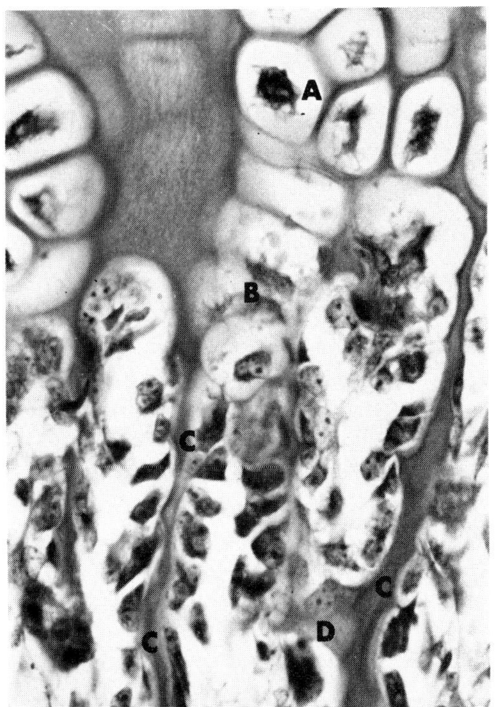

Fig. 3–35. *Growing bone, ulna, dog. Junction of zone of cell maturation and degeneration (A) with zone of calcification (B). The cartilage core (C) is surrounded by immature bone (D). Notice that cartilage degeneration occurs between lacunae, whereas the cartilage between the cell rows remains. H & E. ×420.*

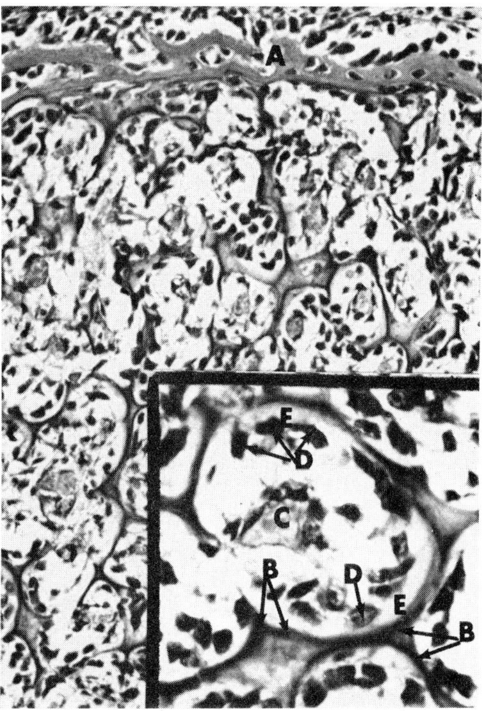

Fig. 3–36. *Trabecular bone, dog. Cross section of bony trabeculae on diaphyseal side of the epiphyseal plate. Bony collar (A). The calcified cartilage core (dark) forms the tube partitions. New bone (light) is deposited inside the tube. H & E. ×175. Inset: one trabecula. Cartilage partition (B) with blood vessel (C) in center. Osteoblasts (D) are forming bone (E) on the inside of tube. H & E. ×570.*

and converted into secondary spongiosa. At the periphery of the disk, however, numerous layers of bone are deposited inside the tubes until only a small endosteal-lined central canal that contains blood and lymphatic vessels and nonmyelinated nerves remains. Thus, complete osteons develop at the periphery of the disk and become part of the compact bone of the metaphysis. The funnel shape of the metaphysis is brought about by continual resorption of bone from the outside of the flared portion, with concurrent increase in bone on the inner portion, which narrows the shaft.

GROWTH IN WIDTH AND CIRCUMFERENCE. The trabecular bone that formed in the original bony collar is converted to compact bone composed of primary osteons. Concurrent periosteal growth and endosteal resorption enlarges the marrow cavity and increases the width of the bone. Because endosteal resorption lags periosteal production, the thickness of the shaft wall slowly increases.

The outer surface of an actively growing bone is uneven, owing to numerous longitudinal ridges and grooves (Fig. 3–38). Osteoblasts from the adherent periosteum deposit bone, so that eventually the shoulders of the groove meet, forming a tube lined with osteogenic cells and enclosing a blood vessel derived from the periosteum. The osteogenic cells produce concentric layers of bone encompassing the blood vessel within the new central canal. In this way, new primary osteons are added to the periphery of an actively growing young bone. Eventually these primary osteons are gradually replaced with more orderly second-

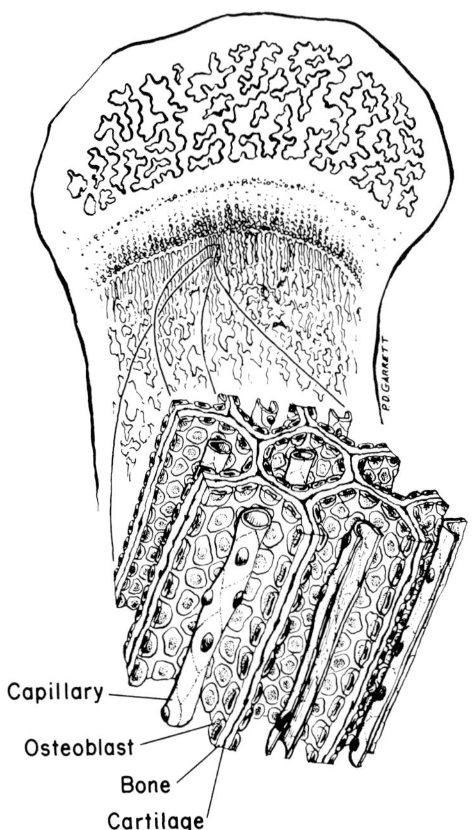

Fig. 3–37. *Schematic drawing illustrating the formation of cartilaginous tubes lined by osteoblasts actively secreting bony matrix. Notice the capillaries that will become the osteon vessels in the center of the tubes.*

ary osteons. Osteoblasts are stimulated to hollow out new tunnels within the primary osteons; they then secrete lamellar bone to form the secondary osteon, resulting in a structually stronger bone shaft.

Finally, the surface growth slows, and appositional growth in the subperiosteal region adds more layers, which smooth the surface. These layers are the circumferential lamellae.

BONE MODELING. The changes in size and shape of bones during the growth process is called *modeling.* The concurrent action of bone resorption and formation on one side of a shaft may move this shaft to the right or left; therefore, some bones may grow eccentrically to satisfy biomechanical demands. This surface motion is called a *drift.* The flaring of the metaphysis and the modification of the cranial curvature are other examples of drifts.

BONE REMODELING. Bone formation and resorption are two continuous and delicately balanced processes that result in the addition of new systems at a rate equal to the resorption of old ones. In cortical remodeling osteoclasts destroy worn-out osteons by forming a resorption tunnel, which is then filled in with lamellar bone from the outer margin inward by osteoblastic activity to form a new osteon. In a longitudinal section these tunnels are cone-shaped, and the advancing end of the cone is called a *cutting cone* lined with osteoclasts. Behind the cutting cone is a *reversal zone,* where resorption is completed. This is followed by the *closing zone,* in which the tunnel is being refilled with lamellar bone. This process has been termed ARF: osteoclastic activation, osteoclastic resorption, and osteoblastic formation. Remodeling of trabecular bone occurs on the surface and does not involve the formation of cutting cones.

FRACTURE REPAIR

After a mid-shaft fracture of a bone, a certain sequence of events occurs during the healing process. Fracture repair involves changes in blood supply that affect cellular proliferation and differentiation as well as bone resorption.

The trauma causing the bone to break also tears the adjacent soft tissues and blood vessels. The blood clot that forms at the fracture site stops circulation and causes necrosis or death of the surrounding tissue. Likewise, the interruption of the blood vessels within the osteons causes cessation of circulation and death of the osteocytes on each side of the fracture site.

New tissue developing at the fracture site forms a bridge between the fragments. This is termed a *callus* and is composed of two parts. The *internal callus* develops between the opposing ends of the bone, and

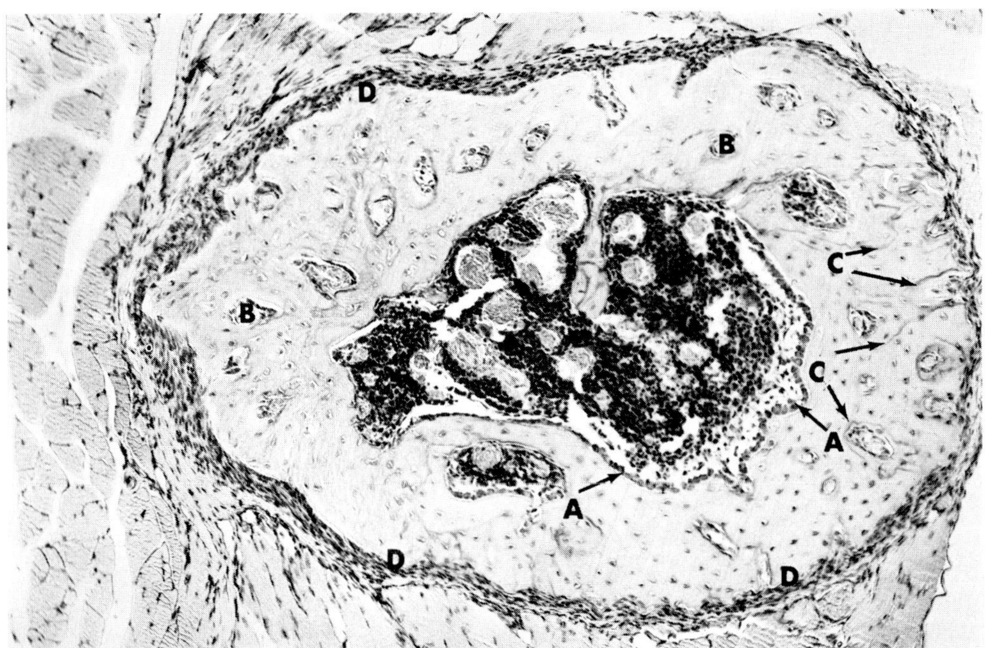

Fig. 3–38. *Whole bone, cross section. Marrow cavity in center is lined with endosteum (A); numerous spaces not yet filled with bone (B); cement lines (C); active periosteum covering irregular bony surface (D). H & E. ×160. (Reprinted by permission from Smith, E.M., and Calhoun, M.L.: The Microscopic Anatomy of the White Rat. Ames, Iowa, The Iowa State University Press, 1968.)*

the *external callus* surrounds the outermost surface of the broken bone. The cells involved in the repair process are osteogenic cells of the periosteum, cells of the endosteum, and undifferentiated bone marrow cells.

Early in the healing process, the cells of the periosteum proliferate to such an extent that the fibrous layer of the periosteum is lifted away from the bone. The endosteal cells proliferate, resulting in a thickened endosteum. The undifferentiated marrow cells increase in number in the same area. Differentiation of these cells takes place in one of two ways and depends on the vascular supply available. Those nearest the bone fragments differentiate in the presence of blood vessels; consequently, they become osteoblasts and form bony trabeculae. Those farther away from the bone proliferate in an area relatively devoid of capillaries; consequently, they form chondroblasts, which produce cartilage in the *external callus*. The cartilage is a temporary tissue eventually replaced by bone, following the same sequence of events that occurs in endochondral ossification. Gradually the callus is remodeled by resorption of the trabeculae at the periphery, until the original outline of the bone is restored.

No external callus develops when a bone fracture results in smooth, even, apposing surfaces that are aligned perfectly, without any space between the fragments, and held rigidly throughout the healing period. Since dead bone extends for some distance on both sides of the fracture line, osteogenic cells and capillaries in the living bone proliferate and grow into the nonliving bone. Simultaneously, osteoclasts invade the area and form resorption tunnels such as those described in bone remodeling. This results in new osteons that cross the fracture line and extend into the bone on the other side.

Fractures that are realigned in direct apposition but have a small space between the two fragments heal similarly, as long as rigid fixation is maintained. The only difference is that the two ends are joined initially by immature bone rather than by new osteons. Remodeling occurs as a secondary event.

Apparently, the rigidity of the fixation prevents osteogenic activity in the periosteum, so that external callus formation does not occur. However, any slight movement between the two ends of the fracture will stimulate callus formation.

Joints

Joints connect two or more bones; the various types of joints are classified according to the type of tissue that makes up the structure and the degree of movement permitted.

SYNARTHROSES

Synarthroses are only slightly movable or nearly immovable. There are four types of synarthroses, classified according to the type of tissue involved in the connection between bones. Those held together by dense connective tissue, either collagen or elastic, are *syndesmoses.* Skull sutures are typical syndesmoses. Joints in which the two bones are connected by cartilage are *synchondroses,* such as those between epiphyseal disks and sternebrae. As the result of aging, syndesmoses and synchondroses become *synostoses,* because the respective connective tissues are eventually replaced by bone. In the *symphysis* joint, the hyaline cartilage caps of adjacent bones are joined by thick fibrous bands. Between the hyaline cartilage and the collagen fibers is a transition zone of fibrocartilage. The pubic symphysis is a good example of this type of joint.

The intervertebral disk is a symphysis that consists of a layer of calcified cartilage covering the vertebral bone, followed by hyaline cartilage. The center of the disk is occupied by the semifluid *nucleus pulposus,* consisting primarily of an amorphous matrix resembling that of hyaline cartilage. The periphery of the nucleus pulposus, the *annulus fibrosus,* is composed of fibrocartilage.

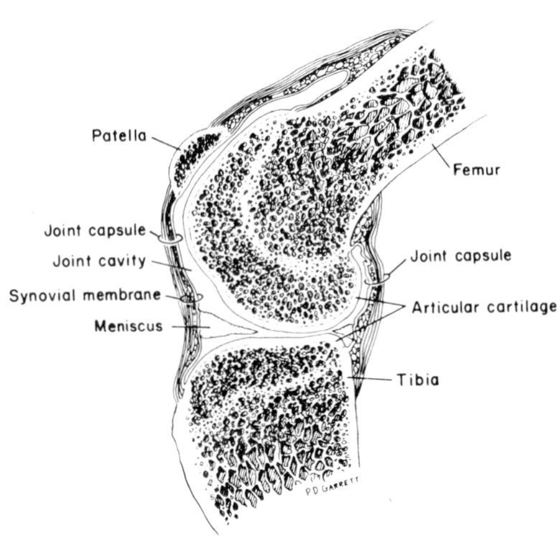

Fig. 3–39. *Schematic drawing of a synovial joint. The joint capsule is continuous with the patellar ligaments.*

SYNOVIAL JOINTS

Synovial joints are characterized by having articular cartilage on the opposing bony surfaces, a fluid within a closed cavity, and a synovial capsule enclosing the entire joint (Fig. 3–39).

The articular surfaces of synovial joints are covered with hyaline cartilage. The cartilage is devoid of a perichondrium, and the arrangement of the collagen fibers delineates three zones. (1) The tangential or superficial zone has flattened cells with collagen fibers oriented parallel to the articular surface. (2) The deep radial zone has larger, more spherical cells, and the fibers are perpendicular to the surface. (3) The transitional zone lies between the other two zones and unites them by means of numerous fibers arranged in overlapping arcades. In addition, fibers from the deep radial zone extend into the calcified area near the epiphyseal bone. This structural arrangement of the fiber bundles has functional significance relevant to compression and shear forces of joints.

The proteoglycans chondroitin sulfate, keratan sulfate, and hyaluronic acid, a small amount of which is in the ground substance of articular cartilage, bind water, causing swelling of the matrix. Compression on the joint surfaces release this bound water, thus lubricating the joint. Conversely, when compression is released the excessive fluid is re-bound. Functionally, these two activities act as an effective pump to transport nutrients and waste matter throughout the articular cartilage.

The joint capsule encloses the entire joint. It consists of an outer fibrous layer of collagen fibers that is continuous with the periosteum, and an inner layer, the *synovial membrane,* which lines the joint cavity except on the articular surfaces (Fig. 3–40). The cells of this membrane are referred to as *synovial cells* which do not form a continuous epithelial lining but are interspersed with collagen fibers. Synovial membranes have blood vessels, lymphatics, and sometimes a substantial amount of adipose tissue. The predominating type of tissue in the synovial membranes varies with the location within the joint. In areas not subjected to strain or pressure, the synovial membrane rests on loose connective tissue (Fig. 3–40). The synovial cells form a distinct lining and are held together by collagen fibers; the underlying loose connective tissue contains many elastic fibers. Those parts of the joint that are subject to stress have fibrous synovial membranes in which the synovial cells form a discontinuous lining, and the intercellular spaces are filled with amorphous ground substance

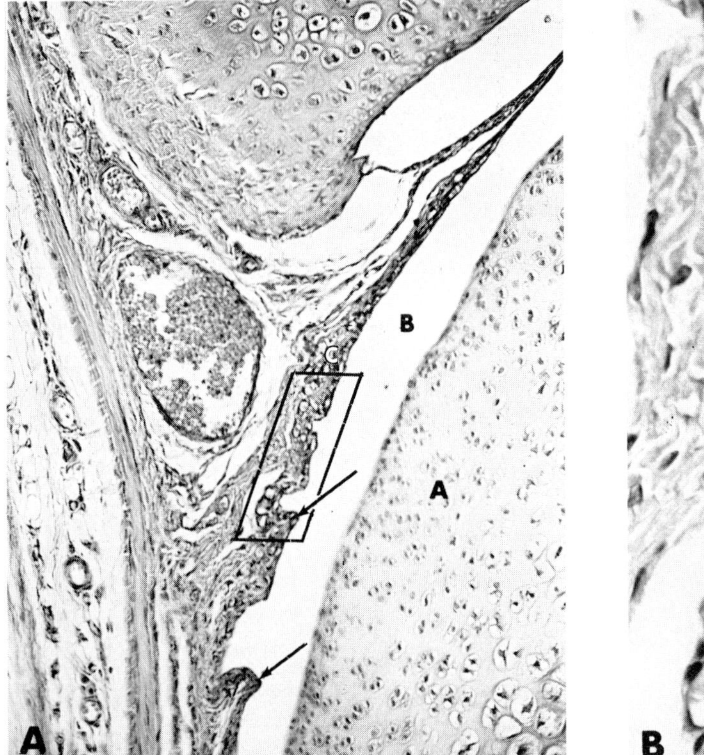

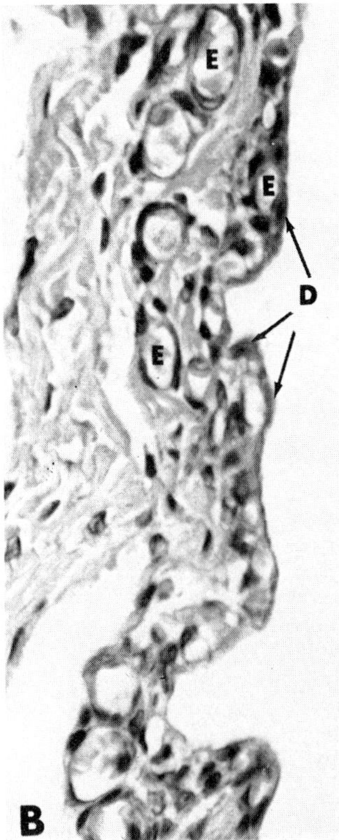

Fig. 3–40. *Stifle joint, rat. A, The articular cartilage (A) is adjacent to the joint cavity (B). The synovial membrane (C) has synovial villi (arrows). ×160. B, Area outlined in A. Synovial cells (D) rest on loose connective tissue containing numerous capillaries (E). H & E. ×750. (Reprinted by permission from Smith, E.M., and Calhoun, M.L.: The Microscopic Anatomy of the White Rat. Ames, Iowa, The Iowa State University Press, 1968.)*

and fibers. In some areas, the membrane is made up of adipose tissue with a single layer of cells resting on thin connective tissue.

Some synovial joints have intra-articular menisci composed of fibrocartilage. Usually they are anchored on one side to the fibrous layer of the joint capsule. If they are removed following traumatic injury, a new structure develops from the fibrous layer of the capsule; however, it is composed of dense collagen rather than fibrocartilage.

The synovial cavity is filled with *synovial fluid,* whose composition is similar to that of tissue fluid, with a substantial amount of polymerized hyaluronic acid. This fluid, derived from both the synovial cells and bound water from the articular cartilage, provides lubrication for the articulating surfaces of the joint.

We gratefully acknowledge D. von Sickle's critical reading of and suggestions for this chapter.

REFERENCES

Frost, H.M.: Bone Remodeling and Its Relationship to Metabolic Bone Diseases. Springfield, Ill., C.C Thomas, 1973.

Göthlin, G., and Ericsson, J.L.E.: The osteoclast. Clin Orthop *120*:201, 1976.

Ibbotson, K.J., D'Souza, S.M., Kanis, J.A., Douglas, D.L., and Russell, R.G.G.: Physiological and pharmacological regulation of bone resorption. Metab Bone Dis Relat Res *2*:177, 1980.

Jee, W.S.S., and Parfitt, A.M. (eds): Bone Histomorphometry. Paris, Société Nouvelle de Publications Médicales et Dentaires, 1981.

Jee, W.S.S.: The skeletal tissues. *In* Histology, Cell and Tissue Biology. 5th Ed. Edited by Leon Weiss. New York, Elsevier Biomedical, 1983, p. 200–255.

Kimmel, D.B., and Jee, W.S.S.: Bone cell kinetics during longitudinal bone growth in the rat. Calcif Tissue Int *32*:123, 1980.

Piez, K.A., and Reddi, A.H. (eds): Extracellular matrix biochemistry. New York, Elsevier Biomedical, 1984.

Rahn, Berton A.: Bone healing: Histologic and physiologic concepts in bone. *In* Clinical Orthopaedics. Edited by Geoff Sumner-Smith. Philadelphia, W.B. Saunders Co., 1982, p. 335–386.

Reddi, A.H. (ed): Extracellular matrix: structure and function. UCLA Symposia on molecular and cellular biology, vol. 25. New York, Alan R. Liss, Inc., 1985.

Ruggeri, A., and Motta, P.M. (eds): Ultrastructure of the connective tissue matrix. Boston, M. Nijhoff, 1984.

Talmage, R.V.: Morphological and physiological consideration in a new concept of calcium transport of bone. Am J Anat *129*:467, 1970.

Weiss, L., and Sakai, H.: The hemopoietic stroma. Am J Anat *170*:447, 1984.

Wilsman, N.J., and van Sickle, D.C.: Cartilage canals, their morphology and distribution. Anat Rec *173*:79, 1972.

4

Blood and Bone Marrow

ESTHER M. BROWN

Blood is a specialized circulating tissue composed of cells suspended in a fluid intercellular substance. Unlike other tissues, the cells do not maintain any permanent spatial relationship with each other, but move continuously from one location to another. The circulation of blood through the body provides a constant environment in which all cells and tissues perform their various functions. Thus, the major function of blood is to maintain homeostasis. The various blood cell types differentiate from stem cells in the bone marrow and become part of the circulating pool according to the needs of the animal.

BLOOD

In general, the total blood volume for most mammals is approximately 7 to 8% of the total body weight. The intercellular substance, *plasma*, comprises 45 to 65% of the total volume and the cellular component makes up 35 to 55%. The cells are of three major types: *erythrocytes* (red blood cells), *leukocytes* (white blood cells), and *thrombocytes* or *platelets*. The red color of fresh blood is due to the hemoglobin pigment within the red cells. Single erythrocytes are yellow in the fresh state. The leukocytes are so named because when large numbers of these cells accumulate the mass appears white. However, isolated leukocytes in fresh blood are colorless. When whole blood is centrifuged, the heavier red cells make up the lower portion of the packed cell volume; the leukocytes form a white layer on top, with the thrombocytes overlying the uppermost surface of the leukocyte layer.

Blood cell structure is studied by several methods, but the most common is to study the stained dry blood film. It is obtained by spreading a small drop of fresh blood across a slide. The smear is air dried and stained with any one of several modified Romanowsky-type dyes. These dyes are polychromatic in that they are a mixture of methylene blue and eosin, and the various cell types and cellular components react with the dyes, producing a differential staining effect. Because Wright's stain is one of the most common Romanowsky-type dyes, all descriptions of cell structure that follow are based on the appearance of cells after they are stained with this dye.

Erythrocytes

SHAPE. Mature red cells of domestic mammals are non-nucleated, biconcave disks (Fig. 4–1). The depth and size of the

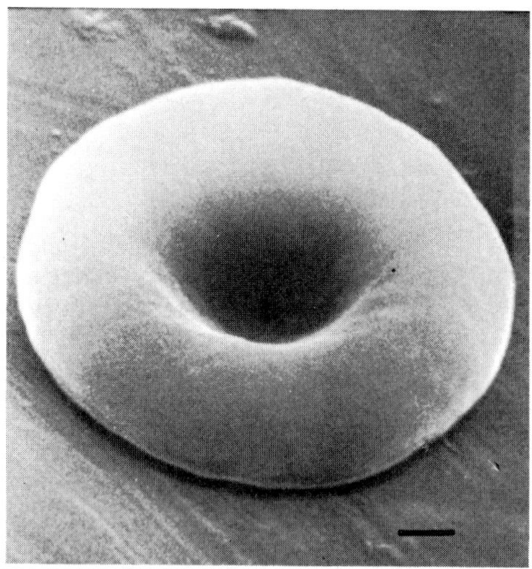

Fig. 4–1. *Scanning electron micrograph of a normal erythrocyte. (From Wintrobe, M.M.: Clinical Hematology. 7th Ed. Philadelphia, Lea & Febiger, 1974.)*

concavity vary with the species. The erythrocytes in the dog, cow, and sheep have a fairly typical biconcavity, and those in the horse and cat have a shallow concavity. The pig and goat have erythrocytes similar to a flattened disk. Cell shape is maintained by spectrin, a contractile protein located beneath the plasmalemma and anchored to it, thereby forming a complete unit membrane. The softness and plasticity are due to the colloidal matrix, which allows the erythrocyte to change shape as it courses through blood vessels, turns corners, and glides through small capillaries without rupturing or tearing the cell membrane.

When a drop of fresh blood is placed on a slide, the cell surfaces adhere to each other and the cells become arranged in long chains similar to a stack of coins. This arrangement, called *rouleaux*, is common in horse and cat blood, occurs occasionally in the dog and pig, and is rarely seen in ruminant blood.

SIZE. The largest erythrocyte is found in the dog (7.0 μm) and the smallest in the goat (4.1 μm). The total number of red corpuscles, expressed in 1 mm^3 of blood, reflects these size differences. For example, the dog has approximately 7 million/mm^3, whereas the goat has 14 million/mm^3. In other words, those species having small erythrocytes have more and those animals with larger red cells have fewer per unit volume. The total number of erythrocytes varies not only for a given species, but with different breeds and with any individual animal's nutritional state, physical activity, and age (Table 4–1).

STRUCTURE AND COMPOSITION. The mature red cell is non-nucleated, and the Golgi complex, centrioles, and most of the mitochondria disappear during maturation, before the cell enters the blood stream. Therefore, adult cells are unable to synthesize proteins, and any enzymes present were there when the cell was nucleated. They must depend on anaerobic glycolysis for their energy in order to maintain hemoglobin in a reduced state. The plasma membrane prevents the escape of the colloidal material and maintains a selective permeability for potassium and sodium ions. More than half (60%) of the red cell volume consists of water, and the remainder (40%) is composed of a conjugated protein, composed of *globin* and the pigment *heme*. Although the pigment makes up a small amount of this conjugated protein (4%), its combination with globin results in the red color, and hence the pigment is referred to as *hemoglobin*.

The complex molecular structure not only is responsible for the shape of the red cell but also is the basis for the physiologic properties that it exhibits. The cell membrane is permeable to water, electrolytes, and some polysaccharides, but it is impermeable to hemoglobin. Therefore, the osmolarity of the erythrocyte is determined by the hemoglobin, and because the osmolarity of plasma equals that of the red cell, the cell and the plasma are isotonic to each other, neither having a tendency to absorb water. However, if red cells are suspended in a solution with less osmolarity than that of plasma (hypotonic), the cells swell owing to imbibition of water. The cell

Table 4–1.
Blood Cell Values of Domestic Animals

	Erythrocytes		*Leukocytes*						
Animal	*Total No.**	*Size (μm)*	*Total No.†*	*Neutrophils (%)*	*Lymphocytes (%)*	*Monocytes (%)*	*Eosinophils (%)*	*Basophils (%)*	*Myeloid: Erythroid Ratio*
Dog	7.0	7.0	12.6	70	20	5.2	4.0	0	1.5:1.0
(range)	5.5–8.5	6.7–7.2	6.0–17.0	60–77	12–30	3.10	2–10	0	
Cat	7.9	5.9	16.0	59	32	3.0	5.5	0	1.6:1.0
(range)	5.0–10.0	5.5–6.3	5.5–19.5	35–75	20–55	1–4	2–12	0	
Cattle	6.3	5.5	7.9	28	58	4.0	9.0	0.5	0.71:1.0
(range)	5.0–10.0	4.5–8.0	4.0–12.0	15–45	45–75	2–7	2–20	0–2	
Sheep	9.5	4.5	7.4	30	62	2.5	5.0	0.5	1.1:1.0
(range)	8.0–10.0	2.5–3.9	4.0–12.0	10–50	40–75	0–6	0–10	0–3	
Goat	14.0	4.1	8.9	36	56	2.5	5.0	0.5	1.2:1.0
(range)	8.0–18.0	2.5–3.9	4.0–13.0	30–48	50–70	0–4	1–8	0–1	
Horse‡	9.5	5.3	9.0	49	44	4.0	4.0	0.5	1.6:1.0
(range)	6.0–12.0	3.8–7.0	5.5–12.5	30–65	25–70	0.5–7.0	0–11	0–3.0	
Horse§	7.5	5.6	8.5	54	35	5.0	5.0	0.5	1.6:1.0
(range)	5.5–9.5	4.0–8.0	6.0–12.0	30–75	15–30	2–10	2–12	0–3.0	
Pig	7.4	6.0	17.1	37	53	5.0	3.5	0.5	1.77:1.0
(range)	5.0–8.0	4.0–8.0	11.0–22.0	28–47	39–62	2–10	0.5–11	0–2	

*Millions per cubic millimeter of blood
†Thousands per cubic millimeter of blood
‡Hot-blooded
§Cold-blooded
The figures in this table represent ranges calculated from values gathered from many sources.

ruptures whenever the amount of water taken in exceeds a critical volume. This is called *hemolysis.* Whenever erythrocytes are subjected to solutions having an osmolarity greater than plasma (hypertonic), the cell volume diminishes owing to water loss. This volume loss causes the surface membrane to fold, and the cells become *crenated.* Occasionally, erythrocytes become crenated from trauma when blood smears are prepared.

Erythrocytes live for approximately 120 days and then are removed from the circulation before completely disintegrating. Old red cells are sequestered in the spleen, bone marrow, and liver by phagocytes. The iron of hemoglobin is salvaged and used in the formation of new erythrocytes. The porphyrin portion of the pigment is used to form bilirubin, a bile pigment.

FUNCTION. The cells and tissues of the body depend on erythrocytes for their supply of oxygen. The absence of a nucleus, the shape, and hemoglobin content all contribute to make the erythrocyte most efficient in oxygen absorption and transport. Hemoglobin has a great affinity for oxygen and becomes readily saturated as the blood courses through the pulmonary alveolar capillaries. When hemoglobin is saturated with oxygen, it is called *oxyhemoglobin;* after the oxygen is released, the remaining hemoglobin returns to its reduced state.

ABNORMAL ERYTHROCYTIC FORMS. Critical examination of dry-stained blood films for changes in red cell shape, size or color provides useful information for the veterinary clinician. Some diseases are characterized by the presence of red cells of various sizes in the peripheral blood, a condition referred to as *anisocytosis* (Fig. 4–2). Excessively large cells are called *macrocytes,* and very small ones are called *microcytes.* These terms are used in the morphologic classification of anemia, a blood disorder characterized by a hemoglobin concentration below normal.

Defects in the hemoglobin structure cause the erythrocytes to assume a variety

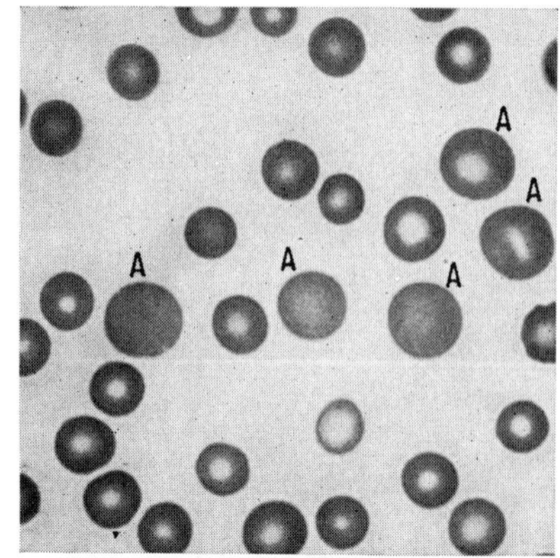

Fig. 4–2. *Blood, dog. Anisocytosis. Macrocytes (A). The smallest erythrocytes are microcytes. Wright's stain.* ×*600. (From Schalm, O.W.: Veterinary Hematology. 2nd Ed. Philadelphia, Lea & Febiger, 1965.)*

of bizarre shapes. Such abnormal cells are called *poikilocytes,* and they may take the form of sickles, burrs, ovals, or spheres.

Normal erythrocytes in a Wright's-stained blood film are brick red with a central pale area. This characteristic color and the width of the central pale area change with alterations in the distribution or in the amount of hemoglobin and are a reflection of excessive blood loss or production, faulty hemoglobin synthesis, or red cell destruction.

Young erythrocytes in the peripheral circulation exhibit a characteristic muddy blue color because hemoglobin has an affinity for acid dye radicals, while residual ribonucleic acids are basophilic. When these cells are treated with a supravital dye, such as new methylene blue (basic blue 24), the remaining ribosomes appear as fine blue-stained threads; therefore, these cells are referred to as *reticulocytes.* It must be understood that this network can be seen only with supravital dyes, whereas with ordinary blood stains such cells exhibit *polychromasia* and are referred to as *diffusely basophilic cells* or *polychromatophilic macrocytes.*

The fact that reticulocytes are usually not seen in blood from healthy cows, sheep, goats, and horses signifies that these cells mature completely in the bone marrow. In contrast, the blood of healthy dogs and cats contains approximately 0.5 to 1% reticulocytes, and that of pigs, nearly 2%.

NUCLEAR REMNANTS. It is not uncommon to find nuclear remnants within the circulating red blood cell. These small, blue-stained fragments may be in the form of granules (1 μm in diameter) called Howell-Jolly (H-J) bodies or blue threadlike rings, the *Cabot ring*. Cabot's rings are probably the result of abnormal mitotic activity, in which an isolated chromosome detaches and does not become part of the next interphase nucleus. Usually, H-J bodies are present whenever there is increased erythrogenesis.

SPECIES DIFFERENCES. The size and total number of red blood cells vary for the different domestic mammals. Likewise, some morphologic features are characteristic for each *species*.

The dog erythrocyte is the largest of all domestic animals' and presents a well-defined central pallor.

The cat erythrocyte stains uniformly throughout with a slight, rather ill-defined central pallor (Plate II–8–12). A peculiar, single blunt process or a small, circular, pale area (0.5 to 1.0 μm) at the edge of the red corpuscle is a unique finding in cat blood. It has been called an *erythrocyte refractile (ER) body* because it has a refractile characteristic when seen in wet films stained with new methylene blue. These ER bodies, however, are actually *Heinz bodies*, which are inclusions resulting from the precipitation of denatured hemoglobin. They occur naturally in healthy cats in about 10% of the erythrocytes because the hemoglobin in the cat is relatively unstable and easily denatured. Some anisocytosis is a normal condition in cat red cells.

The most prominent feature of horse erythrocytes is the marked rouleau formation (Fig. 4–3). This is due to the rapid sedimentation rate characteristic of normal horse blood. Equine erythrocytes exhibit a slight central pale area, but because of the marked rouleau formation there are fewer single cells in the smears.

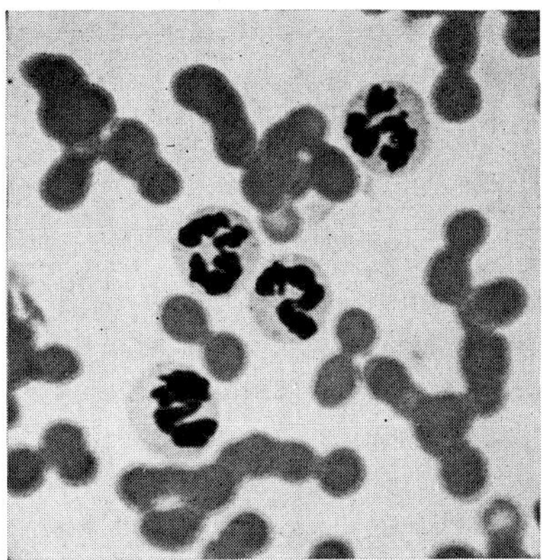

Fig. 4–3. *Blood, horse. Four segmented neutrophils. Erythrocytes in rouleau formation. Wright's stain. ×600. (From Schalm, O.W.: Veterinary Hematology. 2nd Ed. Philadelphia, Lea & Febiger, 1965.)*

Rouleau formation and crenation are common in the blood of normal pigs. Central pallor is inconsistent, as it may be absent in some smears and present to varying degrees in others. In certain disease conditions, the red cell may assume a bowl shape.

The erythrocytes in healthy cattle have an ill-defined central pallor, but in certain diseases they assume a bowl shape. When considerable rouleau formation is present in cattle blood, it is a good indication of a disease condition (Plate I–1). When blood loss is occurring, bovine erythrocytes exhibit marked basophilic stippling along with marked polychromasia. Some anisocytosis is a normal finding in cattle red blood cells.

Normal erythrocytes of sheep exhibit slight anisocytosis, some short chains of rouleaux, and a faint central pallor. In disease, the rouleaux are more marked and the central pallor develops into a "punched-out" appearance. Basophilic stippling is evidence of a normal response in blood loss.

Goat erythrocytes are the smallest among the domestic mammals, with little or no central pallor. Rouleau formation is not a feature of normal goat blood. In immature goats, there is marked anisocytosis and extreme poikilocytosis, with prominent sickle-shaped red cells.

Leukocytes

Leukocytes are typical cells, possessing a nucleus, cytoplasm, and other cell organelles, and all are motile to some extent. Whereas the red blood cells perform their main functions in the blood, the white cells leave the blood and move into the tissues to carry out their functions.

The total number of leukocytes is far lower than that of erythrocytes and varies among the different animal species. For any individual animal, great fluctuations in the leukocyte count occur from any form of stress, circadian influences, exercise, feeding, age, breed, and a wide variety of other conditions. Thus, for total leukocyte counts to be clinically meaningful, they must deviate considerably from the normal values in order for a clinician to evaluate a disease process.

The five different recognizable types of leukocytes are classed into two main groups. Those containing specific cytoplasmic granules are *granulocytes* and those without specific cytoplasmic granules are *agranulocytes*. A meaningful blood evaluation generally includes a differential count, in which the percentage of each of the five different cell types is determined. The blood of the dog, cat, and horse contain a greater percentage of neutrophils than of lymphocytes, whereas in the blood of ruminants, lymphocytes predominate. Pig blood falls between these two groups, having almost equal numbers of both cells but often a few more lymphocytes than neutrophils.

GRANULOCYTES

The three types of granulocytes are named according to the staining reactions of their specific granules. Eosinophils have definite acidophilic granules (stain red with eosin). Basophils possess distinct basophilic (purple) granules, and neutrophils have granules that are neither acidophilic nor basophilic. The staining affinity of the neutrophilic granules varies somewhat among the different animal species. Therefore, the term *heterophil* is another name for the neutrophil, because it indicates that the granules may stain differently from either the *eosinophilic* or the *basophilic* granules but may not be necessarily neutral. Frequently, the neutrophil is called the polymorphonuclear (PMN) leukocyte because of the various configurations of the nucleus.

NEUTROPHIL (HETEROPHIL). The mature neutrophil is approximately 10 to 12 μm in diameter and has fine granules in the cytoplasm and a lobed nucleus. The nuclear chromatin is dense, clumped, and *plaqued*. Definite, fine chromatin strands between the lobes are common in human and ruminant neutrophils, occur occasionally in the cat, horse, and pig, and are absent in the dog (Plate I–1, 8, and 9; Plate II–1 and 8). Because the nuclear constrictions are incomplete, it is difficult to determine definite lobes in neutrophils from animals other than ruminants. Among domestic animals, sheep neutrophils exhibit the greatest number of lobes.

Old cells have more nuclear lobes than young cells. Therefore, neutrophils with V-, U- or S-shaped nonconstricted nuclei are considered to be immature and are referred to as *band* or *nonsegmented* cells. Bacterial diseases usually cause an increase in the number of circulating neutrophils, and many band forms may be present. It is important to record the number of these cells in the differential count, because it is an indication that the bone marrow is releasing new cells to combat the infection. Clinically, this increase in young cells is called a "shift to the left" and is a good prognostic sign. Conversely, an abnormal number of neutrophils with nuclear hypersegmentation is known as a "shift to the right" and may be a poor prognostic sign, or a sign of chronic infection or stress.

In female animals, the neutrophil nucleus formed by constrictions may have a distinct nuclear appendage called the "accessory nuclear lobule" or Barr body (see Chapter 1). This small (1.5-μm) oval lobule, the sex chromatin, is attached to the main lobe by a fine chromatin strand (Plate II–1) and has been reported in females of all domestic mammals. However, it is extremely difficult to delineate in cattle neutrophils because the dense chromatin often masks this lobule. The accessory nuclear lobule is used to determine the genetic sex of an animal in which there may be endocrine dysfunctions or chromosomal anomalies.

The neutrophil cytoplasm is pale grayish blue, containing fine dustlike pink granules. The small individual granules are difficult to distinguish because they blend with the blue cytoplasm, producing a pink-lilac color throughout. Of all domestic animals, the dog neutrophil granules are the smallest, resulting in cytoplasm that has a homogeneous appearance (Plate II–1), whereas the goat neutrophil has the most distinct and deepest-staining granules. Cattle have few neutrophils (30%); therefore, numerous immature cells containing coarse, immature granules may be released rapidly from the storage compartment of the bone marrow.

Ultrastructurally, the neutrophil has only occasional dense mitochondria, few polyribosomes, and glycogen granules. The specific granules are relatively small and well dispersed (Fig. 4–4). During the early stages of cell development, the azurophilic granules are the first to form and are referred to as *primary granules.* Their synthesis ceases with the appearance of the *specific* or *secondary granules.* Therefore, the number of primary granules is reduced by half with each succeeding mitotic division, so that they comprise only about 10 to 20% of the cytoplasmic granules in the adult cell. Conversely, the specific granules predominate since they continue to form with each cell division. Specific granules contain

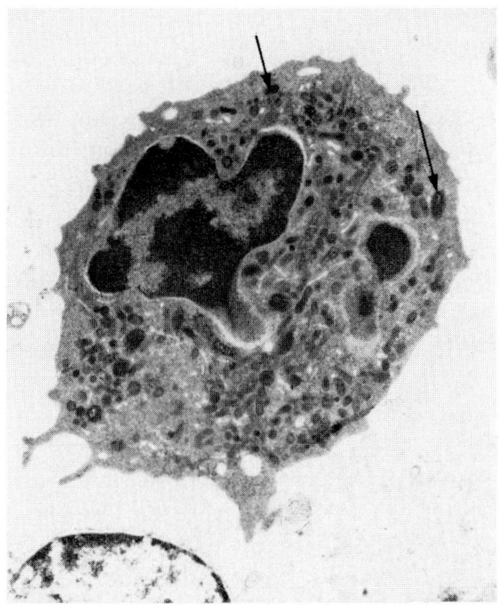

Fig. 4–4. *Electron micrograph, segmented neutrophil, cat. The specific granules predominate with a few primary granules (arrows) still present. ×4000. (Courtesy of Paul Canfield.)*

bacteriocidal lysozyme, an enzyme that hydrolyzes glycosides found in bacterial cell walls. Another important component of specific granules is *lactoferrin,* a protein that binds ferric iron and is bacteriocidal to iron-requiring bacteria. Lactoferrin is also known to inhibit neutrophil production; therefore, this particular activity is the basis of a feedback loop in neutrophil production. Azurophilic granules contain hydrolytic enzymes, lysozymes, and a myeloperoxidase that becomes bactericidal when it complexes with H_2O_2 and releases activated oxygen. These two types of granules work together in the destruction of engulfed foreign matter.

In response to infection, neutrophils move from the blood into the affected area and engulf bacteria and tissue debris. At the same time, the bone marrow is stimulated to release more neutrophils into the circulation, thus producing an elevated white blood cell count, or *leukocytosis,* characterized by an increase in young forms. Neutrophils are considered the first line of defense. Their life span in the bloodstream is about five days.

EOSINOPHIL. Eosinophils account for about 2 to 8% of the leukocytes, are 10 to 15 μm in diameter, have bilobed nuclei surrounded by prominent acidophilic granules 0.5 to 1.0 μm in size, and have a life span of 3 to 5 days. The two nuclear lobes may not always be connected and are often obscured by the granules.

The eosinophilic granules in domestic animals exhibit wide variations in size, shape, staining reaction, and numbers. In the dog, the granules rarely fill the cell, and occasionally only two or three large granules (3 to 4 μm) are present. They stain pale, usually about the same color as the erythrocytes, and never attain the orange hue so typical of eosinophils from other animals (Plate II–4 and 7). Occasionally, small vesicles are seen near the cell membrane, giving the impression that granules have been released. The cytoplasm is pale blue and easily seen between the sparse granule population (Plate II–4 and 7). The cat eosinophil has numerous rod-shaped granules that are not refractile (Plates 1–6; II–11). The eosinophilic granules in ruminants stain bright orange and are numerous and refractile (Plate I–4). The pig eosinophil contains spherical granules that are a dull orange color and usually fill the cell. The nucleus is often oval or kidney-shaped rather than bilobed. The horse eosinophil is so characteristic that it is possible to identify the species by this cell alone (Plate I–7). The granules are large (3 to 4 μm) and so tightly packed that the cell membrane conforms to the granule contour, giving the eosinophil a mulberry-like appearance. These large granules stain bright orange and frequently obscure the bilobed nucleus.

Electron micrographs of eosinophils reveal a Golgi complex with flattened vesicles and small spherical vesicles filled with secretory material. The specific granules are of two types; those granules in the horse and cow eosinophils are homogeneous, whereas the granules in the dog, cat (Fig. 4–5), and goat eosinophils are membrane-bounded and crystalloid and have an electron-dense laminated core surrounded by a less dense homogeneous matrix.

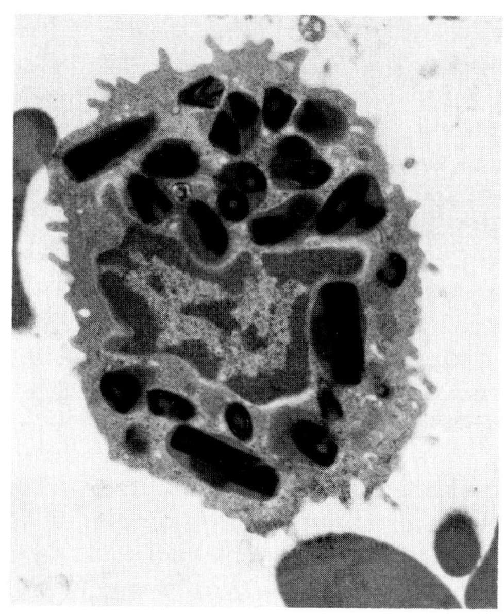

Fig. 4–5. *Electron micrograph, segmented eosinophil, cat. The specific granules are membrane-bound and contain dense laminated structures depicted here as dark areas within the granules. Notice the three rod-shaped granules corresponding to those seen at the light microscopic level. ×4000. (Courtesy of Paul Canfield.)*

Eosinophils play an active role in regulating acute allergic and inflammatory processes, they control parasitic infestation, and they phagocytize bacteria, antigen-antibody complexes, mycoplasma, and yeasts. They contain histaminase, which inactivates histamine and serotonin release from most cells, and they release zinc, which inhibits platelet aggregation and macrophage migration. There is some indication that the eosinophils may augment coagulation and fibrinolysis and may inhibit granulopoiesis.

BASOPHIL. Basophils account for 0.5 to 1.5% of the leukocytes. They are 10 to 12 μm in diameter, with a bilobed or irregularly shaped nucleus. The granules (0.5 to 1.5 μm) are dark blue to purple and often obscure the lighter-stained nucleus.

Basophils are usually rare in the blood of the dog and cat (Plate I–6; Plate II–5, 6, 7, and 12). In the dog, the granules are few in number and the cytoplasm often contains vacuoles, which may be the result of either degranulation or the dissolution of the water soluble granules (Plate II–5, 6, and 7). Cat basophil granules stain a dull purplish blue rather than the typical reddish purple and are elliptical in shape (Plate II–12). Electron micrographs of cat basophils reveal the large, oval, rather homogeneous membrane-bounded specific granules (Fig. 4–6). In the other domestic animals, the granules are large, spherical, or oval, usually fill the cytoplasm, and stain purple (Plate I–7). In the goat, the purple granules have a red halo, which imparts a red tinge to the entire cytoplasm. The pig basophil differs in that the granules are long rods or occasionally dumbbell-shaped.

The granules are metachromatic at low pH due to proteoglycans and sulfated acid mucopolysaccharides (heparin). The fact that cat basophil granules contain little heparin may account for the difference in stain affinity. Ultrastructurally the mature granules appear fairly homogeneous but may have dense particles or filaments. The rER, mitochondria, and Golgi are sparse (Fig. 4–6).

Basophils are involved in a number of important functions, some of which are poorly understood. They release mediators of inflammatory and allergic activities, are involved in triglyceride metabolism, and have receptors for IgE and IgG, which may induce degranulation via exocytosis. The granules contain heparin, histamine, hyaluronic acid, chondroitin sulfate, serotonin, and some chemotactic factors; however, granule content varies with the species. Basophils have a major function in immediate hypersensitivity reactions by secreting vasoactive mediators.

AGRANULOCYTES

The two distinct types of agranulocytes, the *lymphocyte* and the *monocyte,* are devoid of specific cytoplasmic granules but often contain nonspecific *azurophilic* granules. Agranulocytes are further characterized by having a spherical, oval, or indented nucleus.

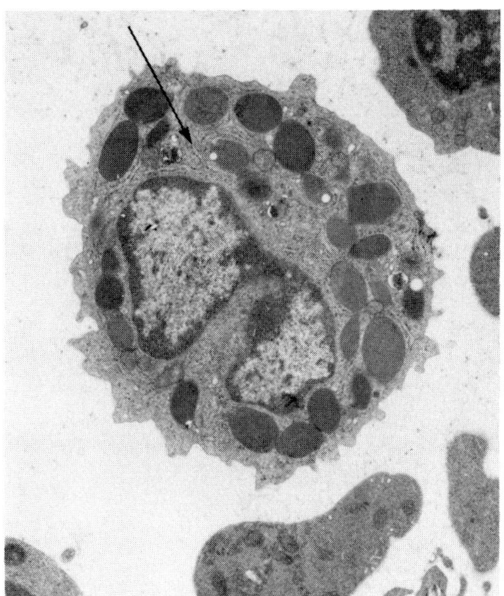

Fig. 4–6. *Electron micrograph, segmented basophil, cat. The specific granules are oval, membrane-bound, with a gray homogeneous content. A prominent endoplasmic reticulum (arrow) is present in the mature stage. ×4000. (Courtesy of Paul Canfield.)*

LYMPHOCYTE. The percentage of lymphocytes in blood is species-dependent: 20 to 40% in the dog, cat, and horse; 60 to 70% in ruminants; and 50 to 60% in the pig. In dry-stained smears there are small and large lymphocytes. The large lymphocytes are a more immature type and are sometimes called *prolymphocytes,* or large "blast" cells.

The lymphocyte displays great morphologic and functional heterogeneity because it is extremely plastic and motile, and it has considerable ability to change size and shape. Lymphocytes move throughout the soft tissues and organs, thereby providing an immunologic defense for the host.

The small lymphocytes, usually about 6 to 9 μm in diameter, have a large dense nucleus surrounded by a thin rim of pale blue cytoplasm (Fig. 4–7). Frequently, the

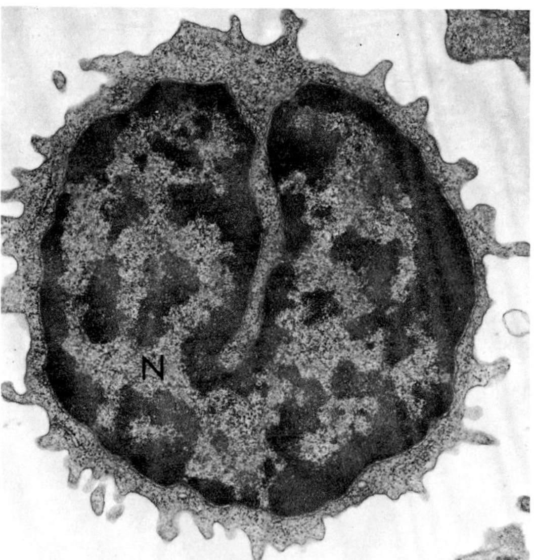

Fig. 4–7. *Electron micrograph of a lymphocyte. Indented nucleus (N); scanty cytoplasm with several small pseudopodia. ×4000. (From Mathews, J.L., and Martin, J.H.: Atlas of Human Histology and Ultrastructure. Philadelphia, Lea & Febiger, 1971.)*

nucleus has a small indentation on one side. In dry preparations, the nucleus is so dense that the nucleolus is not visible; nonetheless, in electron microscopic preparation it is always seen. The scanty cytoplasm contains numerous polyribosomes and a few mitochondria. Whenever azurophilic cytoplasmic granules are present, they usually are in the area of the nuclear indentation.

Large lymphocytes (12 to 15 μm in diameter) have considerably more cytoplasm, and the nucleus is less dense than that of small lymphocytes. Azurophilic granules may be present at the nuclear indentation, and examination with the electron microscope shows a pair of centrioles surrounded by the Golgi complex. Large lymphocytes contain a larger Golgi complex and more nucleoli, mitochondria, and polyribosomes than do small lymphocytes. These features all indicate increased synthesis and secretory activities concomitant with "blast"-type cells.

In the dog and cat most of the lymphocytes are small (Plate II–2 and 10). Azurophilic granules are rare and small (Plate II–2 and 10). Cattle blood has both small and large lymphocytes. The small ones are similar to those of other animals. The large lymphocytes have a pale nucleus with an even chromatin pattern. Often the nucleus has a deep indentation so that it resembles a kidney bean. The cytoplasm is pale and vacuolated; azurophilic granules are frequent and sometimes extremely large and rod-shaped (Plate I–3).

Sheep lymphocytes occur in various sizes, but there are no definite small and large types. The nucleus may be reddish and binucleated, and sometimes the large azurophilic granules are black.

The goat has small, medium-sized, and large lymphocytes, and the nucleus is usually spherical and occasionally kidney-bean–shaped. The azurophilic granules vary in size and often are a red-purple color.

The pig has mostly small lymphocytes in which the nucleus fills the cell, leaving a small rim of cytoplasm that may contain a small azurophilic granule. The large form has a lighter-stained nucleus and exhibits some chromatin plaques.

Most of the horse lymphocytes are small; however, some large lymphocytes may approach the size of monocytes, with smooth nuclear chromatin, pale blue cytoplasm, and a few small, scattered azurophilic granules.

The lymphocyte population in circulating blood includes three major types—T cells, B cells, and null cells—all of which look alike in ordinary light microscopy. However, they possess certain cytochemically distinguishable surface markers. T-lymphocytes and their subsets have a primary role in cellular immunity (see Chapter 8) and probably make up about 70 to 75% of the blood lymphocytes. The B-lymphocytes are few in number, 10 to 12%, and are concerned with humoral immune responses; some of them become precursors of plasma cells (antibody-producing cells). The null lymphocytes may constitute

10 to 15% of the blood lymphocytes, although this number may vary with different species. Null cells have surface markers unlike those of either the T or the B cells; however, these cells are responsible for two types of cell-mediated cytotoxicity: natural killer function (N-K cells) and antibody-dependent cellular cytotoxicity (K cells).

T-lymphocytes produce several factors, called "lymphokines." One of these, the *migration inhibitor factor,* prevents the migration of macrophages. Another is a *lymphotoxin,* which can destroy a wide spectrum of target cells. Other substances elaborated by sensitized lymphocytes include a chemotaxic factor for macrophages, a lymphocyte-transforming substance, and a factor that induces inflammation.

MONOCYTE. The monocyte is the largest of all the leukocytes, 15 to 20 μm in diameter, and makes up 3 to 9% of the total white blood cells (Fig. 4–8). There is considerable difficulty in identifying some monocytes because there are transition forms between the small and large lymphocytes, all of which resemble one another. This is especally true when viewing blood smears from cattle. The following general description refers to the more typical forms; the transitional types will be discussed for each of the different species.

Monocyte cytoplasm is far more abundant than that of the lymphocyte and is pale grayish blue, often with a "grainy" or ground glass appearance. Many times fine dustlike azurophilic granules are present. The nucleus may be oval, kidney-bean–, or horseshoe-shaped. The nuclear chromatin

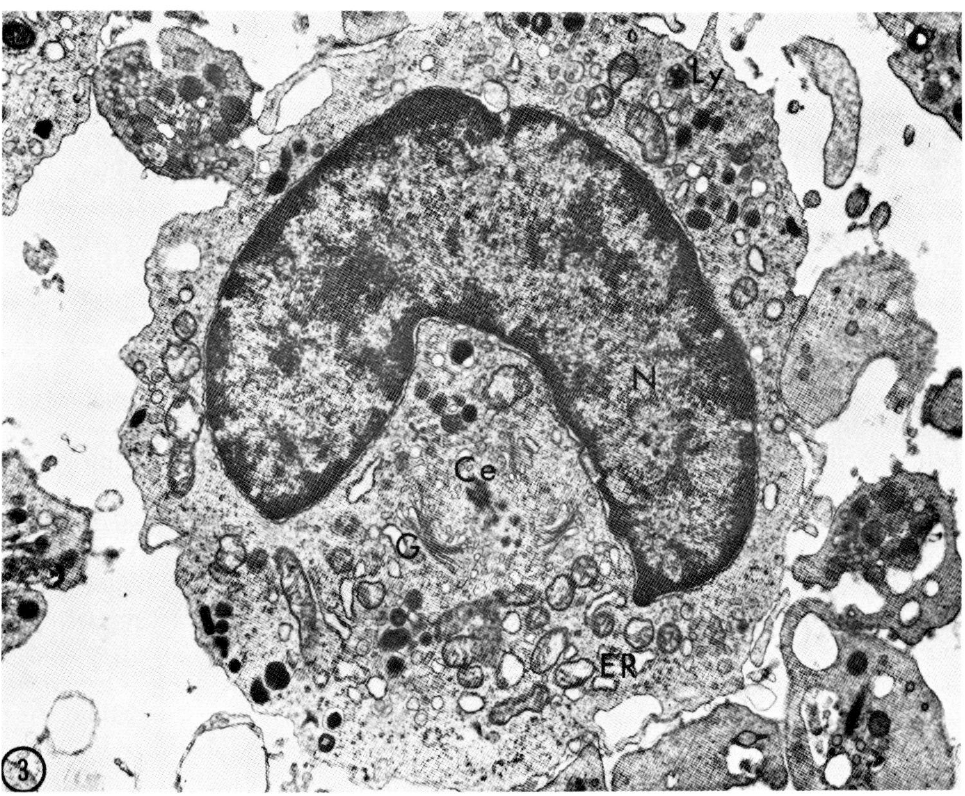

Fig. 4–8. *Electron micrograph of a monocyte. Horseshoe-shaped nucleus (N); centrioles (Ce); Golgi complex (G); azurophilic granules at 7 o'clock position; lysosomes (Ly); rough endoplasmic reticulum (ER). ×12,136. (From Mathews, J.L., and Martin, J.H.: Atlas of Human Histology and Ultrastructure. Philadelphia, Lea & Febiger, 1971.)*

stains lighter than that in the lymphocyte. One to three nucleoli are present, but they are not visible in stained dry smears.

In the dog about 5% of the leukocytes are monocytes with a blue-gray cytoplasm and fine azurophilic granules. The nucleus is usually in a band form and the ends are enlarged or club-shaped (Plate I–10 and Plate II–3).

Monocytes make up 3% of the leukocytes of the cat and contain a few azurophilic cytoplasmic granules (Plate II–9). The nucleus is round with irregular margins and often has folds.

Approximately 4% of cattle leukocytes are monocytes. Unlike in other species, the monocytes are difficult to differentiate from the large lymphocytes, because the nucleus may have many different contours and chromatin patterns. It may be spherical or coiled, with dispersed or clumped chromatin. Prominent azurophilic granules are not a common feature of cattle monocytes (Plate I–2 and 3).

Monocytes in sheep and goats make up only 2.5% of the leukocytes. The nucleus may be oval, slightly indented, or even lobed into three segments, with coarse, stringy chromatin. The gray-blue cytoplasm is abundant and usually has vacuoles in clusters, but azurophilic granules are not common.

Leukocytes in pig blood consist of about 5% monocytes with voluminous blue-gray, mottled cytoplasm. Azurophilic granules are not prominent. The nucleus is folded and the chromatin is lacy or meshlike.

Approximately 4% of horse leukocytes are monocytes, and they appear fairly typical. The nucleus has a kidney-bean or horseshoe shape and a linear chromatin pattern, and often a fold is seen at the closed part of the U. Fine pink azurophilic granules are scattered throughout the blue-gray, homogeneous cytoplasm.

Blood monocytes do not reach their full maturity until they migrate out of the blood into the tissues. They become fixed macrophages in many locations such as the liver sinusoids, bone marrow, pulmonary alveoli, and lymphatic organs. They often lie in close association to vascular endothelium, and in lymphatic tissue, bone marrow, and liver sinusoids they are often attached to the cytoplasmic extensions of dendritic reticular cells. This widely disseminated cell system, which includes the bone marrow stem cells, circulating blood monocytes, and the tissue macrophages, is referred to as the *mononuclear phagocytic system* (MPS).

In addition to its role as a macrophage, the monocyte is important immunologically. The intimate contact between lymphocyte and monocyte surfaces is necessary for the maximal immunologic response.

Thrombocytes

Thrombocytes, or *platelets,* are small irregular bodies, 2 to 4 μm in size, derived from the cytoplasmic portion of large cells in the bone marrow called *megakaryocytes* (Plate III–11). Consequently, they do not contain a nucleus. They are surrounded by a unit membrane and contain a complex microtubule system, lysosomes, a definite canalicular system, mitochondria and a few Golgi vesicles (Fig. 4–9). Because all of these structures are related directly to their adhesive qualities and their hemostatic activities of coagulation and clot retraction, it is logical to consider thrombocytes as functional cells.

The total number of platelets ranges from 350,000 to 500,000/mm^3 of blood. It is difficult to obtain consistent values because thrombocytes tend to clump when they come in contact with glass surfaces. Consequently, unless there is severe loss, total counts are not very meaningful.

In dry-stained smears, two definite areas in the thrombocyte are visible. The outer area stains a pale blue and the central portion appears dark purple. Because of their small size and tendency to clump, it is dif-

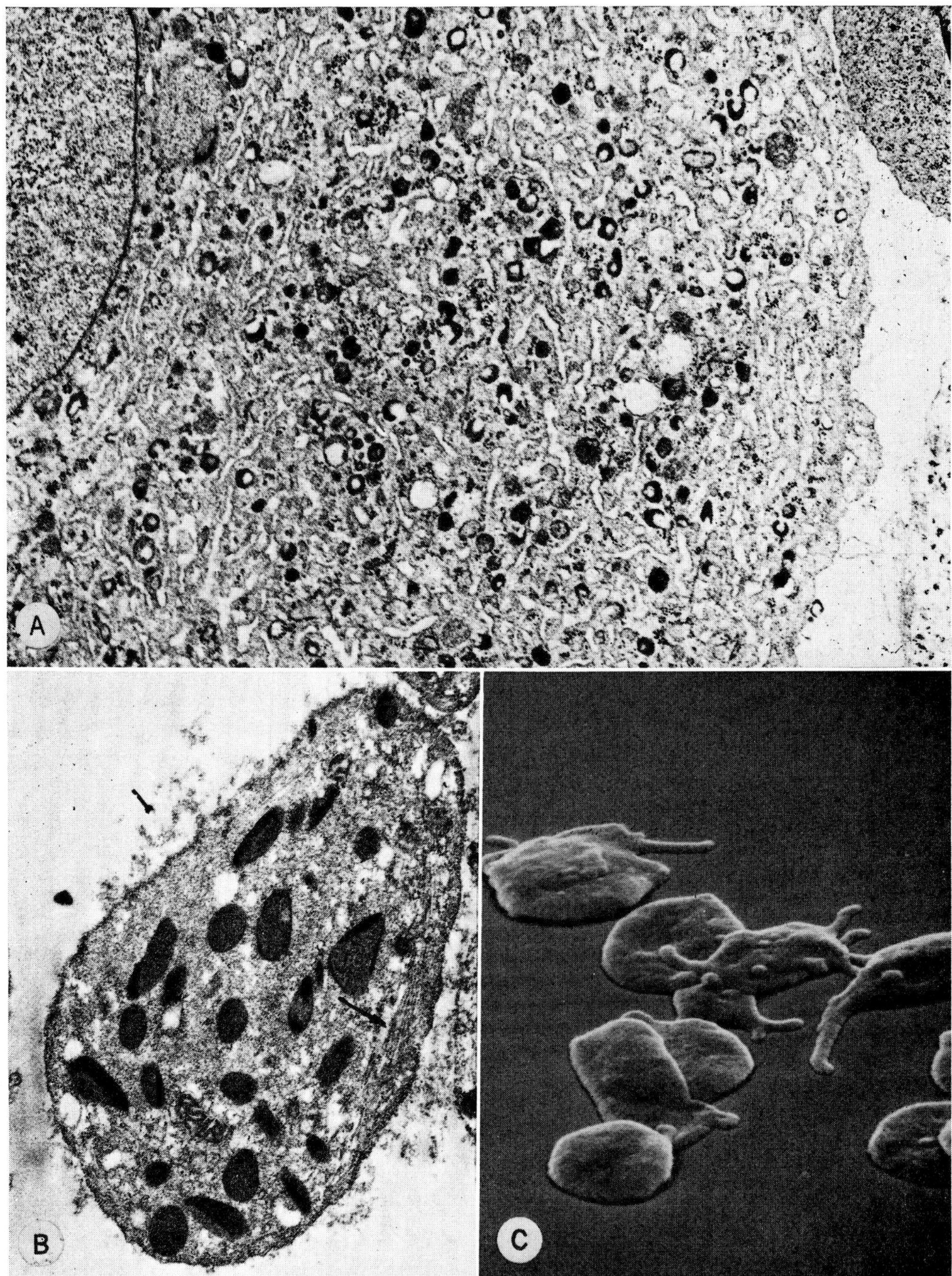

Fig. 4–9. *Megakaryocyte and platelets. A, Portion of a megakaryocyte from canine bone marrow containing numerous granules, membranous tubules and vesicles, and ribosomes. Platelets are formed at the surface as a result of separation of cytoplasmic fragments by membranous channels. Part of the nucleus is also visible at the upper left corner. B, A bovine peripheral blood platelet containing large granules, vacuoles and marginal band of microtubules (right arrow). Indistinct outline of small pseudopodium is also present (left arrow). Such structures are prominent in specimens fixed for scanning electron microscopy. C, A scanning electron micrograph of canine platelets. Small raised areas probably correspond to the internal granules characteristically seen in platelets, and pseudopodia are clearly visible in such preparations. (From Schalm, O.W., Jain, N.C., and Carroll, E.J.: Veterinary Hematology. 3rd Ed. Philadelphia, Lea & Febiger, 1975.)*

ficult to see much detail with the light microscope.

With the EM, three zones are visible: (1) peripheral, (2) sol-gel, and (3) organelle. The peripheral zone is composed of the cell membrane and circularly oriented microfilaments. The sol-gel zone is the pale area seen in stained smears. It contains a circular complex of microtubules and microfilaments, which serves a cytoskeletal function. The organelle zone is the dark center, called the *chromomere* or *granulomere.* It contains granules and dense bodies that are storage sites for the endogenous products secreted by thrombocytes (Fig. 4–9B). These products include, among others, ADP, ATP, ATPase, phospholipids, serotonin, hydrolytic enzymes, glycoproteins, catecholamines, and thrombosthenin. These are but a few of the substances required for coagulation, clot retraction, and the release reaction. A canalicular system extends from the organelle zone through the sol-gel zone, where it becomes continuous with the unit membrane, providing a conduit for the release of the endogenous products to the surface.

In responding to injured endothelium, long, thin dendritic pseudopodia project from the surface of thrombocytes (Fig. 4–9C). These projections, stabilized by the microfilaments, slide between the injured endothelial cells and entwine with adjacent thrombocytes, forming a plug. The sum of all morphologic, biochemical, and functional changes occurring in thrombocytes during the course of the hemostatic plug formation is referred to as "viscous metamorphosis." Occasionally, the pseudopodia are visible in dry-stained smears as thin extrusions.

After plug formation, the dense bodies and granules in the organelle zone release their products into the canalicular system. The microtubules orient the contraction waves produced by the microfilaments, and the coagulation products are extruded. Following this, a complex interaction of coagulation factors that produces fibrin and finally clot retraction takes place.

From the foregoing discussion, it is evident that any change in surface activation, organelle derangement, or abnormal biochemical interactions can contribute to altered thrombocyte function, resulting in hemorrhage or thrombosis. Severe thrombocyte loss is called *thrombocytopenia* and can be induced by drugs, vitamin deficiencies, and poisonous plants, as well as some autoimmune diseases.

BONE MARROW

The bone marrow is the primary site for the production of all blood cells in the adult animal. This complex process, called *hemopoiesis,* involves cell-to-cell interactions within the microenvironment of the marrow, as well as humoral feedback systems from peripheral target tissues. Sustained cellular production depends on a pool of stem cells that self-replicate and differentiate into specific cell lines. Bone marrow is frequently referred to as the *myeloid* or *myelogenous hemopoietic tissue,* to differentiate it from the extramedullary hemopoiesis that occurs in some peripheral organs (lymph nodes, spleen, and thymus).

Histology

The preparation of the bone marrow smears for cytologic examination necessarily destroys the normal marrow architecture. For this reason it is difficult to visualize bone marrow as composed of wedges of hemopoietic cells, supported by a meshwork of connective tissue and blood vessels sequestered within spongy bone (Fig. 4–10). The outstanding vascular feature is the numerous wide sinuses that lie peripherally to a central longitudinal vein into which the sinuses empty. The endothelium-lined sinuses are discontinuous, with wide gaps, and are surrounded by a discontinuous basement membrane to provide easy passage for newly formed blood

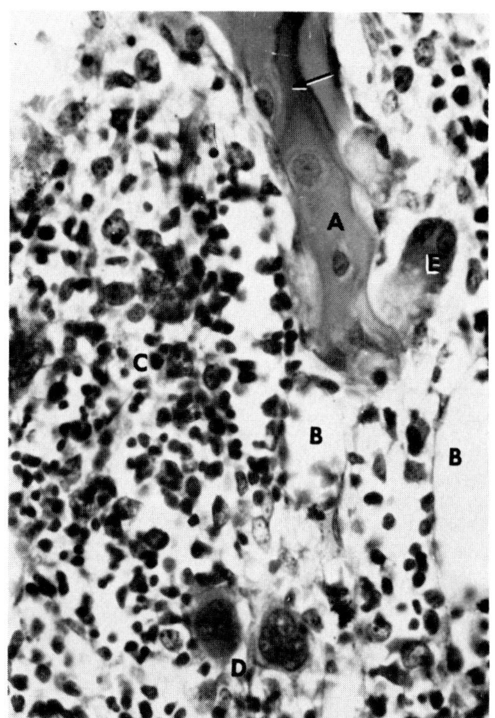

Fig. 4–10. *Bone marrow section, dog. A bony trabecula (A) with cartilaginous core (arrow); sinuses (B) lined with endothelial cells; immature marrow cells (C); megakaryocytes (D); osteoclast (E). H & E. ×420.*

cells into the circulation. The adventitial surface of the sinuses is enveloped by special cells, the *adventitial reticular cells.* These stromal reticular cells are believed to lie upon and secrete reticular fibers, and their wide, flat branches cover the outermost layer of the sinuses. The reticular cell processes apparently control the movements of cells through the gaps in the sinus walls by moving away from the openings whenever there is a call for increased blood cell release. Moreover, these adventitial reticular cells may become filled with fat during times of decreased hemopoiesis, thereby giving the marrow a yellow color and reducing the space available to blood-forming cells. Whenever there is a call for increased hemopoiesis, lipolysis ensues, restoring the hemopoietic volume. Thus, fatty marrow represents a mechanical buffer or filler, which takes up or releases space within the medullary cavity in response to hemopoietic demands. In addition to mechanical support, fatty marrow may have an inductive influence on neutrophil differentiation. During starvation yellow marrow is converted to red marrow; however, this is the result of stress, rather than a response to energy requirements.

In addition to the reticular cells, the bone marrow stroma includes collagen, which not only compartmentalizes the marrow, but probably influences the growth and differentiation of the stem cells as well. Various connective tissue macromolecules are known to have contrasting effects on erythropoiesis and granulopoiesis. Thus, the marrow is organized so that erythropoietic cells and megakaryocytes lie close to the sinus walls and the granulocytes differentiate deep within the hemopoietic wedges. These parenchymal and stomal relationships create an optimal hemopoietic microenvironment for stem cell differentiation.

Bone marrow has an extensive nerve supply that seems to respond to outside pressure. There is some indication that these nerves may adjust blood flow within the sinuses, thereby controlling the release rate as well as the proliferation of cells.

HEMOPOIESIS

PRENATAL HEMOPOIESIS. Very early in embryonic life, mesodermal cells in the yolk sac differentiate into primitive endothelial cells, which proliferate to form hollow buds and ultimately become primitive blood vessels. Within the lumina of these tubes are free, undifferentiated mesenchymal cells called *blood islands.* These cells are the primitive blood cells that develop and proliferate in the yolk sac and later, during gestation, seed the liver. Subsequently, the bone marrow, spleen, and thymus of the embryo are seeded with stem cells from the liver. Prior to the appearance of hemopoietic stem cells in any of these sites, the stromal development is well under way. This is another clue that stromal cells are intimately involved in stem cell growth and differentiation.

POSTNATAL HEMOPOIESIS. At the time of parturition, the bone marrow is the main source of myeloid cells; however, some extramedullary myelopoiesis persists in the liver and spleen for a few weeks after birth, then gradually diminishes. This is more prevalent in ruminants and horses than in carnivores. Red marrow is found in the entire skeleton of newborn animals and gradually is replaced with fat, until in adult animals only the ends of the long bones, the sternum, vertebrae, ribs, skull, and ilia contain active red marrow.

THEORIES OF HEMOPOIESIS. The hemopoietic portion of the bone marrow consists of a pool of stem cells that are self-perpetuating and that range in degrees of specialization from those that are pluripotential to cells committed to only one cell line. The various mitotic steps and maturational changes that take place to bring a multipotential cell to the committed stage are as yet unknown. However, the stem cells of differing potential have a similar morphology and resemble the small- to medium-size lymphocyte.

Because morphologic studies alone proved to be inconclusive in attempting to trace cell lineages, more sophisticated methods involving radiation studies, chromosomal marking, spleen colony techniques, and cell cultures helped to identify the functional capacity of multipotential stem cells to repopulate the bone marrow following hemopoietic injury. Mice were lethally irradiated to destroy their bone marrow cells and then were given a stem cell concentrate from healthy donor mice. After a few days, small colonies of bone marrow cells appeared in their spleens. Histologic studies revealed that some colonies were composed only of erythrocytic cells, others were granulocytes, and some were mixed. Chromosomal examinations confirmed that the colonies were derived from a single pluripotential stem cell; thus, they were clones. The stem cells have been given the name "colony-forming unit"-spleen (CFU-S), and depending upon the stimulus or the microenvironment in which they reside, their progeny will become committed to a single cell line (Fig. 4–11). Such cells are called *committed stem cells*. Kinetic studies indicate that committed stem cells are self-perpetuating for long periods of time. The pluripotential stem cells, on the other hand, exist as a dormant reserve until stimulated into action by signals from the elements of the microenvironment. How such signals are generated and transmitted is still under investigation. The structure of the CFU-S is only inferred from indirect evidence garnered from colony assays. Many investigators believe it to be a null lymphocyte (having neither T nor B receptors), while others prefer to call it a *candidate stem* cell.

CHARACTERISTICS OF CELL MATURATION. Certain morphologic changes are characteristic for most normal blood cells undergoing maturation. A good understanding of these principles helps in identifying the various cell types.

Young, undifferentiated cells are larger than the mature forms, contain no granules, and have a large nucleus and a small amount of cytoplasm. Therefore, the nuclear-cytoplasmic (N/C) ratio is a useful criterion for determining relative cell age. As cells mature, the N/C ratio gradually changes, so that in the mature cell there is more cytoplasm than nuclear material, and total cell size is decreased. The megakaryocyte is the one exception, because it becomes larger as maturation progresses. The nucleus in young cells is pale because the chromatin is more dispersed owing to active DNA synthesis. As maturation continues, the chromatin becomes coarse, clumped, and dense, and stains more intensely. Nucleoli are common in immature cells and tend to disappear as cells become completely differentiated. After the first mitotic division, the nucleolus often appears as a ring because of RNA loss.

Color Plates

PLATE I. *Leukocytes of Various Animal Species (×1800)*

1. *Mature bovine neutrophils. The rouleau formation of the erythrocytes is abnormal and is a response to an inflammatory disease.*
2. *A bovine lymphocyte (cell with round nucleus) and a monocyte.*
3. *A bovine monocyte and a lymphocyte with azurophilic cytoplasmic granules.*
4. *A bovine eosinophil (reddish granules) and a monocyte from the same blood as Plate I–1.*
5. *A bovine basophil.*
6. *A feline eosinophil and two basophils. The eosinophil has reddish rodlike granules, whereas the basophils have faintly stained spherical granules.*
7. *An equine eosinophil and basophil.*
8. *Three mature equine neutrophils in a row and one band neutrophil on the left.*
9. *A mature neutrophil and an uncommon form of canine monocyte with a profuse number of reddish granules.*
10. *Three typical canine monocytes.*
11. *Two monocytes of the Indian elephant. Others have classified these cells as lymphocytes; however, they are peroxidase-positive.*
12. *Peroxidase stain applied to leukocytes of the Indian elephant. A monocyte (left cell) and a neutrophil, both peroxidase-positive.*

(From Schalm, O. W., Jain, N. C., and Carroll, E. J.: Veterinary Hematology. 3rd Ed. Philadelphia, Lea & Febiger, 1975.)

Plate I

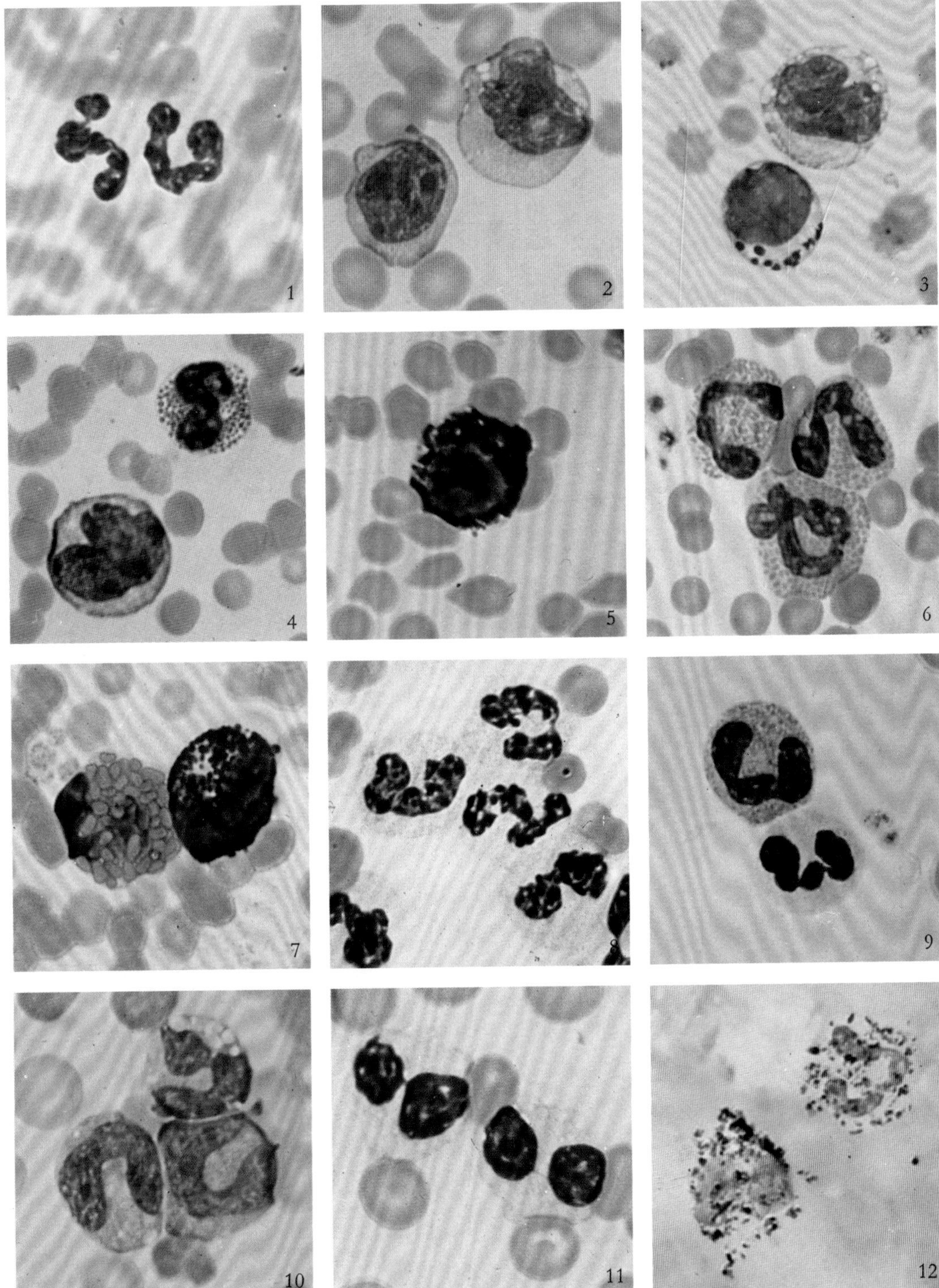

PLATE II. *Leukocytes of the Dog and Cat (×2000)*

1. *Neutrophil, dog. The nucleus has constrictions; the accessory nuclear lobule or "Barr" body is evident on the upper lobule, indicating this cell came from a female dog. The fine, pink specific granules are especially evident at the 2 o'clock position.*
2. *Lymphocyte, dog. This mature cell has definite azurophilic granules at the 2 o'clock position.*
3. *Monocyte, dog. This cell has a typical U-shaped nucleus with numerous azurophilic granules throughout the cytoplasm. Several cytoplasmic vacuoles are present.*
4. *Eosinophil, dog. Various sized specific granules are located in the blue cytoplasm. Numerous vacuoles are evidence of granule release.*
5. *Basophil, dog. In this cell the evenly dispersed specific granules are fairly dense.*
6. *Basophil, dog. Comparing this cell to Fig. 5, there are more granules; however, they are smaller and less dense.*
7. *Basophil and Eosinophil, dog. The basophil (lower left) has few specific granules, and the eosinophil (upper right) has numerous small specific granules and a few vacuoles. Notice the pale blue cytoplasm in the eosinophil.*
8. *Neutrophil, cat. The specific granules are fine and dustlike, imparting an overall pink color to the cytoplasm.*
9. *Monocyte, cat. The nucleus is indented on the left side and there are numerous fine azurophilic granules that impart a pink color to the cytoplasm. Cytoplasmic vacuoles are large and numerous.*
10. *Lymphocyte, cat. This typical cell has sparse light blue cytoplasm surrounding a fairly dense nucleus.*
11. *Eosinophil, cat. The specific granules are rod-shaped and fill the cytoplasm.*
12. *Basophil, cat. The specific granules are oval and stain a dull blue color.*

Notice the difference in the size and shape of the erythrocytes from the dog and cat. The cat erythrocyte appears darker because the concavity is extremely shallow.

Plate II

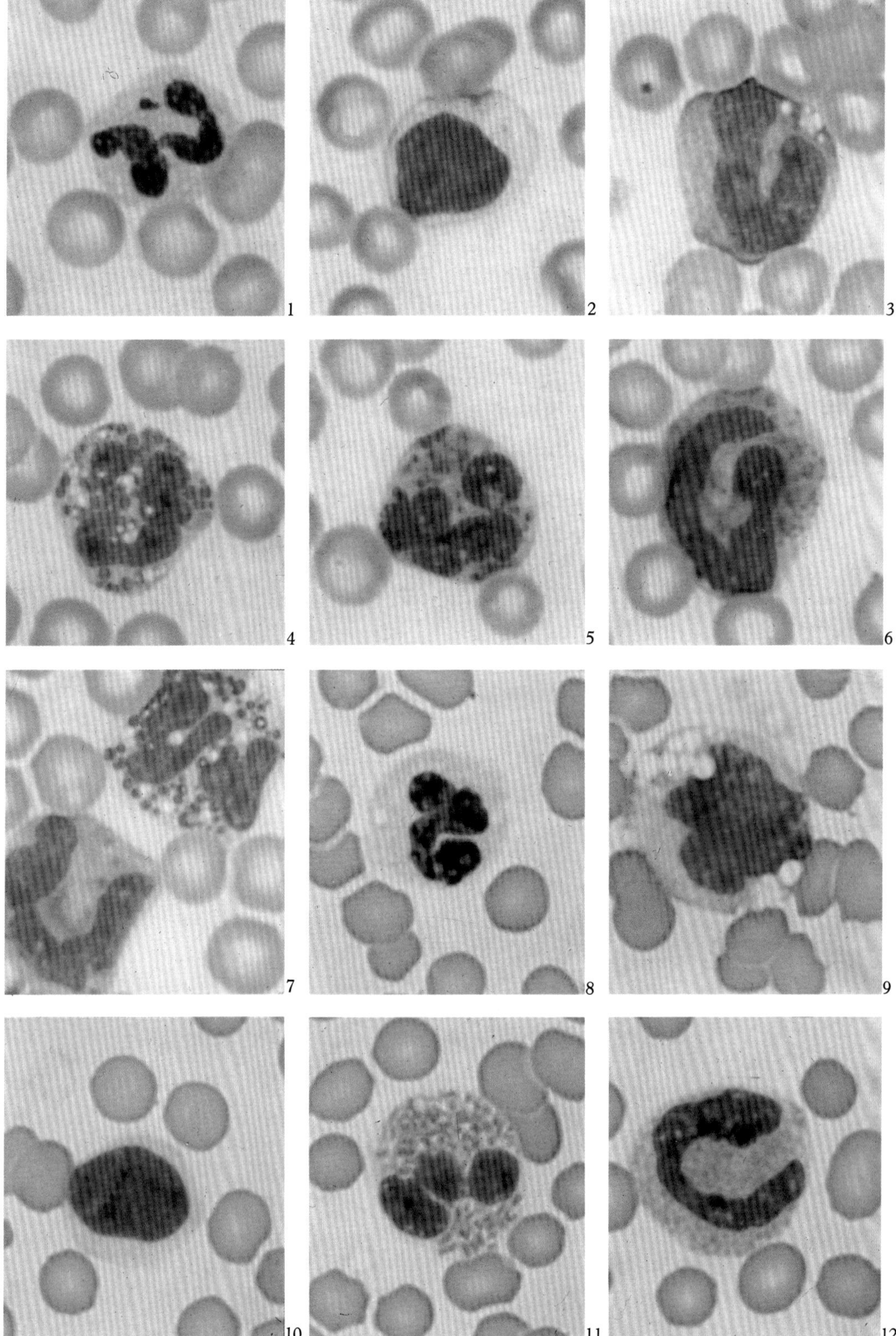

PLATE III. *Bone Marrow Cells (Wright's Stain)*

1. *Rubriblastic island, dog. Cells of the erythrocytic series in various stages of maturation surrounded by one macrophage, M (nucleus, N). 1, Rubriblast; 2, prorubricyte; 3, basophilic rubricyte; 4, polychromatic rubricyte; 5, normochromatic rubricyte; 6, metarubricyte. ×360.*
2. *Rubriblast, dog. The large cell is a rubriblast with an early normochromatic rubricyte adjacent to it. ×360.*
3. *Rubriblast and two mitotic figures, dog. Rubriblast between basophilic rubricytes in mitosis. ×360.*
4. *Polychromatic rubricyte, cow. Two young polychromatic rubricytes. ×360.*
5. *Myeloblast, dog. The immaturity of this cell is indicated by the number of nucleoli visible. ×360.*
6. *Progranulocyte, dog. The large cell is a progranulocyte with characteristic azurophilic granules. ×360.*
7. *Progranulocyte, cow. The progranulocyte is filled with numerous, coarse azurophilic granulocytes. The other cell is a mature eosinophil. ×360.*
8. *Eosinophilic myelocyte, cow. The cell contains a few immature or unripe granules which stain purple. Notice the blue cytoplasm between the granules. ×360.*
9. *Eosinophilic myelocyte, cow. This cell is somewhat more mature than the one in Plate III–8. Notice that all the granules are the characteristic mature color. The nucleus has clumped chromatin. ×360.*
10. *Neutrophilic metamyelocyte, cow. The nucleus is beginning to indent, indicating further maturation. The cytoplasmic granules are evident. ×360.*
11. *Megakaryocyte, dog. The membrane demarcation lines impart a grainy texture to the cytoplasm. There is some evidence of thrombocytes pinching off between the 3 and 5 o'clock positions. ×240.*
12. *Proplasmacyte, dog. This is a fairly immature cell as evidenced by the relatively small amount of cytoplasm. The characteristic Golgi image is seen at the 3 o'clock position. × 360.*

Plate III

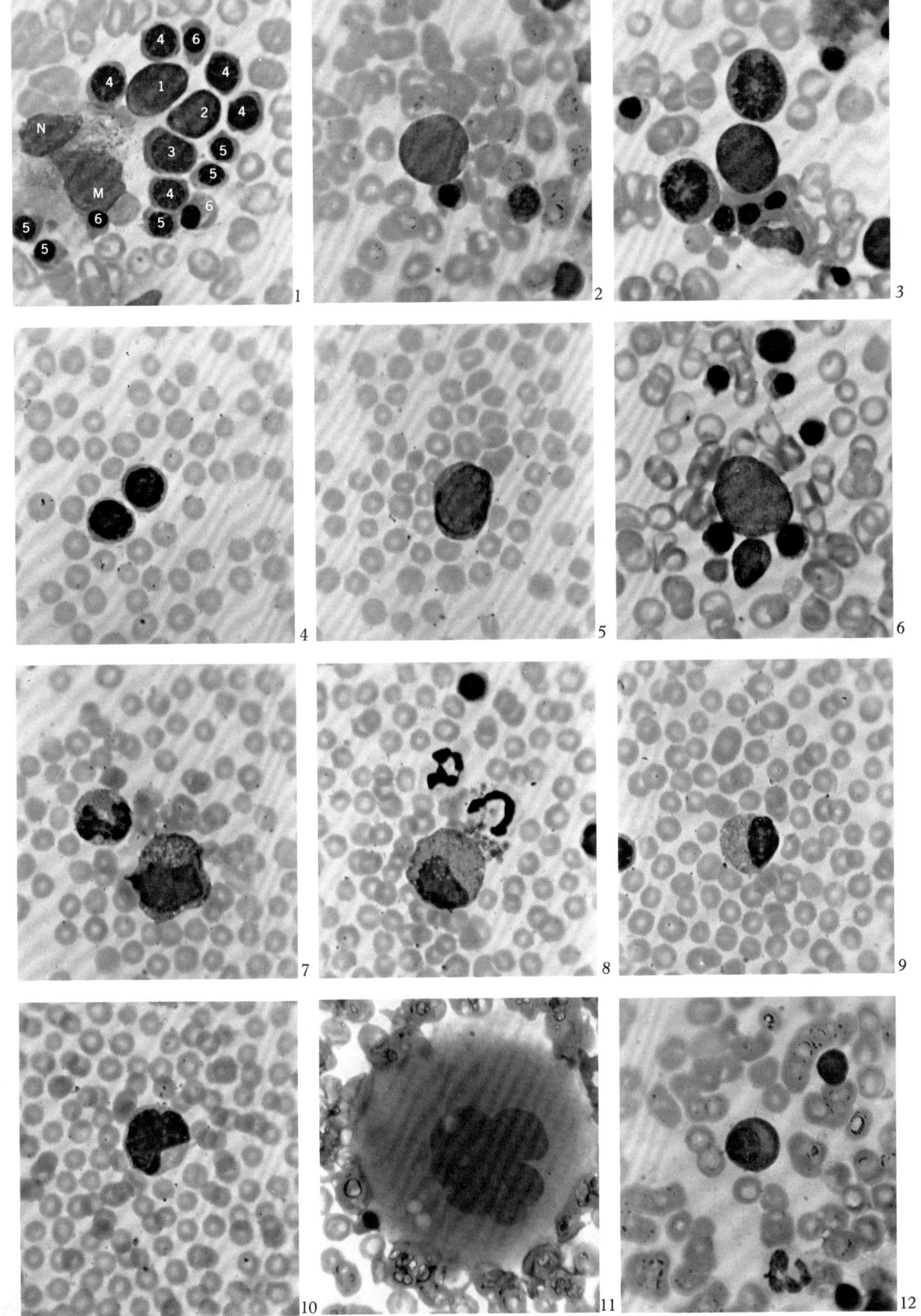

In summary, (1) cells become smaller as they mature; (2) young cells have relatively larger nuclei than do older cells; (3) nuclei in very immature cells have two or more nucleoli or nucleolar rings; (4) the nuclear chromatin in immature cells is euchromatic and with maturity gradually becomes heterochromatic.

As described earlier, mature erythrocytes vary in size among the domestic animals; however, the sizes stated in the following descriptions are for animals whose red cells fall in the 6.5- to 7-μm range. Animals with smaller adult cells likewise have smaller stem cells.

Erythropoiesis

KINETICS

The developmental process of the red blood cell is called erythropoiesis, which encompasses a series of successive morphologic alterations resulting in the production of erythrocytes. The total mass of erythropoietic cells and mature circulating erythrocytes is a functional organ referred to as the *erythron.*

In order for erythropoiesis to occur, the committed erythroid stem cells must be stimulated by erythropoietin, an alpha globulin. Although it is fully accepted that renal hypoxia initiates the production of erythropoietin, there is still some confusion as to where and how this substance is produced. One accepted theory is that decreased oxygen tension stimulates the kidney to release the enzyme erythrogenin; this activates erythropoietinogen, a circulating erythropoietin precursor synthesized by the liver to produce erythropoietin.

As a result of in vitro studies of hematopoietic tissue, two erythrocytic-committed stem cells have been described: *burst-forming units* (BFU-E) and *erythrocytic colony-forming units* (CFU-E). The BFU-E, a direct descendent of the CFU-S, forms bursts or clones of erythrocytic cells and is considered to be the earliest cell committed to the red cell series. A *burst-promoting factor* (BPF) acts on the primitive stem cell (CFU-S) to induce proliferation and receptor acquisition for erythropoietin. The CFU-E forms small clusters of erythrocytic cells and is very responsive to erythropoietin in culture. Neither the BFU-E nor the CFU-E have been identified microscopically; their existence is presumed on the basis of their colony formation in vitro.

The anatomic unit of erythropoiesis is the *rubriblastic (erythroblastic) island* (Plate III–1), which consists of several erythropoietic cells surrounding a macrophage and closely positioned against the outside surface of the sinus wall. These cell clusters are usually seen only in samples teased from the marrow, since aspiration techniques destroy the islands. The rubriblastic cells are enveloped by extensive, slender cytoplasmic processes of the macrophage, where they undergo several mitotic divisions and synthesize neary 80% of the total hemoglobin of the mature erythrocyte. As these erythrocytic precursor cells mature, they move along the macrophage processes so that the mature erythrocyte is in juxtaposition to the sinus wall for entry into the circulation. The macrophage of the rubriblastic island is believed to play the role of a "nurse cell" to the developing erythrocytes by conveying certain undefined nutrients to them and providing the optimal microenvironment for their development. While the macrophage is in close association with the cytoplasmic extensions of the reticular cell, it engulfs the expelled, hemoglobin-coated nucleus of the metarubricyte and salvages the iron and DNA.

MORPHOLOGY OF ERYTHROCYTIC LINEAGE

The rubriblast (pronormoblast), the earliest recognizable cell of the erythrocytic cell line, is oval, 20 to 24 μm in diameter, and has an N/C ratio of 8:1. The spherical, light purple nucleus has a netlike chromatin pattern. There are one to three prominent nucleoli. The cytoplasm has a mottled or splotchy appearance, stains blue-green, and has a lighter blue perinuclear zone. There are no granules of any kind in the cytoplasm (Plate III–2 and 3).

The next stage is the *prorubricyte (early normoblast),* 14 to 19 μm in diameter, with an N/C ratio of 7:1. It appears similar to the rubriblast, except that in the prorubricyte, the nuclear chromatin is beginning to condense and contains no nucleoli or nucleolar rings.

Mitotic division and maturation produce the *basophilic rubricyte (basophilic normoblast).* It is 16 to 18 μm in diameter and has an N/C ratio of 6:1 (Plate III–1 and 3). The nuclear chromatin is clumped and displays a radial pattern. There are no nucleoli. The cytoplasm is a deep greenish blue or dark navy blue owing to the rich content of RNA. Therefore, the basophilic rubricyte exhibits the most intense basophilia among all the bone marrow cells. The perinuclear zone is lighter than in the pronormoblast, and no granules are present.

Further karyokinesis produces the *polychromatic rubricyte (normoblast),* which is 10 to 12 μm in diameter, has an N/C ratio of 2:1 and contains a dark, condensed nucleus with coarse, clumped chromatin (Plate III–1 and 4). The cytoplasm displays a muddy bluish red color owing to the gradual increase in hemoglobin. The mixture of some residual basophilic cytoplasm (RNA) and the orange-red hemoglobin produces this polychromasia.

The *normochromatic rubricyte (orthochromatic normoblast)* is the result of another mitotic division and has an approximate diameter of 8 to 10 μm, with an N/C ratio of 2:1. It possesses a dense nucleus and has more hemoglobin than the polychromatic rubricyte.

The *metarubricyte (late normoblast)* develops by further maturation involving the full acquisition of hemoglobin and nuclear pyknosis. It is 6 to 9 μm in diameter, with an N/C ratio of 1:2. The nucleus may be partially extruded or fragmented, and the cytoplasm varies from polychromatic to normochromatic, depending on the amount of hemoglobin present. After the nucleus is gone, the cytoplasm has a muddy blue color because of the residual RNA. This is the *diffusely basophilic cell,* or *reticulocyte.* The end stage of erythrocyte maturation occurs adjacent to the sinus wall, where metarubricytes begin to squeeze through the endothelial lining, via gaps created by movement of the dendritic reticular cells. As the cell moves into the sinus, the nucleus is at the opposite end of the cell and is extruded and phagocytized by the macrophage. Fully matured red cells assume the characteristic sizes and shapes for each species, as described in the section on blood.

Granulopoiesis

KINETICS

Unlike erythropoiesis, relatively little is known about the mechanisms regulating cellular differentiation and release of granulocytes. Animal experiments designed to elucidate these events necessarily upset the steady state of granulopoietic kinetics, so that attempts to demonstrate these control mechanisms have not been very successful. However, it is well established that bone marrow granulocytes exist in two major compartments: (1) the proliferative (mitotic) compartment, composed of myeloblasts, promyelocytes, and myelocytes, all of which are capable of replication; and (2) the maturation-storage compartment, which includes the metamyelocytes and mature granulocytes, which are nonreplicating. The vast pool of mature granulocytes stored in the marrow is referred to as the *mature granulocyte reserve* and contains more cells than the circulating blood. In addition to the storage pool in the marrow, two granulocyte populations exist in the blood vessels. One of them circulates and the other is a marginated pool out of the blood flow, consisting of white cells lying against the vessel walls. The initial response to a demand for granulocytes is a release of mature cells from the marrow reserve and from the marginated pool rather than a stimulation of proliferative activity.

Tissue culture studies of bone marrow cell colonies have identified committed stem cells for eosinophils (CFU-Eo), basophils (CFU-Ba), megakaryocytes (CFU-Meg) and a committed stem cell that gives rise to both monocytes and neutrophils (CFU-MN), all of which retain a limited capacity for differentiation and cell division. The cells that give rise to all these separate colonies are called *colony-forming units in culture* (CFU-C) and have a limited capacity for self-renewal when compared to CFU-S (Fig. 4–11).

In order for CFU-C to grow and form colonies in tissue culture, a substance termed *colony-stimulating factor* (CSF) must be added to the culture medium. Moreover, it appears that each progenitor responds to a specific CSF. Most agree that CSF is analogous to erythropoietin in that it is an in vivo regulator of granulocyte-macrophage differentiation. CSF has been isolated from macrophages, vascular smooth muscle, and endothelium, and it is known that serum levels increase in animals exposed to bacterial antigens. Exactly how CSF levels are controlled in vivo is not completely understood. One theory is that lactoferrin, a known inhibitor of neutrophil production, may be involved in regulating granulopoiesis by blocking monocyte-produced CSF. However, there are as yet many unanswered questions about CSF control and regulation.

MORPHOLOGY OF GRANULOCYTIC LINEAGE

Maturation of granulocytes involves nuclear and cytoplasmic change as well as granule transformation. Because the morphologic changes are much the same for all types of granulocytes, they will be described together.

The earliest recognizable progenitor of the granulocytic series developing from the CFU is the *myeloblast.* It is an oval cell, 10 to 18 μm in diameter, with an N/C ratio of 6:1 (Plate III–5). The even distribution of purple chromatin imparts a velvety texture to the nucleus. There may be as many as six pale blue nucleoli in this young cell. The cytoplasm is a pale, light blue-green color and forms a complete collar around the nucleus. In pig bone marrow, myeloblasts usually contain several azurophilic granules, whereas in ruminants and carnivores the cytoplasm has a mottled appearance.

The *progranulocyte,* the daughter cell of the myeloblast, is sometimes slightly larger than its progenitor. It is oval or spherical, 12 to 20 μm in diameter, and the pale purple, foamy cytoplasm contains a variable number of large, nonspecific, coarse azurophilic granules (Plate III–6 and 7). The nuclear chromatin has a fine linear arrangement with the little clumping, and two or three nucleoli may be present.

The daughter cell of the progranulocyte is the *promyelocyte* (12 to 18 μm in diameter), an intermediate cell containing some specific granules and a few residual azurophilic granules distributed randomly throughout the pale blue–stained cytoplasm. The type of specific granules present indicates which granulocyte will develop, and because many granules are immature they stain a different color than the mature granules. In *eosinophilic promyelocytes* the granules are brown, purple, or dark blue; in *basophilic promyelocytes* they are fewer in number and usually dark purple, pink, or brown. *Neutrophilic promyelocytes* have pale pink and blue immature granules. In cat bone marrow, the specific granules in neutrophilic promyelocytes are not distinguishable; however, the eosinophilic and basophilic promyelocytes contain a limited number of specific granules along with a few azurophilic (primary) granules. In all cell types, the nucleus is spherical or may have a slight indentation with clumped chromatin. Nucleoli may be present. The N/C ratio is 4:1.

The *myelocyte* is the last stage to form by mitosis from the parent cell. It is 12 to 18 μm in diameter with an N/C ratio of 2:1. At this stage the neutrophilic and eosinophilic myelocytes have all the granules they will ever have, but the basophilic stem cell has only a few specific granules. Regardless of cell type, the granules tend to accumulate near one side of the nucleus in the area of the Golgi complex. This area is particularly prominent in neutrophilic myelocytes and has been described as a "sun burst." Some azurophilic granules may be discernible. The neutrophilic myelocyte contains mature, pale pink specific granules as well as nonspecific azurophilic granules, whereas the eosinophilic and basophilic myelocytes have a mixture of mature and immature specific granules (Plate III–8 and 9). The eosinophilic granules in dog marrow tend to remain brown and never attain a bright orange-red color. For this reason, they are confused with basophils in marrow smears. However, when one considers the rarity of basophils, they need not cause confusion. In all myelocytes, the cytoplasm is pale blue. The nuclear chromatin exhibits definite clumping and may have a slight indentation. No nucleoli are present in the myelocyte, and they are not seen in any subsequent cells.

From the myelocyte stage, the cells go through a series of transformations during which they become smaller, their specific granules mature, and their nuclei attain their final configuration. When the nucleus has a definite indentation, the cell is called a *metamyelocyte* and is 12 to 15 μm in diameter with an N/C ratio of 1.5:1 (Plate III–10). The chromatin is coarse, with definite clumping. A few azurophilic granules are present (10 to 26%) and the specific granules in most cells have their characteristic colors. At the metamyelocyte stage, the basophil has a full quota of granules.

Further nuclear indentation concentrates the coarse, dark purple chromatin into bands of equal diameter, forming C, S, or V shapes without definite constrictions. This is the *band cell* (staff or stab), 10 to 16 μm in diameter, with a 1:2 N/C ratio. In order to differentiate a true band cell from a metamyelocyte, the nuclear indentation must be beyond the central axis of the cell. Granules in the mature cells overlie a pale blue cytoplasm, and because neutrophilic granules are small they blend with the blue cytoplasm, imparting an overall purple hue to the cell. Mature neutrophils may have definite nuclear constrictions and/or lobes, depending on the species, whereas the eosinophil and basophil nuclei usually attain only bilobed configuration.

The preceding descriptions are fairly general. One must remember that there are species differences in granular color and size, as well as in nuclear configuration, discussed in the section on blood leukocytes.

Agranulopoiesis

KINETICS

The existence in the bone marrow of stem cells for monocytes and lymphocytes has been debated for many years. However, experiments involving radioactively labeled cells, chromosomal markings, and tissue culture transformations have given evidence that both cells have a myelogenous origin.

MORPHOLOGY OF AGRANULOCYTIC LINEAGE

MONOPOIESIS. The pool of monocyte precursors in the bone marrow is relatively small, and while there probably is a monoblast, the earliest recognizable cell of this lineage is the *promonocyte.* It is a large cell, 15 to 20 μm in diameter, and has abundant blue-stained cytoplasm containing numerous free polyribosomes, a well-developed Golgi complex, a small amount of rER, and few azurophilic granules. The relatively large oval or spherical nucleus contains two to five nucleoli. As the cell matures, it becomes smaller (12 to 18 μm), and the cytoplasm tends to stain blue-gray. The nucleus may become indented on one side and nucleoli persist, suggesting that adult monocytes retain their ability to synthesize granules containing hydrolytic enzymes. Monocytes enter the blood as relatively immature cells, reaching their full functional potential only when they move into the tissues.

LYMPHOPOIESIS. Chromosomal studies of blood and bone marrow cells indicate that the CFU-S does not give rise to lymphocytes, but that in all likelihood another, less differentiated cell, the CFU-LH, is the progenitor of both the CFU-S and the lymphatic cell line (Fig. 4–11).

The marrow is the major site of production and export of lymphocyte progenitor cells that may become either T- or B-lymphocytes, depending upon their developmental pathway. Relatively immature lymphocytes leave the marrow via the blood and migrate to the thymic cortex, where they proliferate and acquire surface receptors in an antigen-free environment. Upon release from the thymus these *T-lymphocytes* enter the spleen for their final maturation and become part of the long-lived recirculating pool of lymphocytes in the blood and lymph and in certain regions of the peripheral lymphatic organs (see Chapter 8). There are several functional subsets of fully differentiated T-lymphocytes, such as T_H (helper), T_S (suppressor), T_C (cytotoxic), and T_{DTH} (delayed hypersensitive), all of which are described in Chapter 8.

Another lymphocyte population remains in the marrow long enough to acquire certain surface markers and then migrates to the spleen for the final maturation. The cells of this population are *B-lymphocytes* and make up about 5 to 10% of the recirculating lymphocyte pool. They seed certain regions of the secondary lymphatic organs, and it is here that they are antigenically stimulated and differentiate into plasma cells (see Chapter 8).

Lymphocytes and their precursors are difficult to recognize in the marrow. Because of their morphologic and functional heterogeneity, they are classified as either small or large lymphocytes. The large lymphocyte is probably the lymphoblast, measuring 12 to 15 μm in diameter. The nucleus is euchromatic and contains one to three nuclei, depending on the species. The cytoplasm stains intensely basophilic owing to polyribosomes.

The small lymphocytes in bone marrow smears are no different morphologically from those in peripheral blood and probably are the recirculating T- and B-lymphocytes. The two types of lymphocytes are not morphologically distinguishable.

Thrombocyte Development

Thrombocytes originate in the bone marrow as pinched-off cytoplasmic buds from megakaryocytes. The youngest cell of this series is the *megakaryoblast.* It is spherical or oval, measures 25 to 35 μm in diameter, and has a 10 :1 N/C ratio. The cytoplasm is slightly basophilic, and several blunt extrusions give the cell margin an irregular outline. The single nucleus has dispersed chromatin, and several nucleoli are visible. Contrary to other developing cell lines, the daughter cell of the megakaryoblast is larger than the parent cell, with much of the increase in size caused by repeated nuclear divisions without concurrent cytoplasmic divisions.

The *promegakaryocyte* is 25 to 50 μm in diameter, with an irregular outline owing to the numerous cytoplasmic buds. The basophilic cytoplasm has a grainy texture and a few azurophilic granules. The nucleus may be single, indented, or lobulated and is made of clumped chromatin, which often obliterates the one or two nucleoli.

The *megakaryocyte* is the largest cell of this series measuring 40 to 100 μm in diameter (Plate III–11). The nucleus has two or

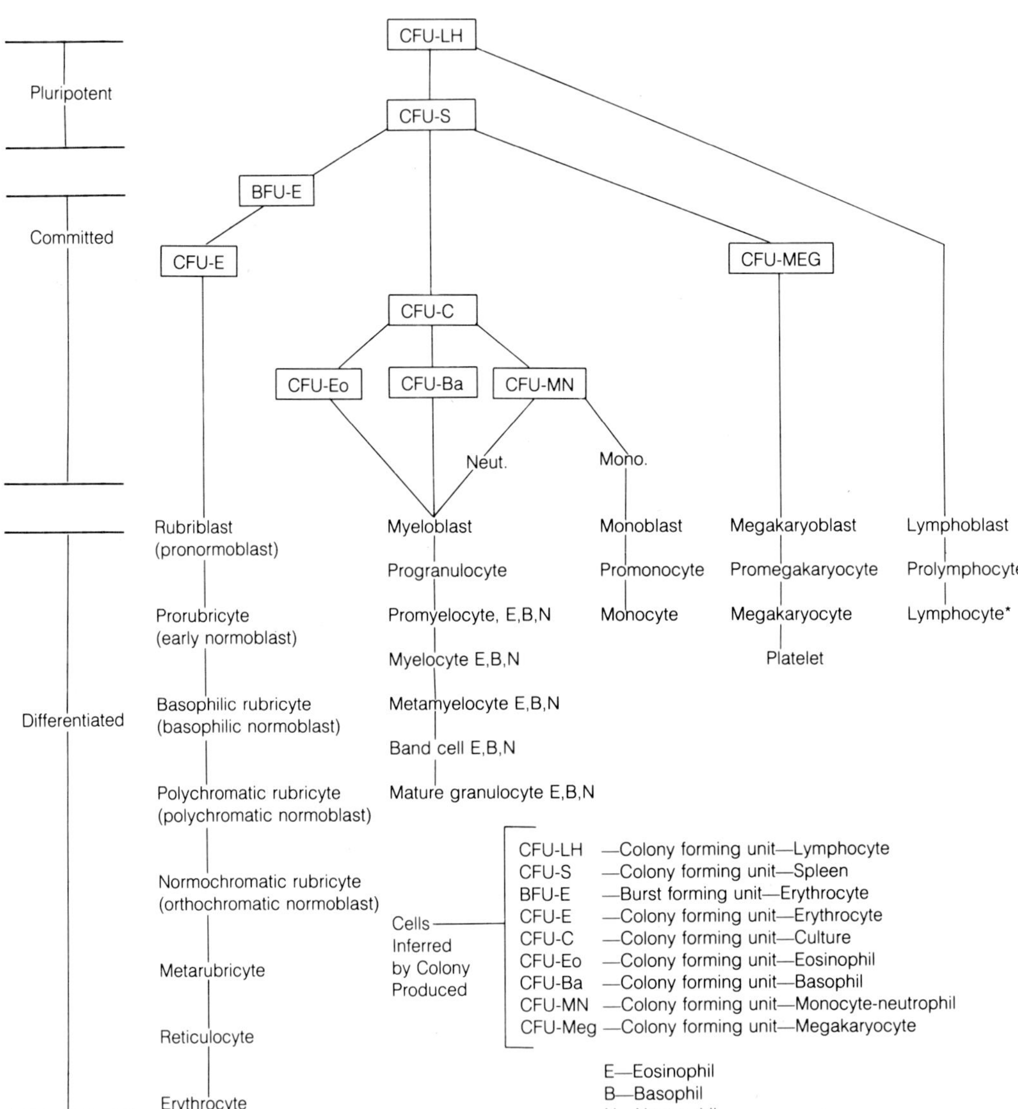

* Bone marrow lymphopoiesis produces B-lymphocytes. Some of these will become plasma cells following antigenic stimulation.

Fig. 4–11. *Hemopoiesis flow chart.*

more lobules, composed of clumped chromatin, and several nucleoli. The abundant blue cytoplasm is rich in ribosomes. There are numerous and large azurophilic granules, which are the membrane-bounded dense bodies seen with the EM. Together with dense bodies, tortuous membranous vesicles, which form a tridimensional network, intersect to partition the cytoplasm into oblong masses. These membranous profiles, visible only with the electron microscope, are called *platelet demarcation membranes* and impart a grainy texture to the cytoplasm (Fig. 4–9A). They are intricate invaginations of the cell membrane. When the thrombocytes are shed from the megakaryocyte, they are completely surrounded by the unit membrane, preserving the integrity of the parent cell membrane.

Plasma Cell Development

Normally, plasma cells are not seen in peripheral blood and comprise only 1 to 2% of the nucleated cells in bone marrow. They are present in almost all of the secondary lymphatic organs (lymph nodes, spleen, tonsils) and are frequent in the lamina propria of the intestine and connective tissues in other sites. The frequent close association of marrow plasma cells and dendritic reticular cells indicates a possible immunologic significance, since these dendritic reticular cells are known to be most effective in antigen presentation.

The most widely accepted theory of plasma cell production is that plasma cells develop from B-lymphocytes that undergo several mitotic divisions and morphologic changes. For this reason, the following description of the plasma cell lineage is included.

The *plasmablast* is 14 to 24 μm in diameter and pear-shaped; it has abundant deep-stained basophilic cytoplasm (N/C = 2:1) with a mottled or splotchy appearance. The color of this cytoplasm is so distinctive that no other cell should be confused with the plasma cell. The nucleus is located eccentrically usually in the narrow end of the cell. The chromatin is coarse and displays two or three nucleoli.

The *proplasmacyte* is not significantly smaller than the plasmablast, and there is little change in the N/C ratio. The nuclear chromatin is somewhat coarser and one or two distinct nucleoli are present. The greatest change occurs in the cytoplasm. The extreme basophilia, indicative of protein synthesis, is still conspicuous, but now the pale juxtanuclear halo is visible (Plate III–12). This area is occupied by the well-developed Golgi complex.

The mature *plasma cell* (plasmacyte) is 8 to 18 μm in diameter at its widest dimension. There is abundant deep blue cytoplasm, and the pale perinuclear halo occupies a large area near the nucleus. Distinct vacuoles are seen near the cell border. The nucleus has dark chromatin clumped in such a manner that spaces between the chromatin give the appearance of spokes of a wheel. This is one of the most distinctive morphologic features of the adult plasma cell.

Other Cells in Bone Marrow

OSTEOBLASTS AND OSTEOCLASTS

Because most of the cells seen in bone marrow lie in close apposition to bony spicules, it is understandable that osteoblasts and osteoclasts may be seen on occasion in marrow smears. They are more prevalent when the marrow is removed from sites where the biopsy needle penetrates a cartilage cap, such as the iliac crest, or areas of new bone formation resulting from previous aspirations. The osteoclast resembles the megakaryocyte more than does any other cell type, because they are both multinucleated, have slightly basophilic, heterogeneous, textured cytoplasm, and are about the same size. The most dependable differentiating feature is the nucleus, which in the osteoclast is separated but in the megakaryocyte is multilobulated with all lobules attached to each other.

The osteoblast and proplasmacyte appear similar because both have a prominent Golgi complex that creates a cytoplasmic pale area. It is not immediately adjacent to the nucleus in the osteoblast, as it is in the proplasmacyte, but occupies an area somewhat away from the nucleus. Also, the basophilia so characteristic of the proplasmacyte is not as intense in the osteoblast.

Clinical Evaluation of Bone Marrow

The identification of the various cellular components of bone marrow and of their characteristic maturation changes provides the veterinarian with useful information. Many disorders occurring in the bone marrow are manifested by changes in the peripheral blood as well as in the bone marrow itself. In any cytologic examination of bone marrow, one should consider the myeloid:erythroid ratio and the cellular composition.

THE MYELOID:ERYTHROID RATIO

The myeloid:erythroid (M:E) ratio refers to the number of myeloid cells seen among all the nucleated bone marrow cells (see Table 4–1). The term "myeloid" is an unfortunate choice here because this actually refers to "marrow," including both the erythrocytes and granulocytes. When used in this context, it actually means the number of *myelocytes,* or granulocytic stem cells, related to the number of nucleated cells in the erythrocytic series. The M:E ratio must be evaluated in relation to the total white blood cell count. If the M:E ratio is elevated and the white blood cell count is normal, depressed erythrogenesis is indicated. Conversely, a decreased M:E ratio occurs whenever there is intensified erythrogenesis as a result of severe blood loss or erythrocyte destruction.

CELLULAR COMPOSITION

The recognition of the cell types seen in aspirated marrow is of value in considering anemia of unknown pathogenesis. Increased erythropoiesis, as indicated by a decreased M:E ratio, may not necessarily increase circulating red cells. In vitamin B_{12} and folic acid deficiencies, a maturation arrest occurs at the basophilic rubricyte stage, resulting in a decreased release of normal red cells into the circulation. Those released are macrocytes. This maturation arrest produces large blue cells, called *megaloblasts,* in the marrow. Iron deficiency anemia causes hyperplasia of the erythrocytic cell series, and the marrow is characterized by an increased number of normochromatic rubricytes. Lack of iron for hemoglobin synthesis causes these cells to continue to divide, and the resulting erythrocyte is microcytic.

Not all hemopoietic disorders require bone marrow studies. Some anemias, caused by hemorrhage or hemolysis or by decreased erythrogenesis secondary to chronic infections, are detectable by red blood cell morphology in most domestic animals. The horse is one exception, in that the peripheral blood usually does not exhibit signs of intensified erythrogenesis in response to red cell destruction or loss.

REFERENCES

Ackerman, G.: Cytochemical properties of the blood basophilic granulocyte. Ann NY Acad Sci *103*:376, 1963.

Ascensao, J.L., Vercellotti, G.M., Jacobs, H.S., and Zanjani, E.D.: Role of endothelial cells in human hematopoiesis: Modulation of mixed colony growth. Blood *63*,(3):553, 1984.

Bagby, G.C., Vasiliki, D.R., Bennett, R.M., Vandenbark, A.A., and Garewal, H.S.: Interaction of lactoferrin, monocytes and T-lymphocyte subsets in the regulation of steady-state granulopoiesis in vitro. J Clin Invest *68*:56, 1981.

Bentley, S.A.: Bone marrow connective tissue and the haemopoietic microenvironment. Br J Haematol *50*:1, 1982.

Broxmeyer, H.E., Bognacki, J., Ralph, P., Dorner, M.H., Lu, L., and Castro-Malaspina, H.: Monocyte-macrophage-derived acidic isoferritins: Normal feedback regulators of granulocyte-macrophage progenitor cells in vitro. Blood *60*:595, 1982.

Burgess, A.W., and Metcalf, D.: The nature and action of granulocyte-macrophage colony stimulating factors. Blood *56*:947, 1980.

Calhoun, M.L.: A cytological study of costal marrow. I. The adult horse. II. The adult cow. Am J Vet Res *15*:181, 1954.

Canfield, P.J.: An ultrastructural study of granulocytic development in feline bone marrow. Zbl Vet Med C Anat Histol Embryol *13*:97, 1984.

Chertkov, J.L., Drize, N.J., Gurevitch, O.A., and Udalov, G.A.: Hemopoietic stromal precursors in long-term culture of bone marrow: II. Significance of initial packing for creating a hemopoietic microenvironment and maintaining stromal precursors in the culture. Exp Hematol *11*(3):243, 1983.

Chikkappa, G., and Phillips, P.G.: Regulation of normal blood neutrophilic, macrophagic and eosinophilic committed stem cell proliferation by autologous blood T-lymphocytes subsets. Blood *63*(2):356, 1984.

Gordon, M.Y., Kearny, L., and Hibbin, J.A.: Effects of human marrow stromal cells on proliferation by human granulocytic (CFC-GM), erythroid (BFU-E) and mixed (MIX-CFC) Colony-forming cells. Br J Haematol *53*(2):317, 1983.

Hann, I.M., Bodger, M.P., and Hoffbrand, A.V.: Development of pluripotent hematopoietic progenitor cells in the human fetus. Blood *62*(1):118, 1983.

Jain, N.C.: Schalm's Veterinary Hematology. 4th Ed. Philadelphia, Lea & Febiger, 1986.

Lipton, J.M., and Nathan, D.G.: Cell-cell interactions in the regulation of erythropoiesis. Br J Haematol *53*(3):361, 1983.

Peter, H.H.: The origin of human NK cells. An ontogenic model derived from studies in patients with immunodeficiencies. Blut *46*(5):239, 1983.

Quesenberry, Petter J.: The concept of the hemopoietic stem cell. *In* Hematology. Edited by W.J. Williams, E. Beutler, A.J. Erslev, and M. Lichtman. 3rd Ed. New York, McGraw-Hill, 1983.

Schryver, H.F.: The bone marrow of the cat. Am J Vet Res *24*:1012, 1963.

Shively, J.N., Feldt, C., and Davis, D.: Fine structure of formed elements in canine blood. Am J Vet Res *6*:893, 1969.

Weiss, L., and Sakai, H.: The hematopoietic stroma. Am J Anat *170*(3):447, 1985.

Williams, W.J., Beutler, E., Erslev, A.J., and Lichtman, M. (eds.): Hematology. 3rd Ed. New York, McGraw-Hill, 1983.

5

Muscular Tissue

GEORGE H. CARDINET, III
JOHN H. VENABLE
H.-DIETER DELLMANN

Muscular tissues produce directed, organized movement. Cells of other tissue types are also capable of movement, but there is little integrated motion. Only specialized collections of cells producing strong, concerted contraction, primarily in one direction, are categorized as muscle.

The specialized cells of muscular tissues have distinct morphologic characteristics directly related to their contractile activity. They are elongate cells with spindle-shaped, fiberlike profiles. Because of their shape, muscle cells are often referred to as muscle fibers or myofibers. Hence, the term "fiber" when referring to muscular tissues has a very different meaning than when referring to the connective tissues, in which "fibers" are extracellular substances rather than cells. There are other terms specific to muscle cell terminology, which use the prefixes myo- (muscle) and sarco- (flesh).

The myofibers are arranged into bundles with their long axes aligned parallel to the direction of their contractions. Within all myofibers are abundant, tightly packed fibrous proteins that make their sarcoplasm compact and are brilliantly stainable with common cytoplasmic stains. In the usual H & E–stained histologic section, the myofibers may be recognized by their brightly stained eosinophilic sarcoplasm. Their sectioned profile in parallel arrays are shaped identically and are characteristic of the particular angle of sectioning. Myofibers sectioned parallel to their long axes appear as long rods or spindles (Fig. 5–1), whereas those sectioned at right angles are polygonal (Fig. 5–2). Random sectioning usually results in obliquely sectioned myofibers, producing various elliptical profiles.

Muscular tissues are present in three principal areas of the vertebrate body: the skeletal muscles, the heart, and the walls of hollow organs (e.g., viscera of the gastrointestinal tract, urogenital tract, blood vessels, etc.). Microscopically, longitudinal sections of skeletal and cardiac muscular tissue reveal that their myofibers have characteristic cross-striations whereas the muscular tissue of hollow organs is composed of myofibers without cross-striations and hence has a smooth appearance. Therefore, three basic types of muscle fibers are recognized: (1) smooth myofibers, which

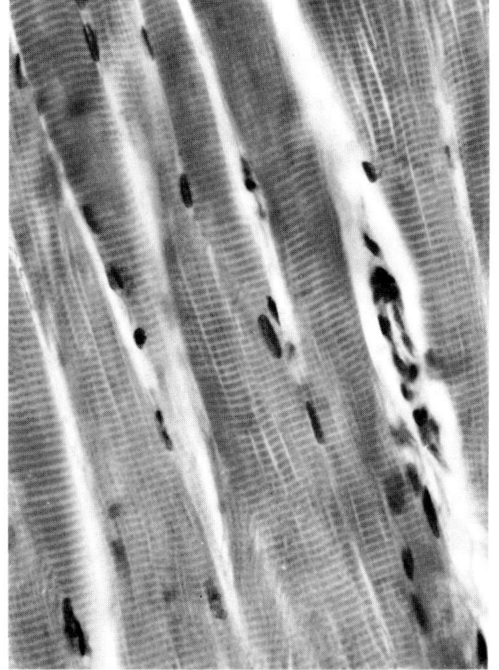

Fig. 5–1. *Skeletal muscle, longitudinal section. Notice the cross striations and the nuclei located in the periphery of the myofibers. H & E.* ×*435.*

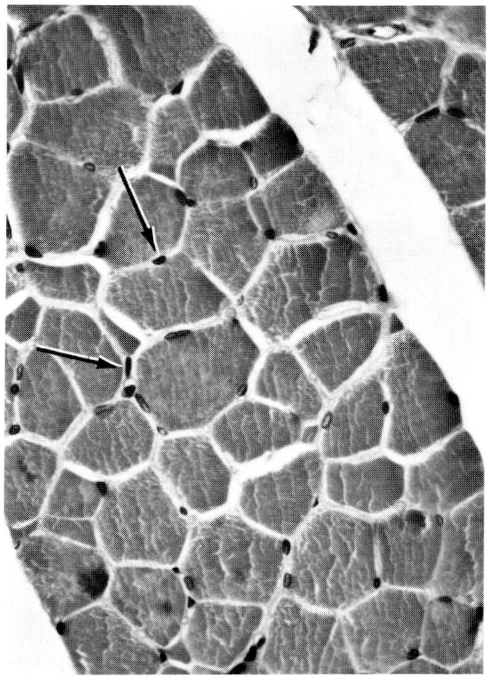

Fig. 5–2. *Skeletal muscle, cross section. The nuclei in the sparse endomysium (arrows) belong to either fibroblasts or satellite cells. H & E.* ×*435.*

form the contractile portion of the walls of most viscera, (2) striated skeletal myofibers, which comprise the skeletal muscles that originate at and insert on the bones of the skeleton, and (3) striated cardiac myofibers, which comprise the walls of the heart.

GENERAL HISTOLOGY

Skeletal Muscle

The extremely long skeletal myofibers vary from 10 to 120 μm in diameter and may course the entire length of one muscle. These long fibers are derived by the fusion of many individual mononuclear cells (myoblasts) into one continuous myofiber. Thus, each myofiber has many nuclei, the majority of which are located normally at the periphery of the myofiber in a subsarcolemmal position in mammals (Figs. 5–1 and 5–2). When viewed in longitudinal section, the transverse striations appear as a regular, cross-banding pattern consisting of repeating arrays of light and dark bands (see Figs. 5–1 and 5–8).

Individual myofibers are bound together into primary bundles or fascicles. Within a primary bundle each myofiber is bound to the other by a sparse, fine web of reticular connective tissue, the endomysium, which ensheathes each myofiber and supports a network of blood capillaries and terminal innervating nerve fibers (Fig. 5–3). Each primary bundle is ensheathed by dense collagen fibers, the perimysium, which binds adjacent bundles and carries blood vessels and nerves passing to the bundles (Fig. 5–3). Also, it is within the perimysium that muscle spindles (skeletal muscle stretch receptors) are located (see Chapter 6). Lastly, the whole muscle is ensheathed by the epimysium, a relatively thick and dense collagenous connective tissue (Fig. 5–3). All of these connective tissues are interconnected and continuous with one another, and they provide the means by which con-

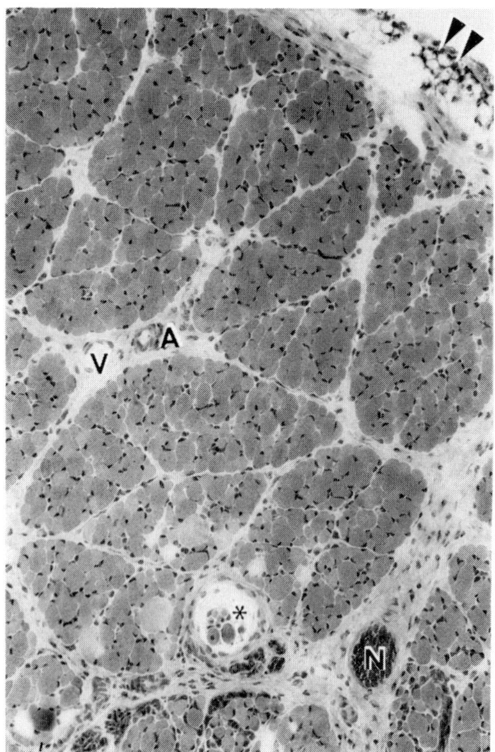

Fig. 5–3. *The myofibers are organized into fascicles (bundles) and separated from other fascicles by perimysium. Within the larger divisions of the perimysium, notice the arteriole (A), venule (V), intramuscular nerve branch (N), and muscle spindle (*) At the margin of the section is a portion of the epimysium (arrowheads).* ×*125.*

tractile forces are transmitted to the tendons of origin and insertion. At the myotendinous junctions of origin and insertion, the terminal portion of each myofiber has villous-like projections that insert into complimentary invaginations of the tendon.

Five primary cell types populate all primary bundles of skeletal muscle: myofibers, endothelial cells, pericytes, fibroblasts, and myosatellite cells (Fig. 5–4). Myofibers predominate. Their thick, platter-shaped nuclei, exhibiting mainly euchromatin and one or two large nucleoli represent over half the nuclei in any field. Nuclei of endothelial cells (capillaries) and fibroblasts are slightly smaller and darker, represent approximately 20% and 15% of the total nuclei, respectively, and are the main cellular components of the endomysium. Pericytes, satellite to capillaries, have small, dark, heterochromatic nuclei and constitute less than 5% of the nuclear types. Myosatellite cells, like pericytes, are mononuclear cells with similar heterochromatic nuclei but lie adjacent to myofibers (Fig. 5–4). In very young animals, they may constitute 20% of the cells in the bundle, but decrease to less than 1% in adults. By light microscopy, their nuclei may be mistaken for unusually dark muscle nuclei. However, with electron microscopy, myosatellite cells are clearly separate from the myofiber but included within the latter's basal lamina (Fig. 5–4).

Other cell types represented include the neurolemmocytes associated with nerves found in the regions of the myoneural junctions (motor end-plates) (see Chapter 6). In the perimysium, all the cells of dense irregular connective tissue are represented.

Smooth Muscle

Each smooth myofiber is a small mononucleated spindle, seldom more than 10 μm in diameter. The length of a smooth muscle myofiber varies between 20 and 500 μm, depending on the organ in which it is located. The nucleus is located in the center of the myofiber (Figs. 5–5 and 5–6). No cross-banding is visible. All myofibers comprising a bundle are packed tightly together with a fine network of elastic and reticular fibers interposed between them (Fig. 5–6). Apparently the connective tissue fibers are produced by the myofibers, because there are no fibroblasts or other cell types within primary bundles. Capillaries and nerve fibers usually lie between muscle bundles. There is no distinct perimysium, since the contractile force from the bundles is not transmitted to tendons or aponeuroses; rather, the contractions usually change the size or shape of the organs of which they are an integral part.

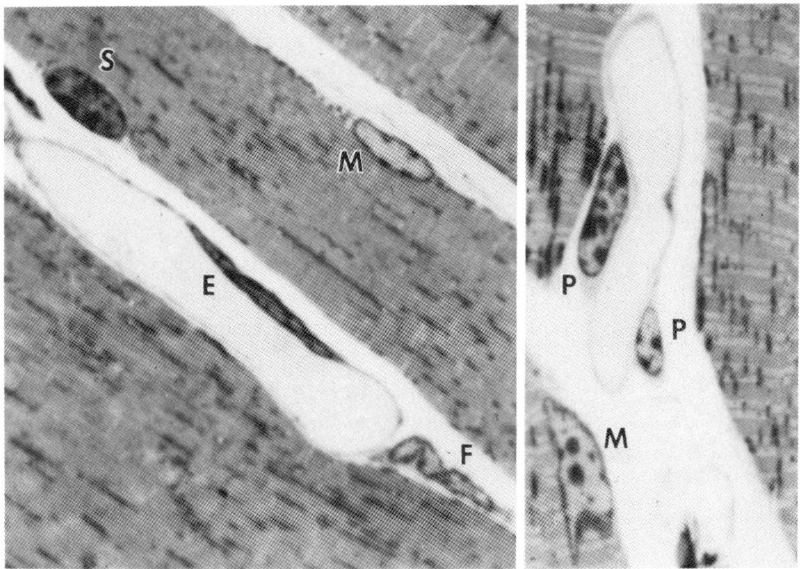

Fig. 5–4. *Primary cell types (nuclei) in skeletal muscle. (E) endothelial nucleus—capillary; (M) muscle nucleus; (P) pericyte nucleus—satellite to capillary; (S) myosatellite nucleus—satellite to muscle fiber, beneath fiber's basal lamina. 0.5 μm sections in epoxy plastic, toluidine blue staining. Dark bodies in fibers are mitochondria. 12-day-old mouse. ×1300.*

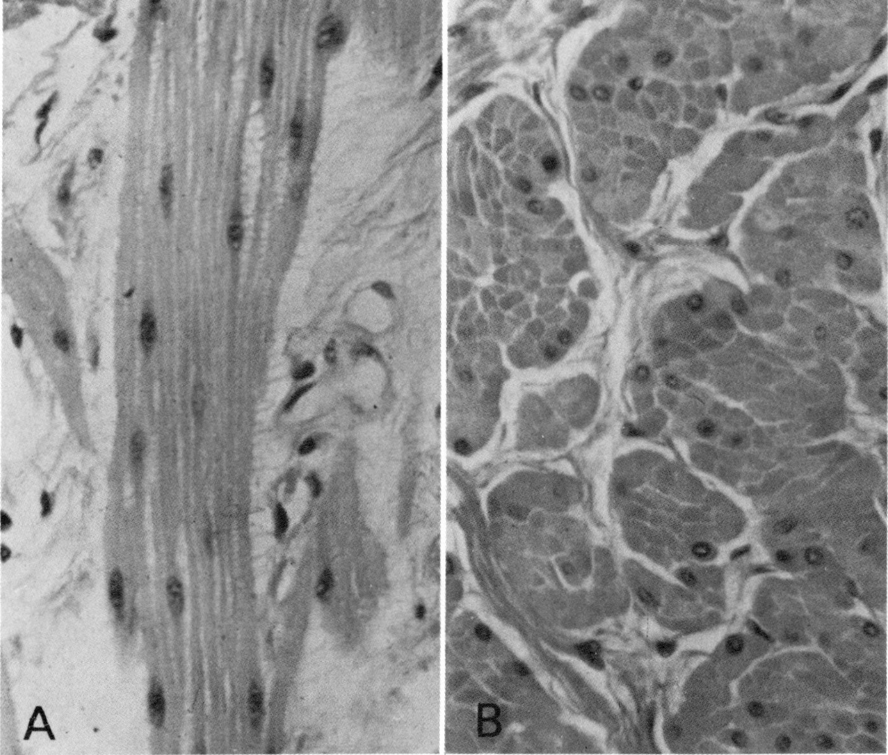

Fig. 5–5. *Smooth muscle, urinary bladder, cat. (A) Longitudinal section showing spindle-shaped myofibers comprising a bundle. (B) Cross-section of bundle showing central nuclei in myofibers cut at midpoint, absence of nuclear profiles in cells cut nearer their ends. H & E. ×400. (Courtesy of R.A. Kainer.)*

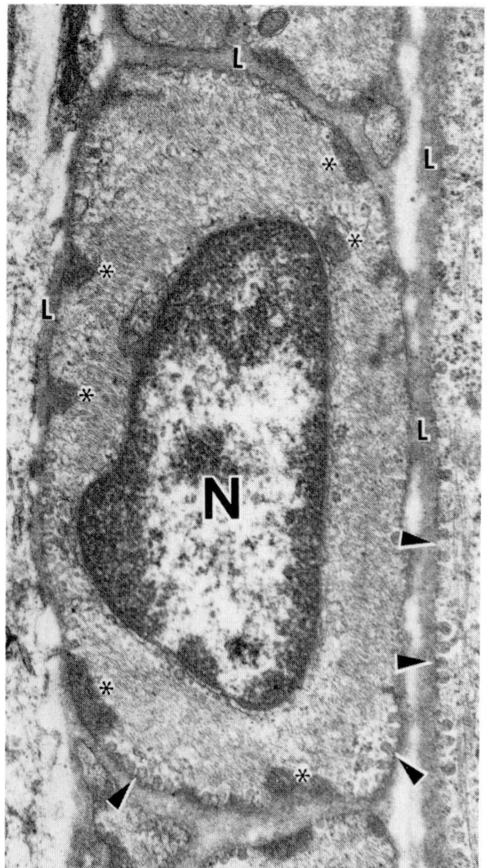

Fig. 5–6. *Electron micrograph of a cross sectioned smooth myofiber, and a portion of a longitudinally sectioned smooth myofiber in an arteriole from a dog. The nucleus (N) is centrally located, and the sarcoplasm contains numerous myofilaments in various orientations. Within the central sarcoplasm and areas adjacent to the sarcolemma, there are electron-dense bodies (*), which are sites of attachment for myofilaments in smooth myofibers (Z-line equivalent). Numerous pinocytotic vesicles are present along the sarcolemma (arrowheads) located just under the prominent basal lamina (L) that surrounds each myofiber. ×23,900. (Courtesy of W.S. Tyler.)*

Cardiac Muscle

Cardiac myofibers are specifically organized for the requirements of the cardiac pump. These cylindric, striated cells are similar in size to small skeletal myofibers but are single cells that branch and anastomose rather than forming long syncytial cylinders (Fig. 5–7). The single nucleus is always positioned in the center of the myofiber (Fig. 5–7). In the ventricular wall, the network of cardiac muscle courses ventrad from the middle of the atrioventricular plate to the cardiac apex, forming the interventricular septum, then spirals back to the plate to form the outer walls of the ventricle. Wavelike contractions following the path of this architecture effectively force blood from the ventricles into the major arteries. The walls of the atria are thinner but are constructed similarly, the network of smaller fibers spreading from the sinus venosus to the atrioventricular plate. There is little uniform division of the cardiac muscle network into bundles, and most of the connective tissue surrounds individual muscle cells.

A profuse capillary network is interposed between the muscle elements in the loose connective tissue. Pericytes and fibroblasts are present, but there are no myosatellite cells. Other details of cardiac structure are discussed in Chapter 7.

MICROSCOPIC STRUCTURE OF MYOFIBERS

Myofibers require a mechanism to transfer chemical energy into mechanical energy. This is achieved through an intracellular complex of filamentous proteins interacting chemically to shorten the total complex. In general, complexes exhibiting quick, exact time-frames of contraction and relaxation are precisely ordered in structure.

Contractile Elements

All types of myofibers possess macromolecular filaments, called *myofilaments,* which pack their sarcoplasm (Figs. 5–6, 5–8, 5–9, and 5–10). The proteins constituting these myofilaments are primarily *actin* or *myosin.* In addition, they contain other proteins involved either in binding the primary filaments together (e.g., actinins, M-line proteins) or in regulating the actin and myosin interaction (e.g., tropomyosin, troponin). Purified actin and

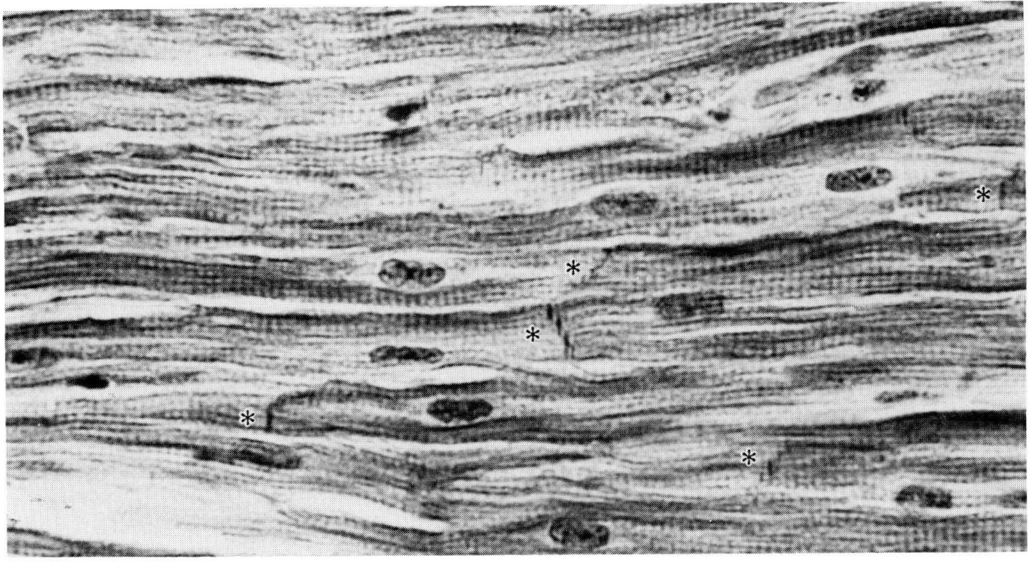

Fig. 5–7. *Cardiac myofibers in longitudinal section. Notice the transverse striations and branching of the myofibers, the central location of their nuclei, and the dark-stained transverse portions of the intercalated disks (*). ×690.*

myosin can be induced to form filaments similar to native myofilaments, and in the presence of ATP and calcium ions, complexes of the two interact and shorten. While structural and functional correlates to this model are present in all myofibers, there exists a spectrum of modifications to the basic design.

STRIATED MUSCLE

The greatest orderliness of myofilaments is found in the striated skeletal and cardiac myofibers, especially the former. The pattern of transverse striations or bands results from the orderly, alternating rectilinear arrays of two types of myofilaments: thick myofilaments, composed principally of myosin, 15nm in diameter; and thin myofilaments, composed principally of actin, 6nm in diameter (Fig. 5–8). The visibly dark (electron-dense) bands contain the thick myofilaments, while the visibly light (electron-lucent) bands contain the thin myofilaments (Figs. 5–8, 5–10, 5–11, 5–12, and 5–13).

Early histologists found that different planes of polarized light were refracted equally (isotropic) when passed through the light band regions, while planes of polarized light were refracted unequally (anisotropic) when passed through the dark band regions. Hence, the light and dark bands were named the isotropic and anisotropic bands, respectively, or merely referred to as the I-bands and A-bands. In the middle of the I-band, these histologists observed a dark line, which they called the Z-line or Z-disk (Fig. 5–8) from the German "Zwischenscheiben" (between disks). When Bowman severed myofibers in the 1860s, the fibrous sarcoplasm splayed out like a brush at the cut ends, demonstrating that the transverse banding pattern was confined to the resolvable intrafiber strands, called myofibrils. With the resolution afforded by electron microscopy, it has been established that the thick and thin myofilaments, collected together, comprise the myofibrils, with the granular sarcoplasm interposed between myofibrils (Figs. 5–9, 5–10 and 5–12).

SARCOMERES. The sarcomere is the interval between two adjacent Z-lines and contains one A-band and one half of two I-bands (Fig. 5–8). The A-band consists of

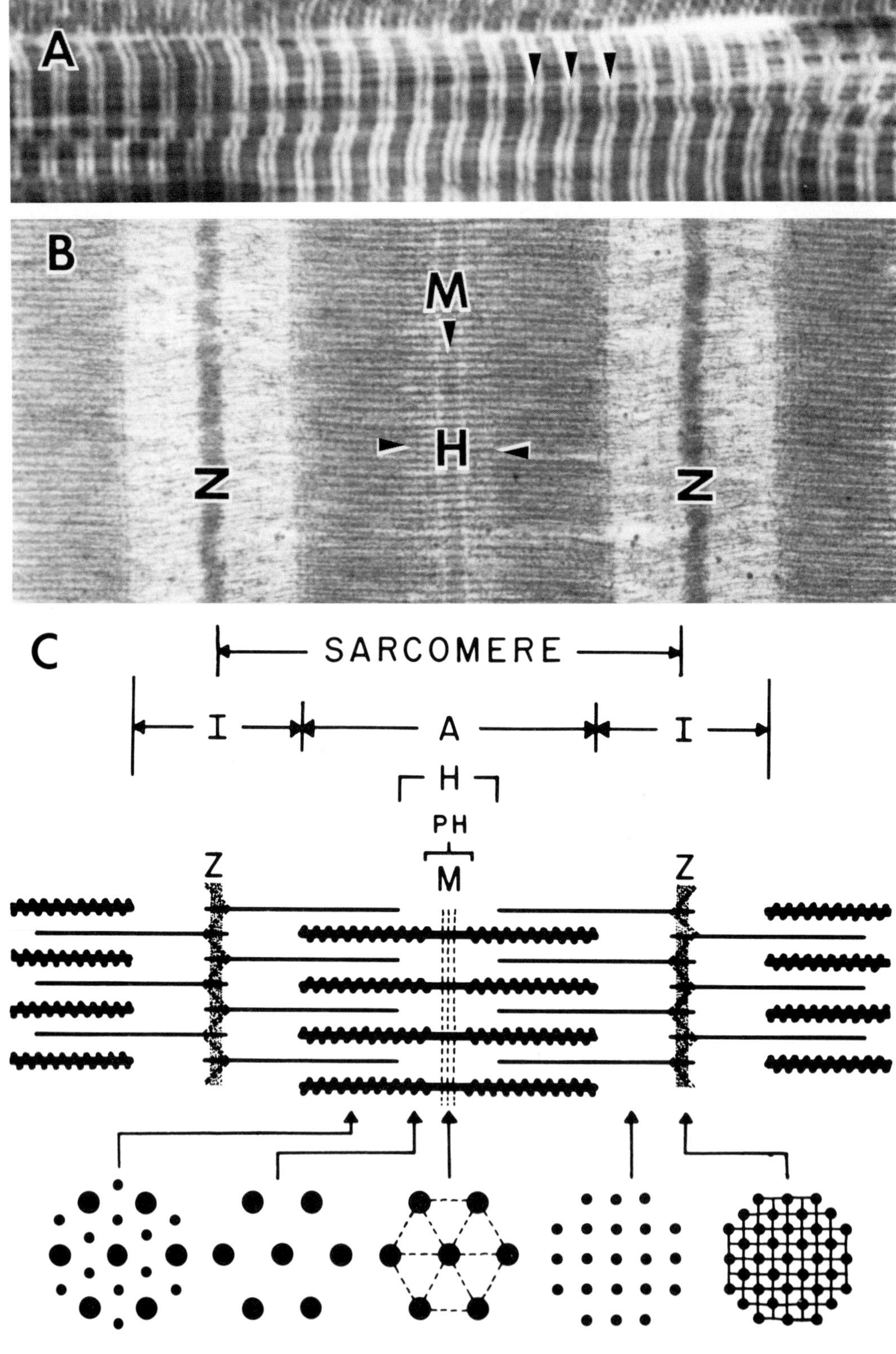

(Legend on Facing Page)

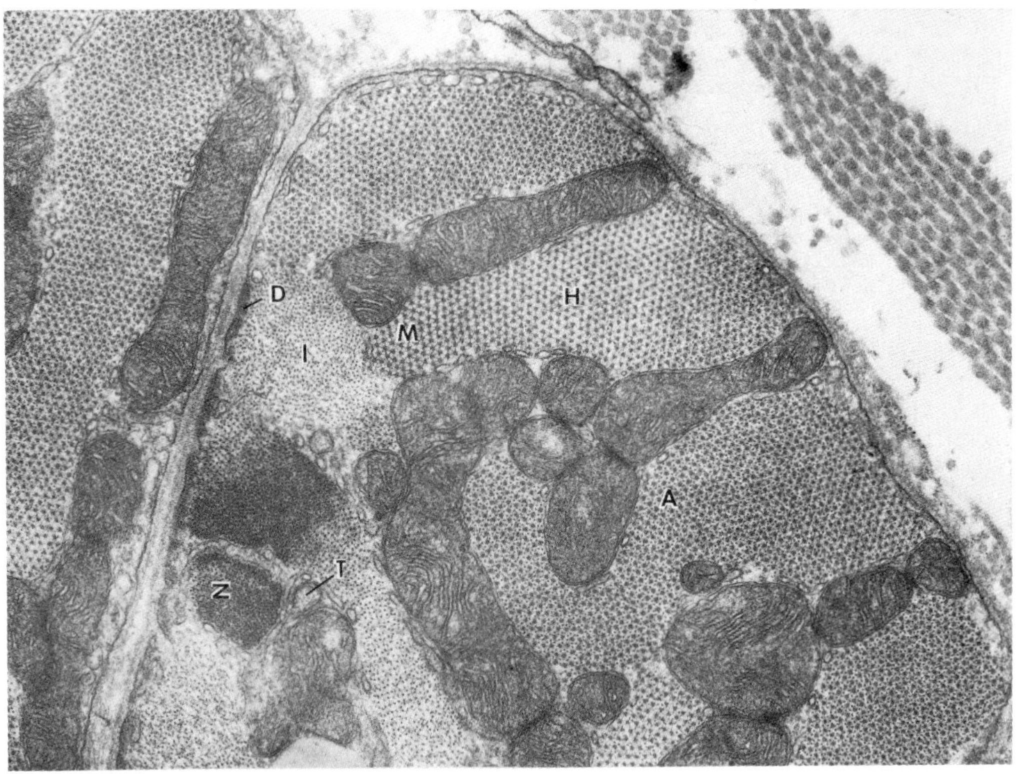

Fig. 5–9. *Electron micrograph of a cross section of adjacent cardiac myofibers. Myofibrils incompletely defined. Section cuts through different bands in different regions: (Z) Z-line; (I) I-band; (A) overlapping thick and thin filaments; (M) M-line; (H) H-line. Other structures: (T) T-tubule; (D) hemidesmosome, probably the edge of an intercalated disk.* ×*35,000. (Courtesy of N.P. Westmoreland.)*

parallel arrays of thick myofilaments while the I-band consists of parallel arrays of thin myofilaments that arise from the Z-line. At their midpoint, each thick myofilament is attached to six adjacent thin myofilaments, aligned in an hexagonal array, by three to five M-line filaments (Fig. 5–8). The name "M-line" is derived from the German "Mittel" (intermediate, or middle). The free ends of thin myofilaments project away from the Z-line and interdigitate between the thick myofilaments for varying distances. Hence, the peripheral regions of each A-band are slightly more electron-dense than the central region because both thick and thin myofilaments overlap,

---

Fig. 5–8. *Light microscopic (image A) and electron microscopic (image B) micrographs of longitudinally oriented sections of striated myofibers, and a schematic representation (figure C) of longitudinal and transverse sections of a single sarcomere. In A, transverse striations consisting of alternating light bands (I-bands) and dark bands (A-bands) can be resolved. Each I-band is bisected by a Z-line (arrowheads);* ×*1150. In B are shown transverse striations consisting of one sarcomere, the interval between two adjacent Z-lines (Z). Each Z-line bisects the electron-lucid I-band composed of thin myofilaments. The A-band is electron-dense and is bisected by the M-line (M-arrowhead), which is composed by M-line filaments connecting adjacent thick myofilaments. On either side of the M-line, notice the fine electron-lucid region where the thick myofilaments are devoid of cross-bridges. The H-band (H-arrowheads) is that portion of the A-band region where there is no overlap of thick and thin myofilaments* ×*22,500. Image C further explains the arrangement of the myofilaments described above. The bottom row represents cross sections through the various portions of the sarcomere, as indicated by the arrows. Large dots represent myosin myofilaments, and small dots represent actin myofilaments.*

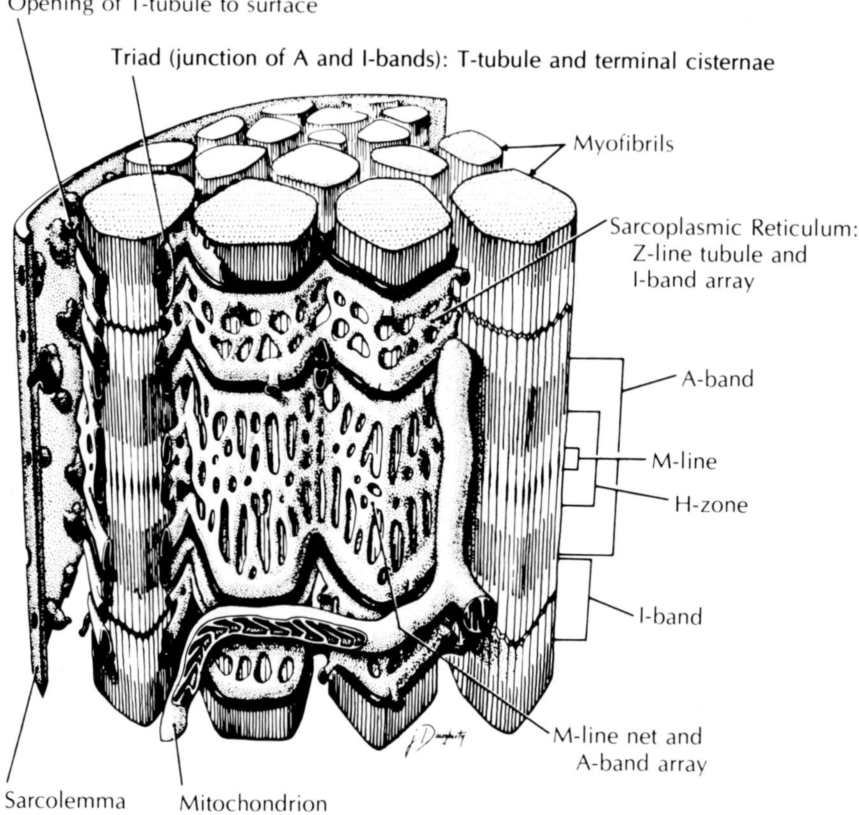

Fig. 5–10. *Diagrammatic illustration of myofibrils, sarcoplasmic reticulum, T-tubules, and sarcolemma of a skeletal muscle fiber.*

whereas in the central region there are only overlapping arrays of thick myofilaments (Fig. 5–8). This central region of the A-band that contains the M-line and only the thick myofilaments is called the H-band. The name H-band is derived from the German "Helles Band" (clear). Within the H-band, on either side of the M-line, there is a thin, electron-lucent region called the pseudo–H-zone. In this central zone, each thick myofilament is devoid of the myosin cross-bridges that project from each thick myofilament for attachment to the six adjacent thin myofilaments. (Fig. 5–8).

In 1957, Hugh Huxley demonstrated that sarcomeres shorten during contraction by the movement of the thin myofilaments into the array of thick myofilaments, and he postulated the "sliding filament model" for muscular contraction. When myofibers are stretched, the sarcomeres (Z-line intervals) lengthen, accompanied by a lengthening of the I-bands. When myofibers are stimulated to contract, the sarcomeres shorten, accompanied by shortening of the I-bands. With both stretching and contracting, the A-bands maintain a constant length; however, within the A-bands the length of the H-band lengthens or shortens in concert with the lengthening or shortening of the I-band and sarcomere, respectively.

BIOCHEMICAL BASIS OF CONTRACTION. An actin filament is a polymer of globular actin (G-actin) forming a double helix (F-actin). In mammalian skeletal muscle, the grooves of the helix contain linear strings

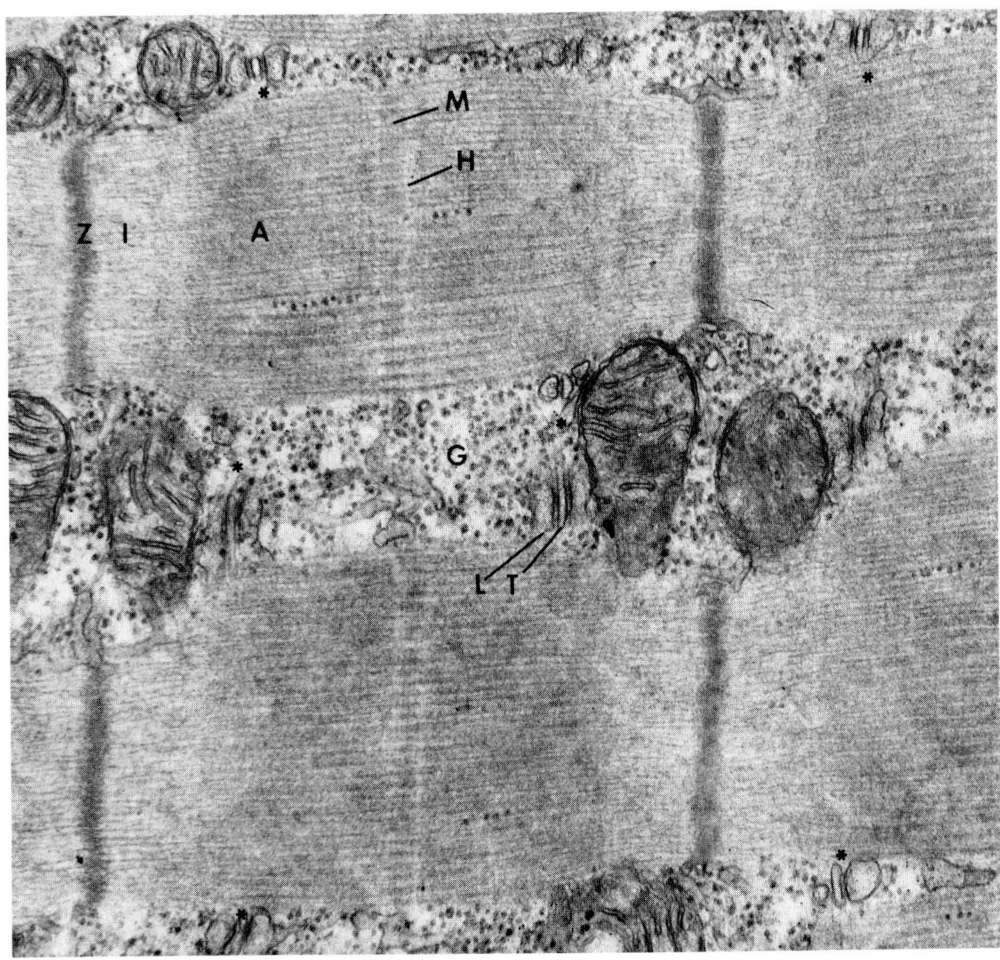

Fig. 5–11. *Electron micrograph of a longitudinal section through a skeletal myofiber. Structures identified include: A-band (A); Z-line (Z); glycogen (G) within the intermyofibrillar spaces accompanied by mitochondria; pseudo–H-band (H); I-band (I); terminal cisternae of sarcotubules (L); M-line (M); T-tubule (T); and triads (*) located within the intermyofibrillar spaces adjacent to the junctions of the A-bands with the I-bands. ×34,000.*

of tropomyosin molecules, which block sites for interaction with myosin molecules. Spaced along the *tropomyosin* and attached to the actin are molecules of *troponin,* which prove to be the trigger molecules that allow actin-myosin interaction and contraction. When calcium ion concentrations exceed 10^{-5} M, troponin undergoes a conformational change that shifts tropomyosin's position enough to expose actin's reactive sites to myosin.

Myosin is a double-headed linear molecule that aggregates under optimal conditions into thick filaments. The tails are oriented toward the M-line and heads are peripheral to the pseudo–H-zone. The thick filaments taper to points at the two ends. The heads are enzymatically active as an ATPase; they can be isolated from the tails as heavy meromyosin, called *H-meromyosin,* as opposed to the light meromyosin in the tails, or *L-meromyosin.* When ATP attaches, the head straightens, pointing toward the thick filaments' tip and cocked like the hammer of a gun, the energy deriving from hydrolysis of the ATP. The hydrolysis products remain attached, requiring the interaction of myosin with actin

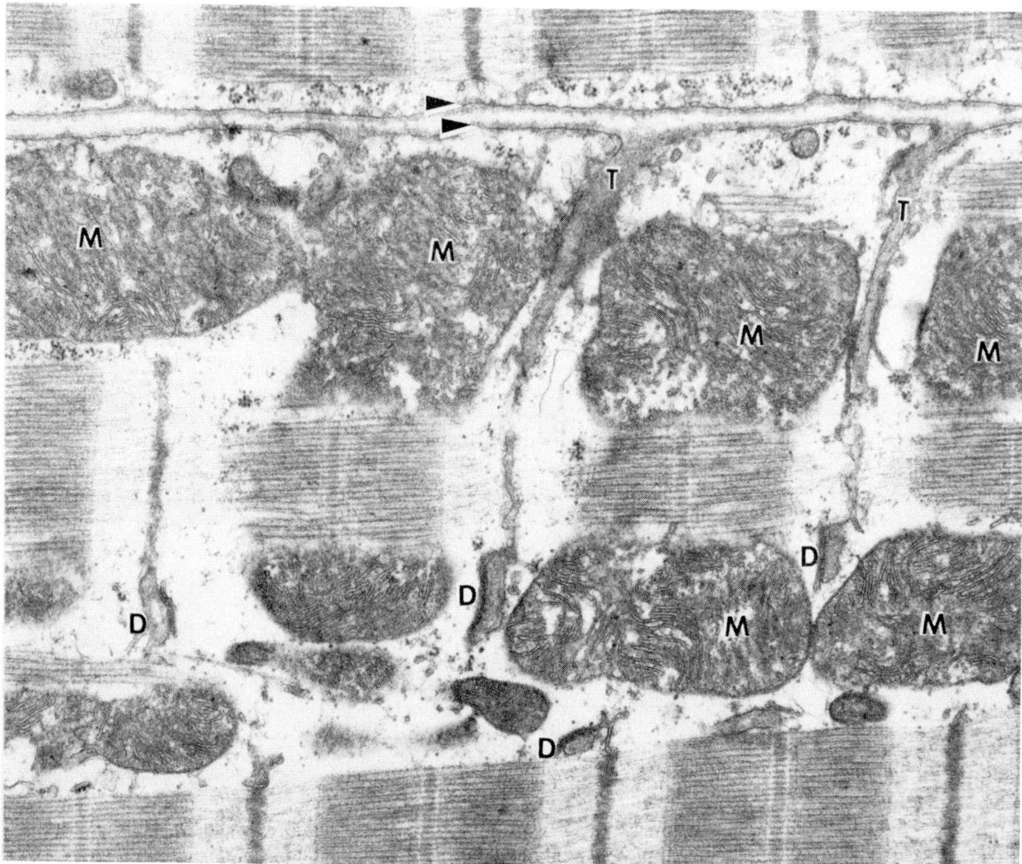

Fig. 5–12. *Electron micrograph of a longitudinal section through portions of two cardiac myofibers. The sarcolemma and basal lamina of each myofiber is identified with arrowheads. Large mitochondria (M) with densely packed cristae are located just under the sarcolemma and within the intermyofibrillar space. Notice the two large T-tubules (T) entering the lower myofiber at the level of its Z-lines and the presence of diads (D) in the intermyofibrillar space at the same level. ×22,500. (Courtesy of W.S. Tyler.)*

before the head can jerk back to its more stable state. When reactive actin sites are exposed by release of Ca^{++} from the sarcoplasmic reticulum, the myosin head attaches to actin and swivels so that the actin filament is pulled toward the M-line. The hydrolysis products are then quickly released, and if ATP is still present in the medium, the myosin head binds a new molecule at ATP and the actin-myosin interaction is broken. The myosin head then becomes reoriented, ATP is hydrolyzed, and if Ca^{++} is present the cycle is repeated. If ATP is not present, the actin-myosin interaction remains stable (rigor). If actin sites are not exposed, the myosin head sits cocked and ready to participate in contraction, but the actin and myosin filaments are unable to slide past one another.

SMOOTH MUSCLE

The contractile apparatus in *smooth myofibers* seems quite different from that of skeletal and cardiac myofibers (Fig. 5–6). There are no cross-striations. Parallel thin filaments are abundant, but thick filaments are rare and usually absent. Scattered filaments of intermediate diameter are common. In all likelihood the thin filaments are actin, since they stream in opposite directions from so-called *fusiform densities* when

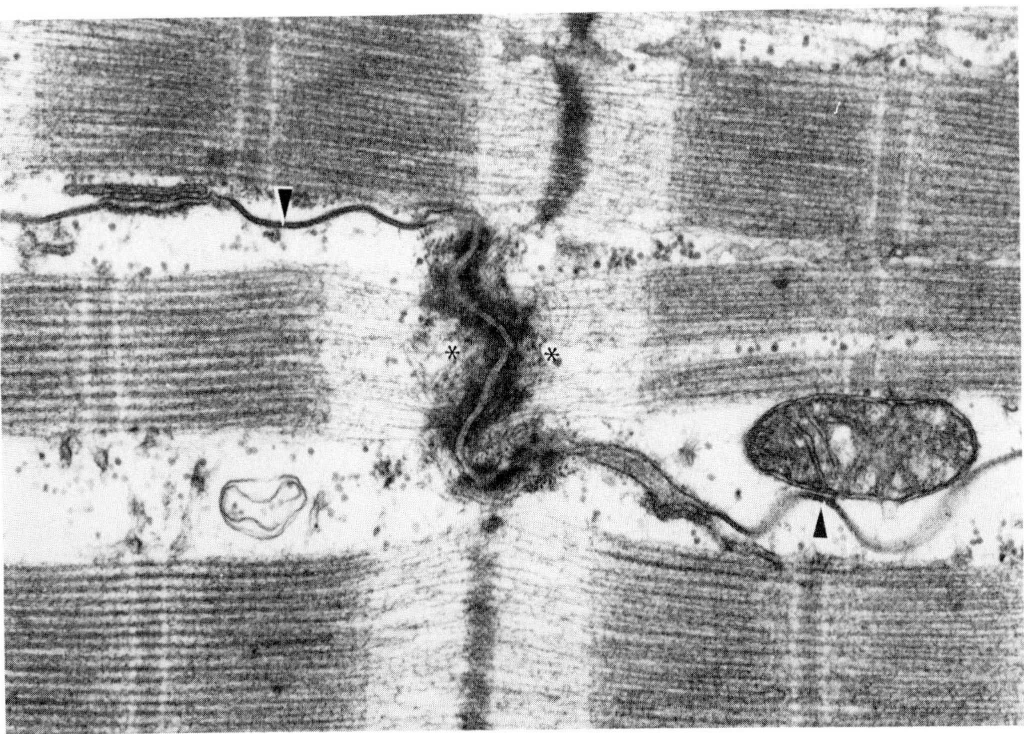

Fig. 5–13. *Longitudinal section through a small portion of an intercalated disk connecting two adjacent cardiac myofibers. Notice the termination of the myofibrils at the fascia adherens junction (*) oriented transversely to the long axis of the myofibrils and to the vectors of force developed during contraction. The terminal sarcomeres end with the insertion of the thin myofilaments into the adherens junction. Located on either side of the fascia adherens junction are two gap junctions (arrowheads) oriented parallel to the long axis of the myofibrils. ×42,100. (Courtesy of W.S. Tyler.)*

"decorated" by purified H-meromyosin. This is analogous to the way actin filaments stream away from Z-lines in striated myofibers. Myosin can be isolated from smooth muscle but at only half the actin-myosin ratio of skeletal muscle; it differs also in activity from skeletal muscle myosin. Some smooth muscle lacks tropomyosin and troponin; thus, while actin-myosin interaction seems to be involved in contraction along with ATP and calcium ions, the mechanisms triggering this interaction must differ and apparently vary in different types of smooth muscles.

The contractile mass is not subdivided in smooth muscle. The thin filament array is actually helical, arising from hemidesmosomes at one end of the cell and spiraling around the nucleus to hemidesmosomes at the other end. The helical mass twists as it shortens, throwing the central nucleus into a spiral. This drawn-out helical organization gives the cell greater potential for shortening than is possible in skeletal muscle. Sarcomeres in the latter can only decrease their length 30%, but mooth muscle cells can shorten to nearly one tenth their resting length and can stretch to a similar degree. This property is uniquely suited to the function of visceral organs such as the urinary bladder and uterus, which must dramatically and forcefully change their dimensions. Contraction and relaxation of smooth muscle may require seconds, minutes, and even hours. They develop constant, increasing, or decreasing tone rather than twitches.

Smooth myofibers actually represent a spectrum of functional types. In the smooth muscle of nictitating membrane, pilomotor muscle bundles, the ciliary body and iris of the eye, and blood vessels, the muscle fibers are less tightly attached one to the other than those in abdominal viscera and have no direct cell-to-cell contacts. In these specialized areas, each fiber has a nerve termination that initiates the contractile process, much like the situation in skeletal muscle. No spontaneous wavelike contractions are demonstrable in these smooth muscles when they are separated from their neural attachments, unless they are bathed in certain pharmacologic agents resembling their normal activating neurotransmitters. Such muscles are called the "multiunit type" in contrast to the "unitary type" in visceral organs, where spontaneous contractility is the rule, independent of neural control. In the unitary type, nerve fibers do not terminate on or even near each muscle fiber. In viscera, the entire muscle bundle acts as a unit. There are direct contacts (gap junctions) between individual muscle fibers within a bundle, and electric resistance between them is low, indicating that electric phenomena associated with the outer membrane of one cell can spread relatively easily to a neighboring cell membrane.

Sarcoplasmic Reticulum and Transverse Tubular System

The myofibrils and their constituent myofilaments comprise the major portion of the sarcoplasm; however, there is also an extensive nonfilamentous sarcoplasm present within the intermyofibrillar spaces, consisting of the membranous tubules of the sarcoplasmic reticulum and the transverse tubular system, mitochondria, and inclusions such as glycogen granules and lipid droplets (Figs. 5–9, 5–10, 5–11 and 5–12). These elements of the nonfilamentous sarcoplasm function in the control and metabolism of the contractile processes carried out by the filamentous sarcoplasm.

In mammals, the sarcoplasmic reticulum of skeletal myofibers consists of two sets of longitudinally oriented sarcotubules that surround each myofibril. One set surrounds each myofibril at the level of the A-band, and at the center of the sarcomere these sarcotubules anastomose to form a network in the M-line region (Fig. 5–10). At the junction of the A- and I-bands within each sarcomere (A-I junctions), these longitudinal sarcotubules become expanded and anastomose to form a terminal cisterna at each A-I junction (Fig. 5–10). The second set of sarcotubules extends between the A-Is junctions of adjacent sarcomeres and surrounds the myofibrils at the level of the I-band. These sarcotubules also form a terminal cisterna at each junction (Fig. 5–10). Hence, at each A-I junction there is a pair of terminal cisternae.

In addition to the sarcoplasmic reticulum, there is a second tubular membrane system, the transverse tubular system (T-system). The T-system is composed of multiple, slender tubular invaginations of the sarcolemma (T-tubules) that pass into the depths of each myofiber at a plane transverse to its long axis. The lumina of the T-tubules are directly continuous with the extracellular space and tissue fluid, and within the depths of each myofiber they freely anastomose with other T-tubules. The T-tubules arise at the level of each A-I junction to pass between, and come into close contact with, the paired terminal cisternae at the A-I junctions (Fig. 5–10). Each T-tubule, flanked by the paired terminal cisternae of adjacent sarcomeres, forms a "triad," i.e., terminal cisternae located on each side of a centered T-tubule (Figs. 5–10 and 5–11). The junctional complex located between the membrane of the T-tubule and the membrane of each terminal cisterna appears to be a low resistance junction similar to a gap junction.

The arrangement of the sarcoplasmic reticulum and T-system in cardiac myofibers differs from that in skeletal myofibers in several important respects. First, the sarcoplasmic reticulum consists of only tubules that do not form terminal cisternae.

Instead, the tubules make individual point contacts with T-tubules, thus forming "diads" (Fig. 5–12) rather than triads. Also, the T-tubules are much larger in diameter than those in skeletal myofibers, and they arise at the level of Z-disks rather than A-I junctions (Fig. 5–12).

Smooth muscle cells lack T-tubules. The sarcoplasmic reticulum is sparse and unorganized and does not subdivide the myofilamentous field. Nonetheless, ends of the sarcoplasmic reticulum do couple with the sarcolemma, and the release of calcium ions by the reticulum after excitation of the cell surface seems to play a major role in triggering contraction.

Both the extracellular space and the sarcoplasmic reticulum contain relatively high concentrations of calcium ions. These are released into the myofilamentous compartment when the sarcolemma is depolarized and diffuse less than 1 μm before triggering the adjacent myofibrils into contraction. Likewise, both the sarcolemma and the sarcoplasmic reticulum contain ATPase-linked transport elements that rapidly pump calcium ions out of the myofilamentous compartment, inducing relaxation. Thus, the finer the network of sarcoplasmic reticulum, the narrower the myofibrils and the faster the contraction-relaxation cycle.

Although 90% of the integral proteins in sarcoplasmic reticular membranes are parts of the "calcium pump," glucose-6-phosphatase and other enzymes associated with glycogen metabolism are also present. Beta-type glycogen granules are in structural and metabolic association with the sarcoplasmic reticulum.

Other Cellular Organelles

Mitochondria appear in all myofibers, but their concentration is variable. There is an inverse relationship between body weight and mitochondrial concentration, correlated with basal metabolic rates. Few mitochondria are present in beef skeletal myofibers, whereas all myofibers of mice are richly endowed (Fig. 5–4). Small animals have more difficulty maintaining body temperature, and muscle mitochondria are a primary source of ATP, from which heat is released during the contraction process. Mitochondria congregate in higher concentration around nuclei, along the sarcolemma, and around motor endplates.

Ribosomes are scattered around nuclei and myofibrils. Protein synthesis is continuous even in adult animals, myofilaments being formed at the margins of myofibrils. Although myofilament degradation also occurs continuously, the sites are not obvious. Apparently the myofilamentous field is continuously resculptured. Muscles atrophy and hypertrophy under various nutritional and working conditions; these processes are reflected solely by increased or decreased diameters of a constant number of muscle fibers. Any change in diameter is accounted for by decreased or increased contractile mass with the same general morphology. However, rapid atrophy is characterized by separated myofibrils, splaying of myofilaments from them, and the accumulation of granular sarcoplasm.

A Golgi complex and centrioles are consistently found around the nucleus in smooth myofibers. They are rarely seen in other muscle types except during myogenesis.

Surfaces of Myofibers and the Sarcoskeleton

The sarcolemma of cardiac, skeletal, and smooth myofibers is reinforced externally by a glycoprotein coat called the basal or external lamina and by reticular fibers (Figs. 5–6, 5–9, and 5–12). Internally, the underlying contractile, filamentous sarcoplasm is harnessed to itself and to the sarcolemma by an extensive sarcoskeletal network of intermediate (10 nm) filaments composed of several different proteins.

In cardiac and skeletal myofibers, intermediate filaments form the sarcoskeleton, a network of transverse and longitudinal filamentous bridges extending within and between the myofibrils. In both skeletal and cardiac myofibers, transverse intermediate filaments containing desmin connect adjacent myofibrils at the level of each Z-line. Other intermediate filaments containing the protein vinculin serve as sarcoskeletal-to-sarcolemmal connections along the length of the myofibers by attaching the peripheral myofibrils to the sarcolemma at the level of each I-band. Vinculin along with a-actinin (a Z-line protein) also serves as a connecting intermediate filament at the myotendinous junctions of skeletal myofibers and at the fascia adherens junctions of intercalated disks in cardiac myofibers (Fig. 5–13) where the thin (actin) myofilaments of the terminal sarcomeres insert into the sarcolemma. Collectively, these internal intermediate filaments provide for the serial and parallel forces developed by the contractile myofilaments to be transmitted to the adjacent connective tissues or other myofibers to which they are attached.

The situation is similar in smooth myofibers. The contractile forces are transmitted to the sarcolemma by intermediate filaments that connect thin actin myofilaments to electron-dense bodies (Z-line equivalent) on the inner side of the sarcolemmal hemidesmosomes, and then to the intercellular reticuloelastic net via the basal lamina surrounding each smooth myofiber (Fig. 5–6).

The mechanical energy of contraction developed by one cardiac myofiber is transmitted to adjacent cardiac myofibers by specialized cell-to-cell attachments called *intercalated disks* (Figs. 5–7 and 5–13). Each intercalated disk is located between two adjacent cardiac myofibers and is composed of multiple junctions consisting of two principal morphologic and functional types: 1) fascia adherens junctions, oriented transversely to the long axes of attached cardiac myofibers, and 2) gap junctions, oriented parallel to the long axes of attached myofibers (Fig. 5–13). The fascia adherens junctions transmit contractile forces from cardiac myofiber to myofiber, whereas gap junctions are low resistance junctions that permit the propagation of depolarization from cardiac myofiber to myofiber.

Gap junctions also occur between most smooth myofibers, facilitating from myofiber to myofiber the spread of membrane depolarization and their subsequent contraction. Skeletal myofibers have no direct contacts with each other. The electrical resistance between skeletal myofibers is high; thus, the excitation of the sarcolemma in one skeletal myofiber does not initiate excitation in adjacent skeletal myofibers.

The sarcolemma of myofibers is found in a variety of forms, indicative of its dynamic nature. The sarcolemma of all myofibers often has vesicles or caveolae (Figs. 5–6 and 5–9). The invaginations may be simple or bizarre, with branching, tubular networks or cloverleaf arrangements. At other times, the sarcolemma appears as an undeviating straight line without invaginations. The simple vesicles represent endo- and exocytotic vesicles, whereas the complex structures appear to be related to the T-tubules, which open into the extracellular space.

Skeletal Muscle Motor Units

Skeletal myofibers are organized into a functional and structural motor unit consisting of a single motoneuron and a variable number of myofibers (10 to 1000 or more) innervated by that single motoneuron. The motoneuron cell bodies are located in the central nervous system (the ventral horns of the spinal cord or the motor nuclei of the brainstem), and their axons pass through a named nerve to enter a given muscle. Upon entering the muscle the axons divide numerous times, with each axon terminal forming a contact (myoneural junction) (see Chapter 6) with one myofiber.

Functionally, three types of motor units have been defined in the cat and are presumed to be present in most other mammals as well. They are: 1) slow-twitch, fatigue-resistant motor units, 2) fast-twitch, fatigue-resistant motor units, and 3) fast-twitch, fatigable motor units. Each of these motor unit types is uniformly composed of a different type of myofiber, which may be identified in sections of skeletal muscles by employing enzyme histochemical methods. The fast-twitch motor unit myofibers have a high myosin adenosine triphosphatase (ATPase) activity when incubated at pH 9.8 and stain dark, while the slow-twitch motor unit myofibers have a lower activity and stain light (Fig. 5–14A). The fatigue-resistant motor unit myofibers derive energy (ATP) for contraction principally from aerobic metabolism of fatty acids and glucose; hence, they have numerous mitochondria and stain dark for succinic dehydrogenase activity (Fig. 5–14D). The fatigable motor unit myofibers have fewer mitochondria and stain light (Fig. 5–14D). The fatigable motor unit myofibers derive ATP for contraction principally from anaerobic glycogenolysis and glycolysis; hence, these myofibers are rich in glycogen and enzymes required for its metabolism. Based on the acid stability or lability of the ATPase reaction, following preincubation of sections in acid media at pH 4.5 and pH 4.3, the fast-twitch fibers may be further subdivided and classified (Figs. 5–14B and 5–14C). A wide variety of classifications have been developed, summarized in Table 5–1. In histologic sections, the classification of myofibers as type 1, type 2A, type 2B, or type 2C is preferred and is used widely in the pathology literature.

Within a whole muscle, individual myofibers from the same motor unit are distributed diffusely. Studies in the cat reveal that only one or two myofibers within a given fascicle normally belong to the same motor unit. Except for the dog, most mammals have muscles composed of type 1, type 2A, type 2B, and/or type 2C myofibers. To date, type 2B myofibers have not been identified in the dog. Also, in mammals most muscles of the body contain a mixture of myofiber types; however, the composition of myofiber types within a given muscle may vary greatly among individuals of the same breed or species, as well as between different species. The muscles of breeds of dogs and horses that have been bred and selected for speed (e.g., the Greyhound and Quarterhorse, respectively) contain more type 2 myofibers (presumed fast-twitch) than the muscles of breeds bred and selected for endurance (e.g., the German Shepherd dog and Arabian horse.)

In the dog and cat, the muscles of mastication and other muscles innervated by the mandibular nerve have a unique type 2 myofiber. In those species, these muscles contain type 2 myofibers that have the histochemical staining pattern of type 2C myofibers; however, they contain a myosin uniquely different from differentiating type 2C myofibers and other type 2 myofibers in limb muscles.

In addition to the histochemical variations, slow-twitch myofibers have wider Z-lines and more M-line filaments than fast-twitch myofibers.

HISTOGENESIS

Cardiac Muscle

All muscle tissue except that in the head arises from mesoderm. Cardiac muscle, one of the earliest forms to differentiate, is a direct modification of the epithelial mesodermal layer of the splanchnopleure. The cells modify their desmosomal-like attachments into intercalated disks, elongate, and form their myofilaments as the heart wall takes shape. They retain the ability to divide both nucleus and cytoplasm, even as the myogenic processes of the cytoplasm are under way. The sources of endothelial cells and fibroblasts of cardiac muscle tissue

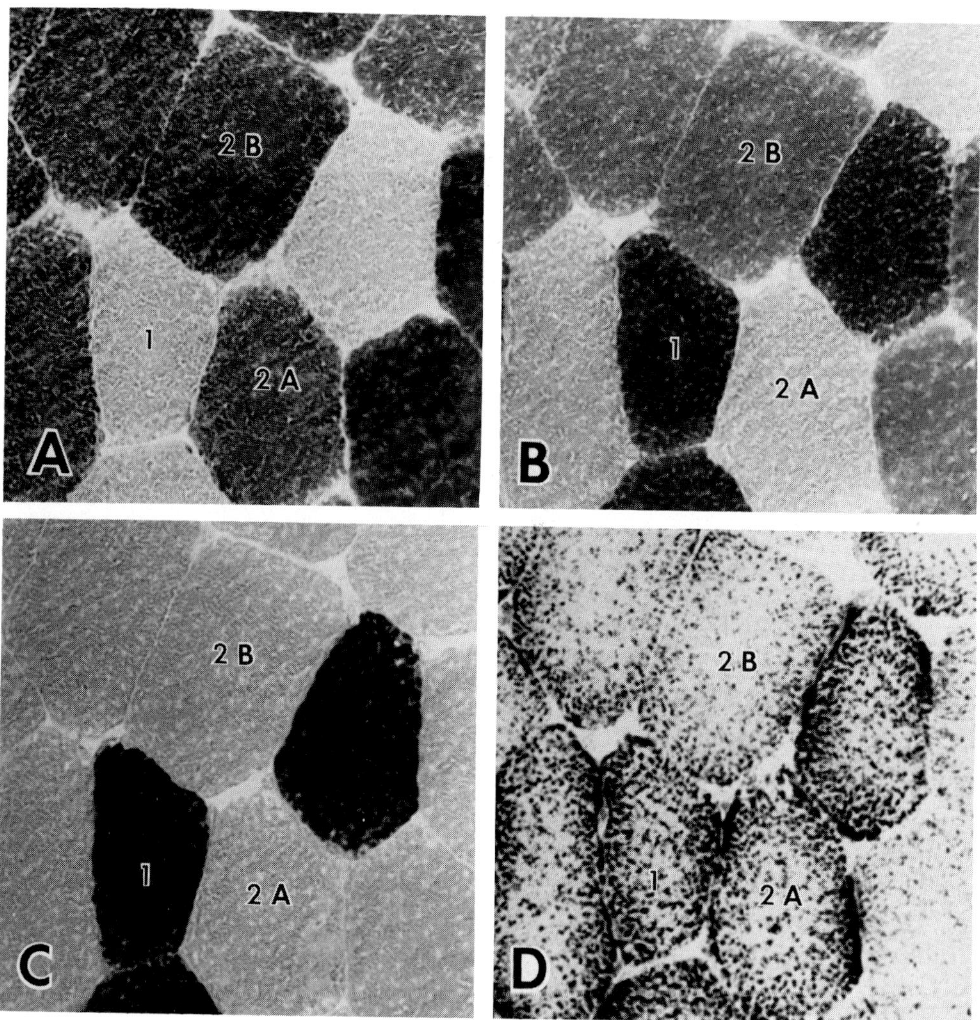

Fig. 5–14. *Serial cross sections of superficial gluteal muscle myofibers in a horse. Sections were stained for myosin ATPase activity at pH 9.8 without preincubation (A), and following preincubation in acid media at pH 4.5 (B) and pH 4.3 (C). Section D was stained for succinic dehydrogenase. Type 1 myofibers (presumed slow-twitch) have lower myosin ATPase activities than type 2 myofibers (presumed fast-twitch) and stain lighter than the type 2 myofibers (A). Following acid preincubation there is a reversal in this staining pattern: type 1 myofibers stain dark while type 2A myofibers stain light after preincubation at both pH 4.5 and pH 4.3 (B, C); type 2B myofibers stain dark after preincubation at pH 4.5 (B) but light after preincubation at pH 4.3 (C). Type 1 and type 2A myofibers are stained dark for succinic dehydrogenase and are presumed to be fatigue resistant, while the lightly stained type 2B myofibers are presumed to be fatigable.* ×450.

are little understood. They probably arise either from the splanchnopleure directly or from the splanchnopleure-derived mesenchyme.

For the most part, the power of cardiac muscle to divide is lost sometime during the early growth period. Enlargement of the heart wall during cardiac insufficiencies from whatever cause is primarily *hypertrophy*, an enlargement of existing cardiac myofibers, rather than *hyperplasia*, an increase in cell number. Damage to a section of the heart wall, with the resultant death of that section, is repaired primarily by proliferation of connective tissue rather than by regeneration of any significant number of new cardiac myofibers. However, the potential for cellular proliferation

Table 5–1.
Physiologic and Histochemical Properties of Motor Unit Myofiber Types

	Histochemical Myofiber Type			
	Type 1	*Type 2A*	*Type 2B*	*Type 2C*
Physiologic Properties				
Twitch contraction	slow	fast	fast	unknown
Fatigability	resistant	resistant	fatigable	unknown
Histochemical Staining Properties				
Myosin ATPase, pH 9.8	light	dark	dark	dark
Preincubation, pH 4.5	dark	light	dark	dark
Preincubation, pH 4.3	dark	light	light	dark
Succinic Dehydrogenase	dark	dark	light	dark
Other Nomenclature				
	I	II	II	II
	β-red	α-red	α-white	—
	S (slow-twitch—oxidative)	FOG (fast-twitch—oxidative-glycolytic)	FG (fast-twitch—glycolytic)	—

of cardiac muscle is always present, if not always expressed, because cardiac muscle transplanted to tissue culture grows and proliferates.

Smooth Muscle

Smooth muscle tissue repairs itself by scar formation similar to repair of cardiac muscle. Although some proliferation of smooth myofibers occurs, it is usually abortive. However, adult animals retain the ability to convert capillaries into muscular arteries when the normal pathways of distributive blood flow are disrupted, presumably by differentiation of primitive perivascular cells (pericytes) into smooth myofibers (Fig. 5–4).

Skeletal Muscle

Histogenesis of skeletal muscle differs from that of the other types of muscle. Studies of young embryos indicate that the earliest skeletal muscle myoblasts arise from a specific region of each mesodermal somite, the *myotome.* From here the cells detach from the epithelial mass and migrate to the locus of the future muscle. Local mesenchyme can differentiate into myoblasts; this is particularly true for the limbs. Because the head lacks somites, the skeletal muscles of this region appear to arise from neuroectoderm or from the mesenchyme migrating into the area.

The first recognition of presumptive skeletal muscle cells is the elongation of the mononuclear myoblasts, their subsequent fusion, and the formation of contractile filaments just beneath the sarcolemma. This results in the formation of a *myotube,* a long cylinder with the myofilaments packed at the periphery under the sarcolemma and a comparatively clear central area containing myonuclei and granular sarcoplasm.

The formation of myotubes occurs in two stages. Initially, a primary generation of myotubes forms, consisting of single myotubes scattered throughout the mesenchymal region that is destined to become a whole muscle. Subsequently, additional myoblasts become aligned along the primary myotubes and fuse to form a secondary generation of myotubes. As a result, the primary myotubes are surrounded by the secondary myotubes to collectively form a muscle bundle, or fascicle. Initially, all myotubes are type 2C; however, innervation of the myotubes initiates their differentiation into either type 1, type 2A, or type 2B myofibers. Differentiation of the primary myotubes occurs first, each be-

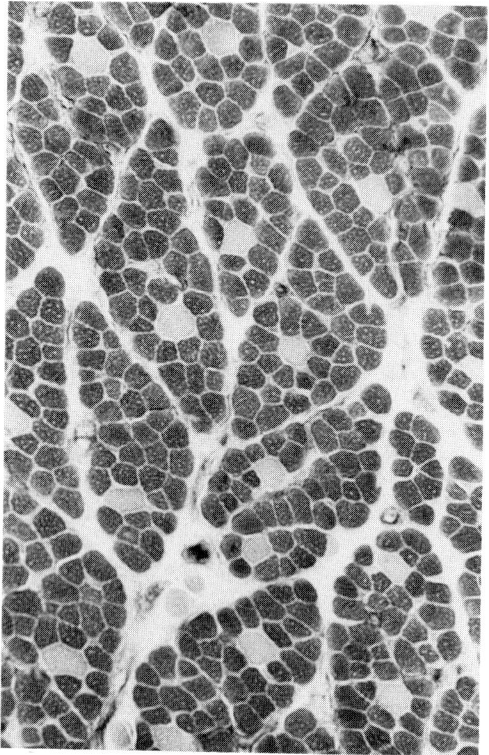

Fig. 5–15. *Transverse section of skeletal myofibers from a day-old dog stained for myosin adenosine triphosphatase (pH 9.8). Notice that each muscle bundle is composed of a single, light-staining type 1 myofiber surrounded by a variable number of dark-staining type 2C myofibers. The type 1 myofibers were derived from primary myotubes, while the type 2C myofibers were derived from secondary myotubes and are not yet differentiated.* ×*360.*

coming a type 1 myofiber (Fig. 5–15), followed by differentiation of the secondary myotubes, which may become type 1, type 2A, or type 2B myofibers. In the dog, differentiation of the primary myotubes occurs by the time of birth, while differentiation of the secondary myotubes does not occur until after 12 to 14 days of age.

The formation of myofibers from myotubes consists of enlargement of the myotubes accompanied by filling of the central region with myofilaments, the migration of the myonuclei from the central regions to a subsarcolemmal position, and the addition of new myonuclei by fusion with myoblasts in the endomysium. Early in the postnatal life of mammals, the total number of myofibers in any one gross muscle becomes established and remains relatively constant thereafter.

Myosatellite cells, whose progeny fuses into the sarcoplasmic mass to form new muscle nuclei, are known to be proliferative in young rats and mice (Fig. 5–4). The fusion process wanes with age, but the number of muscle nuclei in mammals increases slowly throughout life. In many myopathies, myosatellite-like cells proliferate and are apparently myoblastic.

Damaged skeletal muscle fibers can regenerate at any stage in life, but like other muscle tissues, most repair of gross damage is in the form of connective tissue. Degenerating muscle cells have a disrupted sarcoplasm with destruction of the contractile elements. Mononuclear cells proliferate in the damaged area, mostly within the intact sarcolemma. The majority of the cells is derived locally. Some phagocytize the cellular debris and others develop intracytoplasmic filaments, indicative of beginning myoblastic activity. Through fusion, these myoblasts reestablish the continuity of the contractile field.

REFERENCES

Burke, R.E., Levine, D.N., Tsairis, P., and Zajac, F.E.: Physiological types and histochemical profiles in motor units of the cat gastrocnemius. J Physiol *234*:723, 1973.

Cardinet, III, G.H., Leong, C.L., and Means, P.S.: Myofiber differentiation in normal and hypotrophied canine pectineal muscles. Muscle Nerve *5*:665, 1982.

Cardinet, III, G.H., and Orvis, J.A.: Skeletal muscle function. *In* Clinical Biochemistry of Domestic Animals. Edited by J. Kaneko. New York, Academic Press, 1980.

Ebashi, S.: Excitation-contraction coupling. Ann Rev Physiol *36*:293, 1976.

Huxley, H.E.: Electron microscopic studies of the structure of natural and synthetic protein filaments from striated muscle. J Mol Biol 7:281, 1963.

Huxley, H.E.: The structural basis of contraction and regulation in skeletal muscle. *In* Molecular Basis of Motility. Edited by L. Heilmeyer, et al. New York, Springer-Verlag, 1976.

Pardo, J.V., D'Angelo Siliciano, J., and Craig, S.W.: A vinculin-containing cortical lattice in skeletal muscle: transverse lattice elements ("costameres") mark sites of attachment between myofibrils and sarcolemma. Proc Natl Acad Sci USA *80*:1008, 1983.

Peachey, L.D. (ed.): Handbook of Physiology. Section 10: Skeletal Muscle. Maryland, American Physiological Society, 1983.

Tokuyasu, K.T., Dutton, A.H., and Singer, S.J.: Immunoelectron microscopic studies of desmin (skeletin) localization and intermediate filament organization in chicken cardiac muscle. J Cell Biol *96*:1736, 1983.

Wang, K., and Ramirez-Mitchell, R.: A network of transverse and longitudinal intermediate filaments is associated with sarcomeres of adult vertebrate skeletal muscle. J Cell Biol *96*:562, 1983.

6

Nervous System

THOMAS F. FLETCHER

The nervous system provides an animal with sensitivity to environmental energy and thereby awareness of self and surroundings. It initiates and controls movement and most secretions and thus is reponsible for all inborn and learned behavior. Nervous tissue parenchyma consists of neurons and supportive cells, the latter collectively termed neuroglia. Neurons are the structural and functional units of nervous activity; neurons are also trophic units, since they frequently modify and sustain the cells they innervate. Because neurons are incapable of mitosis, they have to last a lifetime. The entire nervous system is a structural and functional cohesive unit; however, it may conceptually be divided into central and peripheral divisions.

The *central nervous system* (CNS) is composed of the brain and spinal cord. Some regions of the CNS appear white while others have a gray appearance. The *white matter* is formed by dense accumulations of nerve fibers individually enveloped by myelin, a white, lipid-protein insulation. *Gray matter* lacks dense accumulations of myelin and is rich in cell perikarya. Gray matter that coats the CNS surface is called cortex, while a gray matter mass within the CNS is generally called a nucleus. In some regions, gray and white matter are intermixed. The entire CNS is enclosed in protective membranes termed meninges.

The *peripheral nervous system* (PNS) consists of spinal and cranial nerves, including associated nerve roots and ganglia. A nerve is a collection of nerve fibers ensheathed or myelinated by neuroglia and divided into one or more fascicles by connective tissue. Ganglia are nerve enlargements produced by the presence of neuronal perikarya. Nerves and ganglia innervating viscera are designated the *autonomic nervous system.*

The nervous system develops from a *neural plate,* thickened ectoderm along the dorsal midline of the embryo (Fig. 6–1). The plate forms a *neural groove* and then a *neural tube* containing a *neural canal.* Cells adjacent to the neural tube proliferate and form a *neural crest.* The crest gives rise to neurons that have perikarya in sensory or autonomic ganglia and to neurolemmocytes, the neuroglial cell of the PNS. The cranial end of the neural tube enlarges to form the brain and the remaining tube forms the spinal cord. The neural canal persists as ventricular spaces in the brain and the central canal in the spinal cord.

Cells that line the neural tube give rise to neurons of the CNS and to neuroglia:

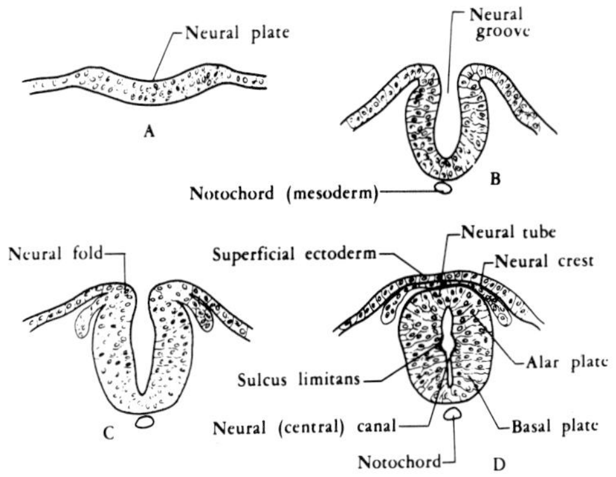

Fig. 6–1. *Schematic diagram of the initial stages of nervous system development, shown in transverse sections. (A) Dorsal ectoderm thickens to form a neural plate. (B) and (C) The plate indents to form a groove that deepens as bilateral neural folds approach the midline and eventually merge. (D) A neural tube containing a canal is formed and detached from superficial ectoderm; between these a neural crest has developed. A sulcus limitans demarcates an alar (sensory related) plate from a basal (motor related) plate. (From Jenkins, T.W.: Functional Mammalian Neuroanatomy. 2nd Ed. Philadelphia, Lea & Febiger, 1978.)*

astrocytes, oligodendrocytes, and ependymal cells. The latter remain in place and line CNS cavities. Some ependymal cells specialize in secreting cerebrospinal fluid. Another neuroglia type, the microglial cell, originates from mesoderm that accompanies vessels when they invade the CNS.

Mesenchyme that surrounds the neural tube develops into protective membranes called meninges. The meninges contain a space filled with cerebrospinal fluid. Thus the CNS is guarded by membranes, shielded by a fluid buffer, and sheltered within bone for protection against the traumas of daily life.

NEURONS

Neurons are specialized in excitability, a membrane phenomenon that requires a voltage gradient across (inside vs outside) the neuron plasmalemma, i.e., a polarized membrane. Excitation is simply depolarization of the plasmalemma, the result of ion flow through protein channels embedded in the plasmalemma.

A typical neuron becomes excited at its input region, conducts excitation to its output region, and transmits excitation, via secretion, to another neuron or to muscle or gland. Since becoming excited and conducting and transmitting excitation all require different protein channels and cellular features, a single neuron has distinct regions: 1) a *dendritic zone,* where excitation is initiated; 2) a *telodendritic zone,* where excitation is transmitted to another cell; 3) an *axon,* which conducts excitation between dendritic and telodendritic zones; and 4) a *cell body* (perikaryon), which nurtures the cell.

These regions have distinct morphologic expressions (Fig. 6–2). A typical dendritic zone features a large surface area produced by highly branched processes called *dendrites.* Alternatively, the dendritic zone may consist of receptors that transform environmental energy into neuronal excitation. The telodendritic zone is also branched and has terminal expansions for storage and release of transmitter molecules. The axon is an elongate cylinder with few branches. The cell body is composed of the nucleus and its surrounding cytoplasm; it is engaged in the synthesis of cell constituents.

Neurons are classified according to the number of processes that emanate from the cell body (Fig. 6–3): A *bipolar* neuron has its cell body located within the axon. Such neurons are found in the retina and the vestibulocochlear nerve. *Unipolar* (pseudounipolar) neurons are initially bipolar during development. The cell body gives rise to a single axon that soon bifurcates. These neurons have cell bodies in spinal and cranial sensory ganglia, and like bipolar neurons they convey sensory information to the CNS. A *multipolar* neuron has its cell body within the dendritic zone. The cell body gives rise to multiple dendrites and a single axon. Nearly all of the billions of neurons comprising the CNS are multipolar, as are the neurons contained in autonomic ganglia. Multipolar neurons

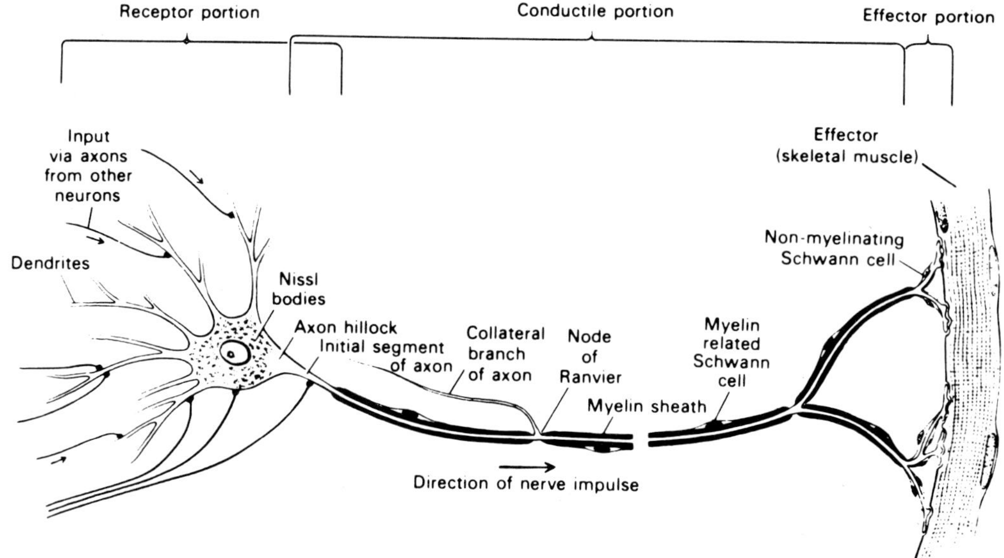

Fig. 6–2. *Schematic illustration of a neuron innervating skeletal muscle. In this neuron the dendritic zone consists of the cell body and the highly branched dendrites arising from it. Telodendria of other neurons synapse on the dendritic zone. The axon, which begins at the initial segment, conducts excitation to telodendria, which synapse on muscle fibers. Neurolemmocytes (Schwann cells) ensheath the telodendria and form myelin sheaths along the axon. When the axon branches it does so at a node between myelin sheaths. Only proximal and distal portions of the axon are shown. (From Kelly, D.E., Wood, R.L., and Enders, A.C.: Bailey's Textbook of Microscopic Anatomy. 18th Ed. Baltimore, Williams & Wilkins, 1984, Fig. 10–2, with permission.)*

can be classified further into those with long axons (Type I neurons) vs those with short axons (Type II neurons).

Neurons assume a great variety of shapes and sizes. Shape is typically compatible with the functional context of the neuron. For example, neurons with extensive dendrites are designed for integrating input from a variety of sources. The orientation of a cell body and its processes is dictated by the connections that have to be made. Size (volume) may be related to the distance over which a neuron extends; however, size is also related to urgency of the information conveyed, since conduction velocity in a cell process increases as its cross-sectional area increases.

Cell Body

The cell body (soma or perikaryon) of a neuron consists of the cell nucleus and the cytoplasm and plasmalemma surrounding the nucleus (Fig. 6–4). Constituents synthesized in the cell body flow distally into the axon and dendrites of the neuron. The portion of the cell body that gives rise to the axon is called the axon hillock.

NUCLEUS. Typically, the nucleus of a neuron is spherical or ovoid, relatively large, and euchromatic. The nucleus appears large because the cell body in which it is found often represents only a minor fraction of the total cell volume. A prominent *nucleolus* is present. In females of some species, a *sex chromatin body* (Barr body) is usually evident in the vicinity of the nucleolus (cat) or the nuclear membrane (primate).

CYTOPLASM. Neuronal cytoplasm is committed to the production of structural proteins (e.g., for microtubules and neurofilaments), of membrane proteins (e.g., for ionic channels and active transport), and of enzymatic proteins (e.g., for glucose metabolism and synthesis of secretion products). Thus, neuronal cytoplasm has a high concentration of rER, free ribosomes, and polyribosomes (Fig. 6–5). In large neu-

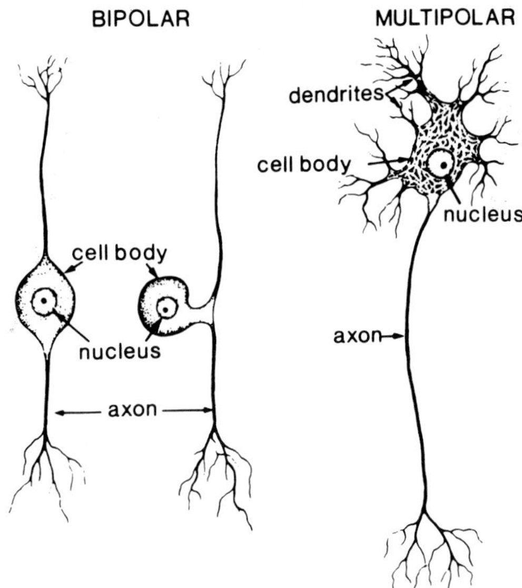

Fig. 6–3. *Schematic illustration of neuron types. A bipolar neuron (left) has its cell body located within the axon. Unipolar (pseudounipolar) neurons develop from bipolar neurons by migration of the cell body (center); a single axonal process will leave the cell body and bifurcate. The cell body of a multipolar neuron (right) gives rise to multiple dendrites and a single axon. (From Ham, A.W., and Cormack, D.H.: Histology. 8th Ed. Philadelphia, J.B. Lippincott, 1979, Fig. 17–2, with permission.)*

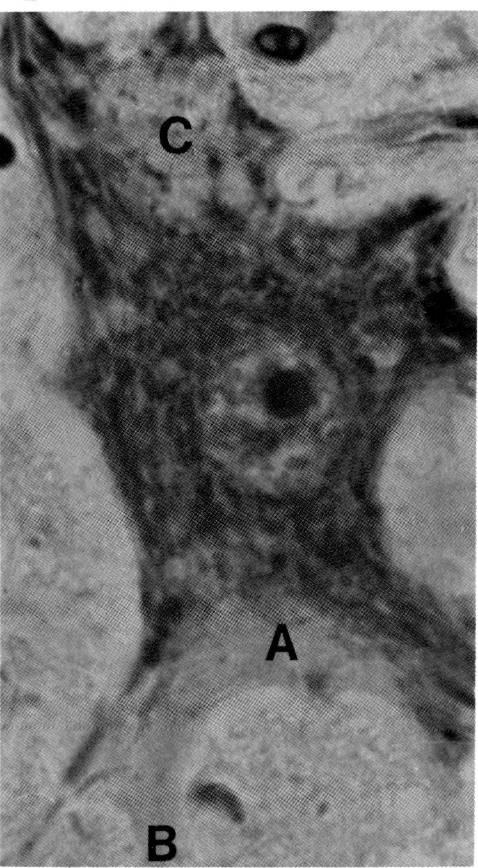

Fig. 6–4. *Light micrograph of a multipolar neuron cell body, spinal cord, horse. The nucleus contains a prominent nucleolus. The cytoplasm features chromatophilic clumps (Nissl substance) that are absent from the axon hillock (A) that gives rise to the axon (B). Lipofuscin inclusions (C) ar present in this cell body. ×1200. (Courtesy of A. Hansen.)*

rons, blocks of stacked rER and ribosomal aggregations are distributed throughout the cell body cytoplasm, including initial dendritic branches but not the axon hillock or axon. The blocks appear as *chromatophilic substance* (Nissl substance) when stained with aniline dyes and examined by light microscopy. In small neurons, aggregations of rER and ribosomes are less dense and the cytoplasmic chromatophilia has a diffuse appearance.

In cases of neuronal injury (e.g., transection of the axon), the cell body swells, the nucleus shifts to an eccentric position within the cell body, and chromatophilic substance disappears except marginally along the plasmalemma *(chromatolysis)*. This response to injury is called the *axonal reaction* (Fig. 6–6). It begins in a matter of days and may persist several weeks in a surviving neuron. It reflects the reaction of a cell body committed to synthesizing constituents for axonal regrowth, since the original distal axon always degenerates as a consequence of isolation from the cell body.

A Golgi complex, which gives rise to secretory and synaptic vesicles, is usually prominent in neurons. *Secretory vesicles* are abundant in cell bodies of certain neurons such as those of the magnocellular hypothalamic nuclei. *Synaptic vesicles* are prominent in the telodendria of nearly all neurons, and in some neurons they are evident in the cell body from which they are transported to telodendria.

Microtubules (25 nm in diameter) and *neu-*

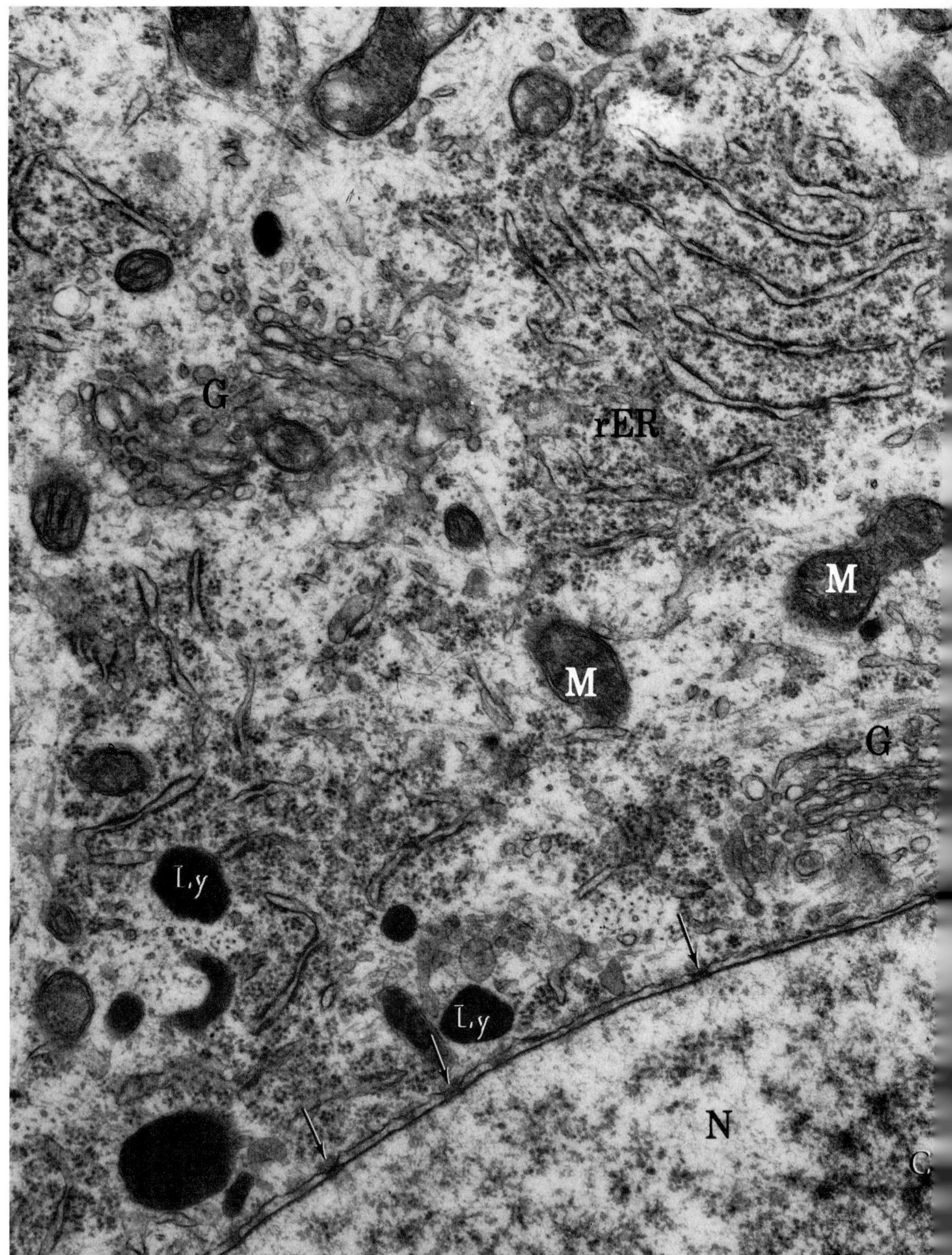

Fig. 6–5. *Electron micrograph of part of a neuron cell body, spinal cord, rat. The nucleus (N) contains chromatin (Chr) and is bounded by a double-layered envelope that has pores (arrows). The cytoplasm features a variety of organelles, including neurofilaments (asterisk), lysosomes (Ly), mitochondria (M), Golgi complex (G), and rough endoplasmic reticulum (rER). Localized densities of rER constitute the chromatophilic substance seen by light microscopy.* ×34,000. *(From Peters, A., Palay, S.L., and Webster, H.DeF.: The Fine Structure of the Nervous System. Philadelphia, W.B. Saunders, 1976, Fig. 2–14, with permisison.)*

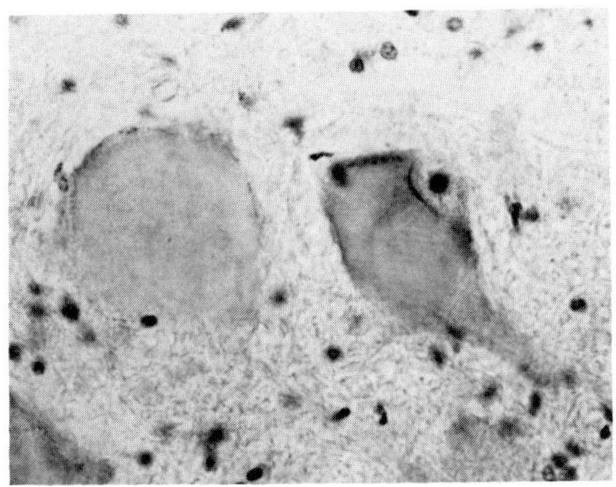

Fig. 6–6. *Light micrograph of chromatolytic cell bodies from a canine spinal cord that had spinal nerves transected. Notice that the cell bodies are swollen, the nucleus is shifted to an eccentric position, and chromatophilic substance is lost except for small amounts accumulated marginally. Nissl stain.* ×374.

rofilaments (10 nm in diameter) are numerous in the cell body. Microtubules play a role in the active transport of proteins and organelles within the neuron. Neuronal cytoplasm also contains *mitochondria, smooth endoplasmic reticulum, lysosomes* in various forms, and lipofuscin granules, which increase with age as a residue of lysosomal activity. Many neurons have a solitary cilium and centriole.

Dendrites, Axons, Telodendria

Dendrites are highly branched processes of multipolar neurons. Treelike, each dendrite emerges as a main trunk that branches repeatedly into smaller and smaller dendritic twigs. The main trunk has an organelle content similar to that of the cell body. Small dendritic branches predominantly feature microtubules (Fig. 6–7), augmented by neurofilaments, mitochondria, smooth endoplasmic reticulum (sER), and occasional clusters of free ribosomes. At multiple sites, dendritic plasmalemma is modified for synaptic activity.

Some neurons have numerous *dendritic spines* (gemmules). Like a bud on a twig, a spine is a short expanded process attached to the dendritic branch by a narrow stalk. Within the spine, a spine apparatus is present, consisting of alternating membranous sacs and dense material. Spines serve a synaptic function.

The *axon* is a usually long, cylindrical process with sparse branches. When present, branches emanate perpendicularly from the axon and are termed collateral branches. The axon originates from the axon hillock of the cell body, a conical region devoid of chromatophilic substance. The hillock is filled with microtubules (neurotubules) and neurofilaments that continue into the axon and constitute its predominant organelles. Axoplasm also features mitochondria and sER.

The *initial segment* of the axon, located just distal to the axon hillock is generally narrower than the rest of the axon. It is the site of lowest threshold for initiating axon potentials in the neuron. Distal to the initial segment, some axons are enveloped in segments of myelin sheath separated by gaps called nodes. Collateral branches of myelinated axons originate at nodes. Electron-dense material is present along the inner surface of the axon plasmalemma at the initial segment and at nodes of myelinated axons.

In addition to a slow flow (1 to 5 mm/day) of cytoplasmic constituents from the cell body to its axon and dendrites, the axon also has an energy-dependent fast transport capability (400 mm/day) involving microtubules. The direction of fast transport is both orthograde and retrograde; the latter conveys organelle remnants from the telodendria to lysosomes in the cell body.

Axons end in a telodendritic zone, typically consisting of multiple, successive branchings. The ultimate telodendritic branches terminate in expansions, called terminal bulbs, each of which contains synaptic vesicles and participates in a synapse.

Interneuronal Synapses

A *synapse* between neurons occurs at a site of morphologic specialization where,

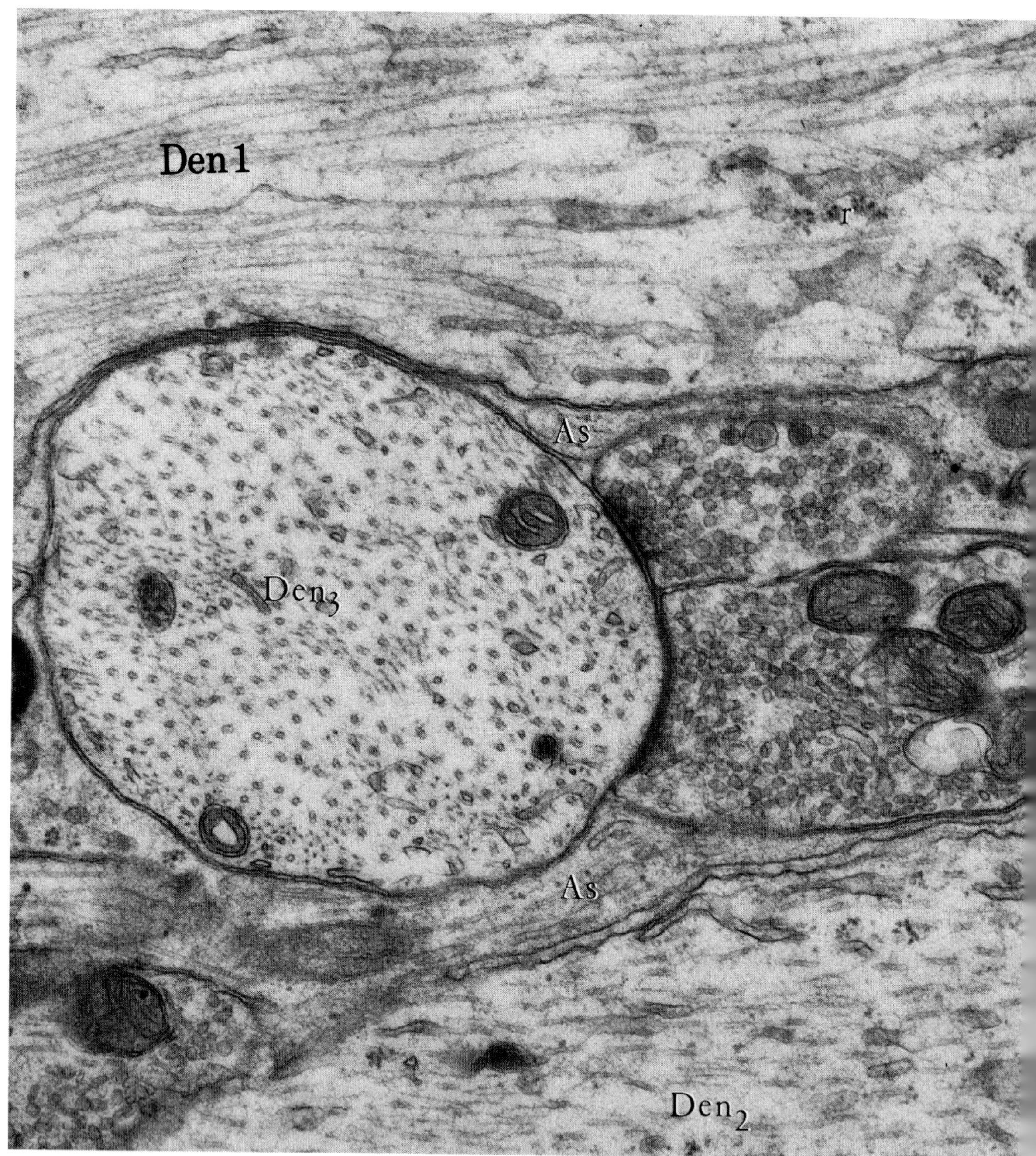

Fig. 6–7. *Electron micrograph of neuropil from rat spinal cord. Dendrites are shown in longitudinal ($Den_{1,2}$) and transverse (Den_3) section. Dendritic cytoplasm features predominantly microtubules, but neurofilaments, mitochondria, and smooth endoplasmic reticulum are also present. Two telodendritic processes, which synapse on Den_3, have abundant synaptic vesicles. The vesicles have electron-lucent cores and are spherical in the upper profile but predominantly flattened in the lower profile. Electron-dense material is associated with synaptic plasmalemma. Astrocyte processes (As) surround the synapses. ×44,000. (From Peters, A., Palay, S.L., and Webster, H.Def.: The Fine Structure of the Nervous System. Philadelphia, W.B. Saunders, 1976, Fig. 3–4, with permission.)*

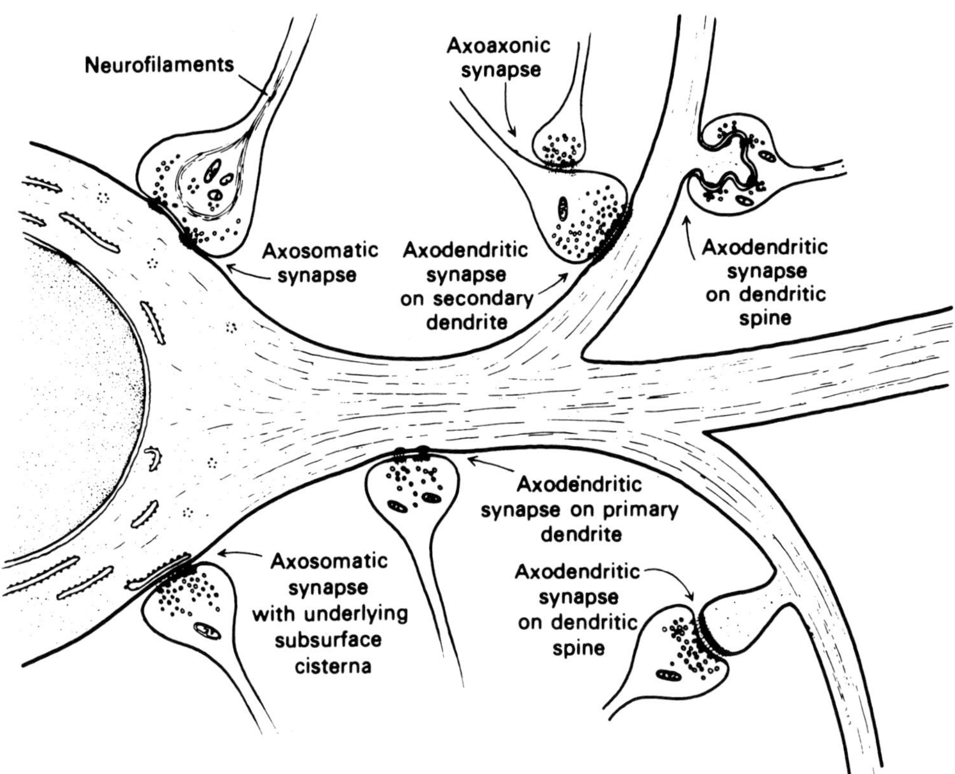

Fig. 6–8. *Schematic illustration of types of synapses. The presynaptic (telodendritic) elements, featuring synaptic vesicles clustered around electron-dense plaques at the plasmalemma, are terminal bulbs except for one terminal calyx. Axosomatic synapses occur on the cell body. Axodendritic synapses occur on dendrites, including dendritic spines. In an axoaxonic synapse one terminal bulb synapses on another to produce inhibition. (From Kelly, D.E., Wood, R.L., and Enders, A.C.: Bailey's Textbook of Microscopic Anatomy. 18th Ed. Baltimore, Williams & Wilkins, 1984, Fig. 10–14, with permission.)*

typically, a telodendritic process influences the excitability of a dendritic zone by releasing a chemical agent. Telodendria generally develop bulbous enlargements at synapses (Fig. 6–8). *Terminal bulbs* (or boutons) are located at the end of each telodendritic branch. Some telodendria have multiple *preterminal bulbs* located periodically on a telodendrite, which can thereby establish multiple synapses along its course. In a few neurons, each telodendrite forms a *terminal calyx* that embraces the postsynaptic structure.

Synapses have been classified according to where the telodendritic process synapses on the postsynaptic neuron. *Axodendritic* synapses are most common, followed by *axosomatic* synapses on the cell body. *Axoaxonic* synapses involve two telodendria (inhibitory effect) or a synapse on the initial segment. Some synapses, such as dendrodendritic synapses, do not involve telodendria.

The essential features of a synapse are the *presynaptic process,* the *synaptic cleft,* and the *postsynaptic membrane.* Nearly all synapses involve chemical transmission with the transmitter molecules stored in synaptic vesicles within the presynaptic process. Presynaptic depolarization leads to an influx of Ca^{++}, which facilitates synaptic vesicle merger with the presynaptic plasmalemma. Transmitter molecules are released into the synaptic cleft, diffuse across it, and bind to protein molecules in the postsynaptic membrane. The protein molecules undergo stereochemical modification, opening ionic channels for depolarization (or inhibitory hyperpolarization) of the postsynaptic membrane. Transmitter molecules then are degraded by enzymatic proteins of the postsynaptic membrane. Synaptic vesicular membrane that was incorporated into the presynaptic plasmalemma is recaptured by endocytosis and reused for synaptic vesicles.

Synaptic vesicles are commonly 40 to 60 nm in diameter (Fig. 6–7). The transmitter molecules they contain are usually synthesized and packaged locally in the presynaptic process. However, in some neurons, vesicles are synthesized in the cell body. Different neurons produce different kinds of transmitter chemicals. Although a broad range of transmitter chemicals has been discovered, there are only three common morphologic types of synaptic vesicles: spherical with electron-lucent cores; spherical with dense cores; and electron-lucent vesicles that become flattened during certain fixation procedures. The latter are usually associated with inhibitory transmitters, while the dense-core vesicles are associated with catecholamine transmitters (norepinephrine or dopamine) or peptides.

In addition to synaptic vesicles, presynaptic processes occasionally contain large dense-core vesicles of unknown significance. Also, large electron-dense secretory vesicles are present in neurosecretory neurons of the the hypothalamus.

The presynaptic plasmalemma has electron-dense plaques along its cytoplasmic surface. Synaptic vesicles tend to cluster around these active regions. The postsynaptic plasmalemma may resemble the presynaptic membrane or it may have thicker accumulations of electron-dense substance. The width of the synaptic cleft may be the same as the typical extracellular gap (20 nm), or it may be 30 nm in asymmetric synapses where the postsynaptic membrane appears thicker than the presynaptic one. The cleft contains a protein-carbohydrate substance that may serve to hold pre- and postsynaptic membranes in apposition.

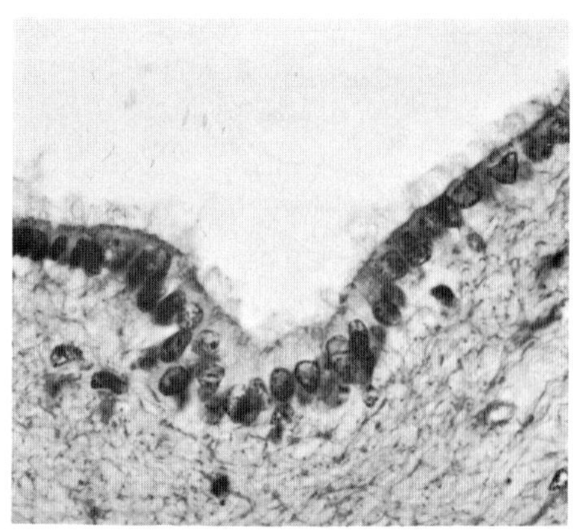

Fig. 6–9. *Light micrograph of ependymal cells lining the fourth ventricle, camel. The cells have motile cilia.* ×*428. (From Dellmann, H.-D.: Veterinary Histology: An Outline Text-Atlas. Philadelphia, Lea & Febiger, 1971.)*

A small minority of synapses utilize electrical rather than chemical transmission. Pre- and postsynaptic membranes form a gap junction (nexus or macula communicans) to establish a low resistance path for intercellular ionic flow. Synaptic vesicles are absent, unless the synapse uses both electrical and chemical transmission.

NEUROGLIA

Neuroglia comprise well over 90% of the cells that make up the nervous system. Neuroglial cells are relatively small; with routine stains only their nuclei and perikarya are evident. Collectively, they provide structural support, form the CNS boundary, ensheath and insulate axons, maintain a narrow extracellular space with a proper ionic milieu, and, in the event of injury, they phagocytize debris and produce "scar" tissue.

Neuroglia cell types in the CNS are *ependymal cells, astrocytes, oligodendrocytes,* and *microglial cells.* In the PNS they are *neurolemmocytes,* which ensheath axons and serve as satellite cells in ganglia.

Ependymal Cells

Ependymal cells line the ventricular cavities of the brain and the central canal of the spinal cord (Fig. 6–9). The luminal surface of each cell has numerous microvilli and multiple motile cilia. Ependymal cytoplasm features glial filaments and mitochondria. Ependymal cells are generally columnar and joined by zonulae adherentes located near the luminal border. Large molecules from the CNS extracellular space can pass between ependymal cells to reach cerebrospinal fluid, which is produced primarily by modified ependymal cells called choroid plexus epithelium. Tanycytes are nonciliated ependymal cells found in the wall of the ventricular system. They have elongate basal processes that terminate at perivascular spaces or in the brain neuropil.

Astrocytes

In routine stains, astrocytes are recognized by their pale, oval nuclei, which are largest among glial nuclei. With silver stains, astrocytes are seen to have numerous processes (Fig. 6–10). In white matter, the processes are long, slender, and moderately branched; in gray matter, the processes appear shorter, thicker, and highly branched. Thus white matter is said to contain *fibrous astrocytes,* while gray matter contains *protoplasmic astrocytes.* Astrocyte processes often terminate in expansions called *end feet.* Collections of end feet form the *glial limiting membrane* at the CNS boundary, including boundaries with vessels that penetrate the brain and spinal cord. End feet also form septa in the spinal cord.

Ultrastructurally, astrocytes feature glial filaments throughout their cytoplasm. Astrocytes provide structural support, take up excess extracelullar K^+, and form diffusion barriers surrounding synapses. Astrocytes are capable of phagocytosis, and they proliferate to form glial scars in the event of CNS injury.

Oligodendrocytes

Oligodendrocytes can be recognized in routine stains by their small, spherical, densely stained nuclei. The cell has relatively few processes, and these are thin and difficult to visualize. The cytoplasm is rich in organelles, especially rER, mitochondria, and microtubules. In gray matter, oligodendrocytes serve as perineuronal satellite cells, but their function is unknown. In white matter, oligodendrocytes form myelin sheaths around axons.

Microglia

Microglia are traditionally regarded as cells of mesodermal origin that invade the CNS when it is vascularized and reside there to proliferate and become phagocytotic in the event of tissue damage. Thus the cells are sparse and difficult to find in normal tissues. They are recognized by their small, elongate, chromophilic nuclei, and with silver stains as small, elongate cells with sparse polar processes.

The traditional concept of microglia is being questioned by neuroscientists, some of whom doubt the existence of microglia as a distinct cell type. In any case, there are several potential phagocytes in the event of CNS damage. In addition to microglia cells, astrocytes and oligodendrocytes can become phagocytic. Pericytes of blood vessels can migrate and become phagocytic. Finally, hematogenous macrophages can invade the CNS.

Neurolemmocytes

Neurolemmocytes (Schwann cells) are gliocytes of the PNS that ensheath axons or encapsulate nerve cell bodies as ganglionic gliocytes or satellite cells. Thus neurolemmocytes provide a protected immediate environment for PNS neurons. Each neurolemmocyte is enclosed within a basal lamina. Neurolemmocytes can become phagocytic in the case of nerve damage.

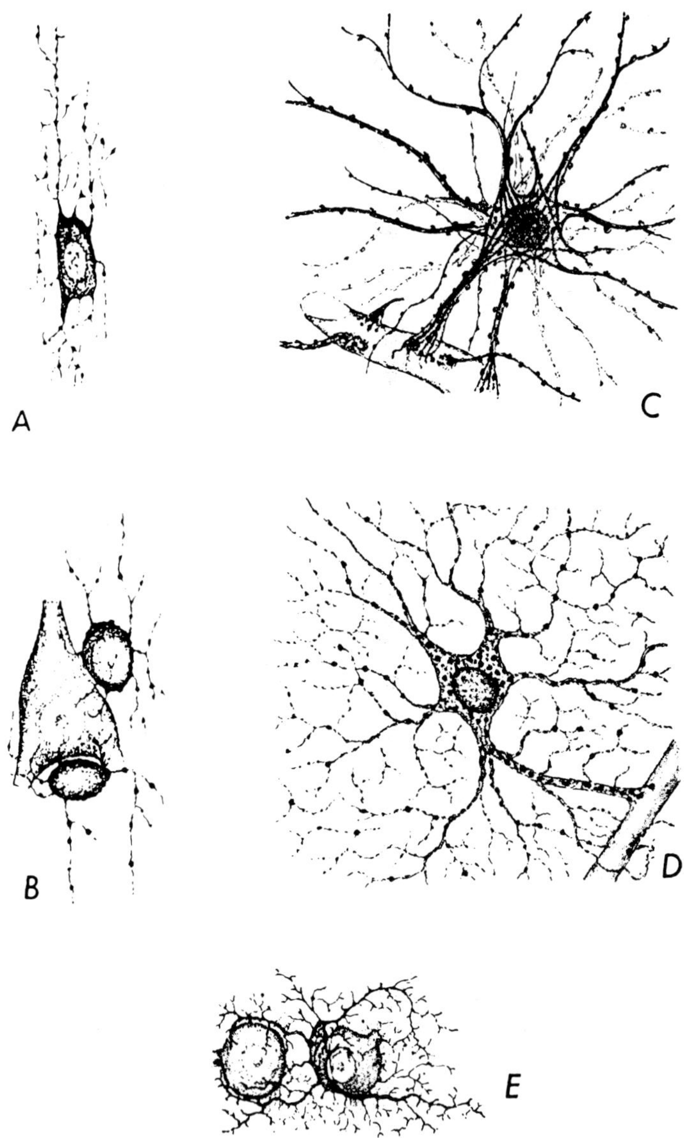

Fig. 6–10. *Schematic illustration of oligodendrocytes, astrocytes, and a microglial cell: (A) oligodendrocyte from white matter; its processes are oriented longitudinally and connected to myelin sheaths (not shown). (B) Two oligodendrocytes serving as perineuronal satellites in gray matter. (C) A fibrous astrocyte from white matter, drawn to emphasize glial filaments. Astrocyte processes terminate in end-feet expansions, shown on a blood vessel. (D) A protoplasmic astrocyte characterized by highly branched processes. (E) An elongated microglial cell in the vicinity of two small neuronal cell bodies. (From Copenhaver, W.M., et al.: Bailey's Textbook of Histology. 16th Ed. Baltimore, Williams & Wilkins, 1971. Redrawn from Penfield. Del Rio-Hortega's modified silver method.)*

In craniospinal (sensory) ganglia, satellite cells form a complete capsule around each unipolar cell body (Fig. 6–11). The satellite cells are continued by neurolemmocytes that ensheath and myelinate the axon. In autonomic ganglia, satellite cells form an incomplete capsule around individual multipolar cell bodies (Fig. 6–12).

Every axon in the PNS is ensheathed along its entire length by neurolemmocytes, except for the most terminal branches in some cases. Since an individual neurolemmocyte is less than 1 mm in length, a tandem series of many neurolemmocytes is required to ensheath an entire axon length. For small nonmyelinated axons, each neurolemmocyte ensheathes a variable number of axons (Fig. 6–13). Each axon is enclosed by a pair of neurolemmocyte processes, which establish a narrow periaxonal space that communicates to the general interstitial space by means of a mesaxonal gap. For axons larger than 1 μm diameter, each neurolemmocyte engulfs a single axon, and its processes produce a myelin sheath (Fig. 6–14).

MYELIN SHEATH

In the PNS, a transverse section of a myelinated fiber viewed by light microscopy reveals an axon enclosed in a myelin sheath surrounded by neurolemmocyte cytoplasm (Fig. 6–15). With electron microscopy, one can see that the neurolemmocyte is within a basal lamina and the myelin sheath is composed of multiple layers of neurolemmocyte plasma membrane (Fig. 6–14).

Myelin formation begins with a neurolemmocyte draped around a solitary axon, establishing a simple mesaxon (Fig. 6–16). Then the neurolemmocyte processes elongate, slide past one another, and continue on to produce multilayered neurolemmocyte wrappings around the axon. Cytoplasm is extruded from the wrappings, leaving concentric lamellae of plasma membrane that constitutes the myelin sheath.

At high magnification, the myelin sheath displays a periodicity of concentric *major dense lines* separated by intraperiod lines. Each major dense line is formed by fusion of plasma membrane inner surfaces as cytoplasm is extruded during myelin sheath formation. An *intraperiod line* is formed where the outer surfaces of adjacent plasma membranes are separated by a minute gap. The gap is continuous with the *inner mesaxon* and the *outer mesaxon,* all of which are derived from the original simple mesaxon. Occasionally major dense lines will appear to split and contain a pocket of cytoplasm. Adjacent pockets of cytoplasm may extend throughout the thickness of the myelin sheath, establishing a *myelin incisure* in the sheath.

A longitudinal view of a myelinated fiber reveals that myelin sheaths formed by adjacent neurolemmocytes are separated by a gap. The gap is referred to as a *node* (of Ranvier), and the myelin between nodes, produced by a single neurolemmocyte, is called an *internode.* The internodal transition region that leads to a node is referred to as a *paranode* (Fig. 6–17). At this region, major dense lines split and cytoplasm is retained in processes that overlap one another as each contacts the axon plasmalemma. The outermost cytoplasmic processes from adjacent neurolemmocytes make contact, thus enclosing the node. A continuous basal lamina is present external to the neurolemmocytes. At the node, the axon bulges slightly and subplasmalemmal electron-dense material is evident.

In the CNS, myelin sheaths are formed by oligodendrocytes (Fig. 6–18). A single oligodendrocyte is known to contribute internodes to as many as 50 myelinated fibers. Outer cytoplasm of the internode is restricted to a single ridge that is connected to the oligodendrocyte perikaryon by a thin process. Nodes and paranodes exist, but nodes are not covered by cytoplasmic processes in the CNS. Internodes are not as thick and nodes are wider in the CNS compared to the PNS.

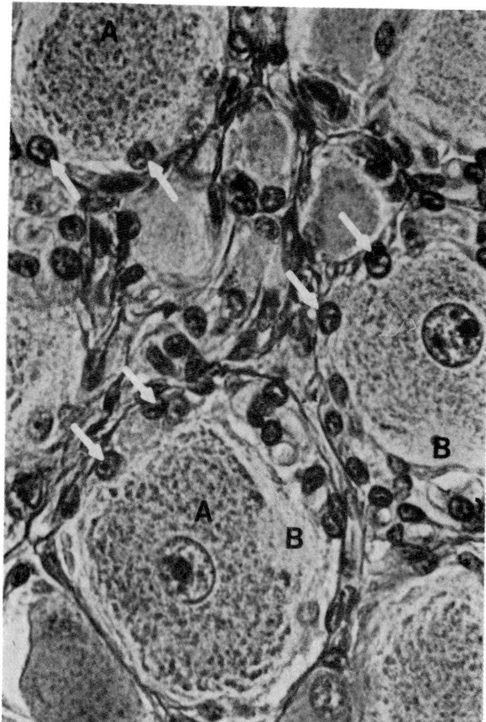

Fig. 6–11. *Light micrograph of a sectioned spinal ganglion, dog. The arrows indicate nuclei of ganglionic gliocytes (satellite cells), which completely encapsulate unipolar neuron cell bodies (A). An axon hillock (B) is evident where Nissl substance is absent. ×625. (Courtesy of E.M. Brown.)*

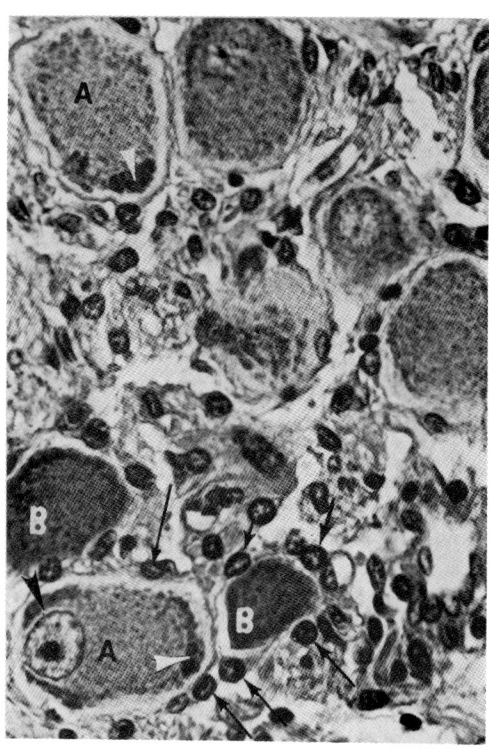

Fig. 6–12. *Light micrograph of a sectioned autonomic ganglion, dog. The thin arrows indicate nuclei of ganglionic gliocytes, which form an incomplete capsule around multipolar neuron cell bodies. Neurons exhibit marginal accumulations of Nissl substance (A, arrowheads) and generalized chromatophilia (B). ×625. (Courtesy of E.M. Brown.)*

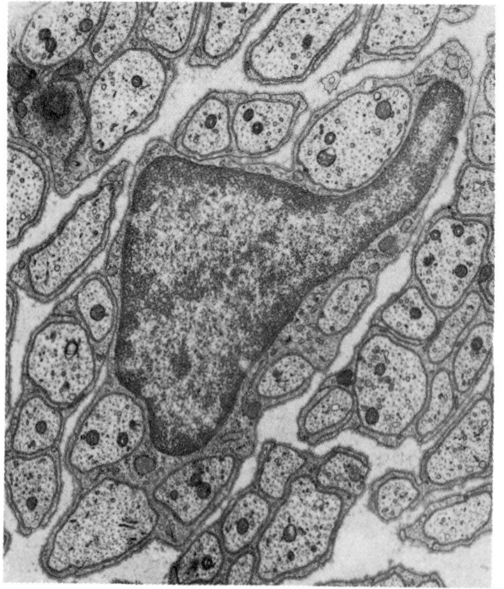

Fig. 6–13. *Electron micrograph of a neurolemmocyte ensheathing nonmyelinated axons of the PNS. All of the axons in the field are enclosed by neurolemmocyte cytoplasmic processes, but mesaxons are not easily seen at this magnification. ×15,600. (Courtesy of H.-D. Dellmann.)*

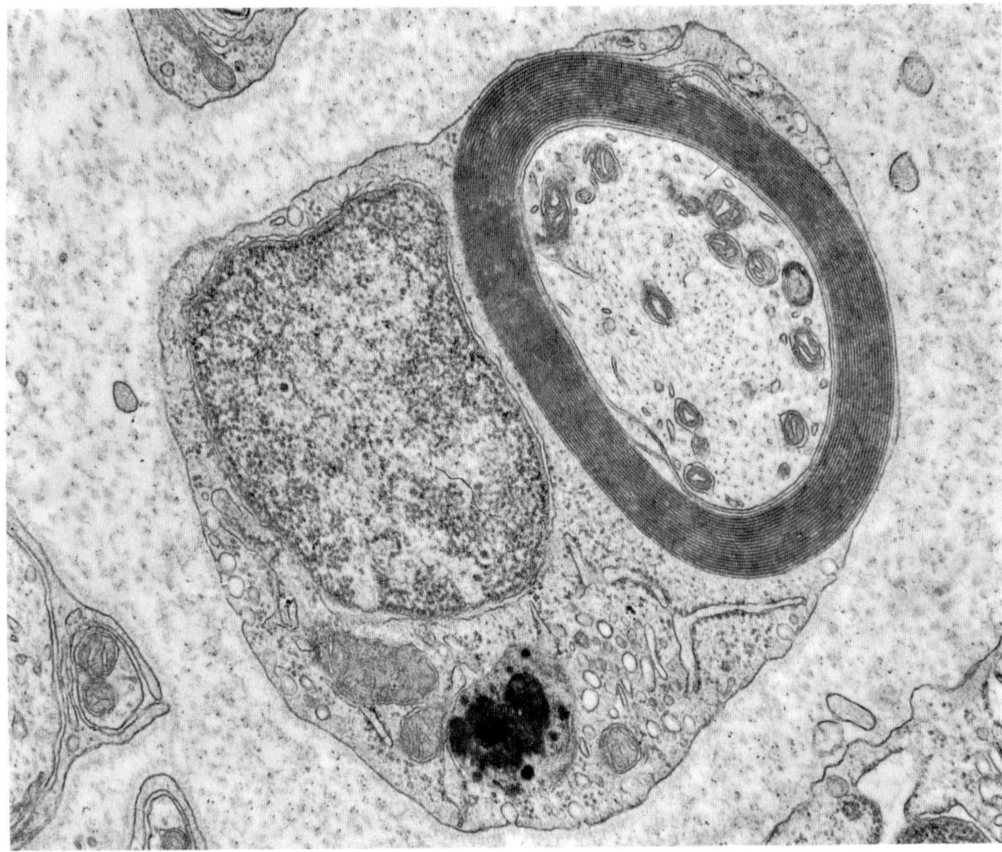

Fig. 6–14. *Electron micrograph of a myelinated fiber of the PNS. A neurolemmocyte has produced a myelin sheath around a single axon. The neurolemmocyte is enclosed by basal lamina, and external to this, collagen fibrils of the endoneurium are evident. (The electron-dense mass in the neurolemmocyte cytoplasm is a lipofuscin inclusion.) The myelin consists of multiple wrappings of neurolemmocyte membrane. An external mesaxon is evident above the myelin sheath, and an internal mesaxon can be seen at the lower left of the axon. The axoplasm features neurofilaments, microtubles, and mitochondria. ×29,325. (From Dellmann, H.-D.: Veterinary Histology: An Outline Text-Atlas. Philadelphia, Lea & Febiger, 1971.)*

Functionally, the myelin sheath provides electrical insulation so the action potential jumps from node to node instead of progressing continuously, as in nonmyelinated axons. The jumping process, called *saltatory conduction,* is much faster than nonmyelinated conduction. The longer the internode, the faster the conduction. Internode length is proportional to myelin sheath thickness, and both are proportional to axon diameter.

PERIPHERAL NERVOUS SYSTEM

The PNS consists of cranial and spinal nerves, including all roots, branches, and ganglia of the nerves. *Cranial nerves* originate from the brain and exit the cranial cavity. *Spinal nerves* originate from the spinal cord and exit the vertebral canal.

A *nerve* consists of usually thousands of axons, each sheathed by neurolemmocytes and all enveloped by connective tissue. A *root* is the proximal region of a nerve where axons are enveloped by neurolemmocytes and meninges. A *ganglion* is an enlargement of a nerve produced by an accumulation of neuron cell bodies. The term "nerve fiber" is somewhat ambiguous; it may refer to a myelinated axon with its associated neurolemmocytes or to a single nonmyelinated axon.

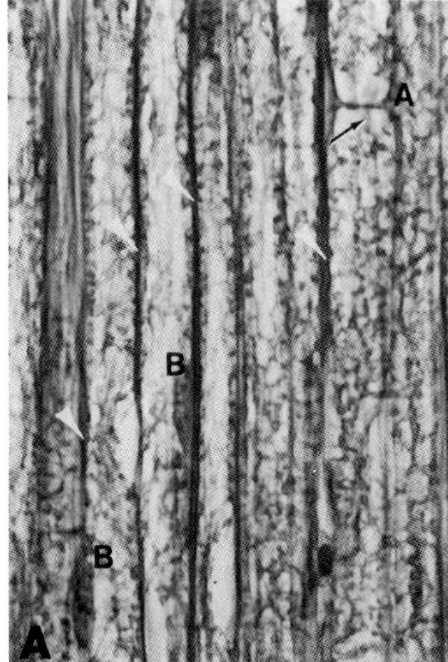

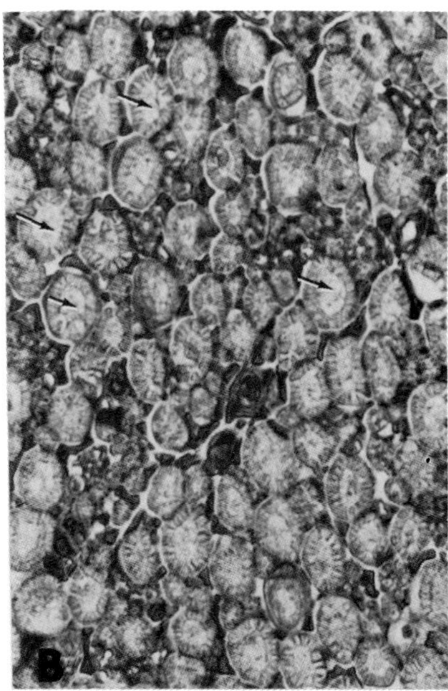

Fig. 6–15. *Light micrograph of longitudinal (image A) and transverse (image B) sections of a canine peripheral nerve. Lipid extraction during tissue preparation disintegrates the myelin sheath, leaving a protein residue (neurokeratin). In A, endoneurium (white arrowheads) surrounds each myelinated nerve fiber; a myelin sheath is interrupted at a node (A); an axon (black arrow) is evident in the center of a fiber; neurolemmocyte nuclei (B) and cytoplasm are present at the surface of each fiber. In B, each myelinated fiber consists of an axon (arrow) surrounded by a myelin sheath (neurokeratin) within a cytoplasmic rim. Nonmyelinated axons are not visible at this magnification, but they are more numerous than the myelinated fibers in the field.* ×625. *(Courtesy of E.M. Brown.)*

Individual nerve fibers may be classified as either *afferent* or *efferent.* Afferent fibers are sensory since they conduct excitation to the CNS. Afferent neurons have unipolar cell bodies in craniospinal ganglia. The dendritic zone of an afferent neuron is composed of receptors, or of synaptic contacts on the sensory epithelium of a sense organ. Efferent axons come from multipolar cell bodies located in the CNS or in autonomic ganglia. Their telodendria excite muscle or gland, or neurons in autonomic ganglia.

Individual nerve fibers are classified also as somatic or visceral. The former innervate skin, skeletal muscles, and joints while the latter innervate cardiac and smooth muscles and glands. Visceral efferent fibers in particular (and often visceral fibers in general) are designated the *autonomic nervous system.* The visceral efferent pathway involves two neurons. The first (preganglionic) neuron has its cell body in the CNS, and the cell body of the second (postganglionic) neuron is located in an autonomic ganglion.

Nerves

A nerve is composed of one to several nerve fascicles (Fig. 6–19). A *nerve fascicle* is delimited by *perineurium,* which has two components: *fibrous perineurium,* an outer shell of moderately dense collagenous connective tissue; and *perineural epithelium,* an inner sleeve of multiple concentric layers of squamous epithelial cells (Fig. 6–20). Collagen fibrils are dispersed between the layers and each epithelial cell is enclosed in a basal lamina. Perineural epithelium forms a continuous sheet from the root-nerve junction to the terminal branches of the nerve, although layers decrease in number as fascicles become smaller. Also,

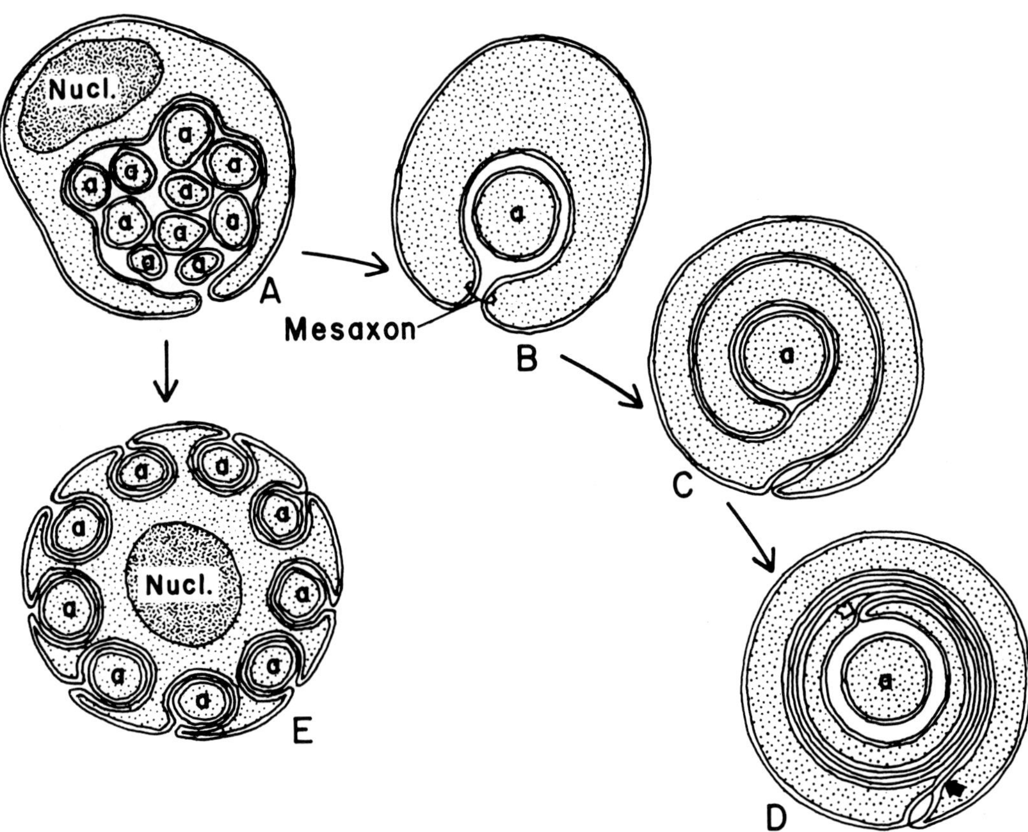

Fig. 6–16. *Schematic diagram showing the ontogenetic relationship of axons (a) to neurolemmocytes in transverse section. (A) Early in development several axons are ensheathed in common by a single neurolemmocyte. (B) Subsequent to neurolemmocyte proliferation, an axon destined to be myelinated is ensheathed individually; a mesaxon is formed where the neurolemmocyte processes meet. (C) The processes elongate and encircle the axon; the original mesaxon is elongated. (D) A myelin sheath is formed, as cytoplasm is extruded from the encircling neurolemmocyte processes. A major dense line is formed where absence of cytoplasm allows adjacent inner surfaces of plasma membrane to unite; an intraperiod line (not shown) is present between major dense lines, representing the elongated mesaxon. An inner mesaxon (white arrow) and outer mesaxon (black arrow) are evident where cytoplasm persists. (E) In the case of nonmyelinated axons, the neurolemmocyte provides multiple invaginations so that each axon is ensheathed in a separate compartment with its own mesaxon. (From Copenhaver, W.M., et al.: Bailey's Textbook of Histology. 16th Ed. Baltimore, Williams & Wilkins, 1971.)*

perineural epithelium proliferates to encapsulate receptors. By serving as a diffusion barrier, perineural epithelium affords peripheral nerve fibers a protected environment, though the epithelium can also serve as a channel for infectious or toxic agents that invade the fascicle.

Within a nerve fascicle, fibroblasts and collagen fibers surrounding neurolemmocytes constitute *endoneurium*. The multiple fascicles of a nerve are bound together by *epineurium*, a connective tissue less dense than fibrous perineurium. Blood vessels supplying a nerve constitute *vasa nervorum*.

Ganglia

Ganglia are accumulations of neuron cell bodies within a nerve fascicle. Spinal ganglia on dorsal roots and cranial nerve ganglia are referred to as *sensory ganglia*, since they contain unipolar cell bodies of afferent neurons (Fig. 6–11) (cell bodies remain bipolar in ganglia of the vestibulocochlear nerve). The unipolar cell bodies are distributed around the fibers of the nerve, which course through the center of the ganglion. Each unipolar cell body gives rise to a single axon that may coil initially be-

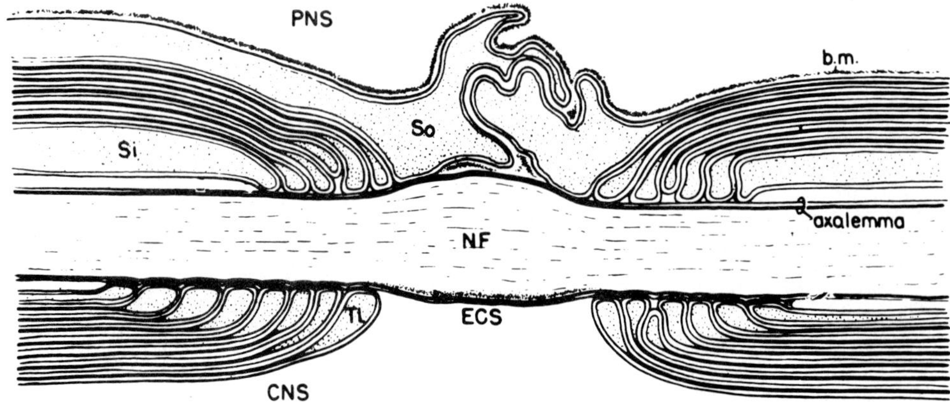

Fig. 6–17. *Schematic illustration of the node and paranodal regions of a myelinated fiber from the PNS (above) and CNS (below). In the PNS, the outer cytoplasm (So) of adjacent neurolemmocytes (Schwann cells) overlaps the node, within a continuous basal lamina (b.m.) At internodes, inner cytoplasm (Si) is generally present inside the myelin sheath, composed of major dense lines separated by intraperiod lines. At each paranode, the major dense lines split to contain terminal cytoplasmic "loops" (TL), which contact the axolemma and impede ionic flow between the node and internode. In the CNS, myelin is formed by oligodendrocytes, and internodes have less cytoplasm than in the PNS. CNS modes are exposed to the general extracellular space (ECS). NF = axon (nerve fiber). (From Bunge, R.P.: Glial cells and the central myelin sheath. Physiol Rev 48:197, 1970, Fig. 12, with permission.)*

fore joining the centrally collected fibers where the axon bifurcates into central and peripheral branches; the peripheral branch may be thicker than the central. Large cell bodies give rise to myelinated axons, and the bifurcation of each axon occurs at a node. Each cell body is encapsulated by satellite cells.

Autonomic ganglia are produced by multipolar cell bodies accumulated within autonomic nerve fascicles (Fig. 6–12). Within visceral organs, there are terminal autonomic ganglia composed of only a few cell bodies. In autonomic ganglia, telodendria of cholinergic preganglonic neurons synapse on the dendritic zones of postganglionic neurons. Postganglionic neurons are classified as *cholinergic* if they synthesize and release acetylcholine and *adrenergic* if their neurotransmitter is noradrenalin (norepinephrine). Adrenergic neurons can be identified by the presence of dense core synaptic vesicles. Some autonomic ganglia contain a few SIF (small intensely fluorescent) cells that contain numerous large dense-core vesicles and release dopamine. Their function is currently unclear.

Efferent Terminations

Somatic efferent neurons innervate skeletal muscle. One such neuron and all of the muscle fibers it innervates is regarded as a *motor unit,* since the muscle fibers it innervates contract as a unit when the neuron is excited. Motor units may have from several to several hundred muscle fibers. Large motor units are innervated by large neurons and are associated with large muscles. An individual muscle fiber belongs to only one motor unit and receives synaptic input at its center.

A neuromuscular synapse consists of a presynaptic motor end-plate overlying the postsynaptic sole plate of a muscle fiber (Fig. 6–21). At the terminal end of a telodendritic branch, a *motor end-plate* is formed by a profusion of short branches within a circumscribed zone (plate). Each end-plate branch is inserted in a corresponding trough of the sole plate with a neuromuscular gap of 40 to 50 nm. The sarcolemma undergoes additional transverse infoldings, creating a series of junctional folds (Fig. 6–22).

End-plate cytoplasm contains many mitochondria and numerous clear synaptic vesicles (40 nm diameter). The vesicles contain acetylcholine, which is released at active sites opposite the junctional folds and then diffuses across the neuromuscular gap and binds to postsynaptic receptor

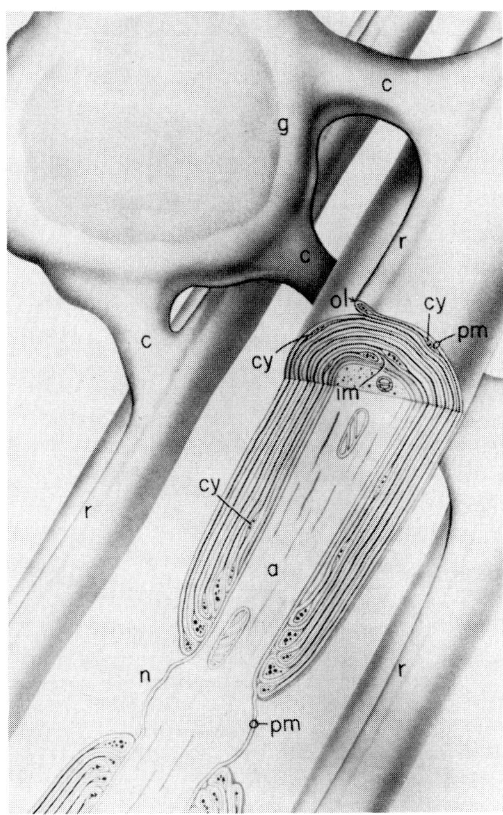

Fig. 6–18. *Illustration of an oligodendrocyte (g) extending thin processes (c) to form myelin sheath internodes. In the CNS, cytoplasm outside the myelin sheath is restricted to a thin ridge (r). (im = inner mesaxon; ol = outer loop; cy = cytoplasm; a = axon; pm = axolemma; n = node) (From Bunge, M.B., et al.: Ultrastructural study of remyelination in an experimental lesion in adult cat spinal cord. J Biophys Biochem Cytol 10:67, 1961, Fig. 18, with permission.)*

sites. Neurolemmocytes cover the endplate and basal lamina extends into the neuromuscular gap and junctional folds.

The *fusimotor* or *gamma motor neuron* is another type of somatic efferent neuron. It innervates small muscle fibers within muscle spindles. These small neurons have myelinated axons that terminate as endplates or trail endings; the latter make multiple synaptic contacts along the muscle fiber surface.

Preganglionic autonomic neurons synapse on postganglionic neurons in autonomic ganglia. The telodendria form end-bulbs typical of interneuronal synapses.

Postganglionic autonomic neurons have nonmyelinated axons that innervate cardiac or smooth muscle or gland. Axon terminations are characterized by a single neurolemmocyte ensheathing one or more telodendria without evidence of perineural epithelium. The telodendria have preterminal bulbs or varicosities featuring synaptic vesicles within a localized enlargement that projects partly beyond the confine of the neurolemmocyte. Ultimately, varicosities are found in isolated telodendria ensheathed by only basal lamina. Thus, transmitter chemical is released from multiple sites (varicosities) and diffuses to bind with receptor sites on effector organs. The diffusion gap may exceed 100 nm, and postsynaptic specializations are not evident.

Receptors

Afferent axons convey information to the CNS from receptors or from sense organs. Sense organs are organized collections of sensory epithelium and neurons that detect visual, auditory, olfactory, or taste stimuli. In contrast, receptors are individual, isolated stimulus detectors widely distributed in the body (Fig. 6–23). A receptor constitutes the dendritic zone of an afferent neuron. Generally, an axon branches repeatedly and a receptor is located at each branch termination. All receptors of a single neuron have the same structure and function.

Receptors are classified in several ways. By location, there are *exteroceptors, proprioceptors,* and *enteroceptors,* which are found, respectively, at the body surfaces, in musculoskeletal structures, and in viscera. According to energy sensitivity, there are mechanoreceptors, chemoreceptors, and thermoreceptors. Based on structure, there are encapsulated and nonencapsulated receptors. The following is a list of common receptors, the first three of which are nonencapsulated:

1. *Free nerve endings* are found throughout the body. They detect stimulation

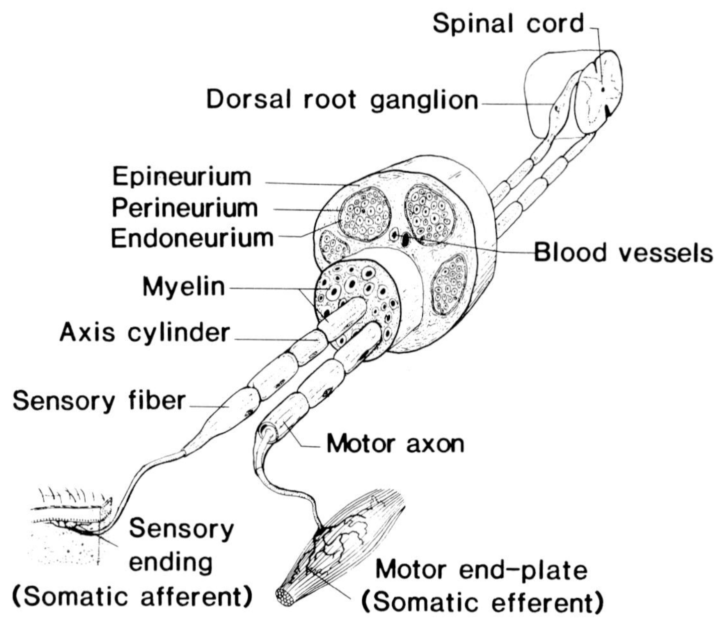

Fig. 6–19. *Diagram of nerve constituents: Five fascicles are joined by epineurium. Each fascicle is encircled by perineurium, which consists of epithelial layers surrounded by fibrous connective tissue. Within a fascicle, endoneurium surrounds individual myelinated fibers. A myelinated fiber consists of an axon (axis cylinder) surrounded by a myelin sheath within a rim of neurolemmocyte cytoplasm; myelin is interrupted by nodes. Somatic afferent and efferent myelinated fibers are diagrammed. (From Jenkins, T.W.: Functional Mammalian Neuroanatomy. 2nd Ed. Philadelphia, Lea & Febiger, 1978.)*

described as pain, warmth, cold, or touch, as well as subconscious stimuli for reflex activity. They are associated with nonmyelinated or thinly myelinated axons that branch extensively to innervate a wide area (receptive field). The receptors are simply unsheathed terminal branches, enclosed by basal lamina.

2. *Hair follicle terminals,* which detect body hairs being displaced, are derived from myelinated axons that branch extensively to innervate hundreds of follicles. Each follicle is encircled by a nonmyelinated plexus that disperses free nerve endings among follicle epithelial cells. (A different situation prevails for tactile hair follicles [vibrissae], each of which receives several myelinated axons giving rise to several kinds of receptors.)
3. *Nonencapsulated tactile corpuscles* are often collected at the base of a slight skin elevation called a tactile pad (Fig. 6–24). Each corpuscle is a terminal expansion embraced by the processes of an epithelioid tactile cell (cell of Merkel) that develops under the trophic influence of the nerve ending. Corpuscles are derived from a myelinated axon that distributes to a restricted receptive field.
4. *Encapsulated tactile corpuscles* (corpuscles of Meissner) are touch receptors found in the dermis of glabrous skin (Fig. 6–23C). Several myelinated axons give rise to dendritic branches that pass through a stack of flattened neurolemmocytes encapsulated by perineural epithelium.
5. *Lamellar corpuscles* (corpuscles of Vater, corpuscles of Pacini) are widely distributed throughout the body. A single terminal branch of a myelinated axon is encased in several layers of flattened neurolemmocytes that are surrounded by a fluid space and multiple concentric rings of peri-

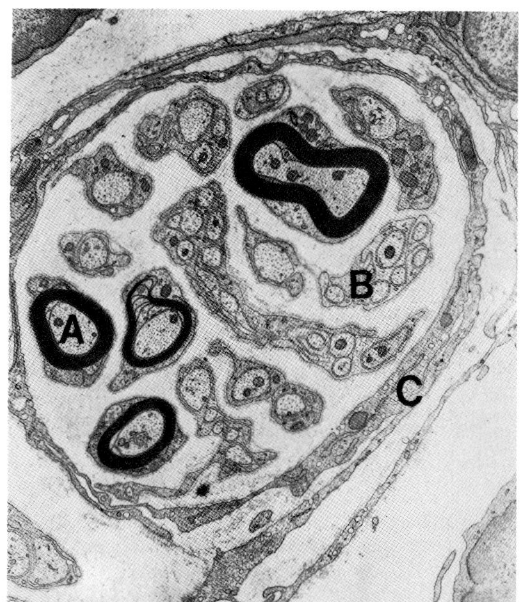

Fig. 6–20. *Electron micrograph of a small nerve (within an organ) consisting of a single fascicle. Four myelinated fibers (A) are present; in one (to right of A), a myelin incisure is evident where major dense lines have split to contain pockets of cytoplasm. Several bundles of ensheathed nonmyelinated axons (B) are seen. Layers of perineural epithelium (C) border the fascicle. ×10,400. (Courtesy of H.-D. Dellmann.)*

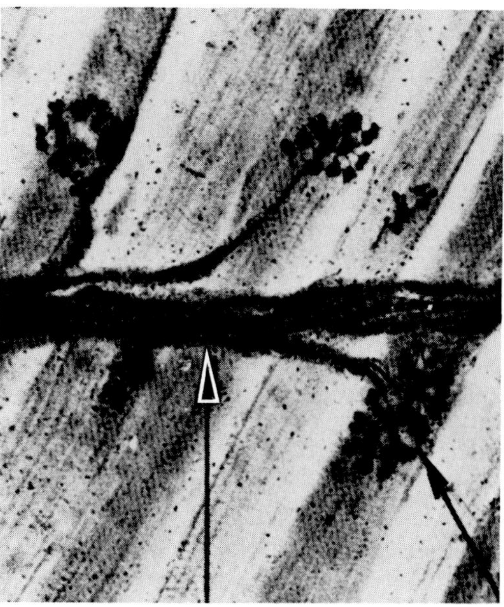

Fig. 6–21. *Light micrograph of somatic efferent nerve fibers (left arrow) innervating skeletal muscle fibers (gold chloride precipitation). A neuromuscular synapse consists of a motor end-plate (right arrow) overlying a muscle sole plate (indistinct). An end plate is formed by a profusion of short, telodendritic branches. (From Kelly, D.E., Wood, R.L., and Enders, A.C.: Bailey's Textbook of Microscopic Anatomy. 18th Ed. Baltimore, Williams & Wilkins, 1984, Fig. 10–48, with permission.)*

neural epithelium (Figs. 6–23D and 6–25). The ellipsoid receptor is large enough to be seen without magnification (0.5 by 1.0 mm). These receptors are sensitive to transient pressure, such as in vibratory stimuli.

6. *Bulbous corpuscles* (corpuscles of Krause, corpuscles of Golgi-Mazzoni, genital corpuscles) vary in location, size, and shape. They are mechanoreceptors derived from myelinated axons having highly coiled terminal branches enclosed in a relatively thin capsule of perineural epithelium.
7. *Neurotendinous spindles* (Golgi tendon organs) are located at muscle-tendon junctions and are activated by tension. Derived from a large myelinated axon, the receptor consists of terminal branches distributed on bundles of collagen fibers within a fluid-filled, thin capsule of perineural epithelium.

   The Ruffini corpuscle found in dermis, fascia, and ligaments is structurally similar to the neurotendinous spindle.
8. *Neuromuscular spindles* (muscle spindles) are so elaborate they could qualify as sense organs. Located in most muscles, the spindle consists of an elongate (1.5 mm) capsule of perineural epithelium containing afferent and efferent innervation and two kinds of intrafusal muscle fibers, designated nuclear bag and nuclear chain fibers (Fig. 6–26).

   A spindle typically has one or two *nuclear bag* fibers. Each of these has a dilated middle zone filled with nuclei; the polar ends of the fiber project beyond the spindle capsule. A spindle has several *nuclear chain* fibers. These are smaller than nuclear bag fibers,

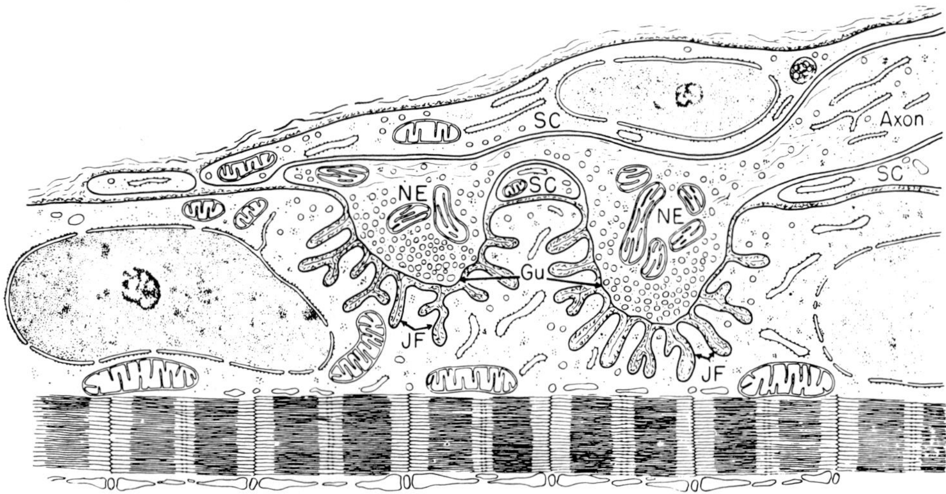

Fig. 6–22. *Schematic illustration of a segment of motor end-plate synapsing on the sole plate of a muscle fiber. Telodentritic branches (NE) featuring synaptic vesicles are in sole plate indentations (Gu). The synaptic cleft is elaborated further by the formation of junctional folds (JF). The cleft contains basal lamina, continuous with that covering the muscle fiber and the neurolemmocytes (Sc) that encase the end-plate. (From Porter, K.R., and Bonneville, M.A.: Fine Structure of Cells and Tissues. 4th Ed. Philadelphia, Lea & Febiger, 1973.)*

are contained entirely within the spindle capsule, and are characterized by a chain of nuclei at the middle of each fiber. The middle, nuclear region of both intrafusal fibers lacks myofilaments and is stretched when the striated regions contract. The striated regions are innervated by fusimotor (gamma) motor neurons that form either end-plate or trail-type neuromuscular synapses. Trail endings establish mutliple synaptic contacts as the telodendria ramify on the muscle fiber surface.

Two types of receptors are found on intrafusal muscle fibers (Fig. 6–26). *Primary endings* are derived from a single, large myelinated axon having dendritic branches that spiral as *annulospiral endings,* around the nuclear region of the intrafusal muscle fibers. *Secondary endings* are derived from myelinated axons having dendrites arranged in annulospiral or flower-spray configurations. The endings are found principally on the nuclear chain fibers, adjacent to its annulospiral ending. Both receptor types are activated by stretch of the nuclear bag and chain zones, when intrafusal muscle fibers contract or the whole muscle is stretched. Information from spindle receptors is subconscious, but it is very important for regulating muscle tone, adjusting posture, and controlling movements.

CENTRAL NERVOUS SYSTEM

The CNS consists of the brain and spinal cord. The brain is divided conveniently into brainstem, cerebellum, and cerebrum (Fig. 6–27). When the CNS is sliced, one can identify white matter, gray matter, and regions where white and gray matter are mixed in an irregular meshwork.

White matter is formed by dense accumulations of myelinated axons. The high lipid content of myelin is responsible for the white appearance. Myelin sheaths are thinner in the CNS than in the PNS, and CNS nonmyelinated axons are not ensheathed by either glial cells or basal lamina. White matter regions are divided functionally into tracts and fasciculi, based on origins and destinations of nerve fibers.

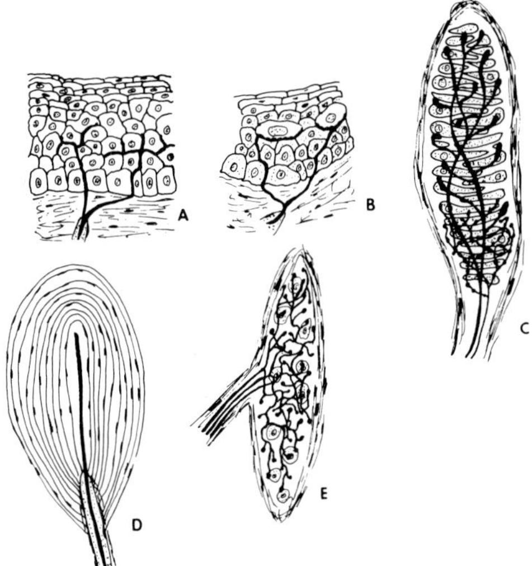

Fig. 6–23. *Schematic drawings of types of receptors: (A) Free nerve endings branching among epithelial cells of the cornea. (B) Two nonencapsulated tactile corpuscles forming relationships with modified epithelial cells. (C) An encapsulated tactile corpuscle consisting of dendritic branches that remify among stacked neurolemmocytes enclosed by perineural epithelium. (D) A lamellar corpuscle composed of a solitary dendritic process encased in flattened neurolemmocytes and perineural epithelium. (E) A spray of dendritic branches within a thin capsule of perineural epithelium; this receptor could be a neurotendious spindle or a Ruffini corpuscle, depending on where it is located. (From Dellmann, H.-D.: Veterinary Histology: An Outline Text-Atlas. Philadelphia, Lea & Febiger, 1971.)*

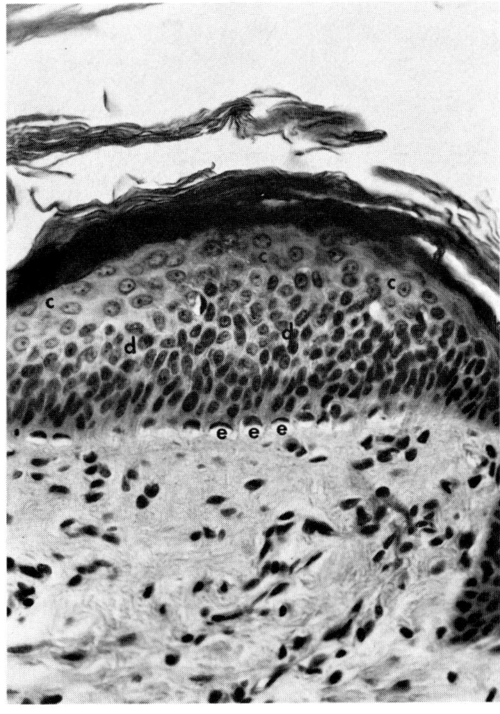

Fig. 6–24. *Light micrograph of a sectioned tactile pad. Tactile corpuscles (e) are associated with cells at the base of the epidermis (d = stratum germinativum, c = stratum granulosum). (From Adam, W.S., et al.: Microscopic Anatomy of the Dog. Springfield, Ill., Charles C Thomas, 1970.)*

An absence or sparsity of myelin results in the gray appearance of nervous tissue. *Gray matter* is rich in neuronal cell bodies, glial cells, and neuropil. *Neuropil* refers to the axons, telodendria, dendrites, and glial processes that form the background matrix for cell bodies seen with the light microscope. Most synapses occur in the neuropil. The neuropil appears dense because the extracellular space in the CNS is uniform and only 20nm wide.

Gray matter on the surface of the cerebellum and cerebrum is called *cortex.* Gray matter accumulations within the spinal cord, brainstem, and cerebellar and cerebral white matter are designated *nuclei.* A typical nucleus receives axons from one or more white matter tracts. The incoming telodendria often synapse on small neurons with short axons. These neurons may

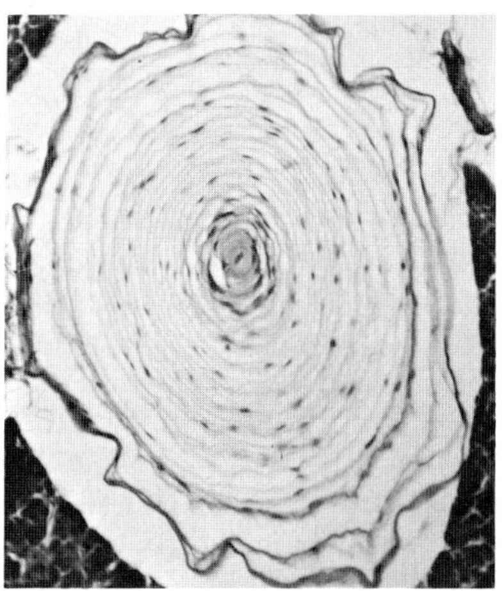

Fig. 6–25. *Light micrograph of a cross-sectioned lamellar corpuscle, pancreas, cat. A single dendritic process is enclosed by a core of flattened neurolemmocytes surrounded by multiple lamellae of perineural epithelium. (From Dellmann, H.-D.: Veterinary Histology: An Outline Text-Atlas. Philadelphia, Lea & Febiger, 1971.)*

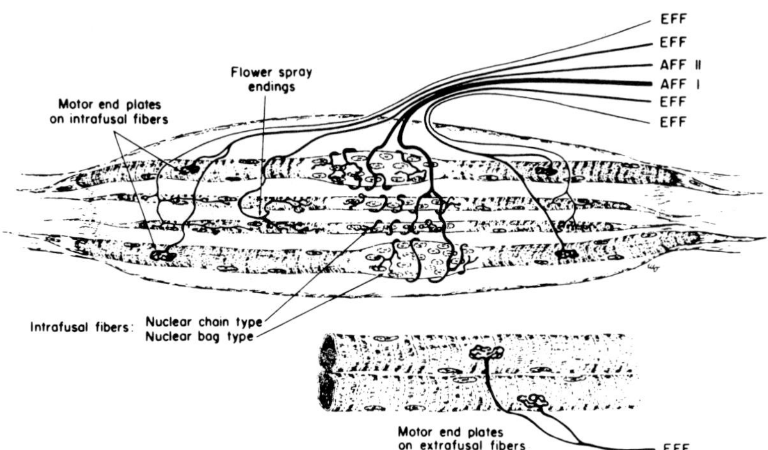

Fig. 6–26. *Diagrammatic illustration of elements comprising a muscle spindle. Within a capsule of perineural epithelium, there are nuclear bag and nuclear chain intrafusal muscle fibers (vs extrafusal muscle fibers that comprise the bulk of the muscle). Annulospinal endings around the nuclear regions constitute the primary ending of a large myelinated axon (AFF I). Flower spray or secondary endings are also shown. Intrafusal muscle fibers are innervated by fusimotor or gamma efferent axons (EFF) that terminate as end-plates or else trail along the fiber surface. (From Ham, A.W.: Histology. 7th Ed. Philadelphia, J.B. Lippincott, Co., 1974, Fig. 28–2, with permission.)*

be called *interneurons,* since they are interposed between the input and output of the nucleus. Interneurons then synapse on large neurons with long axons. These axons leave the nucleus, join a white matter tract, and usually terminate in another nucleus or cortex. It is the interneurons in a nucleus that determine the appropriate output for a particular input.

Cerebral Cortex

The cerebrum is composed of paired cerebral hemispheres. The surface of each hemisphere features *gyri* (ridges) demarcated by *sulci* (grooves). The characteristic neuron of the cerebral cortex has a pyramid-shaped cell body, oriented so the apex is directed toward the outer surface. Dendrites emerge from the apex and basal edges of the cell body, while the axon leaves the center of the base and courses into the white matter.

In mammals, all but the ventral cerebral cortex is designated neocortex, since it is phylogenetically recent. *Neocortex* is divisible into six layers, although the layering is evident in only very thick sections and the depth of the individual layers varies from region to region. From superficial to deep, the layers are (Fig. 6–28):

1. *molecular* (plexiform) layer—consists predominantly of neuropil oriented tangentially, composed of apical dendrites from pyramidal cells and telodendria from input fibers to the cortex
2. *external granular layer*—predominantly small neurons
3. *external pyramidal layer*—medium and large pyramidal neurons
4. *internal granular layer*—the primary receptive layer for modality (sensory) specific input to the cortex; composed of small stellate neurons that form a thick layer in cortical sensory areas (e.g., visual area)
5. *internal pyramidal layer*—medium to very large pyramidal neurons; form a thick layer in the cortical motor area, where electrical stimulation elicits movement
6. *fusiform* (multiform) layer—many spindle-shaped neurons. Deep to this is cerebral white matter composed of

nerve fibers going to and coming from the cortex.

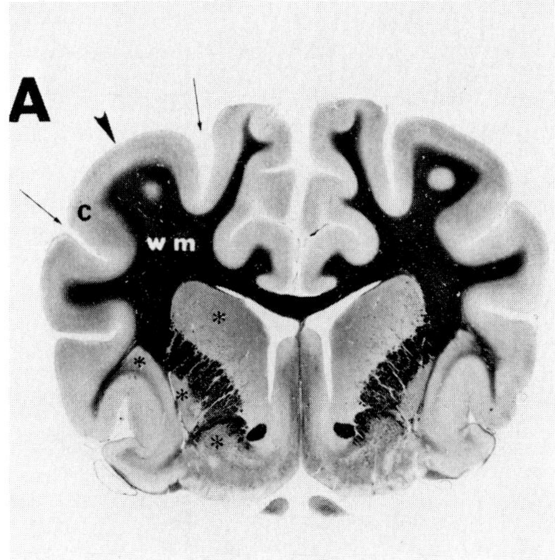

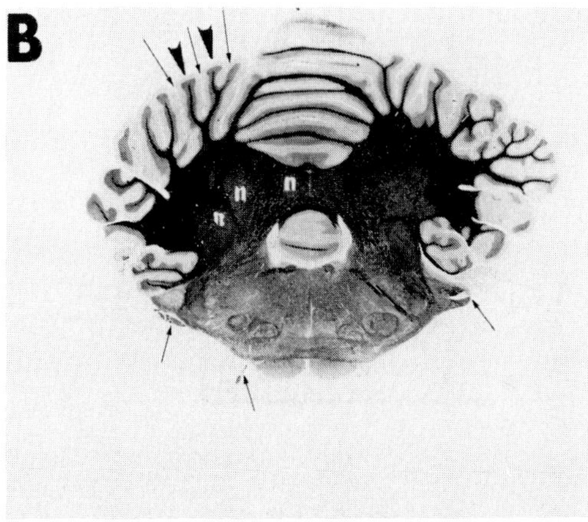

Fig. 6–27. *Transverse sections of the CNS. (A) The cerebrum is composed of two cerebral hemispheres joined across the midline by white matter (corpus callosum). The cerebral surface features gyri separated by sulci (arrowhead = gyrus; arrow = sulcus). Cerebral cortex (c) is gray matter at the surface of the cerebrum; cerebral white matter (wm) is deep to the cortex. Gray matter at the base of the cerebrum constitutes basal nuclei (*) ×2.8. (B) The cerebellum (above) is joined to the brainstem (below). The cerebellar surface features folia (arrowheads) separated by sulci (arrows). Cerebellar cortex, the surface gray matter, appears two-toned because of a cell-sparse molecular layer covering a neuron-dense granule layer. Three cerebellar nuclei (n) are located deep to the white matter bilaterally. The brainstem section exhibits white matter tracts, gray matter nuclei, regions where white and gray are mixed, and cranial nerve roots (arrows). ×2.9.*

The functional unit of the cerebral cortex is a vertical column (about 0.5 mm diameter) extending from the white matter to the cortical surface. The individual cortical columns are not histologically evident, but physiologically, all neurons within a column become active in response to a certain feature of a stimulus and become inactive in the absence of that feature. The anatomical basis for vertical columnar organization is the pyramidal neuron. Having basal dendrites oriented radially within a column, pyramidal neurons establish vertical connections by means of superficially directed apical dendrites and deeply directed axons.

Two types of input fibers enter a cortical column from the white matter. One, which lacks specific information content, ramifies in all cortical layers but especially superficial layers. It produces background excitation and represents a means of alerting selected cortical columns. The other type of input fiber conveys the modality-specific information with which the column is functionally concerned. It synapses on the small neurons of the internal granular layer, which serve as interneurons to distribute excitation throughout the column.

Output from the cortical column is predominantly from pyramidal neurons, which send their axons into the white matter. Superficial neurons send axons to neighboring regions of cortex. Neurons in the deepest two layers send axons to the brainstem and contralateral cerebral hemisphere.

Cerebellum

The cerebellar surface, which features *folia* (narrow ridges) separated by *sulci* (grooves), is coated by cortex. White matter is deep to the cortex, and cerebellar nuclei are embedded within the white matter. The cerebellar cortex can be divided into three

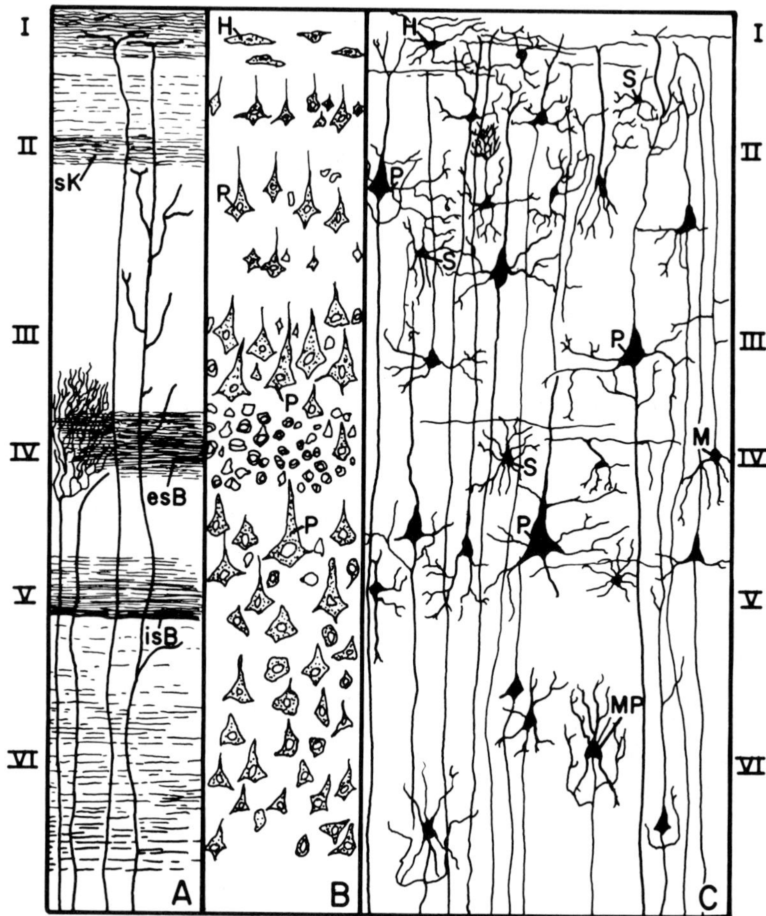

Fig. 6–28. *Schematic illustration of the six layers (I to VI) of cerebral cortex (neocortex), shown in three perspectives. Drawing A illustrates nerve fibers (axons, telodendria, and dendrites) in the cortex. From the white matter, modality-specific input fibers terminate in layer IV; nonspecific input fibers terminate especially in the superficial layers. Drawing B shows neuron cell bodies in the different layers, most of which feature pyramidal neurons. Drawing C displays individual neurons as they might be seen in a Golgi preparation. Notice that pyramidal neurons have an apical dendrite that ascends to the surface, radially oriented basal dendrites, and a single axon that courses into the white matter. (From Crosby, E.C., Humphrey, T., and Lauer, E.W.: Correlative Anatomy of the Nervous System. New York, The Macmillan Co., 1962.)*

layers (Fig. 6–29). The *molecular layer,* composed predominantly of neuropil, is most superficial. The *granule cell layer,* situated adjacent to white matter, features densely packed granule cells—very small neurons with heterochromatic nuclei. Finally there is a single layer of large cell bodies located at the interface of the molecular and granule cell layers. This is called the *piriform cell layer.*

The piriform (Purkinje) cells send axons into the white matter to synapse on neurons of cerebellar nuclei. *Piriform cells* have elaborate dendritic trees that project into the molecular layer (Fig. 6–30). Axons of *granule cells* enter the molecular layer, bifurcate, travel longitudinally within a folium, and synapse on piriform dendritic trees. Another neuron found in the cerebellar cortex is called a *basket cell.* Its cell body is located at the piriform layer and its dendritic tree extends into the molecular layer. The basket cell axon, which courses along the width of the folium, gives

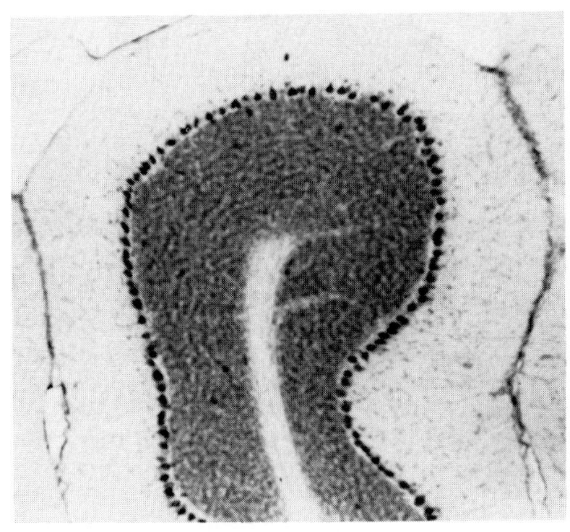

Fig. 6–29. *Light micrograph of a cerebellar folium, pig. A central band of white matter (unstained) is covered by cerebellar cortex that features three layers. From deep to superficial, the layers are: 1) granule cell layer (stained darkly); 2) layer of piriform cells (single row of cell bodies); and 3) molecular layer (relatively acellular, coated by pia mater). Nissl stain. ×38.*

off branches that form telodendritic baskets around the cell bodies and initial segments of piriform cells.

Two types of input fibers enter the cerebellar cortex. One (from the olivary nucleus) has telodendria that climb like vines on piriform dendritic trees, establishing multiple synapses-in-passage upon each dendritic tree. The other input has terminal expansions (mossy endings) in the granule cell layer. Neighboring granule cells send dendrites to synapse with each mossy ending, creating a synaptic complex known as a glomerulus.

The cerebellum regulates muscle tone, posture, and movement so that these are expressed in an appropriate, coordinated pattern. It operates in the following manner: Neurons of cerebellar nuclei are spontaneously active. They send their axons out of the cerebellum to excite brain neurons responsible for initiating posture and movement. Input to the cerebellum comes from these brain neurons and from muscle and joint proprioceptors. Input fibers excite cerebellar nuclei and specific regions of cerebellar cortex. Excitatory granule cells and inhibitory basket cells interact to produce a localized pattern of active piriform cells in the cerebellar cortex. Piriform axons, the only output from the cortex, inhibit neurons of cerebellar nuclei. Thus, the cerebellar cortex continuously compares movement initiation with movement performance and regulates movement execution by selectively inhibiting the generalized excitatory influence of cerebellar nuclei.

Spinal Cord

The spinal cord is divided into segments based on the bilateral emergence of dorsal and ventral roots of spinal nerves. Transverse section of the spinal cord reveals a *central canal*, surrounded by an H-shaped profile of gray matter, which in turn is surrounded by white matter (Fig. 6–31). The spinal cord is bilaterally divided by a *ventral median fissure* and a *dorsal median septum* (the septum is replaced by a fissure in the caudal half of the cord). The spinal cord, and particularly the gray matter, is enlarged at segments supplying limbs because of the increased nervous tissue necessitated by limb innervation.

Spinal gray matter may be subdivided into nuclei, which generally are not very distinct. The gray matter contains interneurons, neurons that project their axons to the brain, and efferent neurons that send their axons into the ventral roots. The *ventral gray column* (horn) of gray matter contains somatic efferent neurons that innervate skeletal muscle. For these neurons, the volume of the cell body is proportional to the volume of its axon and the size of the motor unit being innervated. In a number of segments, the *intermediate gray matter* features a *lateral gray column* (horn) containing visceral efferent neurons that synapse in autonomic ganglia. The *dorsal gray column* (horn) contains interneurons and neurons that project axons to distant segments or to the brain via white matter tracts.

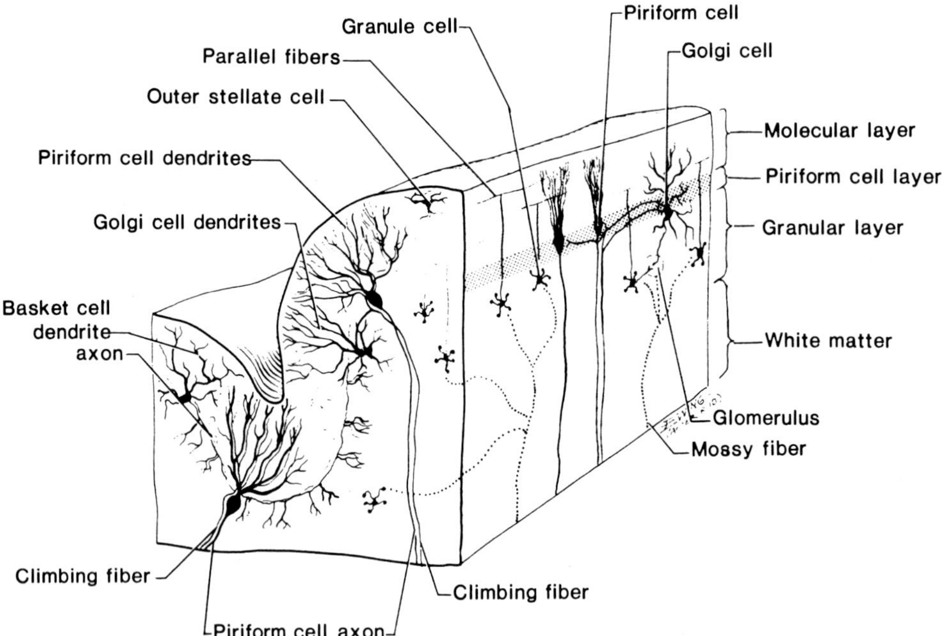

Fig. 6–30. *Schematic diagram of cerebellar cortex. The three layers of cortex and a portion of the white matter are labeled to the right. The white matter is composed of piriform cell axons leaving the cortex and two types of cortical afferents: mossy and climbing fibers. A mossy fiber (shown dotted) makes synaptic contact with granule cell dendrites, forming a glomerulus. Granule cell axons (parallel fibers) course longitudinally in a folium and synapse on piriform dendritic trees, which are oriented with broad surfaces perpendicular to the axons. The axons also synapse on basket cells (left), which inhibit neighboring piriform cells. Climbing fibers form many synaptic contacts per dendritic tree. Other neuron types in the cerebellar cortex are the great stellate (Golgi) cell and the stellate cell. (From Jenkins, T.W.: Functional Mammalian Neuroanatomy. 2nd Ed. Philadelphia, Lea & Febiger, 1978.)*

Spinal white matter is composed of fibers that belong to tracts (fasciculi); additionally, fibers destined for spinal nerves traverse the white matter. Ascending tracts terminate in the brain. Axons of descending tracts come from the brain and synapse on interneurons within the gray matter. Unipolar cell bodies in spinal ganglia give rise to axons that travel in the dorsal root, enter the white matter at the dorsolateral sulcus, and terminate in the dorsal gray column (in some cases, the axons ascend and terminate in the brain). Efferent neurons give rise to axons that exit ventrolaterally as ventral root fibers.

Bilaterally, white matter is regionally divided into a *dorsal funiculus,* between the midline and dorsal root attachments; a *ventral funiculus,* between the midline and ventral root attachments; and a *lateral funiculus,* between dorsal and ventral root attachments.

MENINGES

The brain and spinal cord and the roots of the peripheral nerves are enveloped by membranes called meninges. Meninges also envelop the entire optic nerve, which is actually CNS white matter. Meninges provide a physical and phagocytic barrier and contain cerebrospinal fluid, which attenuates traumatic forces. Traditionally three meningeal membranes are described, from superficial to deep: *dura mater, arachnoid membrane,* and *pia mater* (Fig. 6–32). The latter two are collectively termed *leptomeninges,* since they are delicate and structurally continuous. Dura mater, being thick and strong, has been called *pachymeninx.* A *subarachnoid space,* containing cerebrospinal fluid, separates the arachnoid membrane and the pia mater.

Pia mater coats the entire CNS surface, lining every sulcus and fissure. A basal lam-

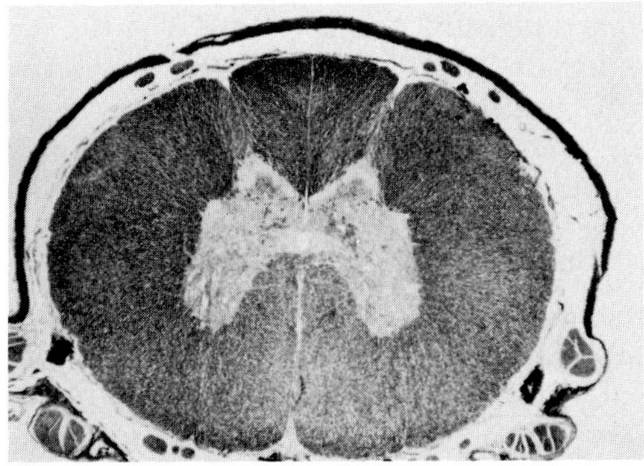

Fig. 6–31. *Photomicrograph of a canine spinal cord transected at the midthoracic region. The central canal is located within gray matter (H-shaped), which is surrounded by white matter (stained dark). Meninges and transected nerve roots are external to the white matter. The spinal cord is divided into bilateral halves by a ventral median fissure and a dorsal median sulcus. In each half, white matter is divided into three funiculi: dorsal, lateral, and ventral. A prominent dorsolateral sulcus, where dorsal roots would enter, separates dorsal and lateral funiculi. The boundary between lateral and ventral funiculi is defined by the emergence of ventral roots. In this thoracic segment, gray matter features a small dorsal horn, a subtle lateral horn, and a large ventral horn, bilaterally. Luxol blue and hematoxylin. ×18.*

ina separates pia mater from the underlying glial limiting membrane. Pia mater has collagenous and cellular components: a variable amount of loosely arranged collagen fibers located adjacent to the basal lamina, and one or more layers of flattened leptomeningeal fibroblasts that cover the surface of collagen fibers. Bilaterally along the midlateral surface of the spinal cord, pial collagen is greatly thickened to form the *denticulate ligament.* The ligament sends processes to the dura mater and thereby serves to suspend the spinal cord within the pachymeninx.

The arachnoid membrane consists of a fine net of collagen fibers coated on both sides by leptomeningeal fibroblasts. *Arachnoid trabeculae* are thin strands of the membrane that traverse the subarachnoid space and join pia mater. The entire subarachnoid space, including the surfaces of nerves and vessels that traverse the space, is lined by leptomeningeal fibroblasts. As vessels penetrate the CNS, an extension of the subarachnoid space extends around the vessel for a short distance, called a *perivascular space.* Macrophages are sporadically distributed on the lining of the subarachnoid space and leptomeningeal fibroblasts can also become phagocytic. Typically, leptomeningeal fibroblasts are flattened and joined by zonulae adherentes.

Dura mater consists of variously oriented planes of collagen fibers that form a thick, strong membrane. Elastic fibers, fibroblasts, nerves, and lymph and blood vessels are also present. The inner surface of dura mater is composed of multiple layers of flattened fibroblasts, to which the arachnoid membrane adheres by surface tension.

Spinal dura mater is surrounded by an ep-

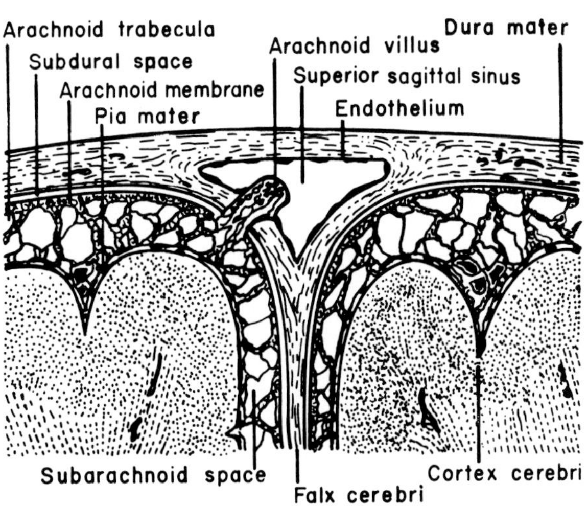

Fig. 6–32. *Schematic diagram depicting meninges at the dorsal midline of the cranial cavity. The internal lamina of dura mater separates from the external and forms a partition (Falx cerebri) between the cerebral hemispheres. A dural venous sinus (Superior sagittal sinus) is formed at the base of the partition. Arachnoid membrane is connected to pia mater by arachnoid trabeculae that traverse the subarachnoid space. Cerebrospinal fluid within the subarachnoid space drains into the dural venous sinus by means of an arachnoid granulation (villus). (From Weed, L.H.: The absorption of cerebrospinal fluid into the venous system. Am J Anat 31:191, 1923.)*

idural space within the vertebral canal. *Cranial dura mater* is formed by merger of two embryologic membranes. The internal lamina is comparable to spinal dura mater and the external lamina serves as periosteum for the cranial cavity. Two laminae are evident only when the inner one separates to form a partition between parts of the brain and a *dural venous sinus* (Fig. 6–32). Venous blood drains into dural venous sinuses, which resist collapse by means of their rigid walls. *Arachnoid granulations* are microscopic pockets of arachnoid membrane that penetrate the venous sinus wall. The granulations act as valves that permit cerebrospinal fluid to drain from the subarachnoid space into the bloodstream. The fluid can also drain into lymphatics of peripheral nerves.

CEREBROSPINAL FLUID

Cerebrospinal fluid (CSF) is produced by choroid plexuses located in brain ventricles. The fluid flows out of the fourth ventricle into the subarachnoid space. Each ventricle has one region where its wall is formed only by ependyma and pia mater; such a region gives rise to an expanded villiferous structure called a *choroid plexus.* The plexus consists of dense microvasculature in loose connective tissue coated by modified ependymal cells, called choroid plexus epithelium. The epithelial cells are joined by zonulae occludentes near the luminal surface. Plexus capillaries are atypical for the CNS in having a fenestrated endothelium.

CSF is produced by active secretion and ultrafiltration. Secretion is correlated with the development of pinocytotic vesicles at the base of each epithelial cell and the migration of the vesicles toward the luminal surface. Besides offering physical protection, CSF compensates for the lack of lymphatics in the CNS. Large molecules can pass from the CNS extracellular space into CSF and eventually into the bloodstream via arachnoid granulations or PNS lymphatics.

REFERENCES

Jenkins, T.W.: Functional Mammalian Anatomy. 2nd Ed. Philadelphia, Lea & Febiger, 1978.

Jones, E.G., and Cowan, W.M.: The nervous tissue. *In* Histology. 5th Ed. Edited by L. Weiss. New York, Elsevier Biomedical, 1983.

Kandel, E.R., and Schwartz, J.H.: Principles of Neural Science. New York, Elsevier/North Holland, 1981.

Kessel, R.G., and Kardon, R.H.: Tissues and Organs: A Text of Scanning Electron Microscopy. San Francisco, W.H. Freeman and Co., 1979.

Palay, S.L., and Chan-Valay, V..: Cerebellar Cortex, Cytology and Organization. New York, Springer-Verlag, 1974.

Peters, A., Palay, S.L., and Webster, H.DeF.: The Fine Structure of the Nervous System, The Neurons and Supporting Cells. Philadelphia, W.B. Saunders, 1976.

Porter, K.R., and Bonneville, M.A.: The Fine Structure of Cells and Tissues. 4th Ed. Philadelphia, Lea & Febiger, 1973.

7

Cardiovascular System

H.-DIETER DELLMANN
JOHN H. VENABLE

Throughout an animal's connective tissues, there is a network of tubular passages, called *vascular systems,* through which the more fluid components of the intercellular milieu flow. The fluids within the vascular tubes vary as to their constituents, but in vertebrates two types are recognized: the highly cellular and viscous *blood,* and the relatively acellular and watery *lymph.* The vascular systems conducting these different fluids are called blood and lymphatic vascular systems, respectively.

Although the vascular systems of animals arise from and are located primarily within the connective tissues, they do invade other types of tissue as well. For example, the embryonic central nervous system does not have connective tissue elements, owing to its ectodermal origin, but must depend on the extensive invasion of blood vascular tubules from the surrounding mesenchyme. Likewise, nervous tissue does not have a lymphatic vascular supply.

The presence of vascular systems and the flow of fluids within them are vital for all but the smallest metazoans. As an animal's mass increases, diffusion can no longer provide adequate exchange of the nutrients available at body surfaces with the metabolic wastes collecting at body depths. Thus, there is a direct relationship between body mass and the number, size, and structure of vascular elements.

The blood vascular systems of vertebrates form circulatory arcs emanating from and returning to the heart, whereas the lymphatic vascular systems form drainage channels, which join the major veins at the thoracic inlet, through which accumulating tissue fluid returns to the circulating blood.

Blood and lymph flow because of the pressure gradients within the lumina of their respective vascular networks. These pressure gradients arise from several forces: the pumping action of the heart, the movements of the muscular and skeletal parts, and gravity. The pressure within the vascular tubes differs from the pressure outside, and the resulting pressure gradients, coupled with the shearing forces of fluid flow, probably determine the structure of the various tubular portions composing the vascular system.

BLOOD VESSELS

Structure-Function Relationships of Blood Vessels

The blood vascular system includes the *heart, arteries, capillaries, sinusoids,* and *veins.*

These five classes of blood vessels are commonly defined by their position in the vascular circuit but are recognized histologically by their individual structures, which reflect the particular forces withstood and the control over vascular function provided by each type.

The arteries, which carry blood from the heart to the tissues, withstand the brunt of the heart's pressure-pulse and the extreme changes in blood velocity, and they control flow to the capillaries and sinusoids. In capillaries and sinusoids, blood flows slowly and can stop intermittently since its pressures are only slightly above or below those of the surrounding tissues. In veins, through which blood returns to the heart, the blood's velocity is back again to at least half that in corresponding arteries, but the pressures are reduced and sometimes reversed. Those portions of the blood vascular system that are visible with the naked eye belong to the macrovasculature. The microvasculature comprises vessels that can be detected only with the microscope, i.e., arterioles, capillaries and sinusoids, venules, and arteriovenous anastomoses.

The greatest impelling force to blood circulation is the phasic contractions of the heart. The thick *elastic, conducting arteries,* such as the aorta, receive the first surge of blood from each contraction, during which both velocity of flow and pressure reach their peaks. The great force of the cardiac blood pumped out during contraction of the cardiac ventricles (systole) is absorbed largely by the stretch of the highly elastic arterial walls; at the time of diastole, release of the wall tension partially maintains blood pressure, and the volume of flow is dissipated into the more numerous *muscular, distributive arteries,* which lead to specific organs or body parts, and eventually into the smallest branches of the arterial tree, the *arteriolar arteries* or *arterioles.* The velocity of flow is reduced in the distributive arteries because their increasing number of branches greatly expands the total volume accepting this flow. Pressure in muscular arteries remains high because of the contractile tone of their walls and the regulated peripheral outflow and overall arterial pressure.

Frequently, the elastic, muscular, and arteriolar arteries are referred to as *large, medium-sized,* and *small,* respectively. On a comparative anatomic basis, the latter nomenclature is confusing, because an elastic artery of a cat may be of smaller caliber than a muscular artery of a large ruminant. Yet within one species, it is valid to assume a relationship between structure and relative size.

From the arterial tree, the vessels open into voluminous networks of small, uniformly thin-walled tubules called *capillaries.* In the liver, the arterioles terminate with large irregular, thin-walled structures called *sinusoids.* The total blood volume in capillaries and sinusoids is so much greater than that in arterioles that the velocity of blood flow decreases from meters per second in the arterial tree to less than a millimeter per second in the capillary or sinusoidal beds. The shearing forces generated by the viscous blood flowing within the narrow arterioles decrease the pressure of the blood until it exceeds that of the surrounding tissue fluid only by 10 mm Hg or less. Thus, capillaries and sinusoids oppose only small-scale forces and have thin walls structured from single cells. It is within the capillary and sinusoidal network as well as within postcapillary venules, which have a comparable structure, that blood-tissue exchanges take place.

Blood from the capillaries and sinusoids returns to the heart via the *veins.* Veins of increasing size, usually classed simply as *small, medium-sized,* and *large,* form inverse trees, analogous to and in most cases parallel with the arterial trees. Consequently, arteries and their accompanying veins are seen together in most tissue sections. Usually a nerve and sometimes a lymphatic vessel are seen along with the paired blood vessels. However, there are specific exceptions, such as in the lung.

Because they receive blood from capillaries, veins oppose little residual pressure from the pumping action of the heart. However, they do withstand pressures caused by gravity and surrounding tissues, particularly muscle. Flow of blood through the veins results from positive pressures in the peripheral tissues in reference to negative pressures, relative to atmospheric pressure, within the thorax. This flow is augmented by a series of valves in the long veins of the extremities, whereby strong forces from adjacent skeletal muscles cause a flow that is directed toward the heart.

The small pressure gradients within the veins provide relatively low velocities of flow as compared to those in arteries. Yet the venous channels are large in comparison to those of the satellite arteries, so that the rate of flow through the two is equal.

Because veins are larger than arteries, they hold nearly half of the total blood volume, and the contractile state of the walls of the larger veins is an important determinant of total vascular volume.

Arteries, then, are the thick-walled contractile and elastic vessels of middle size, structured to distribute blood rapidly under high pressure. *Veins* are the thin, tough-walled larger vessels, structured to store and retrieve blood for use by the heart. *Capillaries* and *sinusoids* are the thinnest vessels, structured for interchange of molecules or cells between the blood and the interstitial spaces.

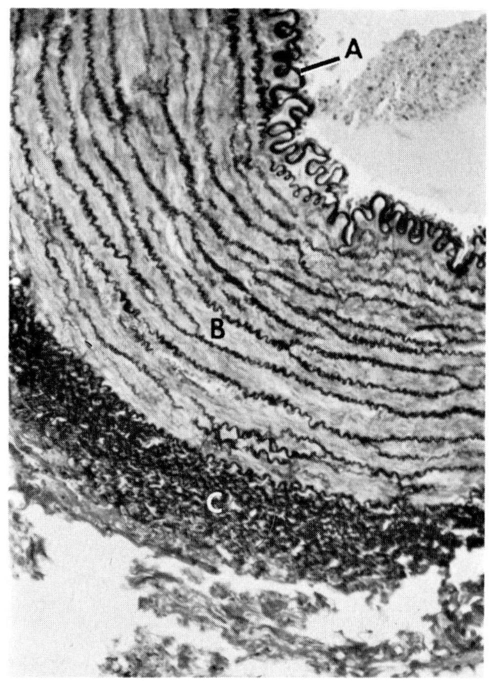

Fig. 7–1. *Cross section through part of the wall of a muscular artery, dog. Tunica intima with prominent internal elastic lamina (A); tunica media with several alternating layers of smooth muscle cells and elastic fibers (B); tunica externa predominantly composed of elastic fibers (C); its innermost elastic layer is the external elastic lamina. Verhoeff's elastic stain. ×130.*

Arteries

When viewed in cross section, arteries are seen to have triple-layered walls: the *external, middle,* and *internal tunics* (Fig. 7–1). The internal tunic or *tunica intima* includes the epithelial inner lining *the endothelium,* and the underlying *subendothelial connective tissue,* which contains collagen fibers or sheets of elastin. Usually, the elements within the tunica intima are oriented parallel to the long axis of the vessel. The middle tunic of arteries or *tunica media* is composed of concentric layers of smooth muscle and/or elastic connective tissue (Fig. 7–1). The elements of this layer are oriented at right angles to the long axis of the vessel. The outer tunic or *tunica externa* (adventitia) is a feltwork of fine elastic and collagen fibers joining the vessel to the continuum of surrounding connective tissue (Fig. 7–1).

ELASTIC ARTERIES. The tunica intima of elastic arteries is often thicker than that of the other types of arteries (Fig. 7–2). The endothelial cells have a bricklike shape and lie on a thin basal lamina. A subendothelial layer contains fibroblasts and a few smooth muscle cells, collagen, and numerous fine longitudinally oriented elastic fibers. In the large domestic mammals this layer is particularly thick. It is avascular and receives nutrients through diffusion and transen-

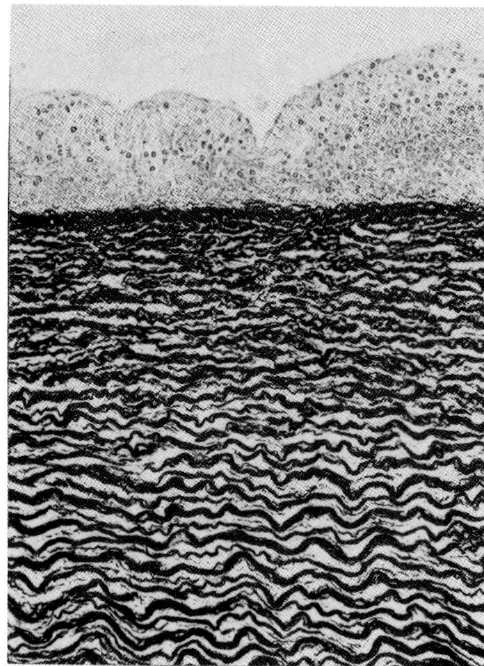

Fig. 7–2. *Cross section through part of the wall of the thoracic aorta, horse. Notice the thick subendothelial layer containing many longitudinally oriented elastic fibers. Elastic fibers predominate in the tunica media. Resorcin-fuchsin-van Gieson's stain. ×50. (Courtesy of A. Hansen.)*

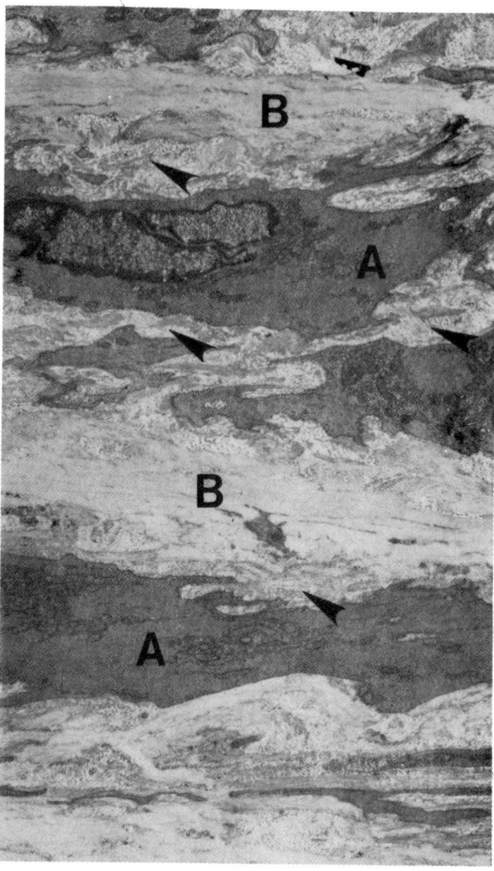

Fig. 7–3. *Part of the tunica media of the aorta, rat. Smooth muscle cells (A) surrounded by collagen (arrowheads) alternate with elastic laminae (B). ×3900.*

dothelial transport. An *internal elastic lamina* is indistinct under the light microscope; thus, a distinct boundary between the tunica intima and tunica media is not always seen. This lamina, however, can readiy be identified by electron microscopy and is often split into lamellae, the deeper parts merging with the underlying elastic laminae of the tunica media.

The tunica media of elastic arteries is the thickest of the three layers and consists primarily of concentrically arranged, fenestrated elastic laminae (Fig. 7–3). Smooth muscle cells, attached to the elastic laminae by collagen and elastic fibers, lie between adjacent laminae. In addition, there are fine elastic fibers and collagen fibers within the interstices between the laminae (Fig. 7–3). The intercellular substance is far more basophilic than that of ordinary connective tissue because it contains a greater amount of sulfated glycosaminoglycans. All intercellular fibers and ground substances of the media are synthesized by the smooth muscle cells.

The amount of smooth muscle is related to the location of the artery with respect to the heart. Generally, vessels farther from the heart have more muscle and less elastic tissue.

An *external elastic lamina* clearly defines the outer limit of the tunica media and is identifiable as a discontinuous lamella only with the EM.

In the tunica externa of elastic arteries, longitudinally arranged bundles of collagen fibers predominate, intermixed with a few elastic fibers and fibroblasts. The interlacing arrangements of the collagen fi-

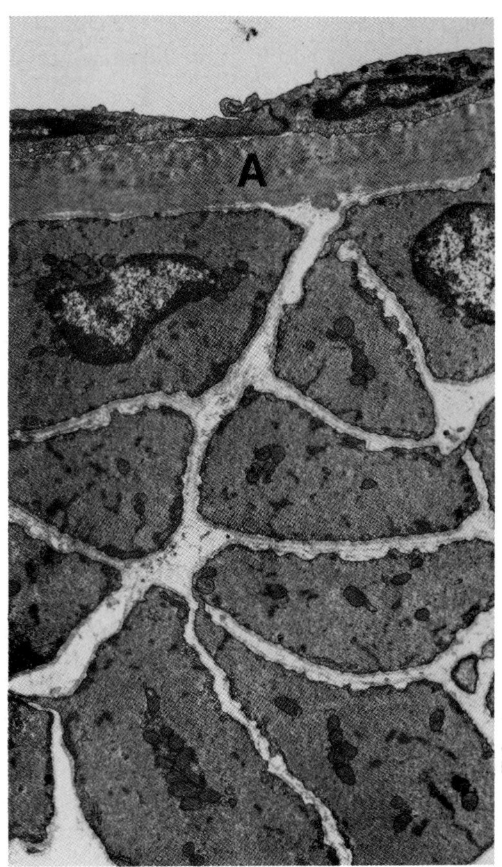

Fig. 7–4. *Longitudinal section through part of the wall of a muscular artery, rat. A thick internal elastic lamina (A) separates the endothelium from the smooth muscle cells of the tunica media that are surrounded by collagen fibers.* × *7800.*

bers limits the elastic expansion of the vessel. Small blood vessels (the *vasa vasorum*), lymph vessels, and fine nerves (the *nervi vasorum*) supply the tunica externa and outer half (approximately) of the tunica media. The remainder of the media receives nutrients through diffusion.

Transition from elastic to muscular arteries may be either gradual or abrupt. In the dog, typical muscular renal arteries arise abruptly at right angles from the elastic abdominal aorta. Carotid, femoral, vertebral, and brachial arteries commonly begin as elastic arteries but gradually transform peripherally into muscular types. The sites of transitional zones vary among species and individual animals.

MUSCULAR ARTERIES. The tunica intima of muscular arteries consists of the endothelium lying on a basal lamina, followed by a thin subendothelial layer composed of collagen and elastic fibers and a few fibroblasts and smooth muscle cells in the larger vessels. With decreasing vessel size, the subendothelial layer gradually becomes thinner and eventually disappears. The thick internal elastic lamina (Figs. 7–1 and 7–4) possesses fenestrations, through which cytoplasmic processes of endothelial cells make contact with the smooth muscle of the tunica media.

Muscular arteries are characterized by a thick tunica media, composed mainly of smooth muscle cells in the form of circular or helical wrappings from 2 to more than 40 cell-layers thick. Interspersed between these smooth muscle cells are their secretory products, i.e., elastic fibers or lamellae, as well as collagen fibers (Figs. 7–1, 7–3, and 7–4). A dense feltwork of elastic fibers adjacent to the tunica adventitia constitutes the often discontinuous and not always clearly defined external elastic lamina (Fig. 7–1). The tunica externa consists of many elastic and collagen fibers and fibroblasts and contains vasa vasorum, nervi vasorum, and lymphatics. In smaller muscular arteries, the amount of elastic fibers is substantially reduced.

When living tissues are prepared for fixation or when an animal dies, the muscular arteries contract considerably, and blood is forced out of the lumina. Consequently, the tunica intima, the underlying internal elastic lamina, and the external elastic lamina are thrown into longitudinal folds. Thus, the cross-sectional profiles of muscular arteries in most histologic preparations possess small lumina containing little blood, and the internal elastic laminae appear scalloped (Fig. 7–1).

ARTERIOLES. The macrovasculature of arteries and veins is connected by the microvasculature, which in its simplest form, comprises afferent arterioles that break up into capillary networks drained by efferent

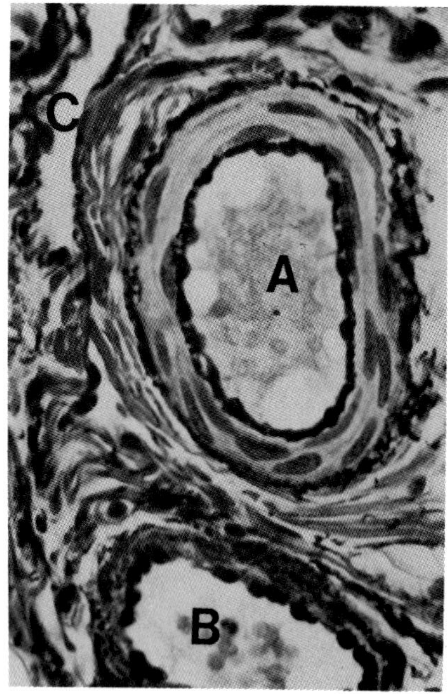

Fig. 7–5. *Cross section through a small artery (A), a venule (B) and a lymph vessel (C) in the submucosa of the esophagus, dog. Resorcin-fuchsin-hemalum-orange-G. ×500. (Courtesy of A. Hansen.)*

venules. Shunts may exist between arterioles and venules in the form of arteriovenous anastomoses and preferential channels. In many organs, the microvasculature possesses unique architectural and structural characteristics that will be discussed with these organs.

The smallest arteries, with tunicae mediae of one or two layers of smooth muscle cells, are referred to as *arterioles* (Fig. 7–5). In all species their diameters are consistently less than 240 μm in the contracted state. The functional change embodied in the arteriole is that contraction of the tunica media effectively restricts flow through the lumen. Although the effective critical closing diameter of an arteriole cannot be stated exactly, it is clear that arterioles with luminal diameters in the range of 100 μm or less bring blood flow near to zero when their diameters are reduced by 50%.

The tunica intima consists of an endothelial lining, its basal lamina, a thin subendothelial layer of collagen and elastic fibers, which is absent in small arterioles, and an internal elastic lamina. The latter is fenestrated and eventually disappears in the smallest arterioles. Basal processes of the endothelial cells cross basal laminae and internal elastic laminae to establish direct contact with smooth muscle cells (Fig. 7–6). In addition to smooth muscle cells, the media may contain collagen fibers.

It is within the capillaries and pericytic venules (see below) that exchange takes place between the circulating blood and interstitial fluid, with water and water-soluble substances leaving the arterial end of the capillaries and reentering at the venous end. Plasma molecules may leave the capillary lumen via endocytosis followed by exocytosis, a process referred to as transcytosis, through temporary transendothelial channels and fenestral diaphragms and by free diffusion (e.g., lipid-soluble substances).

Arterioles are connected directly with either capillaries or metarterioles. At their site of origin from arterioles, capillaries are surrounded by a few smooth muscle cells forming a precapillary sphincter that regulates the blood flow through the capillary bed. Metarterioles are narrow vessels surrounded by isolated bundles of smooth muscle. They give rise to capillaries, again provided with precapillary sphincters, and continue into thoroughfare channels that connect directly with venules.

Capillaries

Capillaries are tubules of uniform diameter, approximately 8 μm wide (ranging from 5 to 10 μm), whose walls are composed of endothelial cells, a basal lamina, and pericytes (Figs. 7–7 and 7–8). Their density is a reflection of the metabolic requirements of different organs. For example, capillaries are most dense in cardiac and skeletal muscle and relatively less dense in tendons. The individual endothelial cells forming the walls are held together by tight junctions (Fig. 7–8); it is not known

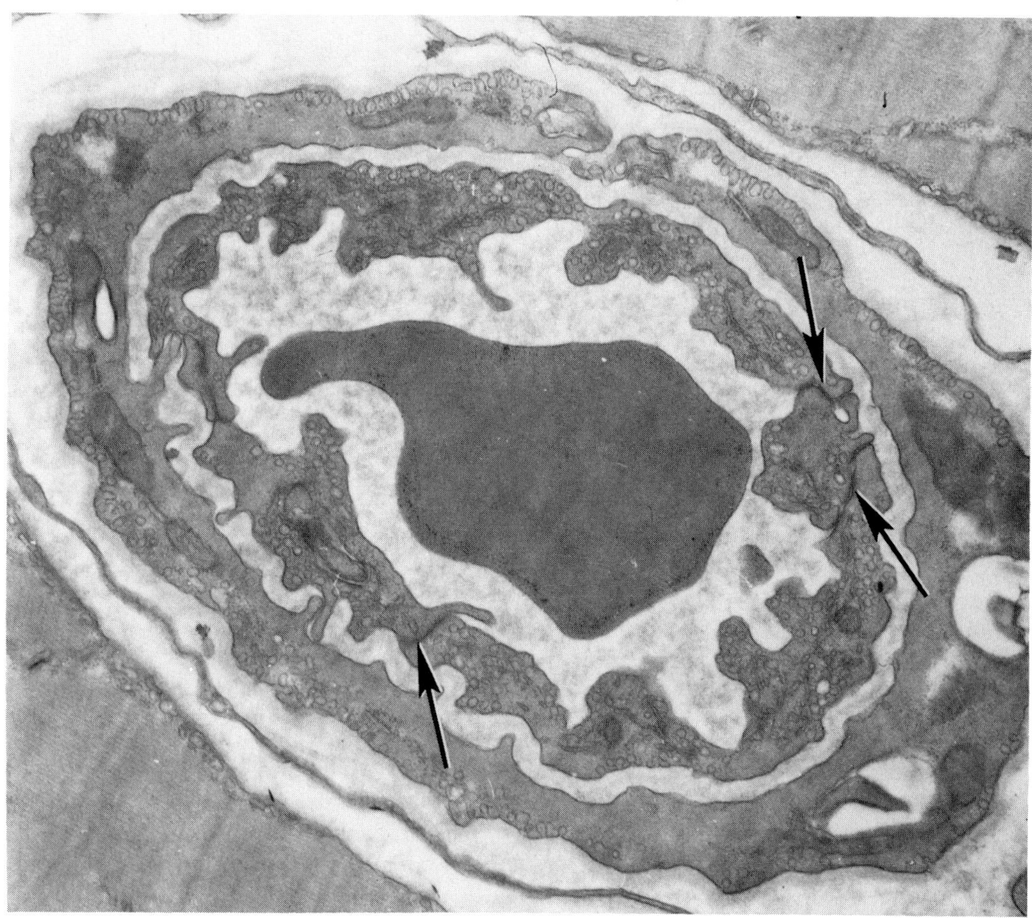

Fig. 7–6. *Electron micrograph of an arteriole with an erythrocyte in its lumen. The endothelial cells are connected by tight junctions (arrows) and contain numerous pinocytotic vesicles. They extend processes into the surrounding basal lamina, which occasionally contact processes of the surrounding single smooth muscle cell. Numerous plasmalemmal vesicles are present at the peripheral surface of the smooth muscle cell. ×19,800. (From Dellmann, H.-D.: Veterinary Histology: An Outline Text-Atlas. Philadelphia, Lea & Febiger, 1971.)*

whether these junctions completely surround endothelial cells. The endothelial tube is ensheathed by a basal lamina, which is continuous yet porous to molecules with molecular weights less than 70,000. Thus, the basal lamina serves as a molecular sieve against larger protein molecules.

Capillary endothelial cells have many unique structural modifications seemingly related to various functional states. Usually, they have minimal development of endoplasmic organelles such as mitochondria, endoplasmic reticulum, ribosomes, and Golgi complexes, primarily because little endoplasm is present. The plasmalemma and associated ectoplasm are often highly modified, and *plasmalemmal vesicles* are a common finding (Fig. 1–9). (Since most of these vesicles do not merge with lysosomes, they should not be referred to as pinocytotic vesicles.) In other regions, portions of the endothelial cells are attenuated and possess circular fenestrae, 60 to 80 nm in diameter, that are closed by thin monolayered diaphragms, facilitating the passage of substances across the endothelium (Fig. 7–9). The diaphragms are absent in the glomerular capillaries of the kidney; thus the endothelial cells are pierced by pores (Fig. 7–10).

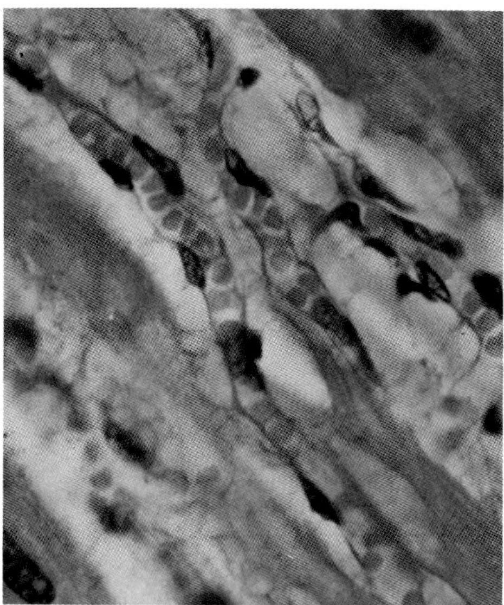

Fig. 7–7. *Capillaries in the myocardium, dog. Notice that the variable widths of the capillaries may be barely greater than or slightly smaller than the diameter of an erythrocyte. It is not always possible to distinguish clearly between the nuclei of endothelial cells and pericytes. H & E. ×750.*

On the basis of these structural characteristics, the following types of capillaries can be distinguished. *Continuous capillaries* are virtually ubiquitous in the organism; they possess either numerous plasmalemmal vesicles, as in muscle capillaries, or very few or no vesicles, as in neural capillaries (Fig. 7–11). *Fenestrated capillaries* (visceral capillaries) (Fig. 7–9) commonly occur in the gastrointestinal tract and in endocrine glands, where they are also referred to as sinusoidal capillaries. *Porous capillaries* are characteristic of the kidney glomerulus (Fig. 7–10). These modifications in structure seemingly correspond to measurable differences in capillary permeability, because fenestrated and porous capillaries have the highest permeability and neural capillaries the least, with that of muscular capillaries lying between these limits.

Capillary "buds" occur during embryonic development, whereas in healing adult tissues, interconnected, solid epithelioid cords arise by mitotic division. These cords eventually develop lumina and become functional capillaries. The endothelial cells of buds and cords have more endoplasm and corresponding organelles, particularly ribosomes, than the fully differentiated type of endothelial cells. Thus endothelium, particularly that of capillaries, has highly vegetative potentials even in adult mammals.

A cell type associated with capillaries is the *pericyte,* or undifferentiated perivascular cell. Pericytes and capillary endothelial cells have a common basal lamina (Fig. 7–8); thus, the pericyte is unmistakably linked, in satellite form, to the capillary. Pericytes have primitive cytologic characteristics, including ease of mitotic stimulation and migration around or away from the capillaries. Evidence suggests that under certain circumstances they transform into a variety of other cell types, including fibroblasts and smooth muscle cells. It is apparently by this means that a capillary can transform into the other types of vascular tubes should the internal flow characteristics change. Indeed, this description is compatible with the method by which arteries and veins develop from simple endothelial tubes during embryogenesis. Some investigators have referred to the population of pericytes around capillaries as the last vestige of embryonic mesenchymal cells available to adult animals. Pericytes also appear in the tunica adventitia of small arteries and veins.

Sinusoids

Sinusoids are present in the liver and differ structurally and functionally from capillaries. They are larger, lack uniformity in diameter, shape themselves to fill space within the confines of the surrounding parenchyma, and are more permeable than capillaries. As indicated previously, blood flow through sinusoids may be slow or nonexistent.

Large openings between and pores in the endothelial cells, with a concomitant discontinuity or absence of the surrounding basal lamina, provide for a maximum ex-

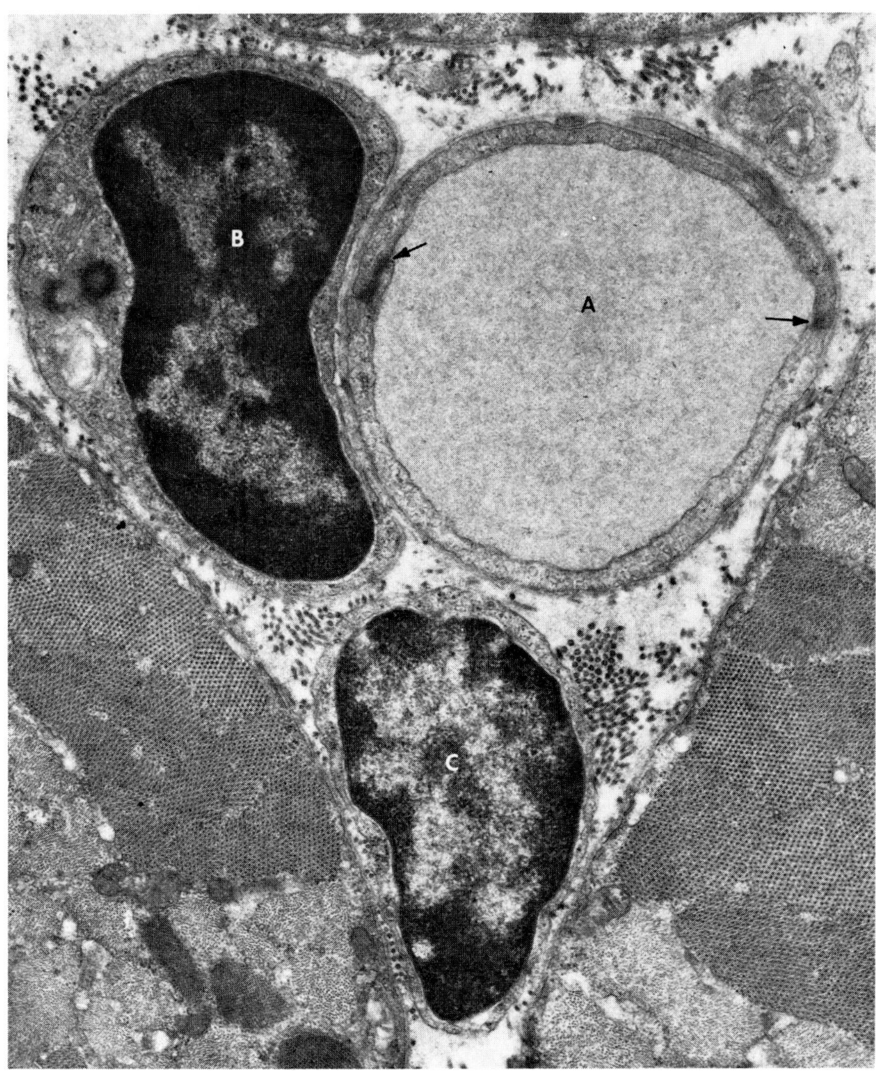

Fig. 7–8. *Electron micrograph of a muscle (continuous) capillary (A). Tight junctions are found between the endothelial cells (arrows) surrounded by a basal lamina that continues around the adjacent pericyte (B) but not around the fibroblast (C). The black dots are cross sections of collagen fibrils.* ×*16,000.*

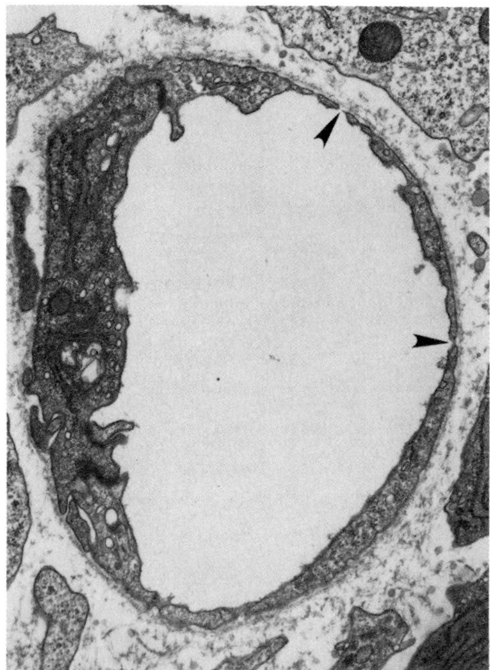

Fig. 7–9. *Fenestrated capillary in the propria of the small intestine, rat. The fenestrae (arrowheads) are closed by a monolayered diaphragm.* ×*15,600.*

change between blood and surrounding parenchyma. Mobile cells appear to pass the barrier of sinusoidal walls with ease.

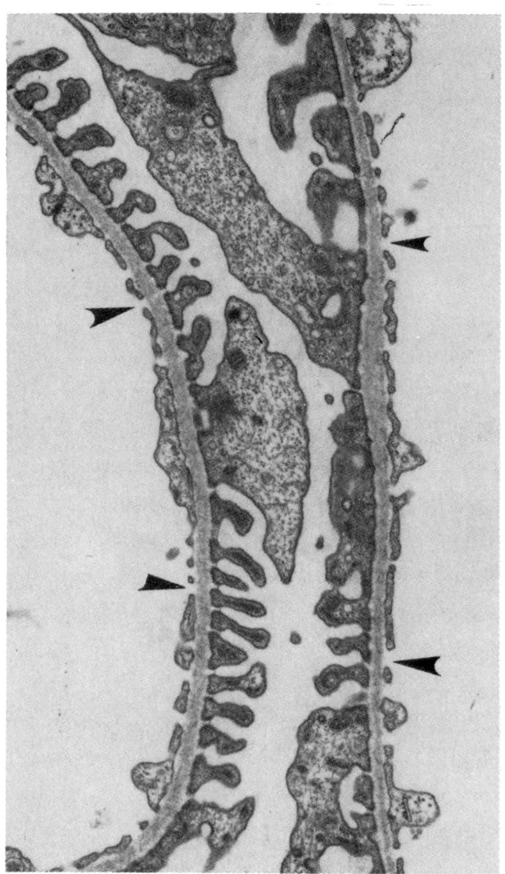

Fig. 7–10. *In the porous glomerular capillaries of the kidney, the endothelial cells are porous (arrowheads).* ×*15,600.*

Sinusoidal Capillaries

The smallest blood vessels of endocrine organs are usually referred to as sinusoidal capillaries, because they possess some characteristics of both sinusoids and capillaries. Indeed, they have a large diameter and adapt their shape to the surrounding parenchymal cells with which they are in intimate contact, separated only by a basement membrane. The endothelial lining of the sinusoidal capillaries is always fenestrated.

Sinuses

The term "sinus" is applied to blood-conducting channels in bone marrow, spleen, and hemal nodes, and to lymph-conducting channels in lymph nodes as well. For more detailed information, see Chapters 4 and 8.

Veins

The structure of veins varies within wide limits and is apparently determined by varying local mechanical conditions. Consequently, a classification of veins is difficult, especially since layers in their walls are often absent or difficult to distinguish.

The terms "small," "medium-sized," and "large" used to classify veins have only relative meaning in any one animal. The large veins of a cat may be smaller than the medium-sized veins of a cow. *Venules* are the

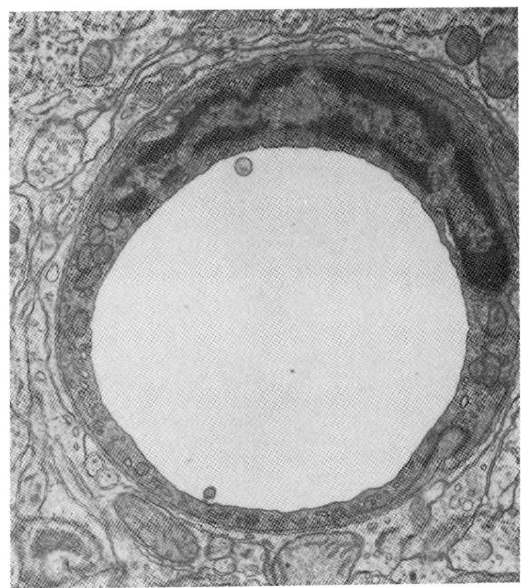

Fig. 7–11. *This neural capillary from the supraoptic nucleus of the rat is an example of a continuous capillary. ×19,500.*

smallest veins leading from capillary beds. The *medium-sized veins* correspond in function and location to the distributive arteries, but are actually *collecting veins,* because blood courses through venous trees in a direction opposite to that in arterial trees. Veins corresponding to the aorta are referred to as the great veins or *large veins,* or simply by their gross anatomic names, such as vena cava and jugular vein.

VENULES. Venules are similar in structure to capillaries but are larger, usually 20 μm in diameter as opposed to the 8-μm diameter of capillaries. The tunica intima is formed by continuous endothelial cells connected by tight junctions, a basal lamina, and a thin subendothelial layer of longitudinal collagen fibers; by occasional fibroblasts; and by numerous pericytes. This type of venule is called a pericytic venule. As the venules increase in size to approximately 30 μm, they first become incompletely surrounded by circularly disposed muscle fibers and subsequently by one to two complete layers of smooth muscle cells. This type of venule is referred to as a muscular venule. A tunica externa, containing elastic and collagen fibers and scattered fibroblasts, becomes evident.

Venules have a functional significance not made evident by simple morphologic studies. The junctions between the endothelial cells are more permeable than those in capillaries and more sensitive to leakage caused by agents such as serotonin and histamine. These compounds play a role in the inflammatory reaction, with the resultant accumulation of excessive extravascular fluid, soluble substances, and blood cells. Venules are a definite site for large molecular exchange between the vascular and connective tissue spaces. Postcapillary venules in many lymphatic organs have a special structure and significance (see Chapter 8).

SMALL VEINS. As venules increase further in diameter, they become small veins, in which appears a distinct media of two to four layers of circularly oriented, continuous smooth muscle cells, interspersed with a varying amount of connective tissue that blends with that of the surrounding tunica externa.

MEDIUM-SIZED VEINS. Because veins of the medium-size range must withstand the physical stresses of gravity and the centrifugal forces of locomotion, they have the typical three-layered wall. Basically, these tunics contain similar components and have the same orientation as those in the corresponding arteries. However, the layers are much thinner, particularly the tunica media. Because there is also considerable variation in position and orientation of smooth muscle components in different veins within the various species, attempts to provide inclusive descriptions are difficult.

The endothelial lining of the tunica intima is followed peripherally by a basal lamina and a thin subendothelial layer of collagen and elastic fibers, which condense into an internal elastic lamina in the larger vessels. Usually, the tunica media consists of two to four layers of smooth muscle with

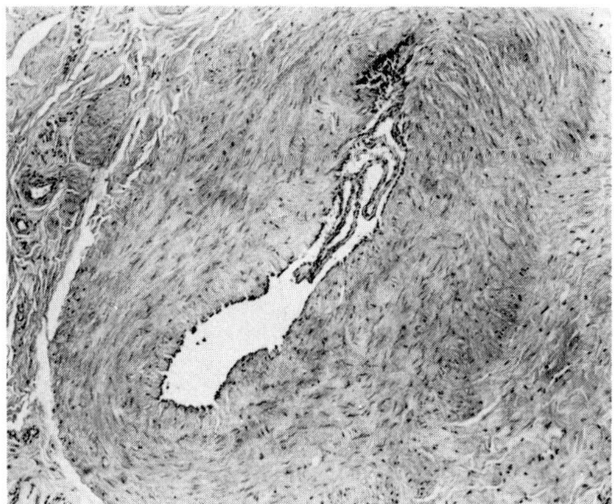

Fig. 7–12. *Cross section through a vein with a thick muscular media, teat, sheep. H & E. ×200.*

associated collagen and elastic networks, commonly arranged as inner circular or spiral and outer longitudinal layers, but there is a high degree of variability to meet particular functions. For example, the veins of the teat are characterized by a particularly thick tunica media, with smooth muscle primarily oriented longitudinally (Fig. 7–12), apparently to counteract the external forces placed on them and to adjust to the changing lengths of the teat. The tunica externa is composed of longitudinally-oriented elastic fibers and more prevalent collagen networks anchored to both the tunica media and the surrounding connective tissue.

LARGE VEINS. The tunica interna of large veins has essentially the same structure as that of medium-sized veins, often with a more prominent internal elastic lamina, the occasional presence of smooth muscle cells, and a slightly thicker, blocklike endothelium. Compared to the size of the vessel or the diameter of the lumen, the tunica media is thin and consists only of a few layers of smooth muscle cells separated by bundles of collagen fibers (Fig. 7–13). This layer may even be absent. The tunica externa, on the contrary, is prominent and composed of longitudinally or spirally oriented bundles of smooth muscle cells, together with collagen and elastic fibers that

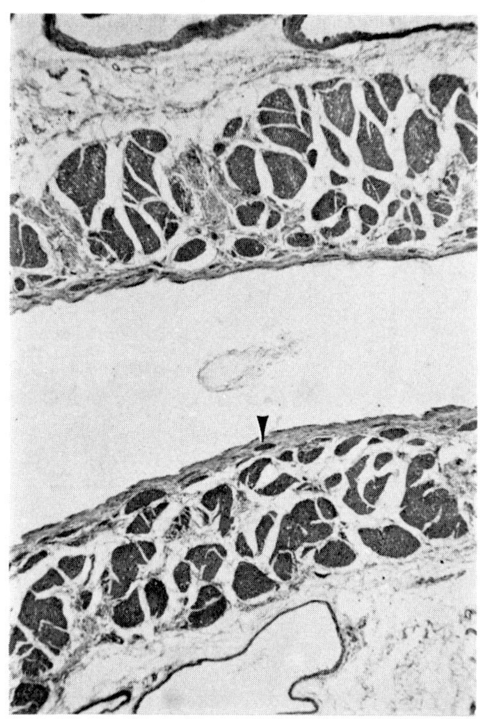

Fig. 7–13. *Cross section through part of the vena cava, sheep. The tunica media consists of a few sparse bundles of smooth muscle cells (arrowhead), whereas bundles of longitudinally oriented smooth muscle predominate in the tunica externa. H & E. ×40.*

maintain the proper tension of the wall. The thickness of this muscle layer depends on the location of the vein and is more pronounced in veins on which greater pressure is exerted by the environment (e.g., in the thoracic and abdominal cavities).

All types of veins, including venules, and especially the small and medium-sized veins of the extremities, are equipped with flap-like, usually paired, *semilunar valves* that close to prevent the backflow of blood. Therefore, blood caught between valves under the force of skeletal muscle contractions moves only toward the heart. The structure of *venous valves* is essentially the same as that of the tunica intima. Covered by endothelium on both sides, they usually have a collagen core continuous with the subendothelial connective tissue, with elastic fibers concentrated toward the luminal side. Occasionally, smooth muscle cells are present. The amount of smooth muscle in the venous wall supporting the valve is less than that found in the wall above and below the areas where the valve originates.

Specialized Blood Vessels

Many blood vessels have special structural features that fulfill specific functions in the regulation of the blood flow. An increase in the thickness of the wall is observed in vessels subjected to unusual blood pressures, such as arteries and veins of the teat, veins of the glans penis, and coronary arteries. Conversely, a decrease in the thickness occurs in protected, low-pressure areas such as the skull (e.g., arteries of the brain, dural venous sinuses), bones, and lungs. Longitudinal muscle bundles that can stop the blood flow occur in the tunica intima in both arteries and veins of the penis, ovary, and uterus. Circular, sphincterlike thickenings of the tunica media of veins perform similar functions in the large intestine, liver, and skin.

Arteriovenous Anastomoses

Because of differing functional requirements, certain areas of the body, e.g., the skin, lips, intestine, salivary glands, nasal mucosa and male and female reproductive tracts, are supplied with special arteriovenous junctions that provide direct communication between arterioles and venules without an intervening capillary bed. These arteriovenous anastomoses are short, usually nonbranched vessels that contain longitudinal, smooth muscle fibers in the tunica media at the transition between the arteriole and venule. These muscle fibers either form a cushion that protrudes into the lumen or are arranged in the form of a sleeve. This area receives a dense vasomotor nerve supply.

Several arteriovenous anastomoses in close topographic relationship and surrounded by a thick connective tissue capsule are called a *glomus*. In a glomus, the thick-walled arterial vessels are convoluted and surrounded by numerous thin-walled veins. Usually these arterial vessels are characterized by the absence of an internal elastic lamina and the presence of numerous, longitudinal, subendothelial epithelioid muscle cells. These cells are distinguished from the surrounding circularly arranged muscle cells by their light-staining cytoplasm and the absence of typical myofibrils. Numerous nerve fibers supply the glomus.

When arteriovenous anastomoses are open, the blood essentially bypasses capillary beds and is shunted directly into the venous system; when they are closed, the blood flow to capillary areas is increased. Arteriovenous anastomoses are found in almost any part of the body and are thus important for the regulation of the blood flow.

SENSORY RECEPTORS

Sensory receptors that monitor changes in blood pressure (baroreceptors) and chemical composition (chemoreceptors) are present in the area of the bifurcation of the carotid artery.

Carotid Body

The carotid body lies dorsal to the bifurcation of the common carotid artery and consists of cell groups surrounded by a dense sinusoidal capillary network derived from the internal carotid artery or the occipital artery. It is surrounded by a connective tissue capsule. Two cell types are commonly described in the carotid body: type I cells or chemoreceptor cells, which contain many granules rich in catecholamines and serotonin, and type II cells or sustentacular cells, which have few or no granules. The type II cells incompletely invest several type I cells (Fig. 7–14). Nonmyelinated afferent and efferent nerve terminals are present on type I cells. It is

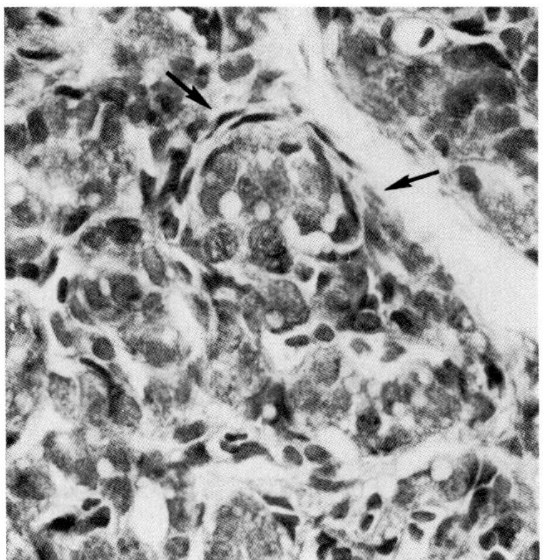

Fig. 7–14. *Carotid body, sheep. Groups of large type I cells are invested by flatter type II cells (arrows) H.& E. ×350. (Preparation courtesy of J. H. Riley.)*

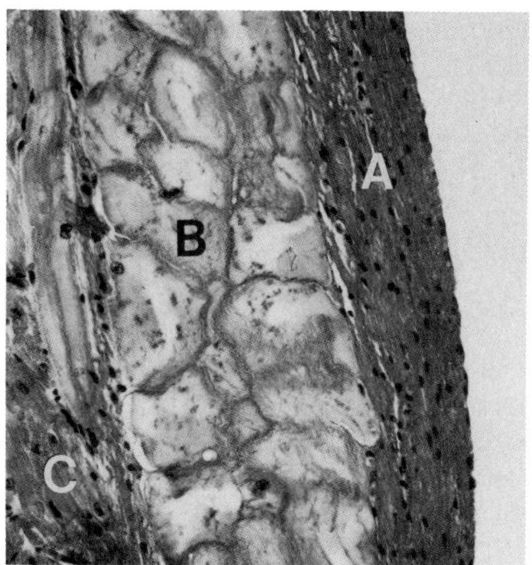

Fig. 7–15. *Horizontal section through part of the heart wall, large ruminant. Notice the thick subendothelium (A), large conducting cardiac fibers (B), and the myocardium (C). Trichrome. ×200.*

probable that changes in the concentrations of blood pH and oxygen and carbon dioxide tension generate action potentials in afferent nerve fibers by mechanisms yet unknown, triggering responsess primarily in the respiratory and cardiovascular systems.

Carotid Sinus

The baroreceptor area of the carotid sinus is a dilatation of the internal carotid artery at the site where it originates from the common carotid artery. At this point, the tunica media is thin and surrounded by a thicker tunica externa that contains many terminals from the sinus branch of the glossopharyngeal nerve. The terminals are mechanoreceptors that, when stimulated by increased blood pressure, cause reflex bradycardia, a fall in blood pressure, and dilatation of the splanchnic blood vessels.

HEART

The heart is that part of the cardiovascular system whose thick wall is composed mainly of cardiac muscle cells, capable of spontaneous rhythmic contraction, which pumps the blood into the vascular system. The inner layer of the heart is referred to as *endocardium* and is continuous with the tunica intima of the large blood vessels leaving and entering the heart. The contractile muscular layer is called the *myocardium* and is by far the thickest layer of the organ, followed peripherally by the *epicardium,* which blends with the visceral layer of the pericardium.

Endocardium

The endocardium completely lines the ventricles and atria, including the cardiac valves and associated structures. The endocardium usually consists of three layers (Fig. 7–15). A continuous endothelium on a thin basal lamina makes up the innermost layer. It is followed by the subendothelium, composed of dense irregular connective tissue with collagen and elastic fibers and occasional smooth muscle cells. The elastic fibers are particularly abundant in the atrial walls and are usually arranged parallel to the endocardial surface. The outermost subendothelial layer is composed predominantly of loosely arranged collagen and elastic fibers. Adipose cells may be present, along with a rich supply of blood and lymph vessels, and in some locations, branches of the impulse-conducting system, the conducting cardiac fibers (Purkinje fibers) (Fig. 7–15). The connective tissue is continuous with that of the myocardium.

Cardiac Valves

The cardiac valves consist of a central layer of dense irregular connective tissue and two peripheral layers of endocardium. The central supporting layer of the atrioventricular valves is composed of collagen fibers that are continuous with the fibrous rings surrounding the atrioventricular openings. Thin layers of elastic fibers are found at both the atrial and ventricular aspects of this layer. The collagen fibers of the central layer are continuous with the collagen fibers of the fibrous cords (chordae tendineae), which in turn continue into the endomysium of the papillary muscles. The semilunar valves of the aorta and the pulmonary artery have a structure essentially identical to that of the atrioventricular valves. Their central connective tissue fibers seem to be predominantly circularly arranged and are reinforced by a thin layer of elastic fibers nearest the vessel and a thick layer of elastic fibers on the ventricular side. The thickening of the free edge of the cardiac valves is due to the presence of loose connective tissue and cartilaginous tissue.

Myocardium

The middle and thickest layer of the heart is the myocardium, composed of bundles and groups of bundles of cardiac muscle cells. They are embedded in loose connective tissue that contain a dense capillary network; the amount of interstitial connective tissue is subject to local variations and is greater in the myocardium of the right than of the left ventricle. The atrial cardiac muscle cells are usually smaller than the ventricular ones and contain numerous granules of unknown significance, especially in the vicinity of the nucleus.

Impulse-Conducting System

The impulse for cardiac contraction is generated in the sinoatrial node, subsequently spreads to the atrioventricular node, and continues in the atrioventricular bundle. The *sinoatrial* node is composed of a network of thin, branching nodal muscle cells that contain numerous ribosomes and mitochondria and scarce myofibrils. These nodal fibers are separated by a large amount of highly vascularized connective tissue, containing many sympathetic and parasympathetic nerve fibers and ganglion cells (vagus nerve). They are continuous with ordinary cardiac muscle fibers of the atrial myocardium.

The *atrioventricular node* has a structure essentially like that of the sinoatrial node, because it is composed or irregularly arranged, small, branching nodal cells that are continuous with the atrial myocardial fibers and the conducting cardiac fibers (Purkinje fibers) of the atrioventricular bundle. In domestic mammals, the conducting cardiac fibers of the subendocardial *atrioventricular bundle* are readily identified by their large diameter, the centrally located large spherical nuclei, the scarce myofibrils, which are usually located in the periphery of the fibers, and a central area rich in glycogen (Fig. 7–15). In longitudinal sections, characteristic cross-striations and intercalated disks are visible. The conducting fibers connect with smaller transitional cells that lack intercalated disks and in turn connect with ordinary myocardial cells.

Cardiac Skeleton

The musculature of the atrial and ventricular walls is inserted into the *cardiac skel-*

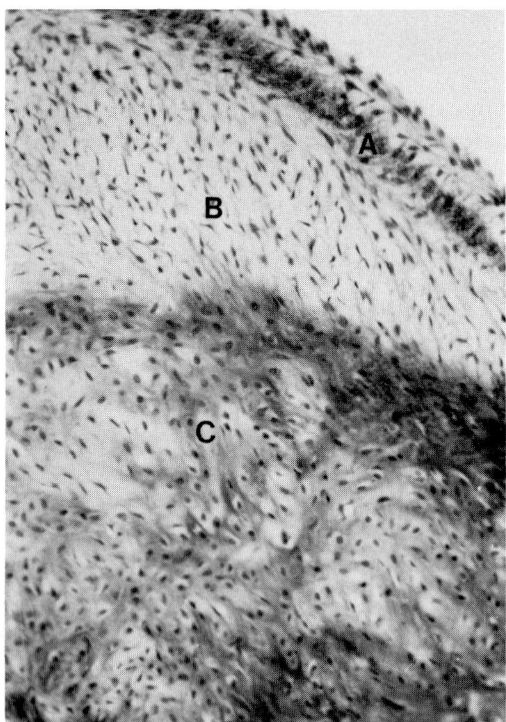

Fig. 7–16. *Horizontal section through the trigonum fibrosum, dog. The innermost endothelial layer is followed by a subendothelial layer of dense irregular connective tissue (A) and a primitive type of connective tissue (B) with many stellate cells and large intercellular spaces. The trigonum (C) is a highly cellular fibrocartilage. H & E. ×130.*

eton, which is made up of three definitive parts: (1) the annuli fibrosi or the fibrous rings, (2) the trigonum fibrosum, and (3) the interventricular septum. The *fibrous rings* are composed of intermingling bundles of collagen and a few elastic fibers that surround the atrioventricular openings and those of the aorta and the pulmonary artery. The *trigonum fibrosum* is the dense irregular connective tissue that fills the space between the atrioventricular openings and the base of the aorta. The type of connective tissue in the trigonum fibrosum varies with the species. In the pig and cat it is predominantly dense and irregular; in the dog it is fibrocartilage; however, the lacunae are often small and do not occur in any regular pattern (Fig. 7–16). It is hyaline cartilage in the horse and bone in large ruminants. Transformation of the dense irregular connective tissue into cartilage and subsequently into bone is possible in all domestic animals and probably is an age-dependent process. The *interventricular septum* consists of collagen fiber bundles.

Epicardium and Pericardium

The myocardium is covered peripherally by the epicardium. It consists of the mesothelial cells of the visceral pericardium and an underlying subepicardial connective tissue layer composed of collagen fiber bundles and elastic fibers crossing each other at various angles forming protective sheaths around blood vessels and nerves. A subepicardial layer of loose connective tissue and adipose tissue is particularly abundant around the large subepicardial (e.g., coronary) blood vessels.

The epicardium becomes continuous with the pericardium at the orifices of the large blood vessels entering or leaving the heart. The pericardium consists of an innermost mesothelial layer resting on a thin layer of loose connective tissue, followed by a thick, resistant layer of collagen bundles and elastic fibers. Like the epicardium, it can readily adapt to the normal continual changes in the size of the heart but provides a limit to overfilling of the heart and will cause cardiac tamponade should the pericardial sac fill with fluid.

Cardiac Blood Vessels, Lymph Vessels, and Nerves

The coronary arteries are thick muscular arteries and often contain bundles of longitudinal muscles and epithelioid muscle cells in the intima that regulate the blood flow within these vessels. From the coronary arteries, a dense capillary network supplies the myocardium, epicardium, the heart skeleton, and the peripheral portions of cardiac valves. Blood is collected by venules and veins that open into the right atrium either through the coronary sinus or by direct openings (venae cordis minimae).

Lymph capillaries begin in the connective tissue of the endomysium, the endocardium, epicardium, and the cardiac skeleton. They are continuous with larger lymph vessels, especially in the subendocardium and subepicardium, which are usually parallel with the blood vessels, especially in the cardiac grooves.

Both sympathetic and parasympathetic fibers of the autonomic nervous system innervate the heart. They are numerous in the atria but infrequent in the ventricles, where mainly sympathetic fibers are represented. They form extensive plexuses that are particularly dense around the sinoatrial and atrioventricular nodes. The parasympathetic (vagus) fibers terminate on ganglion cells, which in turn contribute fibers to the aforementioned plexuses. Both the myocardium and epicardium receive sensory fibers that terminate with club-shaped or platelike enlargements.

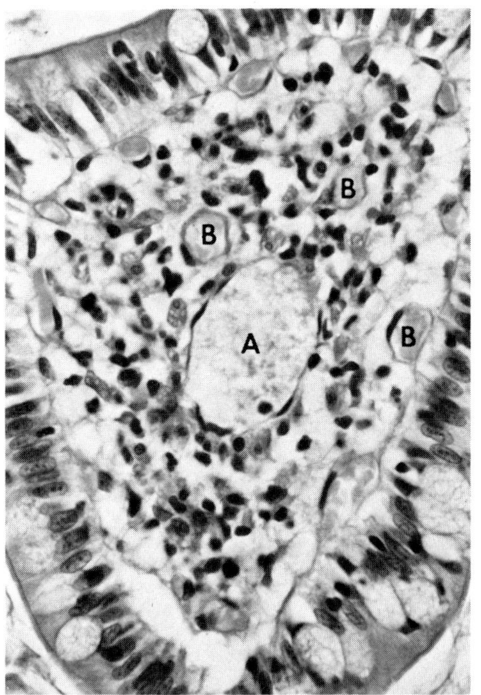

Fig. 7–17. *Cross section through an intestinal villus, ileum, dog. Lymph capillary (A); blood capillaries (B). H & E. ×435.*

LYMPH VESSELS

The lymph vascular system is an integral part of both the circulatory and the defense systems. It originates as a network of anastomosing lymph capillaries in the connective tissue of the organism. It continues with larger lymph vessels that pass through at least one lymph node and even larger collecting ducts that drain the lymph into the venous system.

Lymph Capillaries

Lymph capillaries are endothelium-lined tubes that are usually larger than blood capillaries (Fig. 7–17). Their shape is variable, and the endothelial lining is usually thin. Numerous cytoplasmic projections that protrude into the capillary lumen and into the surrounding connective tissue are observed with the EM (Fig. 7–18). Adjacent endothelial cells are joined either by intimate interdigitations, simple overlap-

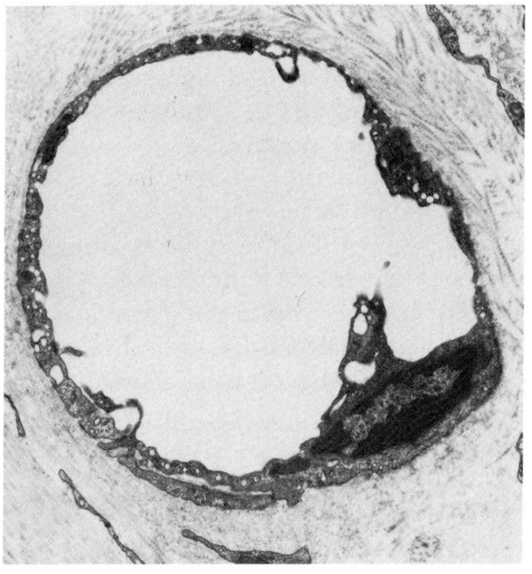

Fig. 7–18. *Lymph capillary from the propria of the small intestine, rat. Notice the thin endothelium with numerous pinocytotic vesicles and microvillous projections, and the absence of a basal lamina. ×13,000.*

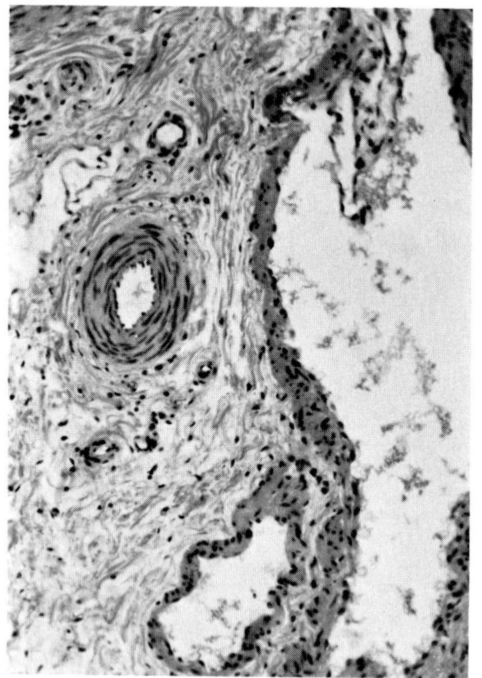

Fig. 7–19. *Longitudinal section through two medium-sized lymph vessels at the hilus of a lymph node, large ruminant. The wall consists of an endothelial lining and a predominantly muscular intima; a distinct tunica externa is absent. H & E. ×110.*

ping, or zonulae adherentes. Frequently, variably sized gaps are observed between adjacent cells. It is likely that these gaps are not stationary, i.e., that they appear and disappear continuously, probably depending on local circumstances.

Lymph capillaries usually lack a basal lamina, which, when present, is discontinuous (Fig. 7–18). Fine anastomosing filaments attach to the outer surface of the endothelial cells on the one hand and the pericapillary collagen fibrils and elastic fibers on the other. These filaments are thought to be responsible for keeping the lumina of the capillaries open, especially when the tissues are edematous.

As a general rule, lymph capillaries are found in conjunction with collagenous connective tissue containing the more fluid ground substances derived from hyaluronic acid. They are absent in organs or parts thereof that lack this tissue, such as the central nervous system, structures within the eye bulb, bone marrow, cartilage, red pulp of the spleen, liver lobules, and tonsils.

Small and Medium-Sized Lymph Vessels

The structure of the walls of these vessels is subject to great variability according to location and the species involved.

The postcapillary lymph vessels differ from the capillaries by their larger diameter and a continuous basement membrane. With increasing diameter, first a thin subendothelial connective tissue layer is present, then one or two layers of smooth muscle and elastic fibers are added. A tunica externa is not distinguishable from the surrounding connective tissue.

Large Lymph Vessels and Collecting Ducts

The walls of these vessels (ducts) comprise three not always well delineated layers. The tunica intima consists of the endothelium resting upon a basement membrane and a layer of longitudinal, interlacing collagen and elastic fibers. An internal elastic lamina is usually absent. The tunica media contains smooth muscle cells, surrounded by many elastic and collagen fibers, whose number and orientation vary with the location and species. The tunica externa is composed of collagen and elastic fibers and may contain muscle cells.

Valves may be present occasionally in lymph capillaries and are a constant feature of all other lymph vessels (Fig. 7–19). They are composed of an endothelial fold with little intervening connective tissue, except at the junction with the vessel wall. Occasional smooth muscle fibers are found in the valves of the larger lymph vessels.

REFERENCES

Bagshaw, R.J., and Fisher, G.M.: Morphology of the carotid sinus in the dog. J Appl Physiol *31*:198, 1971.

Biscoe, T.J.: Carotid body: structure and function. Physiol Rev *51*:437, 1971.

Johansson, B.R.: Size and distribution of endothelial plasmalemmal vesicles in consecutive segments of the microvasculature of cat skeletal muscle. Microvasc Res *17*:707, 1979.

Kaley, G., and Altura, B.M. (eds.): Microcirculation. Vols. 1, 2, 3. Baltimore, University Park Press, 1977–1978.

Leak, L.V.: Lymphatic capillary ultrastructure and permeability. Eur J Physiol *336*:S46, 1972.

Majno, G., and Joris, I.: Endothelium 1977: a review. *In* The Thrombotic Process in Atherogenesis. Edited by A.B. Chandler, et al. Adv Exp Med Biol *104*:169, New York: Plenun Press, 1978.

Maul, G.G.: Structure and function of pores in fenestrated capillaries. J Ultrastruct Res *36*:768, 1971.

Simionescu, N., Simionescu, M., and Palade, G.E.: Structural basis of permeability in sequential segments of the microvasculature. Microvasc Res *15*:1, 1978.

Thaemert, J.C.: Atrioventricular node innervation in ultrastructural three dimensions. Am J Anat *128*:239, 1970.

Verna, A.: Ultrastructure of the carotid body in mammals. Int Rev Cytol *60*:271, 1979.

Viragh, S., and Challice, C.E.: The impulse generation and conduction system of the heart. *In* Ultrastructure in Biological Systems. Vol. 6, Ultrastructure of the Mammalian Heart. Edited by A.J. Dalton and C.E. Challice. New York, Academic Press, 1973, p. 43.

8

Lymphatic Organs

ESTHER M. BROWN
H.-DIETER DELLMANN
LENNART NICANDER

The organism is protected from invading foreign exogenous and abnormal endogenous macromolecules by the immune system. This system includes all the lymphatic organs: thymus, tonsils, spleen, lymph nodes, and hemal nodes, and the diffuse lymphatic tissue and lymphatic nodules in the stroma of various other organs. The circulating lymphocytes and the lymphocytes and plasma cells that are widely disseminated throughout the organism also participate in this protective system.

Two types of functionally distinct lymphocytes are recognized: "thymus-derived" or *T-lymphocytes*, and "bursa-derived" or *B-lymphocytes*. Both types result from antigen-independent proliferation and differentiation of stem cells in the primary lymphatic organs (T-lymphocytes from the thymus and B-lymphocytes from the cloacal bursa in birds and from bone marrow in mammals) from which the lymphocytes seed the secondary lymphatic organs. Within these organs, B- and T-lymphocytes undergo antigen-dependent proliferation and differentiation into effector cells, which cause the disposal of the particular antigens, and into memory cells, which revert temporarily into an inactive state.

The majority of the T-lymphocytes are subtypes that have regulatory functions either as helper cells or as depressor cells necessary in regulating B-lymphocyte and macrophage activities.

THYMUS

The thymus originates as a solid epithelial outgrowth from the epithelium of the third pharyngeal pouch. Spreading of the epithelial cells gives rise to the thymic epithelial reticulum, which becomes invaded by blood vessels from the surrounding mesenchyme. Lymphoblasts, derived from bone marrow stem cells, invade the interstices, filling the spaces between the epithelial cells. The thymus is therefore appropriately referred to as a "lympho-epithelial organ."

Structure

Each thymic lobe is surrounded by a capsule of connective tissue continuous with thin septa that subdivide the lobes into partially separated lobules. The center of each lobule, the medulla, is a branch of medullary tissue that arises from a central stalk in the lobe (Fig. 8–1).

CORTEX. The thymic cortex consists mainly of an epithelial reticulum and lymphocytes. The stellate epithelial cells possess large, pale, ovoid nuclei and long, branching processes that contain numerous microfilaments and are connected to each other by desmosomes. Their organelles are inconspicuous. The epithelial cells form a continuous lining at the periphery of the lobules and around the perivascular spaces. This is an important part of the blood-thymus barrier.

Lymphoblasts and medium-sized lymphocytes predominate in the meshes of the peripheral epithelial reticulum, where they undergo mitotic divisions and subsequently differentiate into small lymphocytes that mainly occupy the deep cortex. Macrophages containing phagocytized lymphocytes or their remnants are abundant, especially in the vicinity of the medulla. Because it contains a greater number of lymphocytes than the medulla, the cortex always stains much darker (Fig. 8–2).

MEDULLA. Some of the epithelial reticular cells in the medulla have the same structure as those of the cortex; however, others are much larger and their epithelial nature is thus more obvious. They contain more mitochondria and have an extensive rER and Golgi complex, as well as granules suggestive of a secretory activity. Medullary epithelial cells characteristically form thymic corpuscles (Fig. 8–3), which consist typically of one or several central calcified or degenerated large cells, surrounded by flat keratinized cells in a concentric arrangement, containing many desmosomes and bundles of microfilaments. The cells in the meshes of the reticular network are predominantly small lymphocytes along with a few macrophages.

Blood Vessels, Lymph Vessels and Nerves

The blood supply of the thymus is derived from arteries that penetrate the parenchyma at the corticomedullary junction by way of the connective tissue septa. The arteries divide into arterioles that course along the junction and give rise to a capillary network that forms arcades in the cortex. These capillaries drain into postcapillary venules located in the medulla or at the junction between the cortex and

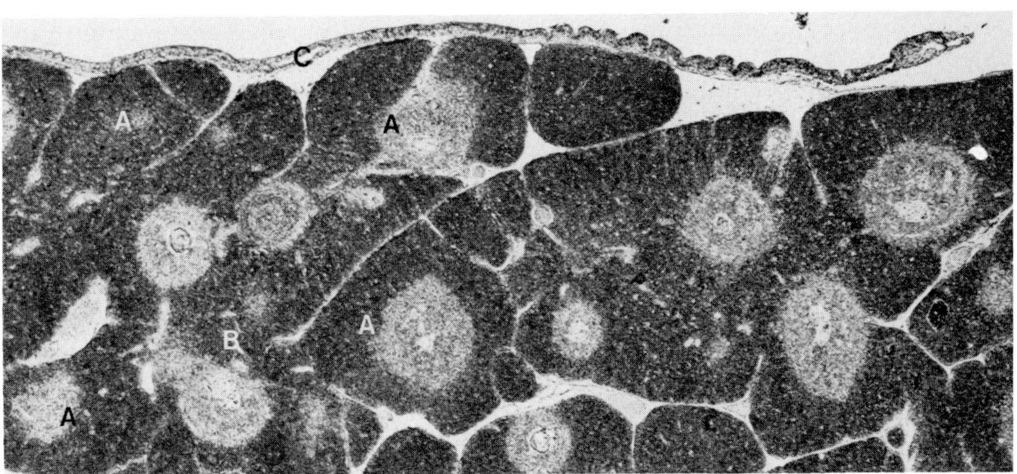

Fig. 8–1. *Thymus, cat. The thymic lobules (A) are all connected to a central lobe (B) Capsule (C). Notice the scarce interlobular and interlobar connective tissue. H & E. ×22.*

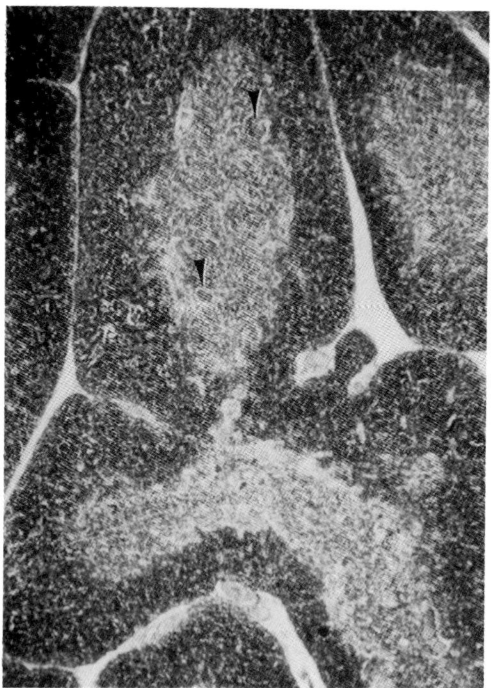

Fig. 8–2. *Thymus, dog. The dark cortex is clearly distinguishable from the light medulla, in which thymic corpuscles (arrows) are readily identified. H & E. ×39.*

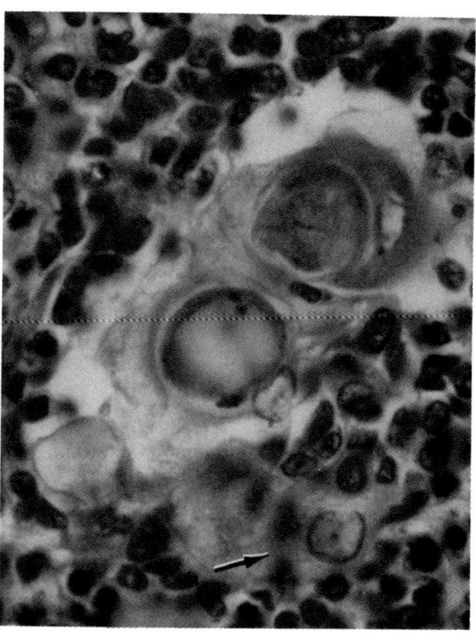

Fig. 8–3. *Thymic corpuscles, thymus, dog. Notice the arrangement of the cells in concentric layers and an enlarged epithelial reticular cell (arrow), which is probably the point of origin of a new thymic corpuscle. H & E. ×735.*

medulla; the postcapillary venules join veins in the connective tissue septa. Thus the cortex is supplied exclusively by capillaries whose continuous endothelium and perivascular space, together with epithelial cell processes, form the blood-thymus barrier. This barrier effectively prevents antigens from reaching the cortical parenchyma and prevents lymphocytes from becoming sensitized. The venules at the cortico-medullary junction, however, which are similar to the high-endothelial venules to be described later with other lymphatic organs, are permeable to blood-borne macromolecules.

The parenchyma of the thymus is devoid of lymph vessels. Efferent lymph vessels drain the capsule and septa. A network of nerve fibers derived from the vagus and sympathetic nerves accompanies the blood vessels.

Functional Morphology

The thymus is particularly active in young animals, and involution of the organ is a normal occurrence during puberty and aging. Involution is characterized by a gradual depletion of lymphocytes especially of the cortex, enlargement of the epithelial reticular cells, and invasion of the parenchyma by adipocytes, originating from the interlobular connective tissue. In adult animals, the thymus consists of narrow strands of parenchyma in which enlarged epithelial reticular cells predominate, surrounded by adipose tissue.

The thymus provides the environment in which precursor cells (stem cells) that migrated from the postnatal bone marrow proliferate and differentiate into T-lymphocytes. This process is promoted by several chemically defined polypeptides produced by the epithelial reticular cells; the exact character of this process is not known. The T-lymphocytes become blood-borne by migrating through the endothelium of postcapillary venules, and they settle within the thymus-dependent regions of the lymphatic organs. They are long-lived lymphotytes, with a specific surface antigen.

The thymus is the first organ in which lymphocytes appear during embryonic development. Since its removal in neonatal animals prevents the seeding of the thymus-dependent regions with T-lymphocytes and has deleterious consequences for a variety of immune responses, the thymus is referred to as a primary lymphatic organ, while all other lymphatic organs are classified as secondary.

LYMPHATIC TISSUE

With the exception of the thymus, lymphatic tissue in the mammalian organism occurs in two distinct forms: as diffuse lymphatic tissue and as lymphatic nodules (follicles).

In addition to lymphocytes and the ordinary connective tissue stroma, several other cell types play a vital role in immune reactions. Unfortunately, many different terms describing these cells appear in the literature. In an attempt to clarify this confusion, the following will be used in this chapter. Accessory cells include 1) mononuclear phagocytes (macrophages) of various types depending on their surface receptors; 2) interdigitating cells that have the capacity to bind antigens or cluster lymphocytes on their surface; 3) follicular dendritic cells, known to retain surface antigens for very long periods of time and located primarily within germinal centers; and 4) dendritic cells in afferent lymph.

Diffuse Lymphatic Tissue

In lymphatic organs, diffuse lymphatic tissue occurs between lymphatic nodules, in the medullary cords and deep cortex of lymph nodes, in hemal nodes, and in the periarterial lymphatic sheaths of the spleen. The stroma of diffuse lymphatic tissue consists of a three-dimensional network of reticular cells intimately associated with reticular fibers that often invaginate the surface of these cells. The reticular cells are stellate (i.e., having numerous long and branching processes) or fusiform. Their light, euchromatic, ovoid nuclei are surrounded by a small amount of eosinophilic cytoplasm that has the fine-structural characteristics of a moderately active fibroblast. The primary function of reticular cells is the synthesis of reticular fibers. There is evidence that this meshwork includes cells with antigen-binding capabilities such as interdigitating cells of germinal centers. The meshes of this reticular network are filled to varying degrees with lymphocytes, plasma cells, macrophages of various types, and other accessory cells.

Diffuse lymphatic tissue is also scattered throughout the loose connective tissues of the body. It consists of an unorganized accumulation of lymphocytes, along with a few plasma cells and macrophages, supported by connective tissue cells and fibers.

Lymphatic Nodules

Spherical aggregations of lymphatic tissue, referred to as *lymphatic nodules,* occur within the loose connective tissue of the body and in all secondary lymphatic organs.

Primary lymphatic nodules consist of a stromal network of reticular cells that have numerous processes and that are associated with reticular fibers. Small, tightly packed lymphocytes are evenly distributed throughout the stromal network.

Secondary lymphatic nodules appear in response to the introduction of antigens into the organism. Secondary nodules have a central, light-staining area called the *germinal center,* in which there is marked lymphoblastic mitotic activity (see Figs. 8–9 and 8–10). The formation of a center in the primary nodule begins with an accumulation of large, basophilic lymphoblasts and of macrophages digesting dead lym-

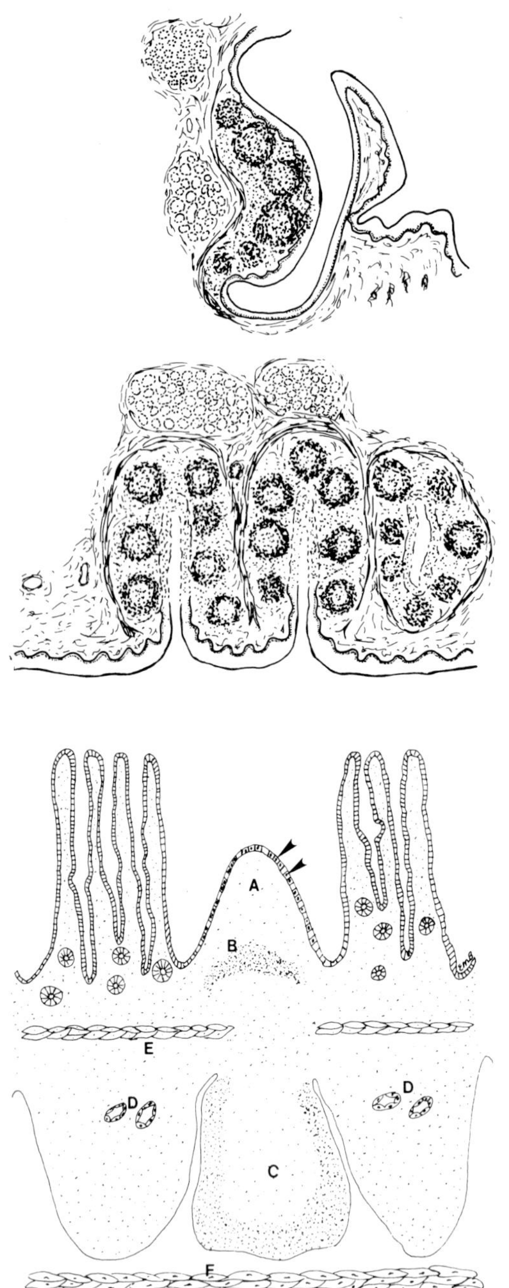

Fig. 8–4. *Schematic drawing of various types of tonsils. (1) Lingual tonsil, horse; (2) Palatine tonsil, dog; (3) Peyer's patch, small intestine. Aggregated nodules illustrating a dome or pseudovillus (A) covered by M-cells with intraepithelial lymphocytes (arrows). A corona (B) of lymphocytes over the lymphatic nodule (C). High endothelial venules (D) are in the submucosa. The lamina muscularis (E) is interrupted by migrating lymphocytes. The tunica muscularis (F) delimits the outer submucosa.*

A single layer of lymphatic nodules is in more (A or B) or less (C) intimate contact with the surface of the epithelium. (Modified and redrawn after T. Landsverk.)

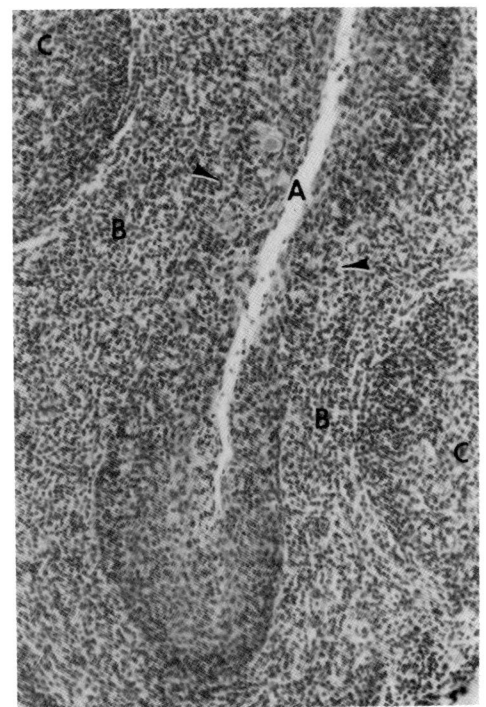

Fig. 8–5. *Lingual tonsil, horse. Tonsillar fossula (A). The lining epithelium is heavily infiltrated with leukocytes (arrows). Notice the subepithelial diffuse lymphoreticular tissue (B) and the solitary lymphatic nodules (C). H & E. ×133.*

phocytes. Modified reticular cells with branching processes, the *follicular dendritic cells,* form the stroma. Antigens retained by these specialized stromal cells are responsible for the ensuing cellular activity. Some time after antigenic stimulation all lymphoblasts accumulate in an area that stains dark. The remaining area stains light because of a population of smaller, less basophiic lymphocytes with few mitoses. This light area faces the subcapsular sinus in lymph nodes and the surface epithelium in mucosal nodules but is usually opposite from the nodular artery in the splenic lymphatic nodules. The dark area is delineated by several layers of flattened reticular cells basally. Laterally they become less distinct. Along the periphery of the light area there is a thin layer of small recirculating B-lymphocytes, which forms the inner layer of the *mantle* of the secondary nodule. The remaining portion of the mantle contains slightly larger lymphocytes, which often form a thicker cap over the apex of the center. When the cellular activity decreases the center gradually fades away because of the loss of lymphoblasts.

The diffuse lymphatic tissue below and around the nodules contains dense accumulations of small T-lymphocytes, mingled with some lymphoblasts (often seen in mitosis) and macrophages. A special type of nonlymphatic cell, the interdigitating cell of bone marrow origin, is characteristic of T domains. In addition, *specialized venules* with high endothelium, to be described with the lymph nodes, are seen here. They are the site at which recirculating lymphocytes leave the blood to enter the lymphatic tissue.

MUCOSA-ASSOCIATED LYMPHATIC TISSUE

Solitary lymphatic nodules as well as aggregates of nodules are common in the subepithelial connective tissue of most mucous membranes. They are especially numerous in the digestive and respiratory systems and are also present in the urogenital tract and around the eye. Organlike aggregated lymphatic nodules are prominent in the intestine and pharyngeal regions. Those in the pharynx and the caudal oral cavity are referred to as *tonsils.*

The tonsil is located adjacent to the lumen of its host organ and is covered by stratified squamous (oropharynx) or pseudostratified columnar (nasopharynx) epithelium. The tonsillar surface may be relatively smooth (e.g., palatine tonsil of the dog and cat) or it may have deep surface invaginations, referred to as tonsillar fossulae (e.g., lingual tonsil in the horse, large ruminants, and the pig; palatine tonsil in the horse and small ruminants) (Figs. 8–4 and 8–5). In the palatine tonsil of large ruminants, the tonsillar fossulae communicate with the mouth cavity via a tonsillar sinus. These invaginations allow for a high

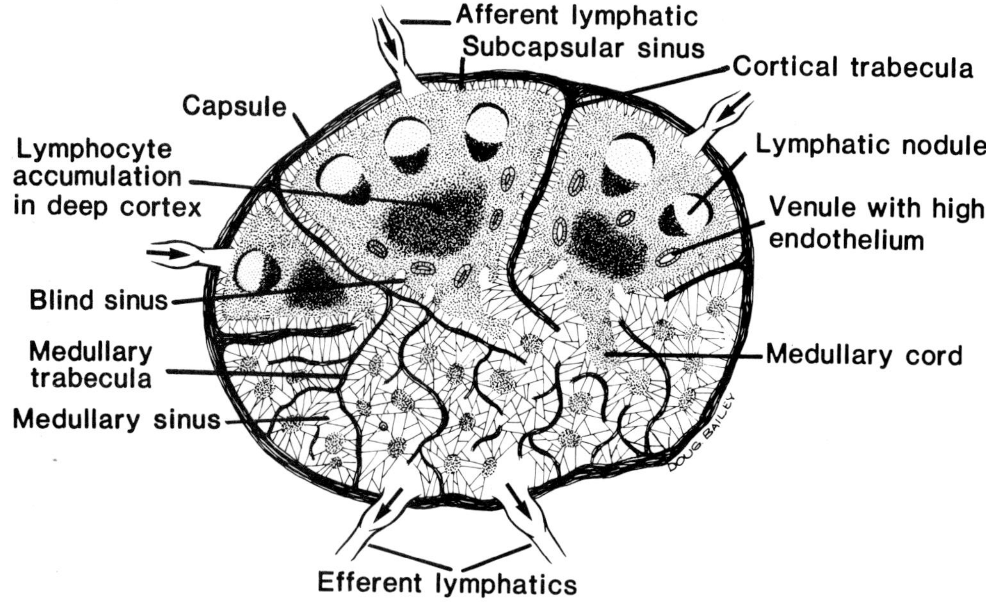

Fig. 8–6. *Schematic drawing of a lymph node.*

concentration of lymphatic tissue in a given area.

The epithelium is usually infiltrated to a variable degree with lymphocytes, polymorphonuclear leukocytes, and macrophages. This infiltration is particularly pronounced in the tonsils of the oropharynx (Fig. 8–5). Lymphocytes and other leukocytes that reach the lumen are referred to as salivary corpuscles. When they are not washed out of the fossulae by secretions from the surrounding salivary glands, these cells, along with microorganisms, may obstruct the fossulae and cause inflammation.

Beneath the epithelium diffuse lymphatic tissue with plasma cells surrounds the lymphatic nodules, which frequently possess germinal centers and a cap of small lymphocytes adjacent to the epithelium (Fig. 8–5). The tonsil is separated from the surrounding tissue by a distinct connective tissue capsule which makes its "enucleation" possible (e.g., pharyngeal tonsil of the dog). Tonsillar blood vessels have essentially the same distribution and character as those of lymph nodes (see p. 173). Afferent lymph vessels are lacking. A plexus of lymph capillaries draining into the larger efferent lymph vessels in the tonsillar capsule is found in the periphery of the tonsil.

The location of the tonsils provides the lymphatic system with the opportunity of an early encounter with infectious agents and other antigens against which antibodies can be produced. This function is thought to be carried out primarily by the local lymphatic nodules.

In addition to numerous solitary nodules, the intestinal wall contains aggregated lymphatic nodules (Peyer's patches). They tend to be most conspicuous in the ileum. Aggregated nodules in ruminants are very large and have germinal centers long before birth. In the ileum of ruminants, individual nodules are especially large and there is very little internodular tissue; the nodules begin to involute at puberty. The secondary nodules within aggregated nodules have all the lymphocytes of the mantle concentrated in a small area at the apex. The subepithelial tissue is similar to that of the tonsil and also forms the core of the

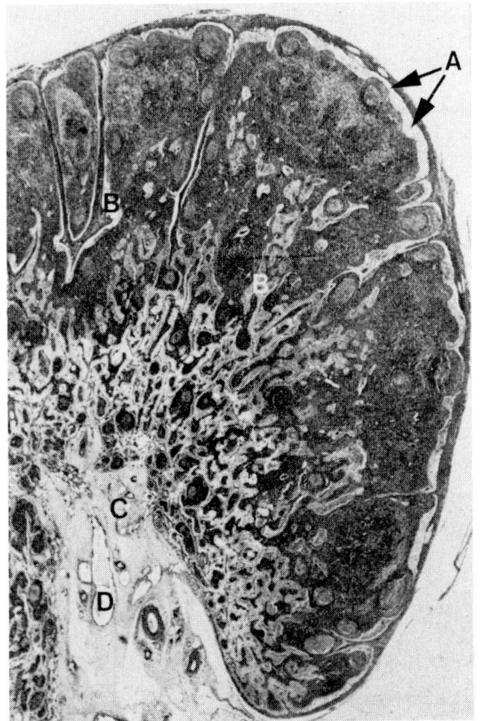

Fig. 8–7. *Lymph node, cow. The dark cortex with lymphatic nodules lies adjacent to the lighter-appearing medulla. Subcapsular (A) and trabecular (B) sinuses drain toward the hilus (C) containing efferent lymph vessels (D). H & E. ×10. (Courtesy of A. Hansen.)*

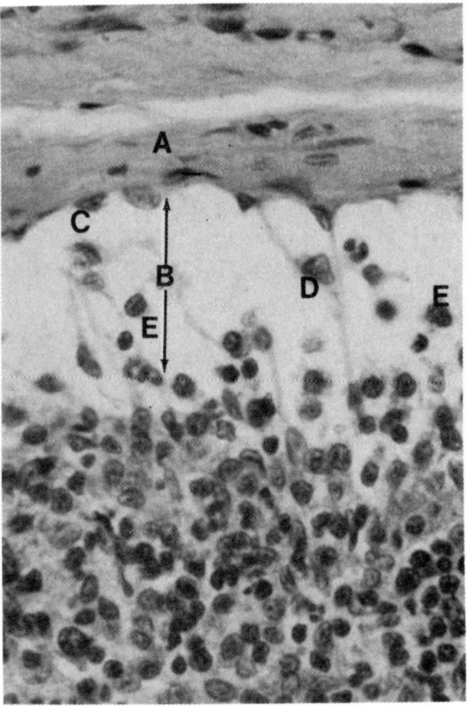

Fig. 8–8. *Lymph node, dog. Beneath the connective tissue capsule (A) is the subcapsular sinus (B) lined with endothelium (C). Reticular cells (D) and lymphocytes (E) are present in the sinus. Crossmon's trichrome. ×600.*

characteristic short dome over each nodule (Fig. 8–4). The intestinal epithelium covering the dome lacks goblet cells but has a special cell, the *M cell.* The surface of M cells has microfolds that enclose antigens and larger particles, including bacteria, from the intestinal lumen and transports them in vesicles towards the intraepithelial lymphocytes clustered at the basolateral cell membrane. From here the antigens and the lymphocytes migrate out of the epithelium into the lamina propria, where they intermingle with the lymphocytes of aggregated nodules. In the large intestine the aggregated nodules have access to the intestinal surface in deep, branching crypts.

LYMPH NODE

Lymph nodes, situated along the course of the extensive lymph vessels, filter the lymph before it is returned to the blood stream. They are the most organized of all the lymphatic organs and are the only ones with both efferent and afferent lymph vessels and sinuses. These organs usually have a slight indentation, the *hilus,* where blood and lymph vessels enter or leave the lymph node. The parenchyma is organized into a cortex of lymphatic nodules and diffuse lymphatic tissue, and a medulla of lymphatic tissue arranged in cords (Fig. 8–6). Lymph nodes provide a unique mechanism whereby lymphocytes are able to respond to lymph-borne antigens.

Structure

Lymph nodes are surrounded by a connective tissue capsule composed primarily of dense irregular collagenous connective tissue and collagen and reticular fibers, with a few scattered elastic fibers. In ruminants, smooth muscle cells are also present. Trabeculae extend from the capsule into the parenchyma as irregular septa (Fig. 8–7). They provide support for the entire node and carry blood vessels and nerves and are surrounded by cortical and medullary sinuses.

STROMA AND SINUSES. The stroma of the lymph node is composed of reticular cells and fibers that permeate the parenchyma in varying densities. Lymphocytes, macrophages, and plasma cells are supported by this reticular meshwork.

The afferent lymph vessels enter the lymph node at its periphery and, after having pierced the capsule, open into the subcapsular sinus. At the hilus, the subcapsular sinus is continuous with the efferent lymph vessel. From the subcapsular sinus arise cortical or trabecular sinuses that accompany the trabeculae and continue into the medullary sinuses. These sinuses form a network of branching and anastomosing channels (between the medullary cords) that converge toward the hilus to open into the efferent lymphatics.

The sinuses are lined by endothelial cells that form a continuous lining toward the capsule and trabeculae but often a discontinuous one toward the parenchyma of the node. The lumina of the sinuses are traversed by a dense network of interconnected reticular cells similar to the lining cells and attached to the sinus walls through numerous slender processes (Fig. 8–8). It is difficult to separate macrophages from the endothelial and reticular cells in the light microscope. For many years it was believed that the latter two cells were extremely phagocytic; thus the term *reticuloendothelial system* was coined. However, it is now firmly established that only the macrophages, not the reticular or endothelial cells, are true phagocytes. This has brought about the term *Mononuclear Phagocyte System (MPS)* described in Chapter 4. In the medullary sinuses, especially in ruminants, the sinus endothelium has marked pinocytotic activity and many inclusions of a lysosomal character.

Lymphocytes, macrophages, and other accessory cells lie free within the stromal mesh and in the sinus lumen. In all probability, the reticular cells function as a baffle to slow lymph flow within the sinuses to facilitate antigen-cell interactions as well as the phagocytic activities of the macrophages.

Lymph percolates into the parenchyma through gaps in the sinus walls. This gives the parenchymal cells access to lymph-borne antigens, cells, and particulate matter.

CORTEX. Most of the outer cortex is made up of typical primary and secondary lymphatic nodules. (Figs. 8–7 and 8–9). The inner cortex is more homogeneous, but in some places many lymphocytes are in juxtaposition to vascular areas. Blind, smooth-walled evaginations of the medullary sinuses extend into the inner cortex (Fig. 8–6). Functionally, the middle-to-deep part of the cortex or paracortical area is referred to as a *thymus-dependent zone,* indicating that the lymphocytes in this region originate from the thymus. This information comes from the results of transplantation experiments. Thymus lymphocytes from thymus tissue transplanted into mice thymectomized at birth migrate to that specific part of the cortex. The significance of this will be discussed with lymphocyte production and immune responses.

MEDULLA. The medulla is much less organized than the cortex. The lymphatic tissue extends from the thymus-dependent cortical zone as *medullary cords,* which branch and anastomose throughout the medulla (Fig. 8–10). These medullary cords are separated by a network of endothelium-lined sinuses and connective tissue trabeculae (Fig. 8–11) and are composed of lymphocytes, plasma cells and macrophages held in a stromal mesh.

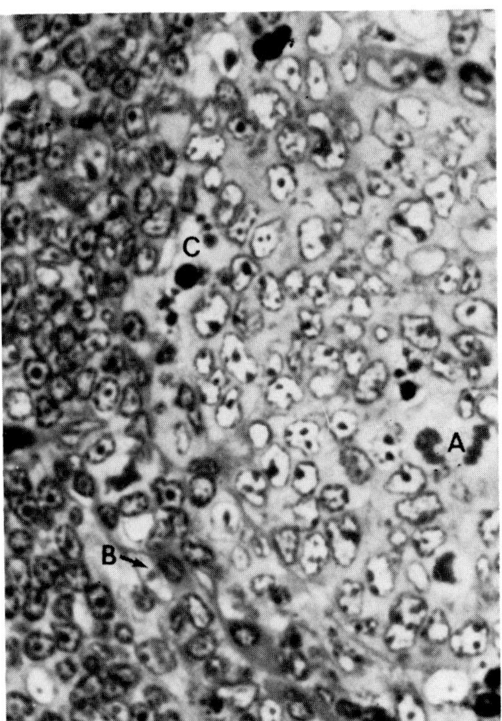

Fig. 8–9. *Part of lymphatic nodule, pig. The light area (right) is the dark part of the germinal center, with lymphoblasts, one in mitosis (A), and macrophages digesting lymphocytes (C). The mantle (left) is made up of small lymphocytes. The nucleus of one reticular cell (B) is evident. Epon. Toluidine blue. ×880.*

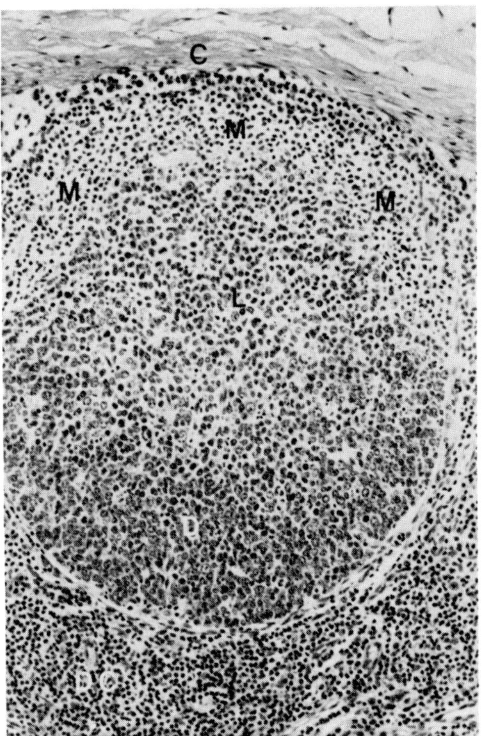

Fig. 8–10. *Lymph node, goat. Secondary lymphatic nodule with germinal center. Dark area (D); light area (L); mantle (M); capsule (C); deep cortex (DC). H & E. ×150.*

Lymph Vessels

Afferent lymphatics penetrate the capsule at several different sites and efferent vessels leave the node at a small indentation, the hilus. There are valves in both the afferent and efferent lymph vessels, thereby ensuring a one-way flow (Fig. 8–7).

As the lymph enters the node through the afferent vessels, it enters the *subcapsular sinus.* From here it may follow one of two possible routes to the efferent lymph vessels at the hilus. Most of it circulates through the subcapsular, trabecular, and medullary sinuses, but some percolates through the cortex and medullary cords to reach the medullary sinuses. Finally, all lymph leaves the node through the efferent lymph vessels (Fig. 8–6).

Blood Vessels and Nerves

The major arteries enter the lymph node at the hilus, whereas smaller vessels penetrate the capsule at various sites. On entering the hilus, the arteries give off some branches that supply the medullary cords directly; other branches enter the trabeculae to supply the connective tissue and capsule. Those supplying the medullary cords give off capillaries along their course, and the main vessels enter the cortex where branches feed capillary networks between and in the nodules. The internodular branches form arcades below the subcapsular sinus and then continue inward to form *postcapillary venules* in the inner cortex. These are long vessels, lined by a cuboidal endothelium. It is here that large numbers of recirculating lymphocytes migrate from the blood into the lymphatic tissue. The lymphocytes slide between the

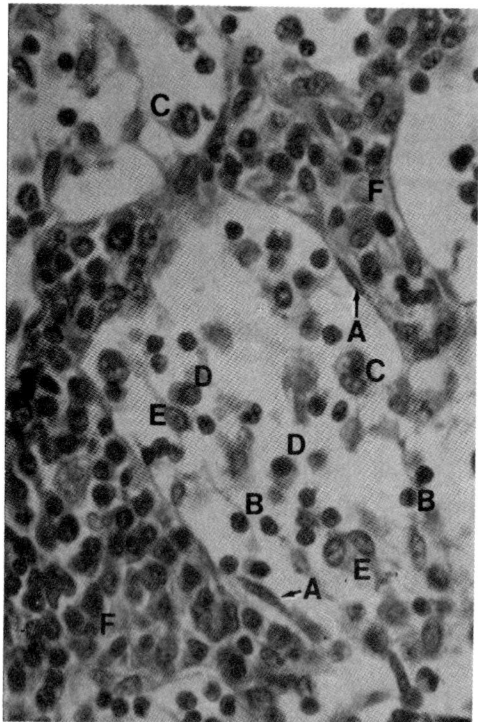

Fig. 8–11. *Lymph node medulla, dog. Endothelium (A) lines the sinus containing lymphocytes (B), macrophages (C), plasma cells (D) and reticular cells (E). Lymphatic cords (F) are composed of lymphocytes, macrophages and plasma cells. Crossmon's trichrome. ×600.*

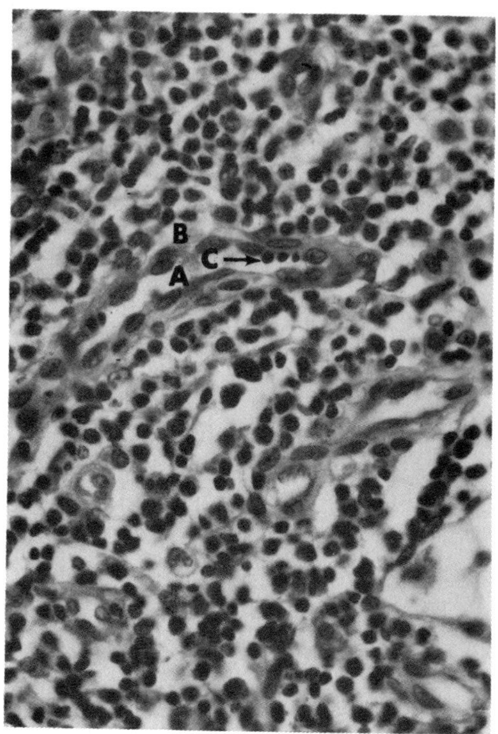

Fig. 8–12. *Lymph node, dog. Postcapillary venule (A), in paracortical area lined with cuboidal endothelium (B), has lymphocytes (C) migrating through the endothelium. H & E. ×425.*

endothelial cells when the intercellular tight junctions open temporarily and then close behind the emigrating lymphocytes before they continue into the subendothelial tissue (Figs. 8–12 and 8–13). The postcapillary venules join veins in the medullary trabeculae, which in turn empty into large veins that leave at the hilus.

Vasomotor nerves form perivascular networks throughout the lymph node. In addition, there are nerve fibers in the capsule and trabeculae that are independent of blood vessels.

Species Differences

Pig lymph nodes are markedly different from those of most other mammals (Fig. 8–14). The cortical and medullary tissues are reversed, with most nodules occupying a deep position along trabecular sinuses. Areas similar to the deep cortex in ordinary lymph nodes, with many high endothelial venules, are seen near the groups of nodules, but the periphery is occupied primarily by a loose unorganized tissue containing macrophages and plasma cells. The sinuses are narrow and medullary cords are absent. Moreover, the afferent lymph vessels enter the capsule at one or more sites and penetrate deep into the area occupied by the lymphatic nodules where they join the trabecular sinuses. The lymph then filters into the peripheral sinuses, which converge and form several efferent vessels at the periphery of the node. Functionally, the flow of the lymph is identical with that in lymph nodes of other animals because the incoming lymph first reaches the lymphatic nodules. However, the ef-

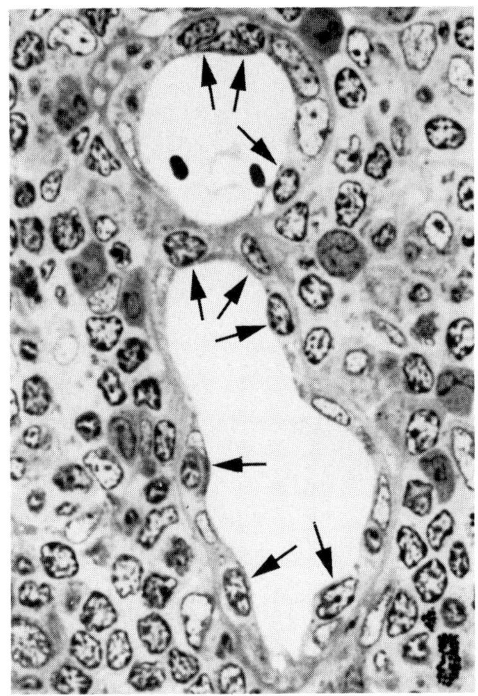

Fig. 8–13. *Lymph node, goat. High endothelium in postcapillary venule with many migrating lymphocytes (arrows). Vascular perfusion, Epon. Toluidine blue. ×1000.*

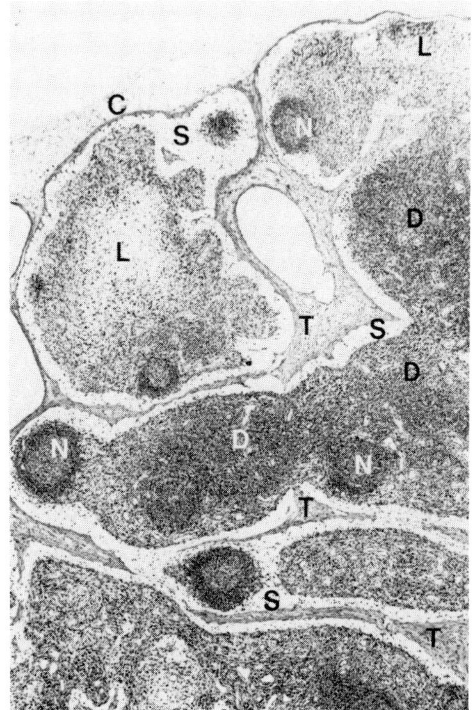

Fig. 8–14. *Lymph node, pig. Capsule (C); trabeculae (T); nodules (N) along trabecular sinuses (S); "deep" cortex (D); loose peripheral tissue (L). Vascular perfusion. H & E. ×100.*

ferent lymph is very poor in lymphocytes compared to that of other species.

The blood vessels enter with the afferent lymph vessels and exit with the efferent vessels. As a result, a definitive hilus may not always be seen; rather, there are microscopic hilus-like indentations wherever afferent lymph vessels enter. It is not uncommon for many small lymph nodes to fuse, forming a large cluster of nodes, and this may account for the fact that a hilus is often difficult to locate in pig lymph nodes.

Functional Morphology

FILTRATION AND PHAGOCYTOSIS. The unique architecture of the lymph node is ideally suited for the lymph to percolate through the coarse mesh where it contacts the lymphocytes, reticular cells, and macrophages. Therefore, any particulate matter in the lymph may be filtered out and engulfed by the macrophages of the medullary sinus. Likewise, antigenic material in the lymph is made available to cortical macrophages and lymphocytes for processing.

LYMPHOPOIESIS AND IMMUNOLOGIC RESPONSES. Although the bone marrow is the chief site of lymphopoiesis in the adult animal, there is considerable lymphocyte production in lymph nodes. The major stimulus that elicits a lymphoproliferative response in peripheral lymphatic tissue is antigenic experience. Any discussion of lymphopoiesis must include the various functional types of lymphocytes produced, as well as their locations within the lymph nodes.

The bone marrow is the anatomical "bursal equivalent" for the production of B-lymphocytes in mammals. During marrow lymphopoiesis, some lymphocytes remain there long enough to gradually develop surface markers characteristic of B-lymphocytes. This cellular maturation occurs without mitotic activity and is antigen-independent.

An immune response is the result of the introduction of an antigen into the organism and requires the cooperation of the lymphocytes with each other and the nonlymphatic accessory cells, the most important of which are *macrophages.* A macrophage has to "catch" and process the antigen before it can be presented to both B- and T-lymphocytes, which are then triggered into activity. In the case of B-lymphocytes, a specific T-lymphocyte is usually necessary for most antigens to trigger the immune response.

In a *humoral* immune response the B-lymphocytes are active. Those that are effector cells, mainly *plasma cells* of varying maturity, produce and secrete humoral antibodies specific for the antigen that initiated the response. The response begins in the outermost cortex just under the subcapsular sinus with proliferation of B-lymphocytes that subsequently differentiate into plasmablasts. These cells migrate into the medullary cords where they become plasma cells (Figs. 8–11, 8–15). Then a *germinal center reaction* begins in the outer cortex, with the formation of memory cells specific for the initiating antigen as its primary function. The outer cortex is populated mostly by B cells and is called the B domain (bursa-dependent region).

During these responses scattered lymphoblasts divide in the paracortex (T domain) and differentiate into effector and memory cells responsible for cellular immune activities. There are three subtypes of effector T cells: 1) cytotoxic T-lymphocytes that kill foreign cells, such as virus-infected cells, cancer cells, and transplants; 2) helper T cells that help B- or T-lymphocytes to respond to antigens and activate macrophages; and 3) suppressor T cells that suppress certain B- or T-lymphocytes. The latter two categories of T cells are referred to as regulatory T cells.

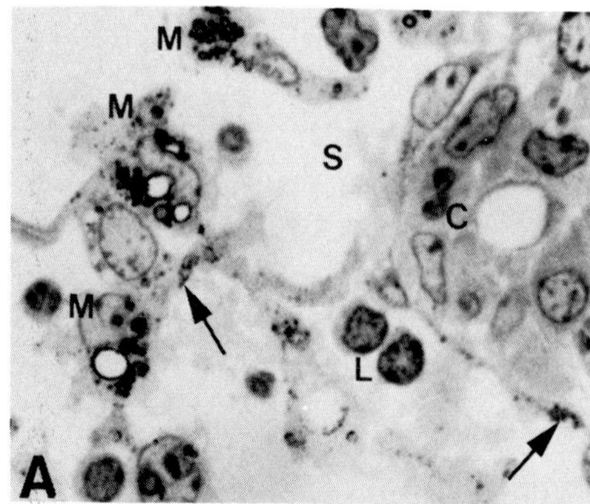

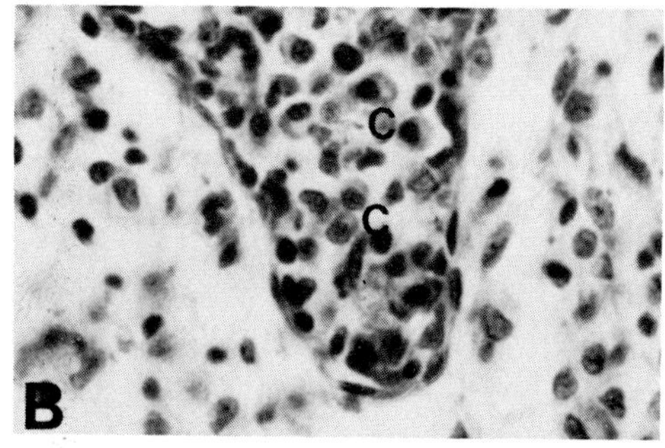

Fig. 8–15. *Lymph node medulla. A, Sheep. Medullary cord (C). Sinus (S) with macrophages (M) containing India ink particles. Lymphocytes (L). Some uptake of ink particles by sinus lining cells (arrows). Epon. Toluidine blue. ×1000. B, Dog. Medullary cord with many plasma cells (C). Crossmon's trichrome. ×600.*

SPLEEN

The spleen is a complicated organ with many functions, some of them not well understood. It serves as a *filter* for the blood and preserves iron for reuse in hemoglobin synthesis. It is involved in immune responses to blood-borne antigens and it stores red cells and platelets.

Structure

CAPSULE AND SUPPORTIVE TISSUE. The spleen is surrounded by a thick connective tissue capsule invested by the peritoneum. The capsule has two ill-defined layers of connective tissue and smooth muscle (Fig. 8–16). The total thickness and relative amount of smooth muscle vary with the species. The horse spleen has the thickest

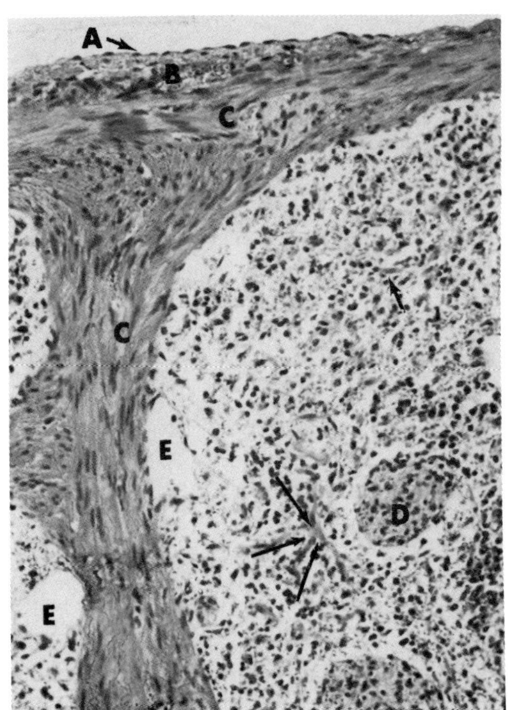

Fig. 8–16. *Spleen, pig. Mesothelium (A) covers capsule of connective tissue (B) and smooth muscle (C), which extends into the trabecula. Ellipsoid (sheathed capillary) (D) is surrounded by red pulp. Venules (E) are distended due to perfusion. Notice isolated smooth muscle cells (arrows) typical of pig spleen. H & E. ×175.*

capsule of domestic animals, with the smooth muscle fibers arranged in two layers oriented at right angles to each other. The outer connective tissue layer is thicker than the muscle layers. The pig and ruminants have moderately thick splenic capsules; however, in the pig most of the capsule is made up of smooth muscle that forms a tridimensional feltwork. Ruminant spleens have two thin layers of muscle fibers interwoven with collagen and elastic fibers. Although the dog and cat have the thinnest splenic capsules, smooth muscle fibers make up more than two thirds of the total thickness. Trabeculae composed of collagen and elastic fibers and smooth muscle cells extend from the capsule and the hilus. The trabeculae contain arteries, veins, lymph vessels, and nerves. The capsule, trabeculae, and reticular fibers support the splenic parenchyma composed of *red* and *white* pulp.

RED PULP. Most of the splenic pulp is red, owing to the vast amount of blood held within the reticular network. The red pulp is composed of pulp arterioles, sheathed and terminal capillaries, venous sinuses or venules, and splenic cords. Two main types of red pulp are seen in mammalian spleens, depending upon the type and amount of postcapillary vessels: *sinusal* and *nonsinusal.* Among the domestic animals only the dog has typical venous sinuses, similar to those in human and rat spleens.

The splenic sinuses are wide vascular channels lined with elongated, longitudinally oriented endothelial cells that contain contractile microfilaments aligned in bands parallel and adjacent to the lateral cell margins. These filaments stabilize the endothelial cells; gaps or slits are created upon contraction, allowing pliant erythrocytes to pass between the cells as they migrate from the splenic cords into the sinus lumen. The lining cells rest upon a fenestrated basal lamina and are further supported by reticular fibers, some of which form hooplike structures encircling the sinus at right angles to the long axis. In the cat and ruminants, venules rather than venous sinuses are present. Their wide lumina are lined with thin endothelium supported by reticular cells and a discontinuous basal lamina. Openings in this wall are common (Fig. 8–17).

The splenic cords situated between the sinuses form a vast three-dimensional network composed of reticular fibers with enmeshed reticular cells, erythrocytes, macrophages, lymphocytes, plasma cells, and other leukocytes. The membranous processes of the reticular cells tend to form channel-like structures that may function to conduct blood toward the interendothelial slits in the sinus walls. In the cat and ruminant spleens, the splenic cords are more extensive. The red pulp of ruminant and pig spleens contains numerous smooth muscle cells, while that of the horse and

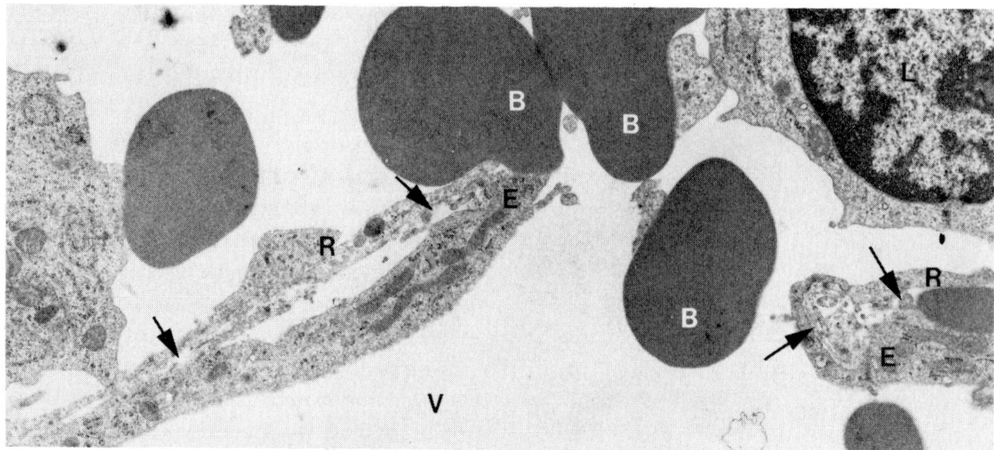

Fig. 8–17. *Spleen, sheep. Electron micrograph of a venule with erythrocytes (B) passing into the lumen (V) through an opening in the wall. Endothelium (E); basal lamina (arrows); reticular cells (R); lymphocyte (L). ×8000.*

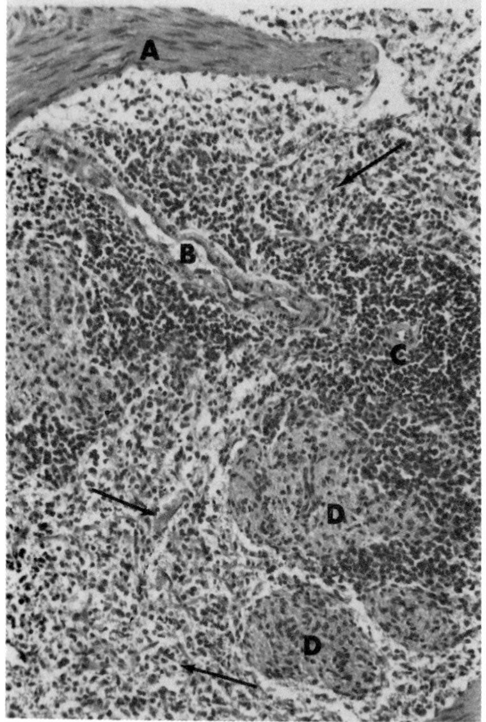

Fig. 8–18. *Spleen, pig. Trabecula (A) and artery (B), ensheathed with lymphocytes, coursing into a nodule to become nodular artery (C). Numerous sheathed capillaries (ellipsoids) (D) surround lymphatic nodule. Isolated smooth muscle cells are at arrows. H & E. ×80.*

dog has myofibroblasts, cells that resemble fibroblasts but have some features of smooth muscle, e.g., actin filaments and dense bodies. It is difficult to visualize all the red pulp constituents, because the spleen collapses at death and many structures are obliterated by compression.

WHITE PULP. White pulp is the lymphatic tissue distributed throughout the spleen as typical lymphatic nodules (splenic nodules) and as periarterial lymphatic sheaths (PALS) (Fig. 8–18). In both locations, the reticular fibers and reticular cells form a three-dimensional stroma containing sequestered lymphocytes, macrophages, and other accessory cells similar to those seen in lymph nodes. The nodules may or may not have active germinal centers, depending on their functional state. The principal cells of the nodules are B-lymphocytes, whereas T-lymphocytes occupy the area immediately around the nodular artery. In the PALS, T-lymphocytes are adjacent to the tunica media and B-lymphocytes comprise the peripheral region of the lymphatic sheaths.

MARGINAL ZONE. At the periphery of the white pulp, the reticulum forms several concentric layers. Immediately adjacent to the last layer is the marginal zone (Figs. 8–19 and 8–20), a reticular network into

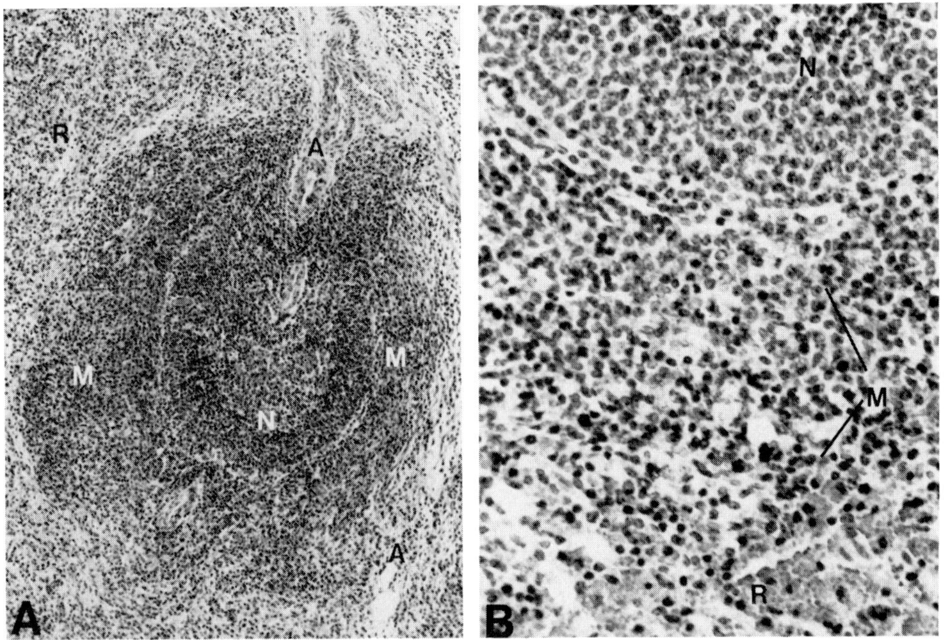

Fig. 8–19. *Spleen, sheep. A, Lymphatic nodule (N) with artery (A), surrounded by marginal zone (M) and red pulp (R). H & E. ×90. B, Marginal zone (M) between mantle of nodule (N) and red pulp with many red cells (R). H & E. ×270.*

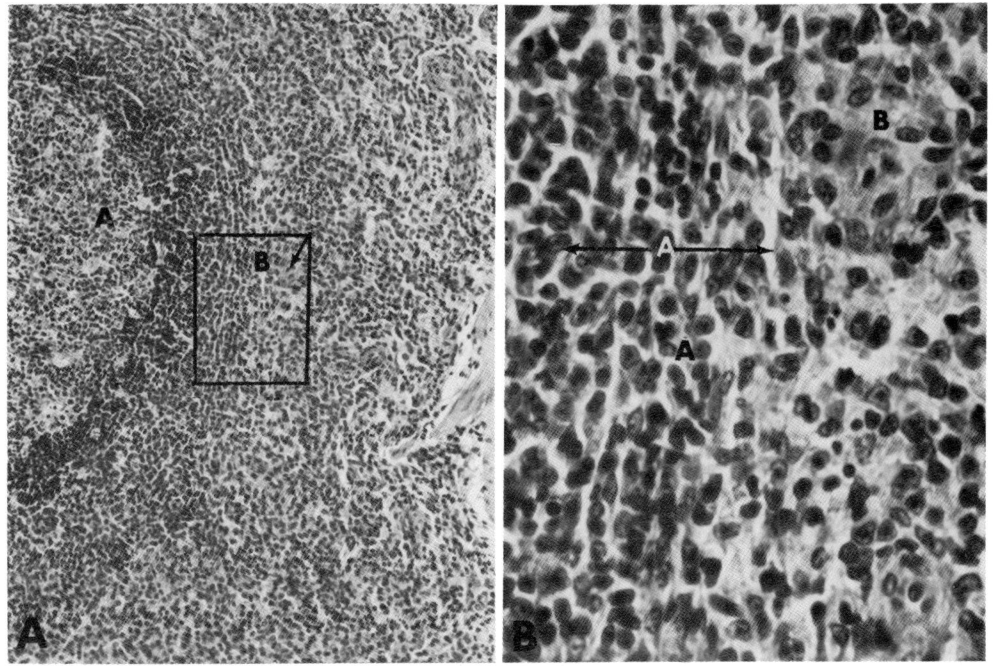

Fig. 8–20. *Spleen, dog. A, Lymphatic nodule with germinal center (A), marginal zone (B) and an ellipsoid at arrow. ×80. B, Enlargement of rectangle in A; marginal zone (A) and an ellipsoid (B). H & E. ×870.*

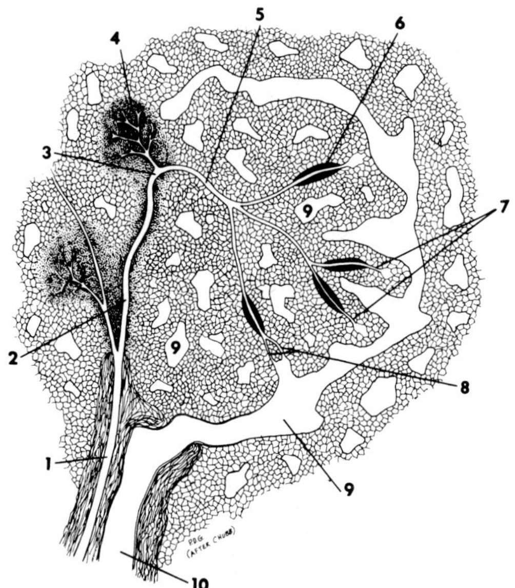

Fig. 8–21. *Diagram of splenic circulation. Trabecular artery (1); artery of the white pulp with lymphatic sheath (2); nodular artery (3); nodular capillaries (4); pulp arteriole (5); sheathed capillary (ellipsoid) (6); terminal capillaries emptying into reticular mesh (open circulation) (7); terminal capillaries emptying into venous sinus or venule (closed circulation) (8); venous sinus or venule (9); trabecular vein (10).*

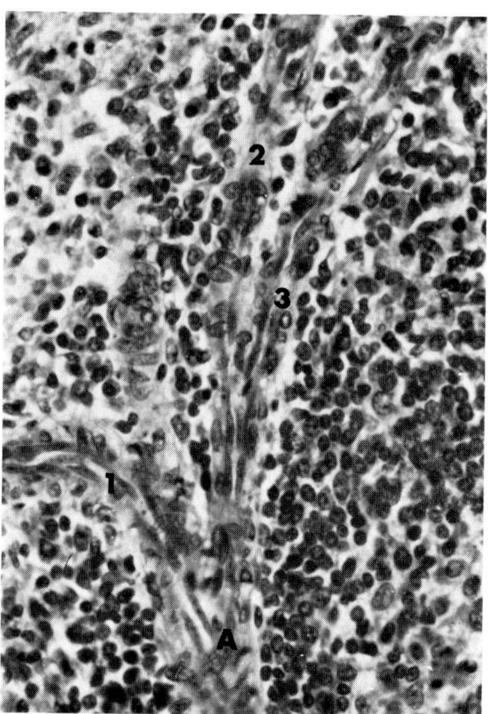

Fig. 8–22. *Penicillus, spleen, pig. Pulp arteriole (A) has three branches (1, 2, 3) before entering ellipsoid. H & E. ×425.*

which open many capillaries from the white pulp and some terminal capillaries of the red pulp. From here the blood is drained slowly towards the venous sinuses or venules of the red pulp. There are many macrophages and a special population of lymphocytes in the marginal zone. All cellular elements of the blood, as well as antigens, are brought into contact with the local macrophages and lymphocytes. Particles suspended in blood plasma are efficiently phagocytized by the macrophages, and conditions are ideal for antigen presentation.

Blood Vessels

The circulation of blood through the spleen has important functional implications, particularly with regard to antigenic stimulation and extraction of hemoglobin and iron from the red blood cells (Fig. 8–21).

Multiple branches of the splenic artery enter the capsule and extend into the large trabeculae. As the artery leaves the trabecula, the externa becomes heavily infiltrated with lymphocytes. The artery is called the *artery of the white pulp*. In certain areas the periarterial lymphatic sheath expands, forming a typical lymphatic nodule, and when a branch enters the nodule it becomes the *nodular artery* (Figs. 8–18 and 8–19A). It is sometimes referred to as the central artery, although it rarely passes through the center of the nodule. Branches of the nodular artery terminate in two principal areas. Some branches feed capillary beds in the nodule and terminate in the marginal zone, while the main branches enter the red pulp, each one forming a *penicillus* (brushlike tuft), composed of two to six straight branches, each with three segments. The initial part, the *pulp arteriole* (Fig. 8–22), is the longest and continues

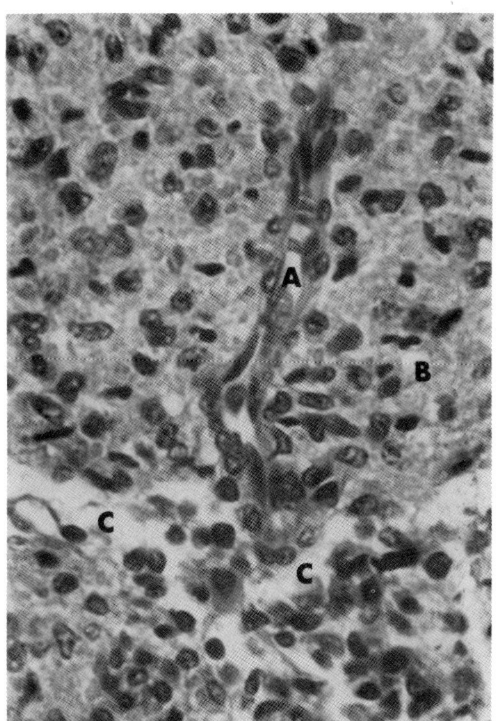

Fig. 8–23. *Spleen, pig. Longitudinal section of sheathed capillary (A), surrounded by its sheath, containing erythrocytes (B), macrophages, and platelets within its meshes. Sinus in the red pulp (C). H & E. ×650.*

into peculiar structures called *sheathed capillaries* or *ellipsoids* (Fig. 8–23). Here the lumen narrows, the endothelium is tall, and the muscle is replaced by a sheath of macrophages sequestered in a reticular meshwork (pericapillary macrophage sheath). Sheathed capillaries continue as wide *terminal capillaries.*

The junction of the terminal capillaries with the venous system is controversial, and currently there are three theories regarding the type of connection. The first theory is that the terminal capillaries expand, form an ampulla, and open directly into the splenic sinuses or venules. This is called the "closed" theory because the connection forms a continuous tubular structure.

The "open" theory suggests that the capillaries open into the spaces between the reticular cells of the red pulp, and the blood enters the venous sinuses through the slits in their walls.

The last theory proposes the existence of both an "open" and a "closed" circulation, depending on the physiologic state. When the spleen is distended, the spaces between the endothelial cells lining the sinuses or venules are pulled apart, and the blood leaks through the open meshwork from the terminal capillaries to the sinuses or venules. In a contracted spleen the cells in the venous sinuses or venules are pushed together, forming a continuous uninterrupted connection with the terminal capillaries. Thus, the circulation is closed. The last theory is widely accepted for sinusal spleens, but nonsinusal spleens seem to have an open circulation. Whatever the exact nature of the capillary-venous junction, the blood in the small vessels eventually drains into the trabecular veins and leaves by the splenic vein.

Lymph Vessels and Nerves

The spleen has no afferent lymph vessels, and the major efferent vessels are in the capsule and trabeculae. They probably penetrate the white pulp for only short distances along the artery of the white pulp and its branches. The trabecular lymph vessels eventually drain into the splenic lymph nodes.

Sympathetic nerve fibers enter the capsule and course in the trabeculae, especially along arteries. Many sympathetic fibers also enter the red pulp to terminate on the smooth muscle cells or myofibroblasts and on the media of arterioles. Many fibers also form free endings in the reticulum.

Species Differences

The spleens of the horse, dog and pig have abundant lymphatic nodules and periarterial sheaths, but in the cat and ruminant spleens the lymphatic tissue is less abundant and occurs mainly as lymphatic nodules; the periarterial lymphatic sheaths are short.

The size and number of the sheathed capillaries vary considerably among the domestic animals. In the pig, and to a lesser degree in the cat, the pericapillary macrophage sheaths are large and abundant and often particularly numerous near the white pulp. They are smaller in the horse and dog and are narrow in ruminants.

Functional Morphology

FILTRATION. The filtration mechanism of the spleen is enhanced by the vast reticular fiber network filled with reticular cells and macrophages. Almost any section of red pulp contains numerous macrophages filled with engulfed red blood cell fragments called hemosiderin. In addition to the ability to remove erythrocytes, sinusal spleens have the ability to remove foreign particulate inclusions (e.g., parasites) from red blood cells without destroying the cells. As the erythrocytes squeeze through the slits in the venous sinus wall, any rigid inclusions are removed in a process called "pitting" and are ingested by perisinusoidal macrophages. The marginal zone is the most important filter encountered by the blood. Indeed, blood-borne foreign particulate matter is first phagocytized by macrophages in the marginal zone. Because of permeable intercellular junctions between endothelial cells of the sheathed capillary and a discontinuous basal lamina, foreign particulate matter, as well as erythrocytes and platelets, have ready access to the pericapillary macrophage sheath and are phagocytized within it.

IMMUNE RESPONSES. The spleen is a lymphatic organ designed to respond immunologically to antigens circulating in the blood. Immune responses are initiated in the marginal zone of nodules and periarterial lymphatic sheaths. The marginal zone provides an ideal situation for blood antigens to make contact with lymphatic elements, because so many capillaries terminate here. Lymphoblast activity at the periphery of the white pulp is the first indication of early humoral immune responses. Germinal centers develop somewhat later and plasma cell precursors move out into the red pulp along the penicilli. Responses to cellular antigens are seen in the central part of the periarterial lymphatic sheaths where there is increased lymphoblastic activity.

BLOOD STORAGE. Large numbers of erythrocytes are stored in the red pulp of horse spleens and to a lesser extent in dog spleens.

HEMOPOIESIS. The major hemopoietic activity of the spleen in adult animals is lymphopoiesis. Erythropoiesis is a major function of the spleen during gestation and persists in newborn horses and ruminants for several weeks post partum.

HEMAL NODE

Hemal nodes seem to be unique to ruminants. They are generally small, brown to dark red organs, but their size, number, and histologic characteristics vary within wide limits. They develop during fetal life from lymph node primordia that lose all their lymph vessels. Therefore, they receive all of their cells and antigens from the blood.

In young animals there is a distinct accumulation of lymphocytes, as in the inner cortex of a lymph node, but few nodules are present (Fig. 8–24). In healthy adults the whole node is generally filled with red blood cells. As a result of antigenic stimulation many nodules may form and only a few red blood cells are present (Fig. 8–25). There is no typical medulla. The sinuses are wide, with very few macrophages and small numbers of lymphocytes. The diffuse lymphatic tissue contains relatively few lymphocytes but has many macrophages that digest erythrocytes and granulocytes.

The vascular supply is similar to that of lymph nodes, but the many venules have a lower endothelium. Many lymphocytes

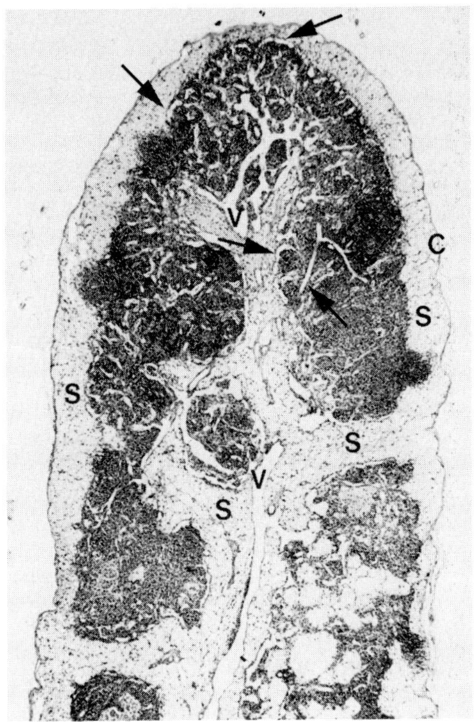

Fig. 8–24. *Hemal node, young goat. Wide sinuses (S) under capsule (C) and around central veins (V). Many small venules (arrows) in lymphatic tissue. Vascular perfusion. H & E. ×35.*

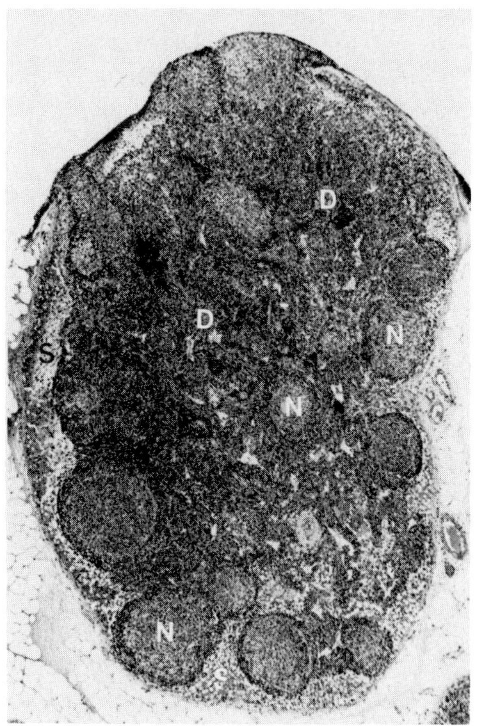

Fig. 8–25. *Hemal node, infected sheep. Sinuses (S) filled with red blood cells compressed by numerous nodules (N) with large germinal centers. Deep cortex (D). H & E. ×40.*

pass through this endothelium just as they do in the postcapillary venules of lymph nodes. They are followed by erythrocytes, which thus leak out of the blood vessels. No openings are present in the walls of the blood vessels. The functional significance of the hemal node is unknown.

CELL TRAFFIC IN THE LYMPHATIC ORGANS

All lymphatic tissues receive recirculating lymphocytes from the blood through their high endothelial venules. Precursors of accessory cells, especially macrophages, or mature accessory cells, also reach these tissues through the blood or lymph. The continuous *recirculation* of an immense number of small clones of antigen-specific lymphocytes, both virgin and memory cells, is the essence of *immunological surveillance.* This creates optimum possibilities for an early encounter of a lymphocyte with its specific antigen. The most advanced arrangement is seen in the lymph node, where tissue fluid from large peripheral areas is drained into a small central area where large numbers of recirculaitng lymphocytes are present in an environment containing many accessory cells.

T-lymphocytes migrate through T domains, but some also reach germinal centers and other B domains. B-lymphocytes have a slower passage through lymph nodes and spleen. They migrate through the outer cortex of lymph nodes and tend to accumulate in the innermost mantle of secondary nodules in all lymphatic tissues. Recirculating lymphocytes are thought to leave the lymph node by efferent lymphatic vessels. In the pig it is believed that they leave the lymph nodes via the blood because porcine lymph has very few lymphocytes. It appears that most splenic lymphocytes migrate by way of the blood vessels in the red pulp.

Lymphocytes produced in a lymph node also leave by way of the sinus system. Some of them are lymphoblasts that home-in in other lymphatic tissues or in mucous membranes. Most of the lymphocytes migrate from aggregated lymphatic nodules to the mesenteric lymph nodes, where they proliferate and differentiate. They then migrate to mucous membranes, both in the digestive tract and in other areas and some even to the mammary glands. They may proliferate at their final destination. Most produce immunoglobulin A, which is then combined to a secretory component that mediates transcellular transport and exocytosis of IgA-secretory-component complex into the lumen.

Lymphocytes that reach a secondary or tertiary lymph node via the afferent lymph generally penetrate the inner wall of the cortical sinuses, then migrate through the whole cortex and into the medullary sinuses. This movement allows many possibilities for interactions with other cell populations.

REFERENCES

Bélisle, C., and Sainte-Marie, G.: Topography of the deep cortex of the lymph nodes of various mammalian species. Anat Rec *201*:553, 1981.

Bienenstock, J., and Befus, D.: Gut- and bronchus-associated lymphoid tissue. Am J Anat *170*:437, 1984.

Binns, R.M.: Organization of the lymphoreticular system and lymphocyte markers in the pig. Vet Immunol Immunopathol *3*:95, 1982.

Blue, J., and Weiss, L.: Electron microscopy of the red pulp of the dog spleen including vascular arrangement, periarterial macrophage sheaths (ellipsoids), and the contractile, innervated reticular meshwork. Am J Anat *161*:198, 1981.

Duijvestijn, A.M., and Hoefsmit, E.C.M.: Ultrastructure of the rat thymus: The micro-environment of T-lymphocyte maturation. Cell Tissue Res *218*:279, 1981.

Nieuwenhuis, P., and Opstelten, D.: Functional anatomy of germinal centers. Am J Anat *170*:421, 1984.

Owen, J.J.T., and Jenkinson, E.J.: Early events in T lymphocyte genesis in the fetal thymus. Am J Anat *170*:301, 1984.

Paul, W.E.: Fundamental Immunology. New York, Raven Press, 1984.

Snook, T.: A comparative study of the vascular arrangements in the mammalian spleens. Am J Anat *87*:31, 1950.

Veerman, A.J.P., and van Ewijk, W.: White pulp compartments in the spleen of rats and mice. A light and electron microscopic study of lymphoid and non-lymphoid celltypes in T- and B-areas. Cell Tissue Res *156*:417, 1975.

Wenk, E.J., Orlic, D., Reith, E.J., and Rhodin, J.A.G.: The ultrastructure of mouse lymph node venules and the passage of lymphocytes across their walls. J Ultrastruct Res *47*:214, 1974.

9

Respiratory System

C.G. PLOPPER
D.R. ADAMS

The primary function of the respiratory system is to provide for the exchange of respiratory gases (oxygen and carbon dioxide) between the organism and the environment. The conducting airways (nasal cavity, nasopharynx, laryngopharynx, larynx, trachea, bronchi, and bronchioles) provide a series of air passages for moving air to and from the gas exchange area in the lungs. The conducting airways also serve a protective function by conditioning incoming (inspired) air. This conditioning includes heating the air to body temperature, saturating it to 100% relative humidity, and filtering out noxious gases and particles such as bacteria and dust. The conducting airways also conserve body heat and water by extracting them from the air during expiration. The mucociliary blanket, which covers the mucosal surface of conducting airways, serves to trap inhaled particles and conveys them and cellular debris out of the system. A number of other structures such as the nasolacrimal duct, vomeronasal organ, paranasal recesses and sinuses, and the auditory tube and equine guttural pouch are associated with the conducting airways.

The gas exchange area constitutes most of the lung tissue. This area occurs in those sites where a very thin membrane forms a barrier between pulmonary capillary blood and respired air. The thinnest blood-air barrier occurs in the walls of small air pockets, or alveoli. The alveoli connect to the most distal conducting airways by a series of air passages, the alveolar ducts and alveolar sacs. An extensive pulmonary capillary bed receives the entire output of the right ventricle of the heart and serves to filter and chemically alter the blood.

The two internal layers of most hollow organs are the tunica mucosa and tela submucosa and are separated by the deepest layer of the mucosa, the lamina muscularis mucosae; however, such a smooth muscle layer is not present in the mucosa of the nasal airways, larynx, trachea, and bronchi. The connective tissue layer between epithelium and underlying cartilage, bone, or adventitia may be subjectively divided into a superficial lamina propria mucosae and a deeper tela submucosa.

NASAL CAVITY

Nasal Vestibule

The nasal cavity is composed of right and left passages, each of which is divided ros-

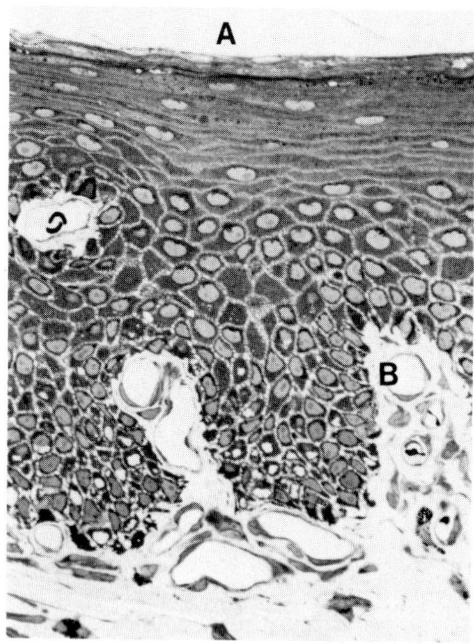

Fig. 9–1. *Stratified squamous epithelium, nasal vestibule, dog. Airway lumen (A); dermal papilla (B). 1 μm. Azure II. ×385. (From Adams, D.R., and Hotchkiss, D.K.: The canine nasal mucosa. Zbl Vet Med C Anat Histol Embryol 12:111, 1983, Fig. 4, with permission.)*

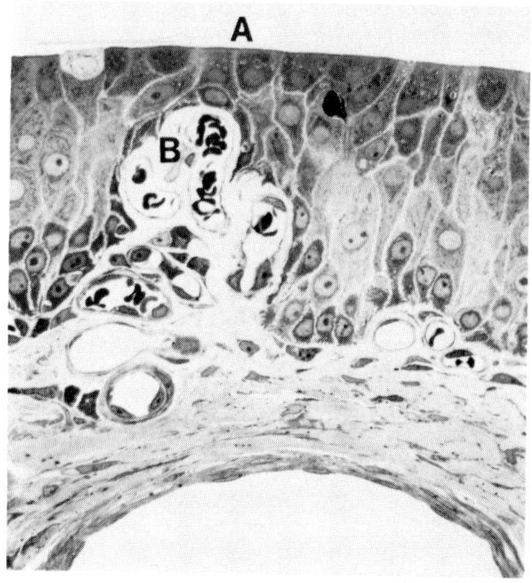

Fig. 9–2. *Transitional mucosal zone, dorsal concha, dog. Stratified cuboidal to columnar epithelium. Airway lumen (A); connective tissue papillae (B). 1 μm. Azure II. ×385. (From Adams, D.R., and Hotchkiss, D.K.: The canine nasal mucosa. Zbl Vet Med C Anat Histol Embryol 12:113, 1983, Fig. 6, with permission.)*

trally into nasal vestibule and caudally into nasal cavity proper. Each vestibule is partially subdivided by the alar fold of the ventral concha, which projects dorsomedially into the lumen. The nasolacrimal duct opens through the ventrolateral wall of the vestibule at the base of the alar fold, and the duct of the lateral nasal gland opens through the dorsolateral wall of the nasal vestibule.

The skin of the nasal apex is continuous through a tissue gradient with the mucous membrane of the nasal cavity proper. Rostrally, the cutaneous region of the nasal vestibule is lined by a pigmented, relatively thick keratinized stratified squamous epithelium. At midvestibule the epithelium is thinner and nonkeratinized (Fig. 9–1). Superficial cells have microridges on their free surface. The caudal portion of the nasal vestibule and rostral third of the nasal cavity proper are a transitional zone surfaced by an epithelium that varies from stratified cuboidal to nonciliated pseudostratified columnar. Surface epithelial cells in the transitional zone contain multilobated nuclei, possess microvilli on their free surface, and are frequently spherical (Figs. 9–2 and 9–3). Connective tissue in the dermis of the nasal vestibule interdigitates via papillary pegs with the basal region of the epithelium. The papillary layer contains small vessels and numerous free cells including mast cells, plasma cells, lymphocytes, macrophages, and granulocytes. Lymphocytes are also frequently observed in the basal portion of the epithelium. The deeper portion of the dermis contains bundles of collagen fibers, blood vessels, and serous glands.

The following specializations occur in the nasal vestibule of domestic mammals. The rostral portion of the equine nasal vestibule is lined by an integument containing vibrissae, sebaceous glands, and sweat glands. A nasal diverticulum lined with skin, present lateral to the nasal passage, opens into the rostral portion of the equine nasal vestibule. A second ostium of the na-

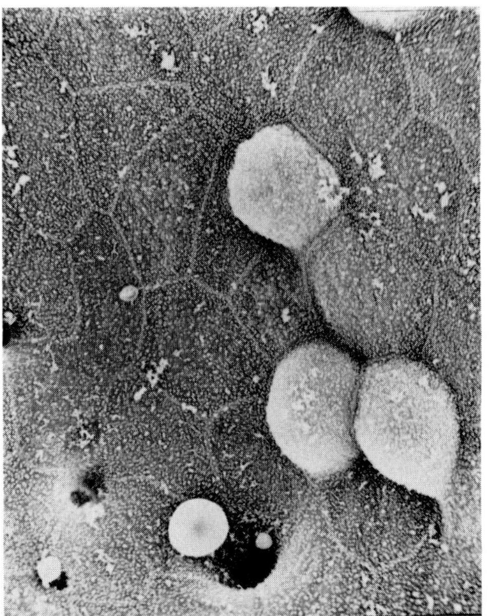

Fig. 9–3. *Scanning electron micrograph of stratified cuboidal to columnar epithelium, nasal septum, calf. ×1800.*

solacrimal duct is frequently present in the caudolateral surface of the ventral concha of dog and pig; the portion of the porcine nasolacrimal duct leading to the nasal vestibule is vestigeal in adult animals. A lateral nasal gland and duct are not present in cattle. The papillary stratum of the vestibular dermis in the dog has particularly numerous papillae and capillary loops.

Nasal Cavity Proper

The constricted portion (nasal limen) of the passage between nasal vestibule and nasal cavity proper contains the rostral tip of the dorsal concha and the junction between alar fold and caudal portion of the ventral concha. The lumen of the nasal cavity proper is subdivided by lamellae of the ventral, dorsal, and ethmoid conchae. Epithelium lining much of the caudal half of the nasal cavity proper is ciliated pseudostratified columnar. That lining the middle nasal meatus is thinner and contains fewer ciliated and goblet cells. Olfactory mucosa is present over a portion of the caudal surfaces of the ethmoid conchae and the nasal septum.

The nonolfactory ciliated epithelium (Figs. 9–4 and 9–5) of the nasal cavity contains a number of cell types including basal, ciliated, secretory, and brush cells. *Basal cells* are electron-dense columnar cells attached at the base of the epithelium to the basal lamina by hemidesmosomes. By division and differentiation these cells may replace other epithelial cell-types lost through attrition. The cytoplasm of basal cells contains numerous bundles of tonofilaments and free ribosomes. Individual *ciliated cells* have 200 to 300 motile cilia and numerous microvilli projecting into the nasal lumen; the cilia are anchored to the apical cytoplasm by basal bodies and the microvilli, sometimes branched, contain microfilaments that extend down into the cytoplasm. The supranuclear portion of the cell contains numerous mitochondria and a Golgi complex; small strands of granular ER are scattered throughout the cell. Defects in the microstructure of cilia may result in immotility or ineffective ciliary beat. Immotile cilia syndrome is a condition in which respiratory tract infections persistently recur as a result of congenital ciliary abnormality. Animals with this syndrome often have a left/right reversal in position of thoracic and abdominal viscera ("situs inversus totalis"). The structure of secretory cells, which occur either as *goblet cells* or as slender mucus-secreting cells, varies with both secretory phase and location within the nasal cavity. *Goblet cells* have their nuclei pressed to the base of the cell by a supranuclear mass of large, relatively electron-lucent secretory granules. Organelles usually present in the perinuclear region include a Golgi complex, granular ER, and slender mitochondria. The luminal surface of the cell has short microvilli. Goblet cells of most species are thought to secrete primarily a sulfated acid glycoprotein as a major component of mucus. *Brush cells* have long, thick microvilli containing bundles of microfilaments, and a cytoplasm

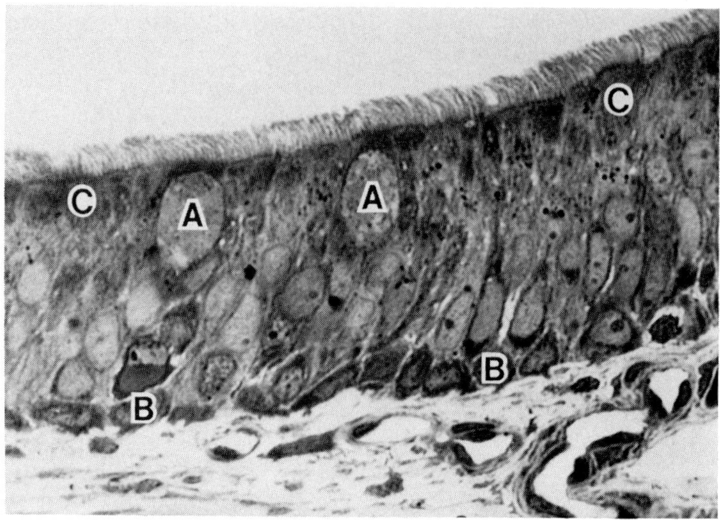

Fig. 9–4. *Ciliated pseudostratified columnar epithelium with goblet cells, ethmoid concha, dog. Goblet cells (A); basal cells (B); ciliated cells (C). 1 μm. Azure II. ×590.*

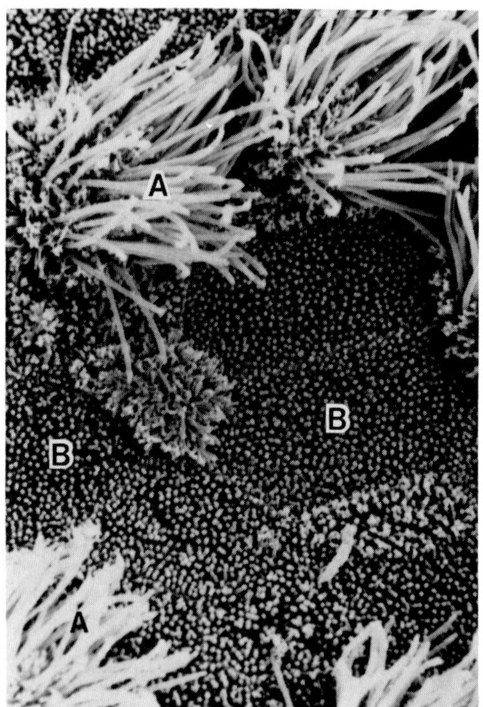

Fig. 9–5. *Scanning electron micrograph of ciliated pseudostratified columnar epithelium, nasal septum, calf. Ciliated cells with microvilli (A); nonciliated columnar cells with apical microvilli (B). ×3500.*

containing mitochondria, granular ER, and a large number of filaments. These cells may be sensory receptors associated with endings of the trigeminal nerve. Another nonciliated cell type in the nasal mucosa has surface microvilli and contains much smooth endoplasmic reticulum and little secretory material; this unnamed cell type is thought to function in the metabolism of xenobiotic compounds (see pp. 189, 199).

The caudal, nonolfactory mucosa of the nasal cavity is more highly vascular than that in the vestibular, transitional, or olfactory regions. The submucosal layer is called the *cavernous stratum* (Fig. 9–6). The cavernous stratum of the dog is more vascular than that of other domestic mammals, consisting of 35% vessel lumen. Simple branched tubuloacinar nasal glands are situated between veins of the cavernous stratum (Fig. 9–7). In domestic mammals such glands discharge through the epithelium at all levels within the nasal cavity. The *lateral nasal gland* (Fig. 9–8) is a relatively large compound gland in the mucosa adjacent to the opening between the middle nasal meatus and the maxillary recess or sinus. It secretes via a long duct into the

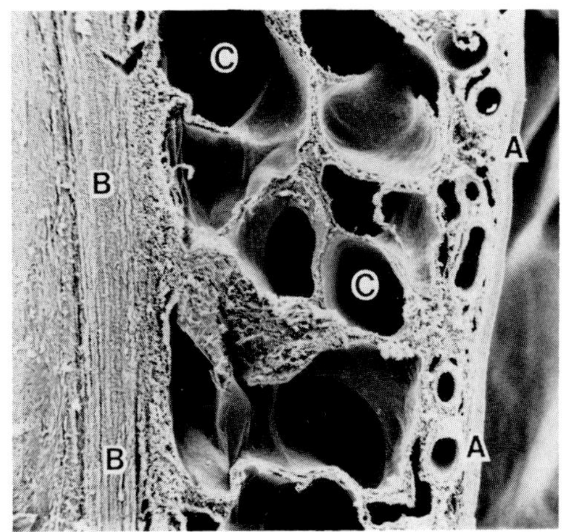

Fig. 9–6. *Scanning electron micrograph of a section of mucosa, nasal septum, calf. Epithelium (A); perichondrium (B); lumina of blood vessels (C) in the cavernous stratum. ×40.*

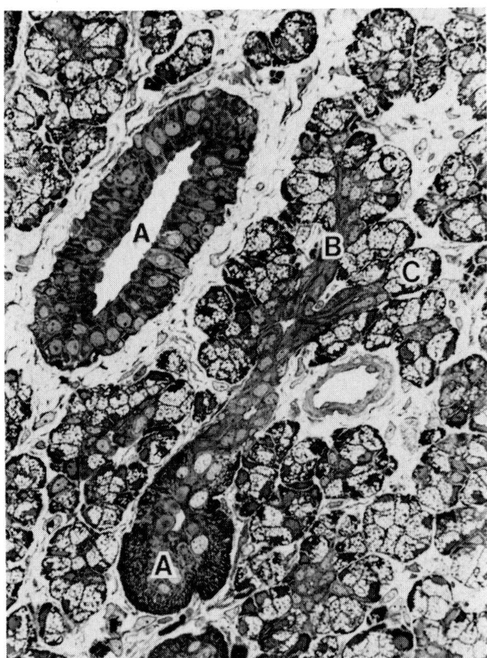

Fig. 9–8. *Mucosa of maxillary recess, lateral nasal gland, dog. Striated ducts (A); intercalated duct (B); acinar cells (C). 1 μm. Azure II. ×425.*

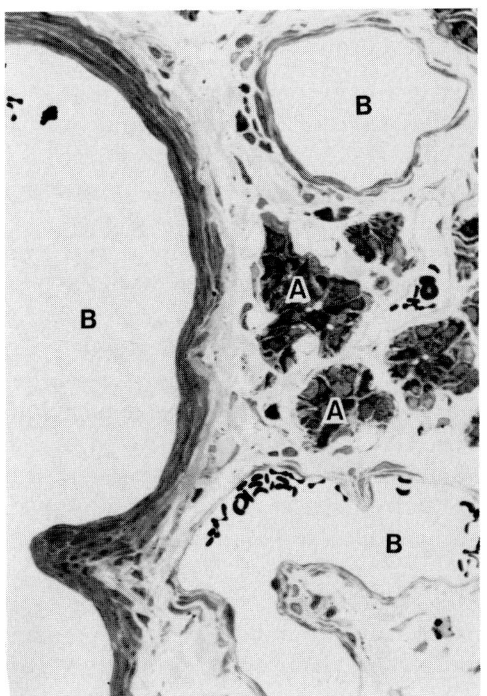

Fig. 9–7. *Nasal glands, dog. Gland acini (A); lumina of veins (B). 1 μm. Azure II. ×425.*

nasal vestibule. In the lateral nasal gland and the nasal mucosa, cytochrome P-450-dependent monoxygenase enzymes actively metabolize endogenous compounds, such as progesterone and testosterone, as well as a number of inhaled pollutants. These enzymes convert lipid-soluble exogenous compounds to water-soluble metabolites, some of which are highly toxic (such as formaldehyde and acetaldehyde). A number of metabolically active exogenous substances (xenobiotics) remain for a lengthy period in the nasal tissues by binding firmly to tissue elements.

OLFACTORY ORGAN

The *olfactory tunica mucosa* covers the caudodorsal portion of the nasal cavity including some of the surfaces of the ethmoid conchae, dorsal nasal meatus, and nasal septum. Pigment granules in the olfactory epithelium make the mucosa appear yel-

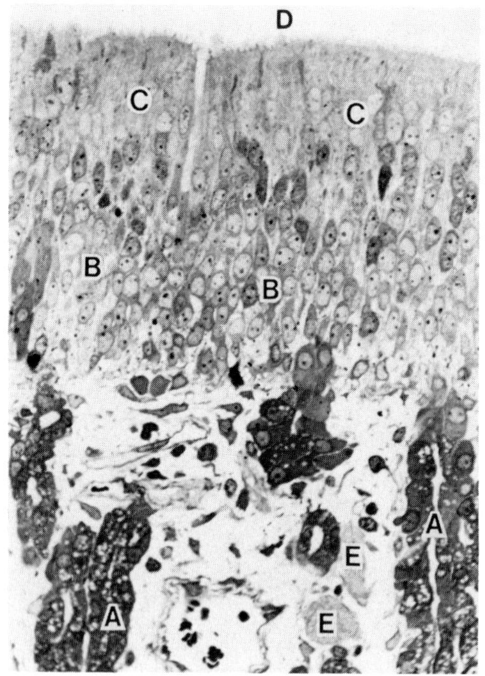

Fig. 9–9. *Olfactory mucosa, ethmoid concha, dog. Olfactory glands (A); nuclei of neurosensory cells (B); nuclei of sustentacular cells (C); lumen of the ethmoid meatus (D); olfactory nerves (E). 1 μm. Azure II. ×410.*

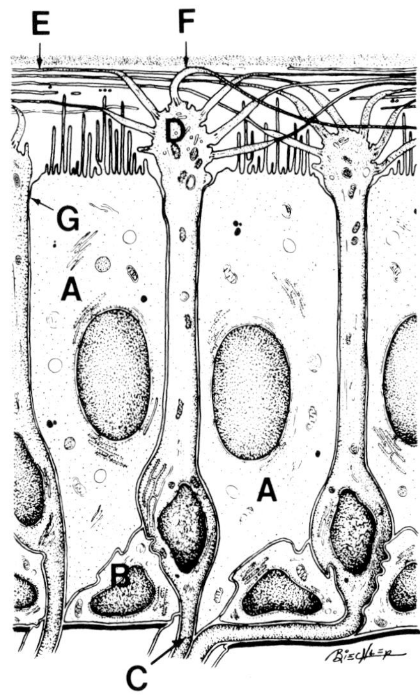

Fig. 9–10. *Schematic drawing of the olfactory epithelium. Sustentacular cell (A); basal cell (B); axon of the receptor cell (C); dendritic bulb (D); thin distal portion of cilium (E); thick proximal portion of cilium (F); junctional complex between receptor and sustentacular cells (G).*

low- to green-brown, grossly distinguishable from the adjacent nonolfactory area. Microscopically, olfactory mucosa may be discerned from adjacent nonolfactory mucosa because it has a thicker epithelium, numerous slender, vertically oriented glands, and numerous bundles of nonmyelinated nerve fibers in the lamina propria.

The olfactory mucosa is lined by a ciliated pseudostratified columnar epithelium consisting of three primary cell types: basal, neurosensory, and sustentacular (Fig. 9–9). *Basal cells* are similar in structure to those of the nonolfactory epithelium.

Mature *neurosensory olfactory cells* are bipolar neurons with perikarya in a wide basal zone of the epithelium, dendrites reaching the nasal cavity lumen, and axons reaching the olfactory bulb of the brain. A club-shaped apex, the *dendritic bulb*, protrudes from each dendrite into the lumen (Fig. 9–10); the dendritic bulb contains numerous microvesicles and supports 10 to 30 cilia. Each cilium is 50 to 80 μm long, consisting of a wide short basal portion and a long, thin, tapering distal portion. The number of microtubules decreases from the typical 9 + 2 arrangement in the basal portion of olfactory cilia to singlets of 1 to 4 microtubules distally. The slender dendritic portion of the neurosensory cell contains neurotubules and elongate mitochondria. The perikaryon is an ovoid, darkly stained body containing a nucleus, granular ER, free ribosomes, and Golgi complex. The slender axon contains longitudinally oriented neurotubules. Individual axons converge as they pass into the lamina propria forming bundles of nonmyelinated nerve fibers. Neurosensory cells are continuously replaced during the life of the animal by cells derived from basal cells.

Sustentacular cells taper from a narrow

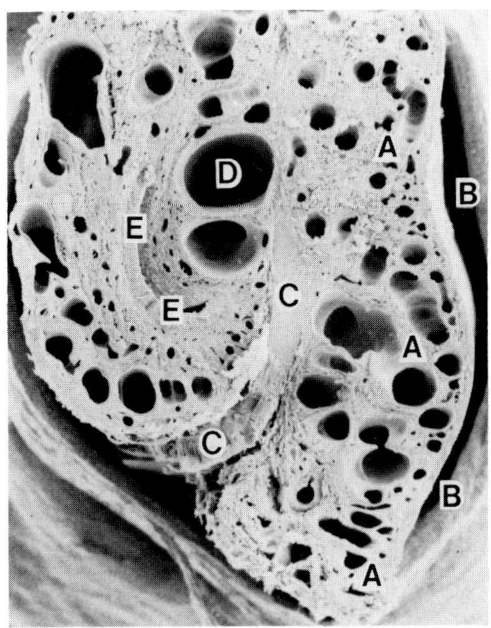

Fig. 9–11. *Scanning electron micrograph of the right vomeronasal organ, dog. Ventral mucosa of nasal septum (A); lumen of nasal cavity (B); vomeronasal cartilage (C); lumina of vomeronasal blood vessels (D); vomeronasal epithelium (E). ×20. (From Adams, D.R., and Wiekamp, M.D.: The canine vomeronasal organ. J Anat 138:773, 1984, Fig. 3, with permission.)*

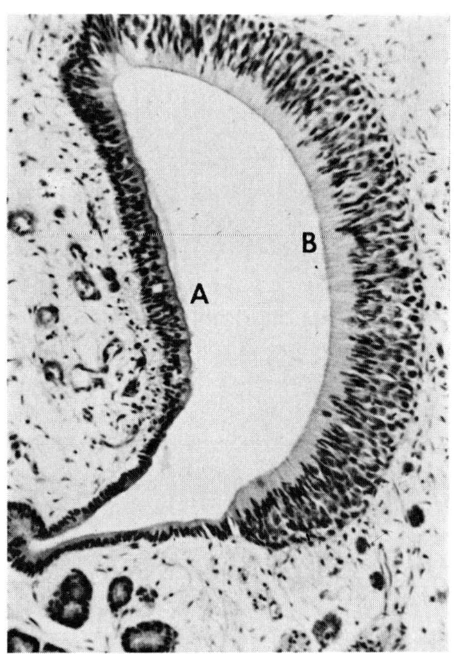

Fig. 9–12. *Vomeronasal duct, dog. The lateral epithelium (A) includes ciliated and nonciliated cells, whereas the medial epithelium (B) contains neurosensory and sustentacular epithelial cells. ×158. (Courtesy of A.W. Stinson.)*

base at the basal lamina to a wide apical portion. Their lightly staining nuclei are more superficial than those of neurosensory cells. Granular ER and Golgi complex are present in the supranuclear zone; smooth ER is present throughout the cytoplasm. Microvilli, often branched, cover the luminal surface of sustentacular cells. Juxtaluminal junctional complexes occur between sustentacular cells and the adjacent dendritic portion of neurosensory cells. Sustentacular cells are replaced by gland cells.

Gland density is higher in olfactory than in nonolfactory mucosa. *Olfactory gland* acini are composed of light serous and dark mucous secretory cells. The ducts pass through the epithelium as a tube lined by squamous cells. Pigment granules are present in the infranuclear portion of sustentacular cells and in olfactory glands.

VOMERONASAL ORGAN

Located in the mucosa of the ventral portion of the nasal septum, the tubular, blind-ending vomeronasal organ consists of an external cartilaginous support, a middle lamina propria that is both highly glandular and vascular, and an internal epithelial duct (Fig. 9–11). Right and left *vomeronasal ducts* open into ipsilateral incisive ducts. The hyaline *vomeronasal cartilage* is J-shaped, enclosing all but the dorsolateral portion of the organ. Epithelium passes through a transition from a stratified cuboidal lining rostrally near the incisive duct to a ciliated pseudostratified columnar epithelium over much of the caudal portion of the vomeronasal duct. The vomeronasal duct is crescent-shaped in transverse section with a lateral convex and a medial concave mucosal wall. The medial epithelium is a pseudostratified columnar epithelium of basal, sustentacular, and neurosensory cells (Fig. 9–12). The dendritic portions of vomeronasal neurosensory cells are different from olfactory neurosensory cells in that they lack dendritic bulbs and have microvilli instead of cilia on their apical surfaces. An abundance of mitochondria, basal bodies, and ciliary precursor bodies are present in the apical cytoplasm. Neurosensory cells are periodically replaced in the adult mammal. The lateral epithelium is a pseudostratified columnar epithelium of basal, nonciliated columnar, ciliated columnar, and goblet cells.

Structural diversity is considerable in vomeronasal epithelium from one species to another. The vomeronasal neurosensory cells of the dog have nonmotile cilia on their apical surface.

Leukocytes are frequently observed in the lateral epithelium or on its luminal surface. *Vomeronasal glands* secrete into the vomeronasal organ most commonly through the commissures between lateral and medial mucosal walls. Secretory granules of the acinar cells contain neutral glycoproteins.

The vomeronasal organ functions in the chemoreception of liquid-borne compounds of low volatility. Sensing of these compounds is thought to function in sexual behavior of both the female and male, in maternal behavior of the female, and in the interaction of the fetus with its uterine environment. The vomeronasal organs and the accessory olfactory bulbs, into which vomeronasal neurosensory cells project, are somewhat independent of the olfactory mucosa and olfactory bulbs. The vomeronasal organ is associated with the lip-curl type of facial grimace (Flehmen) action used by some male mammals to sample substances in the urine of the female; odorant particles may reach the incisive duct of other mammals with inhaled air, through contact with the tongue, or during passage through the mouth with food or water. These substances, dissolved in fluid in the incisive duct, are sucked into the vomeronasal lumen by constriction of blood vessels within the cartilaginous capsule of the vomeronasal organ. In a number of mammals, vomeronasal detection of the odor of a female results in an elevation of plasma testosterone in the male. The equine incisive duct is blind-ending ventrally, opening into the nasal cavity but not the oral cavity.

PARANASAL SINUSES

The mucosae lining the paranasal sinuses are thinner than those of the nasal cavity with which they are continuous. Few subepithelial glands or blood vessels are in the mucosal walls of the various sinuses. The epithelia are low, ciliated, pseudostratified columnar containing few goblet cells. The ciliary beat carries mucus toward openings connecting the sinuses with the nasal cavity.

The maxillary recess of dog and cat is lined by a mucosa-containing acini of both the lateral nasal and maxillary recess glands. The lining is a tall, ciliated, pseudostratified columnar epithelium containing few goblet cells. Maxillary recess glands secrete neutral glycoproteins into the recess.

BLOOD VESSELS, LYMPHATICS, AND NERVES

Within the nasal mucosa, arteries and large thin-walled veins are oriented rostrocaudally in the cavernous stratum; the veins, which occur at several levels from superficial to deep, interconnect profusely. The large, thin-walled veins are called capacitance vessels because they determine the degree of mucosal congestion and, inversely, nasal patency. Constriction of nasal blood vessels is effected by alpha adrenergic stimulation via the sympathetic nervous system. Periods of vascular engorgement varying from 30 minutes to 4 hours followed by periods of decongestion normally occur in the cavernous stratum of mammals; during this nasal cycle the vascular activity in one side of the nose alternates with that of the other side. Small branches arise from deep arteries and supply the glands and basal region of the epithelium with blood. Such small superficial vessels, adjacent to the basal lamina of the surface epithelium, are abundant in the rostral half of the nasal cavity.

Nerves in the nasal mucosa include sensory fibers of the terminal, olfactory, vomeronasal, and maxillary division of the trigeminal nerve, and efferent fibers of the autonomic nervous system. Nerve endings are frequently observed within the epithelium, adjacent to the juxtaluminal junctional complex between adjacent cells. Lymphatic nodules are commonly present in the caudal part of the nasal cavity, adjacent to the opening between nasal cavity and nasopharyngeal meatus.

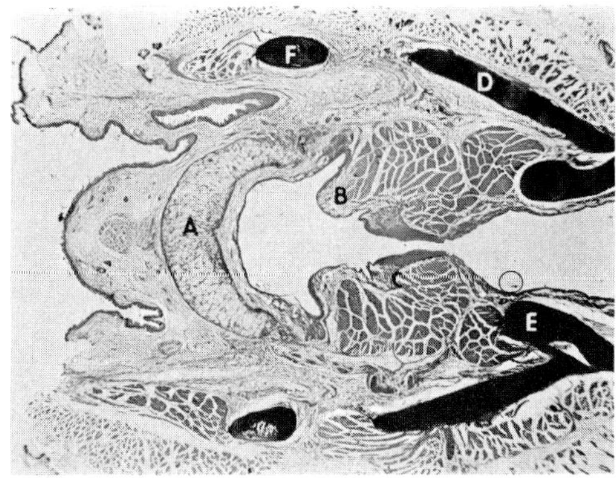

Fig. 9–13. *Horizontal section through the larynx, cat. Epiglottis cartilage (A); ventricular ligament (B); vocal ligament (C); thyroid cartilage (D); cricoid cartilage (E); stylohyoid bone (F). H & E. ×8.3. (From Dellmann, H.-D.: Veterinary Histology: An Outline Text-Atlas. Philadelphia, Lea & Febiger, 1971.)*

NASOPHARYNX

The nasopharynx is that portion of the pharynx located dorsal to the soft palate and extending from the nasal cavity to the laryngopharynx. The lining of the nasopharynx consists mostly of ciliated, pseudostratified columnar epithelium with goblet cells. The lining of the caudodorsal portion of the soft palate, which makes contact either with the dorsal wall of the nasopharynx during deglutition or with the epiglottis, is stratified squamous. The lamina propria consists of loose connective tissue characterized by a relatively dense infiltration of lymphocytes and granulocytes. Lymphatic nodules are particularly prominent in the dorsal portion of the nasopharynx, in the median line of which they aggregate as the pharyngeal tonsil. Simple branched tubuloacinar glands are present in the lamina propria.

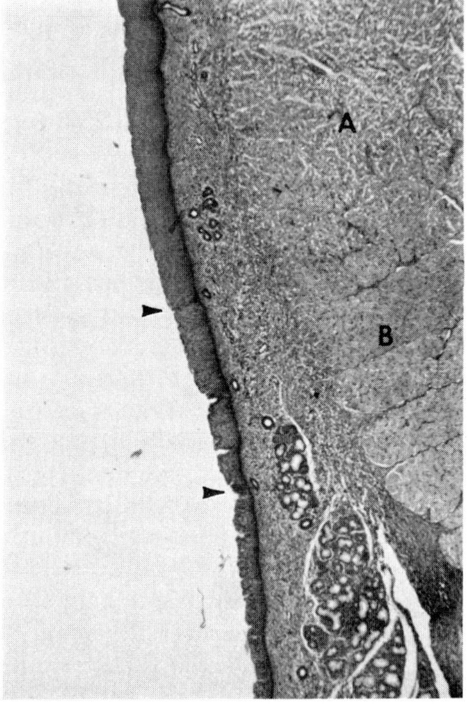

Fig. 9–14. *Horizontal section through the caudal portion of the vocal fold, cat. Vocal ligament (A); vocal muscle (B). Notice the thick stratified squamous epithelium on the vocal folds and its gradual decrease in height toward the trachea. After a short transitional zone (between arrows) the epithelium becomes respiratory in nature. H & E. ×39.*

LARYNX

The larynx opens rostrally into the laryngopharynx and is continuous caudally with the trachea (Fig. 9–13). It is lined by mucosa and supported by cartilage. The laryngeal cartilages are connected to each other, to the trachea, and to the hyoid apparatus by ligaments. Extrinsic skeletal muscles move the larynx during swallowing; intrinsic skeletal muscles move individual laryngeal cartilages during respiration and phonation.

The mucosa of the epiglottis, laryngeal vestibule, and vocal folds is lined by a nonkeratinized stratified squamous epithelium; the laryngeal epithelium caudal to the vocal fold grades into a ciliated pseudostratified columnar type with goblet cells (Fig. 9–14). A ciliated pseudostratified columnar epithelium is also present lining the equine laryngeal ventricle. The epithelium on the laryngeal surface of the epiglottis, aryepiglottic folds, and arytenoids may contain taste buds in all species except the horse. Nerve receptors in the laryngeal epithelium respond to fluids such as water, milk, gastric fluid, and saliva; stimulation of these receptors results in apnea with the sensory limb of the reflex passing through the cranial laryngeal nerve.

The lamina propria beneath the stratified squamous epithelium is a dense irregular connective tissue; that beneath the ciliated pseudostratified columnar epithelium is a loose connective tissue. It contains numerous elastic fibers, leukocytes, plasma cells, and mast cells. Diffuse lymphatic tissue or solitary lymphatic nodules are frequently observed. In the pig and small ruminants a paraepiglottic tonsil is present on either side of the base of the epiglottis; this tonsil occurs occasionally in the cat. Simple branched tubuloacinar glands (Fig. 9–14) occur in the lamina propria and submucosa; glands are absent in the vestibular and vocal folds. Numerous elastic fibers are present in the vocal ligament and, to a lesser extent, in the vestibular ligament.

Most of the laryngeal cartilages are of the hyaline type, the perichondrium of which blends with the adjacent submucosa. The epiglottis, the cuneiform and corniculate cartilages or processes, and the vocal process of the arytenoid cartilage contain elastic cartilage. The epiglottis of carnivores often consists of a peripheral cartilaginous wall enclosing adipose tissue, strands of elastic fibers, and small areas of elastic cartilage. A loose connective tissue forms the tunica adventitia surrounding the laryngeal cartilages and muscles.

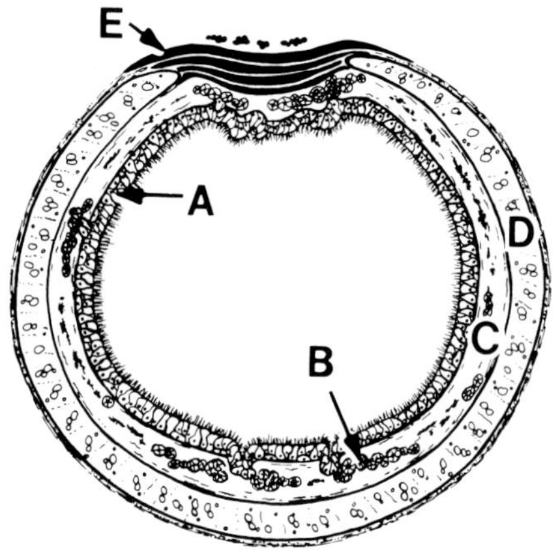

Fig. 9–15. *Schematic drawing of cross section of trachea. Pseudostratified epithelium (A) lines the lumen. Glands (B) in the lamina propria and submucosa (C). Cartilage (D) and a band of smooth muscle (E), the trachealis muscle, form the majority of the wall.*

TRACHEA AND EXTRAPULMONARY BRONCHI

The trachea provides the air passageway between the larynx and the bronchi. It is a semiflexible and semicollapsible tube in the ventral portion of the neck that extends from the larynx into the thoracic cavity. Histologically, the wall of the trachea (Figs. 9–15 and 9–16) is organized in four layers or tunics: mucosa, submucosa, muscle and cartilage, and adventitia.

The mucosa of the trachea is composed of pseudostratified ciliated columnar epithelium and its lamina propria (Fig. 9–17). The following seven epithelial cell types have been identified in the lining epithelium of the trachea: basal cells, goblet (or mucous) cells, ciliated cells, brush cells, serous cells, Clara cells, and neuroendocrine cells. *Basal cells* are oriented with long axes parallel to and in contact with the basal lamina. The cytoplasm, containing many

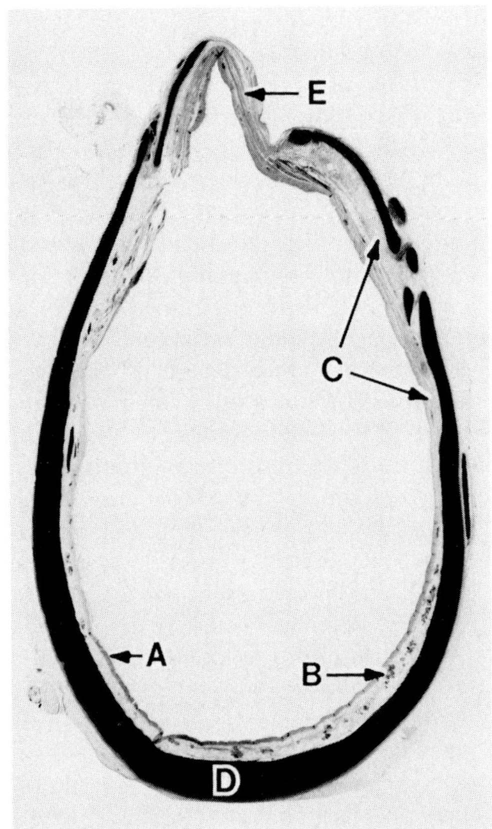

Fig. 9–16. *Cross section of trachea, sheep. Epithelium (A); glands (B) in submucosa (C); cartilage (D). Trachealis muscle (E). High iron diamine–Alcian blue. ×3.*

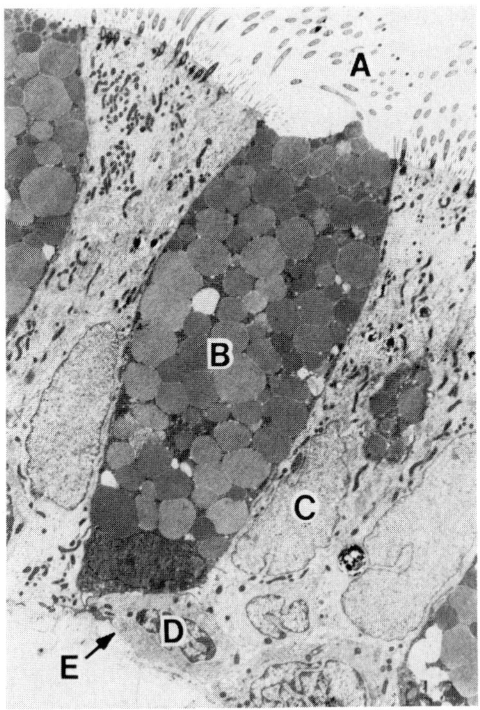

Fig. 9–17. *Electron micrograph of tracheal epithelium, cat. Airway lumen (A); mucous goblet cell (B); ciliated cell (C); basal cell (D); basal lamina (E). ×2750.*

filaments and few organelles, is usually small in relation to the size of the nucleus. This cell is thought to be the progenitor cell for the other epithelial cell types. *Goblet, ciliated,* and *brush cells* of the trachea are similar to those in the upper respiratory system. *Serous cells* have basal, lobated nuclei and apical microvilli; they contain abundant granular ER and apical electron-dense secretory granules. The structure of the *Clara cell* is described on page 199. *Neuroendocrine cells,* also known as Kultschitzky-like cells (K cells) or amine precursor uptake decarboxylation (APUD) cells, are typically pyramid-shaped with their bases on the basal lamina and contain dense-cored, argyrophilic granules, abundant ER, Golgi complex, ribosomes, and many filaments. These cells are more abundant in young animals and are sometimes associated with nerve endings. Other *indifferent cells* represent a very small proportion of the epithelial cell population and are characterized by a generalized cell structure with none of the individual specific characteristics of the seven cell types described. A variety of *migratory cells* are also observed in the epithelium. These include lymphocytes, globule leukocytes, and mast cells. *Globule leukocytes* are mononuclear cells containing acidophilic, metachromatic granules. They have been studied more thoroughly in the intestinal epithelium where they are associated with parasitic infestations.

There is great interspecies variation in the composition of the mucosal epithelium in the trachea. Goblet cells are the predominant secretory cell type in domestic mammals (horse, cow, sheep, pig, goat, dog, and cat), while Clara or serous cells are the major secretory cell of other species. Other variations between species include the relative abundance of brush cells, neurosecretory cells, and basal cells.

The lamina propria consists of a basal lamina, fine collagen fibers in a dense, irregular meshwork, and a dense, irregular band of longitudinally oriented elastic fibers. The lamina propria also contains small blood and lymph vessels and nerve endings.

Tracheal glands are extensions of surface epithelium into subepithelial connective tissue. They are tubuloacinar seromucous glands that remain connected to the surface by a series of ducts, some of which are lined by a ciliated epithelium. The primary cell types of the ducts include ciliated cells, mucus-secreting cells with granules in their apical portion, and various intermediate cells. The majority of the secretory portions of these glands are located within the submucosal region, with proximal portions composed of tubules and lined by mucus-secreting cells, and with distal portions composed of acini and lined primarily by serous secretory cells. The mucus-secreting cells lining the tubules generally secrete sulfated acid glycoproteins. Serous cells are the major secretory cells of the glands in most species; their secretory product is a neutral glycoprotein that is sometimes sulfated. The serous cells that produce this protein have small, dense, discrete granules and a cytoplasm filled with large amounts of granular ER. Acini and tubules are surrounded by myoepithelial cells. Nonmyelinated nerve fibers and nerve endings are generally adjacent to the secretory portions of submucosal glands. Migratory cells in the vicinity of the glands include lymphocytes, plasma cells, globular leukocytes, and mast cells. Tracheal glands are thought to provide most of the secretory material that lines the ciliary surface in the trachea. These glands are abundant in the proximal portions of the trachea of virtually all domestic mammalian species.

The most distinctive feature of the trachea are the cartilages (Figs. 9–15 and 9–16), which in most species are roughly "C"- or "U"-shaped pieces of hyaline cartilage that are incomplete dorsally. The number of cartilages in the wall of the trachea varies, not only among different species, but among different individuals of the same species. In some individuals they are fused in places so that instead of being separate, distinct entities, they form a continuum. The trachealis muscle is a band of smooth muscle whose fibers extend transversely between the dorsal free ends of the cartilage, along the entire length of the trachea. In the majority of species, except the dog and cat, the smooth muscle attaches to the dense, irregular connective tissue of the perichondrium on the interior side of the rings, generally at some distance from the ends of the cartilage (Fig. 9–16). In carnivores (Fig. 9–15) this attachment is on the external surface of the cartilage. Nerves and large blood vessels are generally associated with the smooth muscle band.

A dense, irregular connective tissue meshwork of large collagen fibers and elastic fibers surrounds the outside of the cartilage rings. The distal portion of the trachea continues into the thoracic cavity where it terminates by bifurcating into two primary bronchi. A triangular-shaped cartilage forms a ridge separating the openings of right and left primary bronchi; this ridge is named the tracheal carina. Distal to the bifurcation, the primary bronchi provide branches that enter the lungs.

LUNG

Most of the thoracic cavity is occupied by the right and left lungs. Subgrossly, the lung of mammals may be divided into intrapulmonary conducting airways, parenchyma, and pleura. The intrapulmonary airways *(bronchi* and *bronchioles)* compose

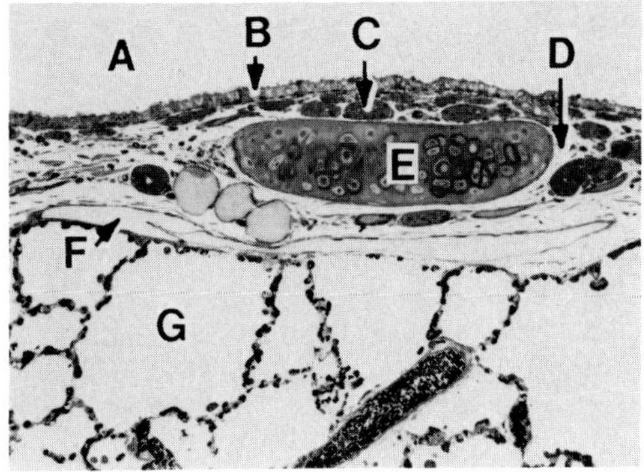

Fig. 9–18. *Portion of wall of medium-sized bronchus, cat. Airway lumen (A); pseudostratified epithelium (B); glands (C) in submucosa (D); cartilage plate (E); peribronchial lymphatic with valve (F); alveolar airspace (G). Toluidine Blue. ×110.*

approximately 6% of the lung. The *parenchyma,* or gas exchange area, consisting of alveolar ducts, alveolar sacs, and alveoli, makes up approximately 85% of the lung. A *transitional zone* joins small bronchioles with gas exchange tissue. The lung is encapsulated by a layer of connective tissue and mesothelial cells termed the *visceral pleura.* Along with the pleura, the intrapulmonary nervous and vascular tissue (pulmonary arteries, pulmonary veins, and bronchiole arteries) make up the remaining 9 to 10% of the lung.

Bronchi

The bronchial tree is formed by a primary bronchus and the various orders of airways that it supplies. The largest segments of the intrapulmonary conducting airways are called *lobar bronchi,* each of which is a branch of a primary bronchus and enters a lung lobe at its hilum. Each of the lobar bronchi divides into two smaller branches, each of which divides again. These branches also divide, and this process continues until the gas exchange area is reached. This system of division is called pseudodichotomous branching because one daughter branch is larger in cross-sectional area than the other and because each of these branches exits the parent branch at a different angle. The number of times the bronchial tree branches before the gas exchange area is reached varies from species to species, from lobe to lobe in the same species, and by position within any particular lobe. The number of generations of branching between the trachea and the parenchymal airspace can vary in the same lobe from as few as six for gas exchange areas closest to the hilum to as many as 28 or 30 for gas exchange areas located in the most distal portion of a lobe. Each of the first two or three generations of branching from a lobar bronchus supplies portions of the lung lobe called bronchopulmonary segments. Each succeeding generation of branching is made up of a greater number of airways and has a larger total cross-sectional area than the generation before it.

The histologic appearance of a bronchus (Figs. 9–18 and 9–19) is generally similar to that of the trachea except that the various layers are thinner. Bronchi are lined by a pseudostratified columnar epithelium composed primarily of secretory cells, ciliated cells, and basal cells. Fewer total cells and proportionally fewer secretory cells line the proximal bronchi than the trachea. The composition of the epithelium changes in a proximal to distal direction in a single species (Fig. 9–20). Proximal bronchi have more epithelial cells and more basal cells per unit surface area than do more distal bronchi. In species in which mucous cells are the predominant surface secretory cell type, the percentage of the population composed of mucous cells decreases and that for Clara cells increases in more distal airways. The epithelial height and the thickness of the lamina propria progressively decrease proximally to distally. Submucosal glands are fewer and smaller in proximal bronchi as compared to the trachea; in those species in which glands are sparse or nonexistent in the distal trachea, submucosal glands do not occur in intrapulmonary bronchi. Intrapulmonary bronchi contain glands in carnivores,

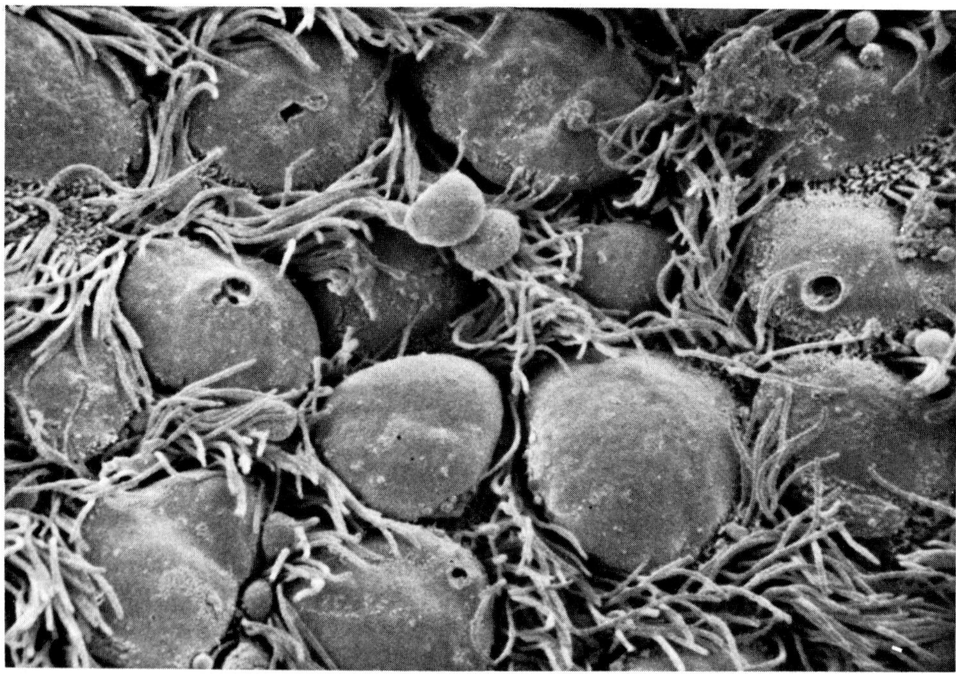

Fig. 9–19. *Scanning electron micrograph, small bronchus, horse. The goblet cells are surrounded by cilia, some of which support debris or remnants of the mucous layer. Microvilli are found at the periphery of the goblet cells and at the base of the cilia. Notice the openings in the luminal surfaces of four goblet cells, probably for the discharge of the mucigen granules. ×2850. (From Tyler, W.S., Gillespie, J.R., and Nowell, J.A.: Modern functional morphology of the equine lung. Equine Vet J 3:84, 1971.)*

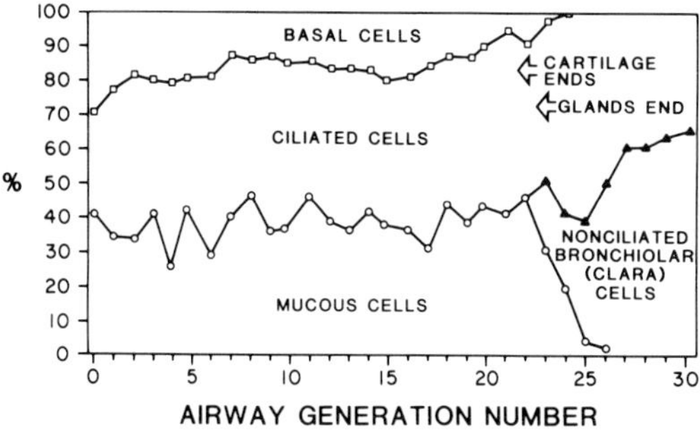

Fig. 9–20. *Graph of relative abundance of epithelial cell types in the tracheobronchial tree of the sheep. Left cranial lobe. Trachea (generation numbers 0 and 1). Lobar bronchus (generation number 2). Intrapulmonary bronchi (generation numbers 3 through 23). Bronchioles (generation numbers 24–30).*

ruminants (cow, sheep), the horse, and the pig. The structure of bronchial submucosa varies in a proximal to distal direction, with bronchial glands being less abundant in distal bronchi. The hyaline cartilage of the proximal bronchi is in the form of irregular plates, instead of "C"- or "U"-shaped pieces (Fig. 9–18), and the smooth muscle is interspersed either between the plates or on the luminal side of the plates. The muscle cells are generally arranged in a circular fashion perpendicularly to the long axis of the airway. The amount of cartilage decreases in more distal bronchial generations while the relative abundance of smooth muscle increases. The extent of bronchial cartilage within the tracheobronchial tree varies greatly from species to species. In the sheep, for example, cartilage plates are in more than 20 generations of bronchi (Fig. 9–20). The connective tissue external to bronchial cartilage in the adjoining adventitia is primarily loose, with many collagen fibers and variable numbers of elastic fibers. Many of the fibers are oriented longitudinally while others are oriented perpendicularly to the long axis of the airway. Small groups of myelinated and

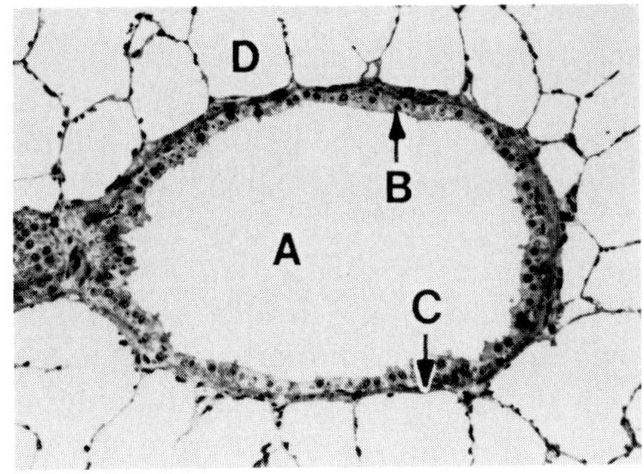

Fig. 9–21. *Cross section of a bronchiole, sheep. The airway lumen (A) is surrounded by a wall composed of simple cuboidal epithelium (B) and smooth muscle (C). Alveolar airspaces (D) surround the bronchiole. Toluidine blue. ×135.*

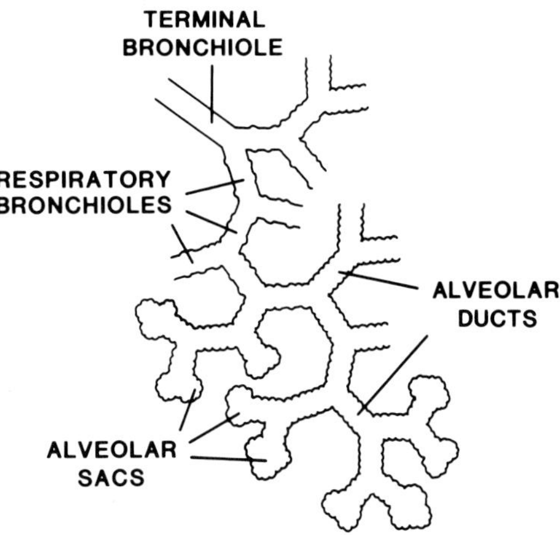

Fig. 9–22. *Schematic diagram of the organization of a pulmonary acinus. All of the gas exchange tissue (alveoli, alveolar sacs, alveolar ducts) join one terminal bronchiole by a series of respiratory bronchioles.*

nonmyelinated nerves and parasympathetic ganglia are in the adventitia and submucosa of the bronchi. Nerve endings have been identified within the surface epithelium and surrounding the glands. Adjoining the periphery of the adventitia of intrapulmonary bronchi are alveoli of the gas exchange area.

Bronchioles

The most distal intrapulmonary air passages are the *bronchioles.* The bronchioles (Fig. 9–21), whose cross-sectional profiles are roughly circular, may be distinguished from bronchi histologically. In general, walls of bronchioles are composed of epithelium, smooth muscle, and small amounts of connective tissue without glands or cartilage. Bronchioles without alveoli (see p. 202) opening directly through their walls are said to be nonalveolarized. Several generations of nonalveolarized bronchioles are present in the horse, ox, and sheep; generally only one or two generations of nonalveolarized bronchioles are in the lungs of the dog and cat. The most distal conducting airway free of alveoli is the *terminal bronchiole.* Its lining epithelium is a simple columnar or cuboidal epithelium composed of ciliated cells and Clara cells. The *Clara cells* (bronchiolar exocrine cells) have characteristics of both secretory cells and cells capable of metabolizing xenobiotic compounds. The secretory granules are discrete, membrane-bounded, electron-dense structures thought to contain neutral glycoprotein. These cells have a large number of mitochondria scattered throughout their cytoplasm and a variable amount of agranular ER and glycogen. Agranular ER is very abundant within Clara cells in the horse and sheep and is minimally present in the dog, cat, cow, and pig. Glycogen, the predominant cellular feature of Clara cells in the cow, dog, and cat, is rarely observed in most other species. The Clara cell is restricted to the most distal generations of airways in domestic mammals. In the dog and cat, epithelium of the most distal nonalveolarized bronchioles consists of ciliated and Clara cells in a 1:19 ratio.

The thickness of the lamina propria and submucosa is extremely reduced compared to bronchi. The smooth muscle is in separate fascicles that branch and anastomose such that the fibers course both circularly and obliquely. The surrounding connective tissue includes collagen fibers oriented in all directions and elastic fibers oriented circularly or obliquely. Numerous nerve fibers occur in the area immediately below the epithelium and interspersed between muscle fascicles.

There are two exceptions to the structure of distal nonalveolarized bronchioles as described. In marine mammals and macaque monkeys, cartilage is present in the walls of terminal bronchioles. In addition, the epithelium lining these airways is pseudostratified, containing basal cells, ciliated cells, and mucous cells.

Transition Zone

The *transition zone,* or area where small air passages of the tracheobronchial tree join the gas exchange area, is the focus of most lung pathologic conditions. This transition occurs by the formation of outpocketings of gas exchange tissue in the walls of bronchioles. Such bronchioles that are alveolarized are termed *respiratory bronchioles.* Their histologic appearance is very similar to that of terminal bronchioles, with the exception that the epithelium is interrupted by alveoli (Figs. 9–22 and 9–23). The smooth muscle is arranged in fascicles that underlie the simple cuboidal or columnar epithelium. The alveolae open between these muscle bundles.

The organization of the transitional zone is highly variable among species with two extremes described. In one, the transition is abrupt (Fig. 9–24), with the respiratory bronchiole being very short or absent such as occurs in some rodents and many domesticated animals, including the horse, cow, sheep, and pig. The other condition is one of extensive alveolarization of the distal bronchioles (Fig. 9–23), with the number of alveolar outpocketings per generation of branching generally less proxi-

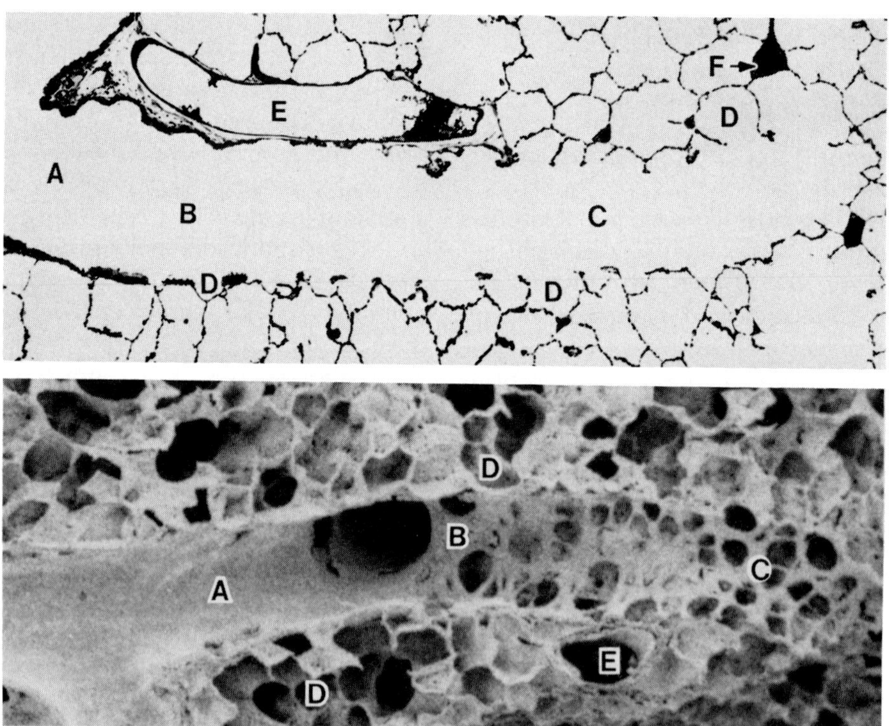

Fig. 9–23. *Histologic (upper) and scanning electron microscopic (lower) appearance of the terminal airspaces of the cat. Terminal bronchiole (A); respiratory bronchiole (B); alveolar duct (C); alveoli (D); pulmonary arteriole (E); pulmonary venule (F). Upper: Methylene blue/Azure II. ×55. Lower: ×70.*

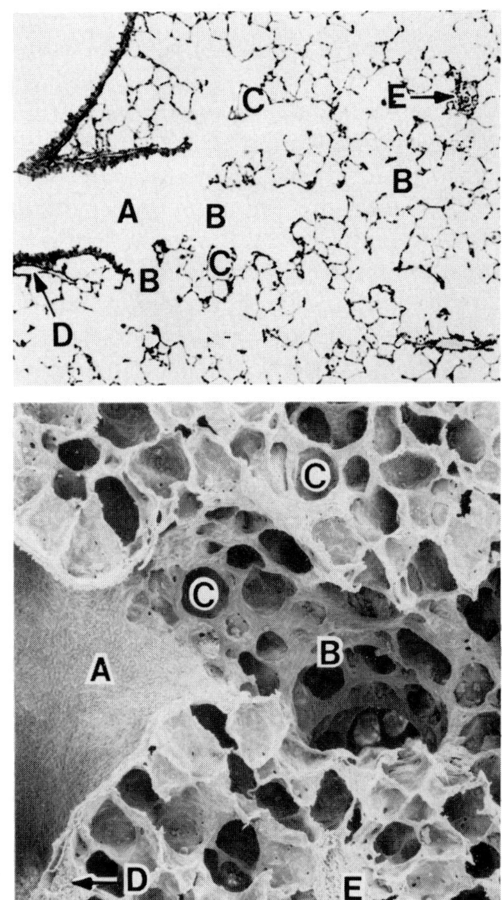

Fig. 9–24. *Histologic (upper) and scanning electron microscopic (lower) appearance of the terminal airspaces of the mouse (upper) and the rat (lower). Terminal bronchiole (A); alveolar duct (B); alveoli (C); pulmonary arteriole (D); pulmonary venule (E). Upper: Toluidine Blue. ×85. Lower: ×110.*

mally and greater distally. This is the organization typical of dogs and cats. In these species the epithelium in respiratory bronchioles consists almost entirely of Clara cells.

Respiratory Area

The respiratory area, where gas exchange takes place, is often called the *parenchyma;* parenchyma consists of alveolar ducts, alveolar sacs, alveoli, and the air spaces contained within these structures.

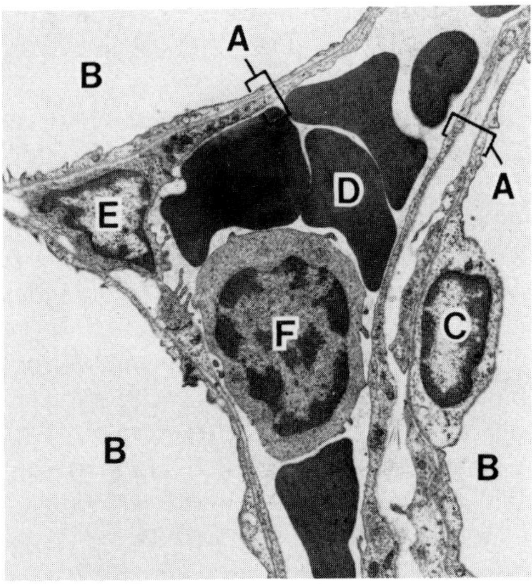

Fig. 9–25. *Electron micrograph, rat, of interalveolar septa showing the blood-air barrier (A). The alveolar airspace (B) is lined by the squamous (or type I) alveolar epithelial cell (C). The capillary containing red blood cells (D) is lined by endothelial cells (E). Lymphocyte (F). ×4300.*

In the inflated lung of most species, the parenchyma occupies approximately 85% of the volume, of which 70% is airspace and 30% is gas exchange tissue surrounding the airspace. This tissue includes epithelium, some connective tissue, arterioles and venules, and the pulmonary capillary bed. The gas exchange membrane, or *blood-air barrier* (Fig. 9–25), is a vast surface with capillary bed on one side and air on the other. The surface area of this gas exchange membrane ranges from less than 0.02 m^2 in the tiny shrew (*Suncus etruscus,* average body weight: 0.003 kg) to 2450 m^2 in the domestic horse (average body weight: 510 kg). The surface area of the capillary side of this membrane is only slightly less than that of the air side. This vast surface, which is approximately twice the size of a football field in an adult horse and about the size of a tennis court in an adult human, is packed into a small lung volume (0.1 ml in the shrew, and 38,000 ml in the horse). This is accomplished by the development of numerous small air passages with *alveoli.* Gas exchange generally occurs on both sides of tissue septa that separate the alveoli. These septa are called *interalveolar septa.*

The air passages of the parenchymal tissue are organized into units. The functional unit of the gas exchange area is called the *acinus,* or *terminal respiratory unit* (Fig. 9–22). The acinus includes all of those airspaces distal to one terminal bronchiole. This includes all of the respiratory bronchioles branching from one terminal bronchiole and all alveolar ducts, alveolar sacs, and alveoli joined to these respiratory bronchioles. Unoxygenated blood is supplied to this unit by a *pulmonary arteriole* (Figs. 9–23 and 9–24), which courses in the connective tissue associated with a terminal bronchiole.

In many species, acini are separated into groups, called *lobules.* The lobule is a structural unit rather than a functional unit. It comprises a cluster of acini that is separated from adjacent clusters by connective tissue septa. These connective tissue septa are termed *interlobular septa* and are composed of collagen and elastic fibers and blood vessels. Both *bronchial arteries* and *pulmonary veins* are situated in interlobular septa. The interlobular septa, when complete, extend from the connective tissue of the visceral pleura to the connective tissue surrounding major bronchi and blood vessels. The lungs of the cow, sheep, and pig are highly lobulated and have complete septa. The lungs of the horse have incomplete septa and are considered poorly lobulated. The septa in this species extend into the gas exchange area from the pleura but do not come in contact with the connective tissue surrounding large airways and vessels. Most species, including the dog and cat, do not have interlobular septa.

Alveolar Ducts, Alveolar Sacs, and Alveoli

The vast majority of the parenchyma is organized either as tubular or saclike structures. The tubular structures are termed *alveolar ducts* (Figs. 9–23 and 9–24). They are comparable to hallways lined by doorless rooms on all sides. Each of these doorless rooms is a single pocket or alveolus. Between one and five generations of alveolar ducts are supplied by a single respiratory bronchiole. The walls of an alveolar duct are composed of the open sides of alveolar airspaces and the terminations of the interalveolar septa that separate these alveoli. Spiraling bands of smooth muscle and elastic fibers, perpendicular to the long axis of the alveolar ducts, occupy space deep to the epithelium at the terminations of the interalveolar septa.

The alveolar ducts terminate in clusters of alveoli called *alveolar sacs* (Fig. 9–22). A shared space into which a number of alveolar sacs open is called an atrium. The basic unit for gas exchange in the pulmonary parenchyma is the alveolus (Fig. 9–26). Alveoli are essentially spheroidal airspaces that open into an alveolar sac, alveolar duct, or the lumen of a respiratory bronchiole. Thin sheets of tissue called *interalveolar septa* separate adjacent alveoli.

The interalveolar septa are sheets of connective tissue containing a capillary plexus and covered on both sides by a layer of epithelium (Fig. 9–25). Two epithelial cell types line the interalveolar septa, forming the air side of the blood-air barrier. The *squamous,* or *type I, alveolar epithelial cell* (respiratory epithelial cell) is a very flat cell with a centrally placed nucleus (Fig. 9–25). It has the appearance of a fried egg. The flat sheet of cytoplasm that composes the majority of the cell has few organelles. There are a small number of mitochondria, minimal amounts of granular ER, and a moderate number of endocytotic vesicles. This cell type covers approximately 97% of the interalveolar septal surface in all the species studied thus far yet forms only 45% of the cells lining the alveolus. The average surface area of a type I cell ranges from 5000 to 7000 μm^2. The tissue side of this vast sheet of cells is lined by a continuous basal lamina.

The second type of epithelial cell (Fig.

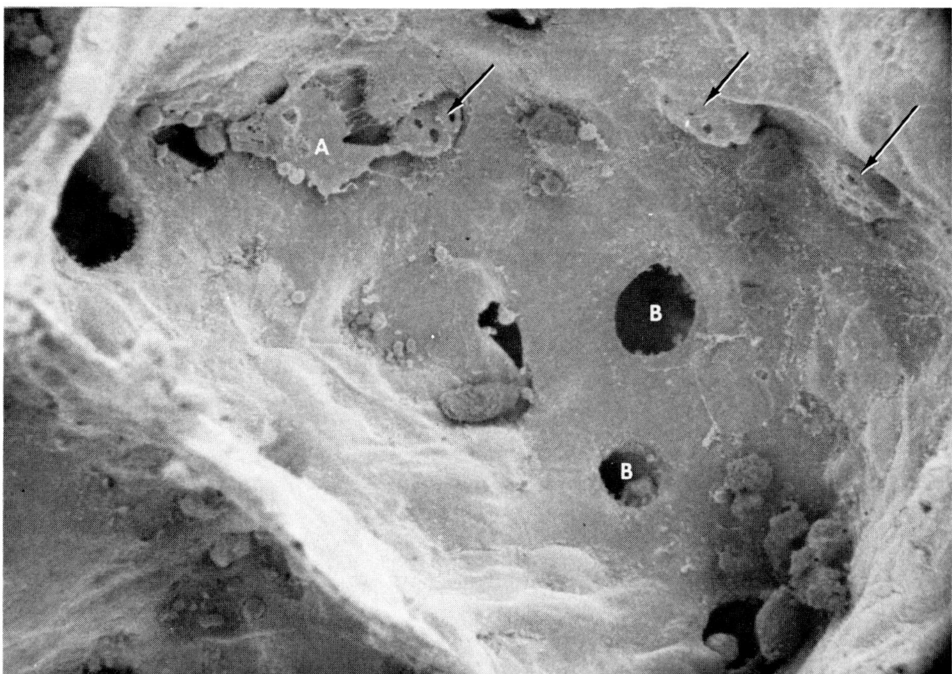

Fig. 9–26. *Scanning electron micrograph of portion of an alveolus, horse. Cuboidal alveolar epithelial cells (type II cells) are seen to bulge into the lumen (arrows). On the left is a pulmonary alveolar macrophage (A). Notice the pores in the interalveolar septum (B).* ×*1232. (Courtesy of W.S. Tyler.)*

9–27) is the *granular,* or *type II, alveolar epithelial cell (great alveolar cell).* It is a cuboidal cell with a central nucleus. This cell type covers the remainder of the interalveolar septal surface area (approximately 3%). The alveolar type II cell constitutes approximately 12% of the cells composing the canine interalveolar septum. Its average cell surface ranges from 100 to 280 μm^2 per cell. This cell is filled with large numbers of organelles, including mitochondria, granular ER, microvesicles, and a Golgi complex. The alveolar surface has large numbers of microvilli. Its characteristic feature is the presence of large numbers of osmiophilic, laminated vesicles called lamellar bodies. These lamellar bodies are thought to be primarily phospholipid and to be the source of the phospholipids that compose the *pulmonary surfactant* that lines the airspaces. The type II alveolar cell is thought to function as the progenitor cell for both type I and type II cells.

Another cell found on the air side of the interalveolar septa is the *pulmonary alveolar macrophage* (Fig. 9–28). These cells make up approximately 2 to 9% of the cells in the lung parenchyma. As active phagocytic cells they are part of the macrophage system distributed throughout the body.

The capillary bed of the interalveolar septa is an intermeshed network of short, branching vessels. Interalveolar capillary blood volume in mammals ranges from 0.01 ml in the shrew to 2800 ml in the adult horse. Capillary *endothelial cells* resemble endothelial cells in other organs (Fig. 9–25). Endothelial cells are characterized by small numbers of organelles and relatively large numbers of endocytotic vesicles. The average surface area of an endothelial cell is approximately 1000 μm^2. Endothelial cells are attached to a continuous basal lamina. The intercellular junctions tend to be of the loose or leaky variety with the tight junctions having few parallel

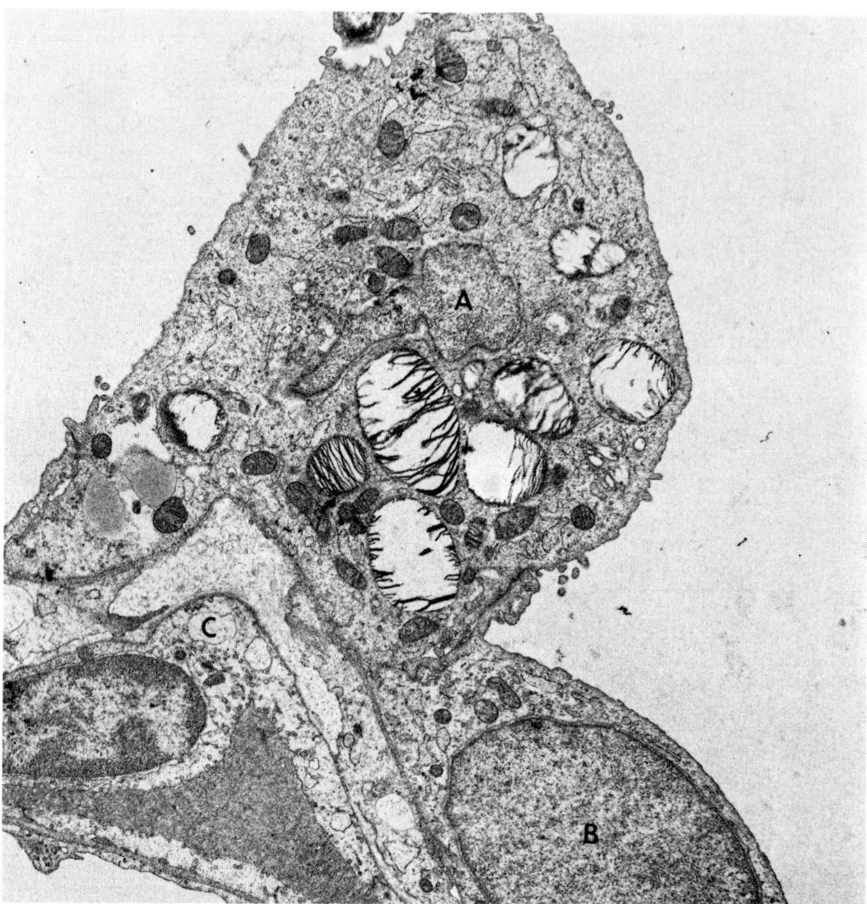

Fig. 9–27. *Electron micrograph of a cuboidal alveolar epithelial cell (A) and a squamous alveolar epithelial cell (B). Notice the numerous characteristic lamellar cytosomes in the cuboidal alveolar epithelial cell and endothelial cell (C) of a capillary. ×8200. (From Tyler, W.S., Gillespie, J.R., and Nowell, J.A.: Modern functional morphology of the equine lung. Equine Vet J 3:84, 1971.)*

arrays of contact. The surface area of the gas exchange capillary bed is between two thirds and three fourths of the surface area of the air side of the interalveolar septa. Individual capillary beds traverse the walls of from three to seven alveoli in passing from a pulmonary arteriole to a pulmonary venule. Most of the endothelial cells surrounding the capillaries have one side with a very thin extension of cytoplasm. The side faces the epithelial cells lining the air portion of the blood-air barrier. In these attenuated areas, the basal laminae fuse. The endothelium of the opposite side of the capillary is separated from the lining epithelial cell by a band of elastic and collagen fibers.

The space between alveolar epithelial and endothelial cells within the interalveolar septum, termed the *interstitium,* contains a variety of cells and collagen and elastic fibers. The majority of the cells in the interstitium are fibroblasts. Other cells include pericytes surrounding capillary endothelial cells, monocytes, lymphocytes, plasma cells, and contractile or fat-storing interstitial cells.

In the living animal, the alveoli contain a small amount of fluid within the airspace. This fluid consists of a biphasic layer of plasma filtrates overlaid by a thin layer of phospholipids called pulmonary surfactant. It is the pulmonary surfactant that reduces the surface tension in these small

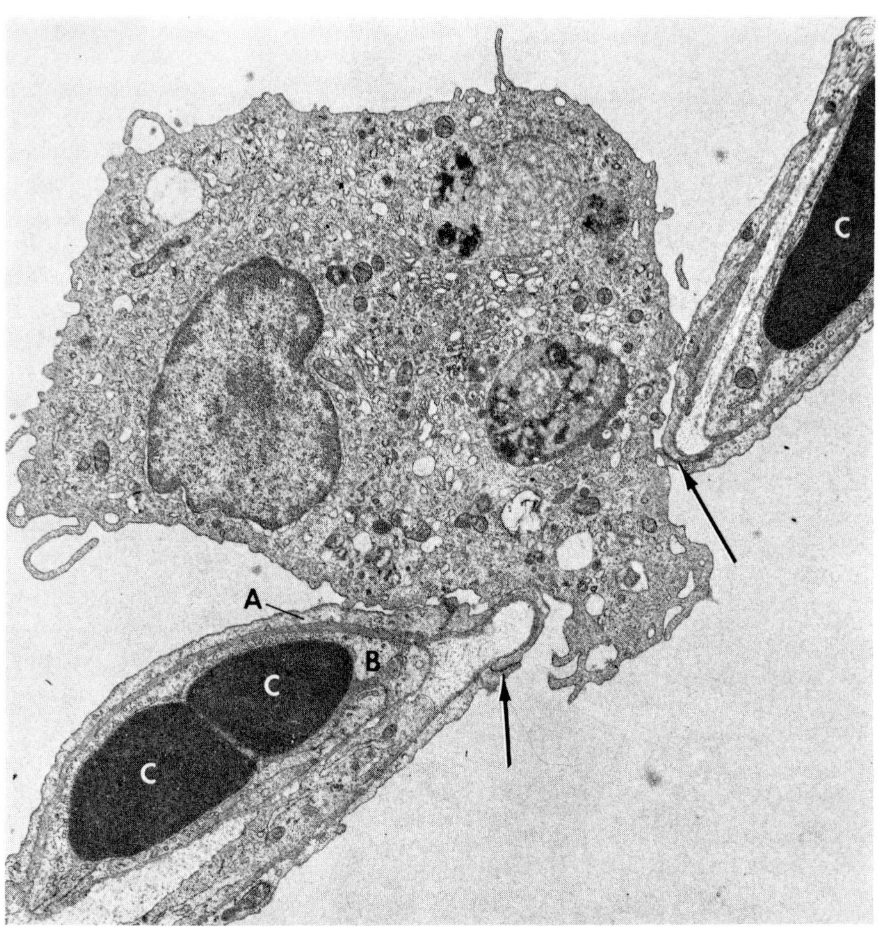

Fig. 9–28. *Electron micrograph of an alveolar macrophage projecting through an alveolar pore, lung, horse. The macrophage has numerous filopodia, lysosomes and digestive vacuoles. The very thin layer of cytoplasm of the squamous alveolar epithelial cells (A) is separated by a basal lamina from the capillary endothelium (B). Erythrocytes (C) are in the capillary lumen. The dark lines (arrows) are tight junctions between adjacent squamous alveolar epithelial cells.* ×*8100. (From Tyler, W.S., Gillespie, J.R., and Nowell, J.A.: Modern functional morphology of the equine lung. Equine Vet J 3:84, 1971.)*

pockets of air to prevent them from collapsing. The blood-air barrier (Fig. 9–25) serves to prevent the massive release of fluid filtrate from endothelial cells into the airspace. The average thickness of this barrier is 1.5 μm in most species. At its thinnest, the blood-air barrier (Fig. 9–25) consists of the surface lining layer of pulmonary surfactant and fluid, the thin cytoplasm of an alveolar type I cell, fused basal laminae of the alveolar epithelial cell and the underlying capillary endothelial cell, the capillary endothelial cell, and the plasmalemma of a red blood cell. The thickness of the thinnest areas, which is significant in gas diffusion, ranges from 0.2 to 0.7 μm. At its thickest, this barrier consists of the above-mentioned layers and interstitial connective tissue and cells between the basal laminae of epithelial and endothelial cells. Openings in the interalveolar septa interconnect adjacent alveoli. These openings, called *alveolar pores* (Fig. 9–26), are lined by epithelial cells and permit air and alveolar macrophages to pass from one alveolus to another.

Pleura

The *visceral,* or *pulmonary, pleura* completely covers both lungs except at the hilum and the pulmonary ligament. The pleura is a serous membrane consisting of mesothelial cells that vary from squamous to cuboidal and a layer of varying amounts of dense irregular connective tissue and elastic fibers. Deep to the pleura, a layer of pulmonary capillaries supplies the superficial portion of the gas exchange area. At the periphery of the lung the connective tissue of interalveolar septa is continuous with the pleura. At its thickest, the pleura's connective tissue elements consist of two or more layers of elastic laminae, many dense irregular bundles of collagen fibers, pulmonary capillaries, and two additional sets of vessels. These two sets of vessels include capillaries and small arterioles from the bronchial circulation and lymphatic vessels. There is variation in the thickness of the pleura from species to species and within different regions of the same species. The thinnest pleura is found in the dog and cat. In these species the subpleural connective tissue is minimal and the only circulation derives from the pulmonary artery. The pleura is very thick in large domestic mammals. In those species with interlobular septa, the septa are connected to the pleural connective tissue. Pleural mesothelial cells are joined by tight junctions and covered by a microvillar surface and contain large amounts of granular ER and mitochondria.

Pulmonary Circulation

Blood is supplied to the lungs through two different circulations, *pulmonary* and *bronchial.* The vast majority of the blood flow to the lungs comes from the pulmonary arteries. The entire output of the right ventricle flows into the two pulmonary arteries as unoxygenated blood. The pulmonary circulation is a low-pressure system, as large, medium, and small arteries have thinner walls than vessels of comparable size in the systemic circulation. They have fewer elastic and collagen fibers and fewer smooth muscle cells. The pulmonary arterial circulation shares its connective tissue adventitia with that of the tracheobronchial tree.

The bronchial arteries are under high pressure as a part of the systemic arterial circulation. The blood vessels in this circulation have the same wall structure as those of other systemic arteries of the same size. It is a very low flow system, with less than 1% of the left ventricular output entering the bronchial arteries. In all species, the bronchial artery supplies blood to the walls of the large bronchi, the major pulmonary vessels, and the pulmonary lymph nodes. In the dog and cat, the bronchial artery also supplies blood to the walls of bronchioles as far distal as the terminal bronchioles. In species with a thick pleura (the horse, cow, sheep, and pig), the bronchial artery also supplies blood to the pleural connective tissue and interlobular septa. In the horse the bronchial artery also supplies capillaries in the interalveolar septa. Anastomoses between bronchial and pulmonary arterial circulations have been identified in the walls of medium-sized bronchi and bronchioles of the horse, cow, and sheep. The bronchial arteries are dispersed within the connective tissue of the walls of the bronchial tree, pulmonary arteries, and pulmonary veins.

All blood from the lungs is carried back to the heart by the *pulmonary veins,* a low-pressure system. The intima is composed of endothelium and an internal elastic lamina. The tunica media is composed of irregularly arranged smooth muscle and elastic and collagen fibers. There is no clear demarcation between the media and the externa. In most species the pulmonary vein is located at the periphery of lobules and courses to the hilum in parenchymal gas exchange tissue or interlobular septa. In the cow, horse, pig, and sheep, the pulmonary veins accompany the bronchial tree on the side opposite the pulmonary arteries. The pulmonary veins have thin fibrous walls with little smooth muscle in the dog, cat, horse, and goat. Pulmonary veins with large muscle bundles are present in the cow and pig. In the cow, pulmonary veins often have clumped, circularly arranged bundles of smooth muscle.

The *pulmonary lymphatics* (Fig. 9–19) provide a unidirectional drainage system that collects excess tissue fluid from the interstitial spaces of interalveolar septa, pulmonary vessels, and airways. Pulmonary lymphatic capillaries, located throughout the interstitium, except for that of interalveolar septa, are similar in structure to lymphatic capillaries in other organ systems. They have a discontinuous basal lamina. Anchoring filaments that insert on connective tissue are numerous. Adjacent endothelial cells overlap and have large intercellular clefts. The majority of the cytoplasmic organelles common to other cells (Golgi complex, mitochondria, microtubules, and ER) are present in the perinuclear cytoplasm of lymphatic endothelial cells. The remainder of the cell is greatly attenuated and contains numerous endocytotic vesicles. Collecting lymphatic vessels are found in all connective tissue spaces of the lung with the exception of alveoli, alveolar sacs and ducts, and respiratory bronchioles.

Innervation

The structure of the nervous tissue within the lung is similar to that in other organs. The innervation is from two sources: the *vagus nerve* (parasympathetic innervation) and the *sympathetic system.* General visceral afferent sensory fibers from pulmonary tissue are also contained in the vagus nerve. Both vagus nerves intermingle to form a plexus along the walls of the airway tree and the pulmonary vasculature. Individual nerve fibers are distributed irregularly over the wall of arteries, veins, and airways. There is considerable interspecies variation in the nature of the innervation. In general, as in dogs and cats, there are cholinergic excitatory fibers and noradrenergic inhibitory fibers. Few morphologic studies have been done in other domestic species. Free intraepithelial nerve endings have been observed near glands, within smooth muscle bundles, and in the interalveolar septa. Parasympathetic ganglia are present in the peribronchial connective tissue of large airways.

REFERENCES

Adams, D.R., and Hotchkiss, D.K.: The canine nasal mucosa. Zbl Vet Med C Anat Histol Embryol *12*:109, 1983.

Adams, D.R., and Wiekamp, M.D.: The canine vomeronasal organ. J Anat *138*:771, 1984.

Berendsen, P.B., Ritter, A.B., and DeFouw, D.O.: An ultrastructural morphometric comparison of the peripheral with the hilar air-blood barrier of dog lung. Anat Rec *209*:535, 1984.

Breeze, R.G., and Wheeldon, E.B.: The cells of the pulmonary airways. Am Rev Respir Dis *161*:705, 1977.

Crapo, J.D., Young, S.L., Fram, E.K., Pinkerton, K.E., Barry, B.E., and Crapo, R.O.: Morphometric characteristics of cells in the alveolar region of mammalian lungs. Amer Rev Respir Dis *128*:S42, 1983.

Frasca, J.M., Auerbach, O., Parks, V.R., and Jamieson, J.D.: Electron microscopic observations of the bronchial epithelium of dogs. I. Control dogs. Exp Mol Pathol *9*:363, 1968.

Gladysheva, O., and Martynova, G.: The morphofunctional organization of the bovine olfactory epithelium. Gehenbaurs Morph Jahrb *128*:78, 1982.

Jacobs, V.L., Sis, R.F., Chenoweth, P.J., Klemm, W.R., and Sherry, C.J.: Structure of the bovine vomeronasal complex and its relationships to the palate: tongue manipulation. Acta Anat *110*:48, 1981.

Jeffery, P.K.: Morphologic features of airway surface epithelial cells and glands. Am Rev Respir Dis *128*:S14, 1983.

Kay, J.M.: Comparative morphologic features of the pulmonary vasculature in mammals. Amer Rev Resp Dis *128*:S53, 1983.

Leak, L.V., and Jamuar, M.P.: Ultrastructure of pulmonary lymphatic vessels. Amer Rev Resp Dis *128*:S59, 1983.

Mariassy, A.T., and Plopper, C.G.: Tracheobronchial epithelium of the sheep: I. Quantitative light microscopic study of epithelial cell abundance and distribution. Anat Rec *205*:263, 1983.

Mariassy, A.T., and Plopper, C.G.: Tracheobronchial epithelium of the sheep: II. Ultrastructural and morphometric analysis of the epithelial secretory types. Anat Rec *209*:523, 1984.

Mariassy, A.T., Plopper, C.G., and Dungworth, D.L.: Characteristics of bovine lung as observed by scanning electron microscopy. Anat Rec *183*:13, 1975.

McLaughlin, R.F.: Bronchial artery distribution in various mammals and in humans. Amer Rev Resp Dis *128*:S57, 1983.

Phalen, R.F., and Oldham, M.J.: Tracheobronchial airway structure as revealed by casting techniques. Amer Rev Resp Dis *128*:51, 1983.

Plopper, C.G.: Comparative morphologic features of bronchiolar epithelial cells: The Clara cell. Am Rev Respir Dis *128*:S37, 1983.

Plopper, C.G., Mariassy, A.T., and Lollini, L.O.: Structure as revealed by airway dissection: A comparison of mammalian lungs. Amer Rev Respir Dis *128*:S4, 1983.

Plopper, C.G., Mariassy, A.T., Wilson, D.W., Alley, J.L., Nishio, S.J., and Nettesheim, P.: Comparison of nonciliated tracheal epithelial cells in six mammalian species: Ultrastructure and population densities. Exp Lung Res *5*:281, 1983.

Reid, L., and Jones, R.: Bronchial mucosal cells. Fed Proc *38*:191, 1979.

Stratton, C.J.: Morphology of surfactant producing cells and of the alveolar lining layer. *In* Pulmonary Surfactant. Edited by B. Robertson, L.M.G. Van Golde, and J.J. Batenberg. Amsterdam. Elsevier Science Publishers, 1984, pp 68–118.

Tandler, B., Sherman, J.M., and Boat, T.F.: Surface architecture of the mucosal epithelium of the cat trachea: I. Cartilaginous portion. Am J Anat *168*:119, 1983.

——— II. Structurae and dynamics of the membranous portion. Am J Anat *168*:133.

Tyler, W.S.: Comparative subgross anatomy of lungs: Pleuras, interlobular septa and distal airways. Amer Rev Resp Dis *128*:S32, 1983.

Wysocki, C.J.: Neurobehavioral evidence for the involvement of the vomeronasal system in mammalian reproduction. Neurosci Biobehav Rev *3*:301, 1979.

10

Digestive System

AL W. STINSON
M. LOIS CALHOUN

The digestive system is made up of a series of tubular organs and associated glands whose main function is to break down the ingested food into smaller units that can be absorbed into the tissues and utilized for the maintenance of the organism.

Morphologic adaptations to specialized functions are characteristic of the digestive systems of many domestic species. Considerable variations in the teeth, stomachs, and large intestines result mainly from the variety of food consumed. The forestomach of ruminants and the cecum and colon of horses reflect structural variations that facilitate the digestion of rough fibrous food, while the teeth of carnivores are especially adapted for tearing flesh.

All epithelial components of the digestive system, except those of the oral cavity, are derived from endoderm. Ectoderm gives rise to the epithelial structures of the oral cavity, and mesoderm is the origin of the muscular and connective tissue components of the entire system.

There is a general structural pattern for all tubular organs of the digestive system (see Fig. 10–31). Familiarity with this general pattern is helpful in understanding the specific characteristics of each organ. The layer next to the lumen is the *tunica mucosa* or mucous membrane. A mucous membrane lines all organs that communicate to the outside of the body and is protected by a layer of mucus, a viscous secretory material produced by specialized glands. The mucosa is composed of an *epithelium,* a *lamina propria* consisting of a thin bed of connective tissue, and a *lamina muscularis* (muscularis mucosae), composed of one or more thin layers of smooth muscle. In some organs the lamina propria contains glands that are referred to as *mucosal glands* because they are confined to the mucosa. The *tela submucosa* is a layer of connective tissue that may contain glandular units *(submucosal glands).* In those organs without a lamina muscularis, the lamina propria and submucosa blend together without a clear line of demarcation. The *tunica muscularis* is the layer of muscle responsible for the movement of the ingesta through the tract.

There are usually two layers of muscle in the tubular organs of the digestive system. The muscle fibers of the inner layer are oriented circularly or in a tightly coiled pattern, whereas the outer layer is composed of longitudinally or loosely coiled muscle fibers. The outermost layer is the *tunica serosa* or serous membrane. The se-

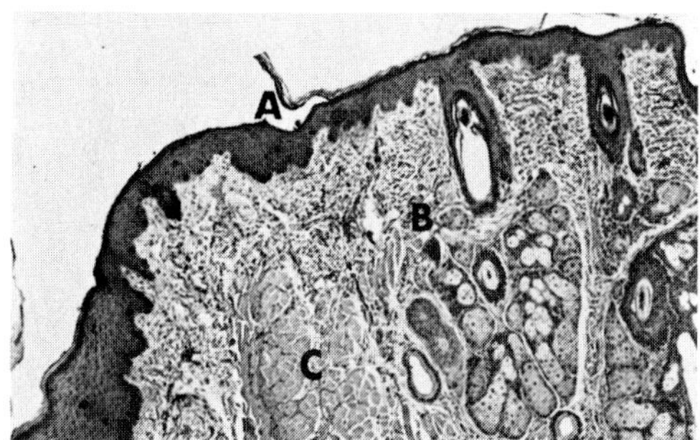

Fig. 10–1. *Lip, cat. Junction of keratinized stratified squamous epithelium of skin and mucous membrane (A); junction of dermis and lamina propria of lip (B); orbicular muscle (orbicularis oris) (striated) of lip (C). H & E. ×45.*

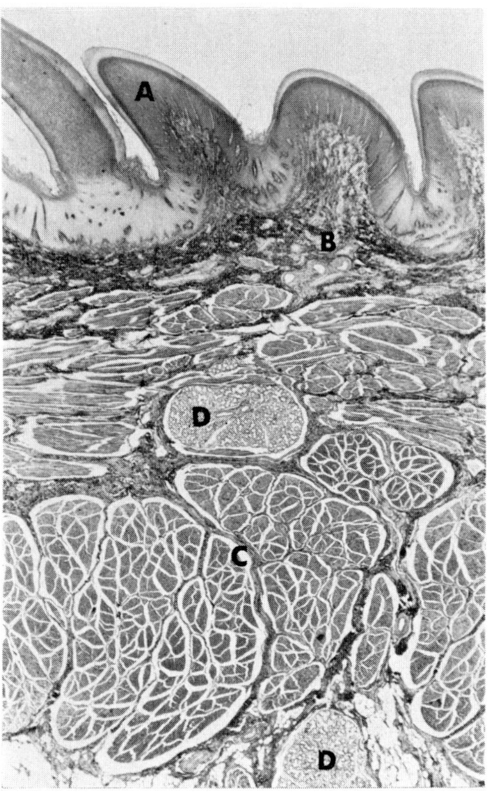

Fig. 10–2. *Buccal wall, cow. Conical buccal papillae covered with keratinized stratified squamous epithelium (A); lamina propria (B); striated muscle (C); buccal glands (D). H & E. ×12.*

rosa is composed of connective tissue with a covering of mesothelium. Those organs enclosed within the thoracic, pericardial, and abdominal cavities are surrounded by serosa, whereas those located outside the cavities, such as the cervical portion of the esophagus, do not have a mesothelium, and the connective tissue, called a *tunica adventitia,* blends with the surrounding fascia (see Fig. 10–31).

Although the large accessory digestive glands—pancreas, salivary glands, and liver—are located outside of the tubular portion of the digestive system, they originate as epithelial evaginations from the digestive tube. Their main ducts penetrate the walls of the tubular organs and empty their secretory products into the lumina. Two types of ganglionic nerve plexuses of the autonomic nervous system are found in the wall of the tubular organs. The *submucosal plexus* is in the submucosa, whereas the *myenteric plexus* lies between the two layers of the tunica muscularis.

ORAL CAVITY

Lips

The junction between the integument and the digestive system occurs on the lips. They are covered on the outside by skin and on the inside by a mucous membrane. Near the junction of the skin with mucous membrane, the skin is devoid of hair follicles, and the epidermis is thicker, with a more elaborated interdigitation with the underlying connective tissue (Fig. 10–1). The inner side of the lips is covered by stratified squamous epithelium that is keratinized in ruminants and the horse but nonkeratinized in the carnivores and pig. The lamina propria and submucosa blend together without a clear junction. Aggregates of labial glands, usually serous or seromucous, are distributed in the propria-submucosa. The tunica muscularis consists of striated muscle fibers of the orbicular muscle (orbicularis oris).

Cheeks

The cheeks, like the lips, are composed of an external covering of skin, a middle

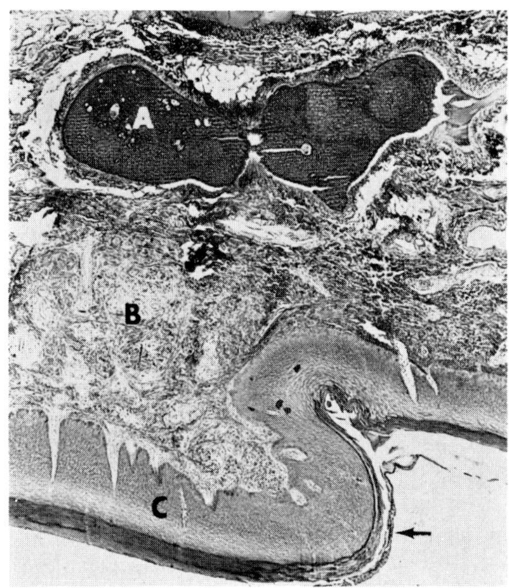

Fig. 10–3. *Hard palate, sheep. Large veins (A); lamina propria (B); keratinized stratified squamous epithelium (C); posterior surface of transverse ridge (arrow). H & E. ×30.*

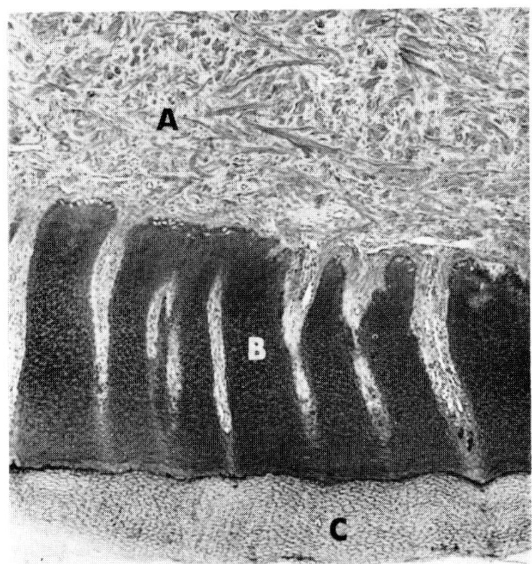

Fig. 10–4. *Dental pad, sheep. Lamina propria (A) with papillae extending into the stratified squamous epithelium (B); stratum corneum (C). Trichrome. ×48.*

uscular layer, and a mucous membrane lining. The buccal mucosa is lined with stratified squamous epithelium that may or may not be keratinized, depending on the particular area or species. In ruminants, the mucosa is studded with conically shaped macroscopic papillae that facilitate the prehension and mastication of food (Fig. 10–2). The buccal glands are minor salivary glands located in the submucosa and among the striated muscle bundles of the cheek, with some secretory units penetrating into the dermis. The glands are compound tubuloacinar glands and may be serous, mucous, or seromucous, depending on the location and the species.

Hard Palate

The roof of the rostral portion of the oral cavity is covered by a mucous membrane overlying the bony structures. The mucosa has keratinized stratified squamous epithelium, which is particularly thick in ruminants (Fig. 10–3). The stratum corneum of the rostral portion of the hard palate is also especially thick in ruminants and forms the dental pad *(pulvinus dentalis)* (Fig. 10–4). The lower incisor teeth press against the pad, forming a tight grip on forage during grazing. The lamina propria has a well-developed papillary layer that blends with the submucosa without an intervening lamina muscularis. The submucosa is composed of a dense network of collagen and reticular fibers and blends with the adjacent periosteum. A dense network of capillaries and large veins permeates the lamina propria and submucosa. Branched tubuloacinar mucous and seromucous glands are located in the caudal part of the hard palate in all domestic animals except the pig.

Soft Palate

The soft palate is formed by a fold of the mucous membranes of the oral and nasal cavities, with a core of striated muscle fibers. The oral surface is covered by a stratified squamous epithelium, whereas the nasal mucosa has a ciliated, pseudostratified columnar epithelium. A zone of transition between these two types of epithelia occurs on the nasal surface at varying and often considerable distances from the free margin of the soft palate. The propria and submucosa contain branched tubuloacinar mucous and seromucous glands. Diffuse and nodular lymphatic tissues occur in the mucosa of both the oral and nasal sides. Longitudinally oriented striated muscle fibers and connective tissue hold the two mucous membranes together.

Tongue

The tongue is a muscular organ covered by a mucous membrane. It is important in the prehension, mastication, and swallowing of food.

The epithelium is stratified squamous with varying thicknesses of the stratum corneum. It is thickest on the dorsal surface and thinnest on the ventral surface, where it may be nonkeratinized. The dorsal surface contains numerous *macroscopic papillae.* These may serve either a mechanical or a gustatory function. The filiform, conical, and lenticular papillae facilitate the movement of ingesta within the oral cavity; the fungiform, vallate, and foliate papillae contain taste buds, which are responsible for mediation of the sense of taste. These papillae differ somewhat in shape and are named according to their morphologic characteristics.

The *filiform papillae* are the most numerous type. They are slender, sharp-pointed structures that have a mechanical function in the movement of food into and within the oral cavity. They project above the surface of the tongue and are covered by a keratinized stratified squamous epithelium with a thick stratum corneum. They are supported by a highly vascularized connective tissue core. Equine filiform papillae have thin cornified threads projecting above the surface (Fig. 10–5). The connective tissue core ends at the base of the cornified thread. In ruminants, a keratinized cone projects above the surface and the connective tissue core has several sec-

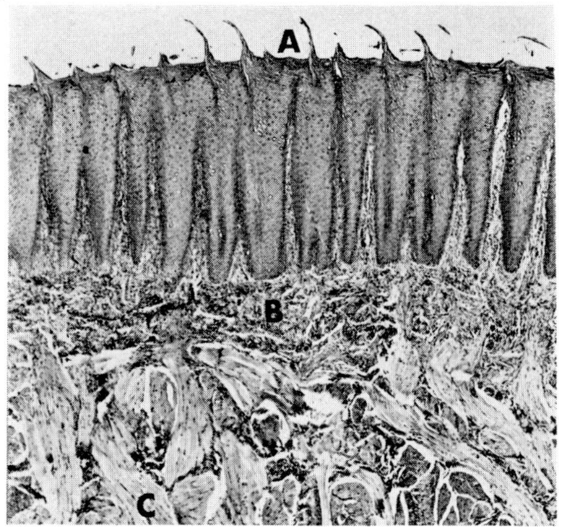

Fig. 10–5. *Tongue, horse. Filiform papillae extending from the surface of the stratified squamous epithelium on the dorsum of the tongue (A); lamina propria (B); striated muscle (C). H & E. ×26.*

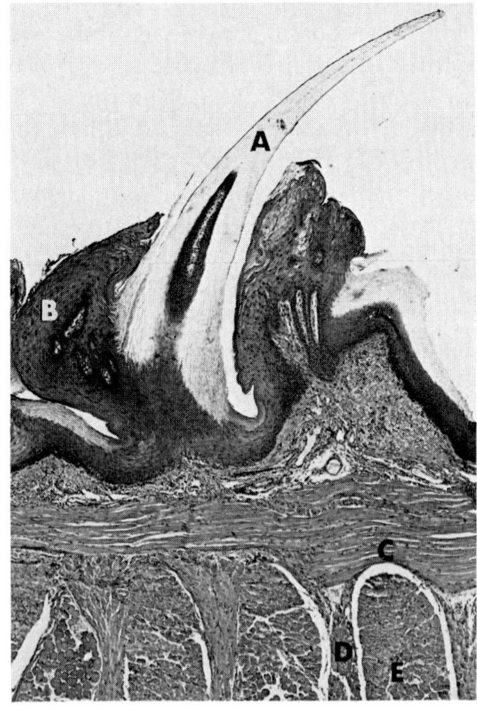

Fig. 10–6. *Tongue, cat. Filiform papilla with a caudally directed keratinized spine arising from the caudal prominence (A); supporting rostral papilla (B); tongue muscles: longitudinal (C), vertical (D), transverse (E). H & E. ×35.*

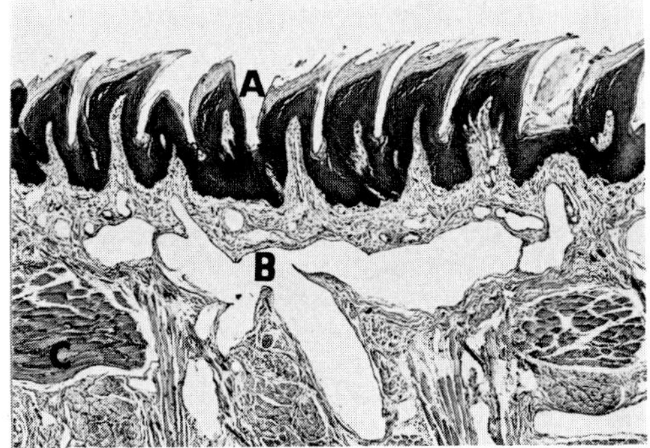

Fig. 10–7. *Tongue, dog. Filiform papillae (A); large veins (B); longitudinal striated muscle (C). H & E. ×28.*

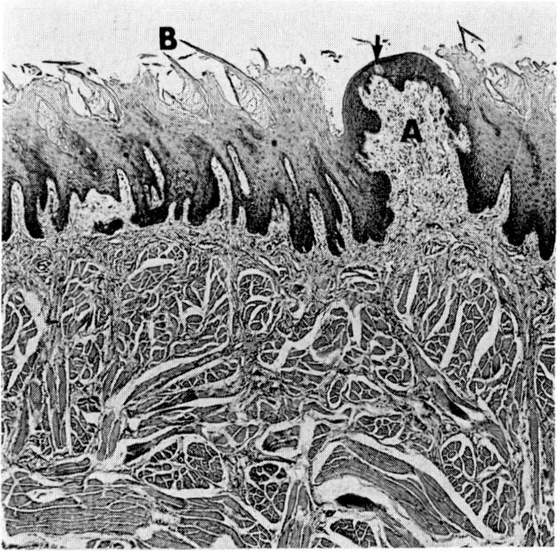

Fig. 10–8. *Tongue, pig. Fungiform papilla (A) with taste bud (arrow); filiform papillae (B). H & E. ×30.*

ondary papillae. The cat has large papillae with two prominences of unequal size (Fig. 10–6). The caudal prominence is especially large and gives rise to a caudally directed keratinized spine, supported by a more rounded rostral papilla with a thinner stratum corneum. The filiform papillae of the dog may have two or more apices; the caudal one is larger and has a thicker stratum corneum than the other (Fig. 10–7).

Conical papillae occur on the root of the tongue in the dog, cat, and pig, as well as on the cheek and floor of the oral cavity of other species. They are larger than the filiform type and usually are not highly keratinized. They have both primary and secondary connective tissue papillae.

Lenticular papillae are flattened lentil-shaped projections of the tongue surface and occur mainly in ruminants. They are covered by stratified squamous epithelium and have a core of dense irregular connective tissue.

The *fungiform papillae* are scattered among the filiform papillae and have a dome-shaped upper surface in the horse and pig (Fig. 10–8). The shape is suggestive of a mushroom, a type of fungus, and thus the name fungiform. The papillae are covered by a nonkeratinized stratified squamous epithelium containing one or more taste buds on the upper surface. The taste buds (see below) are sparse in these papillae in the tongue of horse and cattle, more numerous in those of sheep and swine, and abundant in those of carnivores and the goat. The connective tissue core is rich in blood vessels and nerves.

The *vallate papillae,* located on the dorsum and rostral to the root of the tongue, are large, flattened structures completely surrounded by an epithelium-lined cleft or moat (Fig. 10–9). They extend only slightly, if at all, above the lingual surface and are covered by a stratified squamous epithelium. The epithelium on the papillary side of the moat contains many taste buds, and deep to the moat lie groups of gustatory serous glands whose ducts open into the moat at various levels (Fig. 10–9). Mucous glands may also be found beneath the papillae, but their secretory products are emptied onto the lingual surface. The connective tissue core is rich in blood vessels and nerves.

The *foliate papillae* are parallel folds of the lingual mucosa located on the lateral border just rostral to the palatoglossal arch. The folds are covered with stratified squamous epithelium, with taste buds located in the epithelium on the sides of the folds. The papillae are separated by gustatory furrows into which the taste buds open (Figs. 10–10 and 10–11). Deep to the fur-

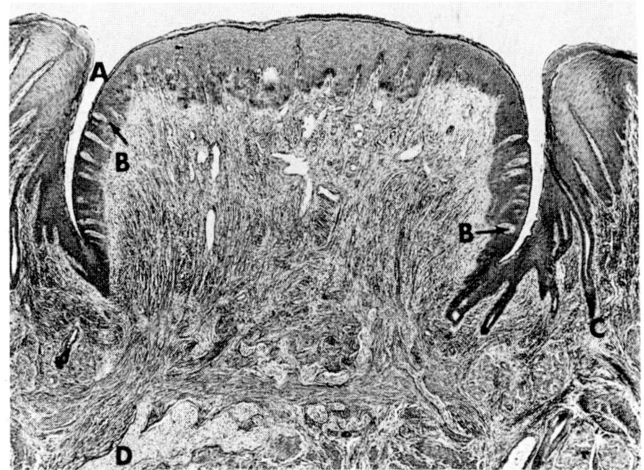

Fig. 10–9. *Tongue, cow. Vertical section of a vallate papilla with surrounding gustatory furrow (A); taste buds in the epithelium (B); a gland duct opening into the furrow (C); gland (D). H & E. ×30. (From Stinson, A.W., and Brown, E.M.: Veterinary Histology Slide Sets. East Lansing, Mich., Michigan State University, Instructional Media Center, 1970.)*

rows lie serous gustatory glands, the ducts of which empty into the furrows. Foliate papillae are absent in ruminants and are rudimentary and without taste buds in the cat.

The *taste buds* are ellipsoid clusters of sensory taste cells embedded in the stratified squamous epithelium of the fungiform, vallate, and foliate papillae of the tongue (Fig. 10–12). They also occur widely dispersed in the soft palate, epiglottis, or other areas of the mouth and throat. The taste bud consists of a cluster of three different cell types located within the surface squamous epithelium and extending from the basement membrane to a small opening, the *taste pore* (Fig. 10–13). The *neuroepithelial taste cells,* located in the center of the bud, are spindle-shaped and studded with microvilli *(taste hairs)* that project into the taste pore. Located toward the periphery and between the taste cells are spindle-shaped supporting or sustentacular cells. The third cell type is the *basal cell,* located near the basement membrane. It is thought that this cell type gives rise to the other two types, since cell degeneration occurs continuously within the taste bud. The average life span of the cells in the taste bud is about 10 days. Nerve fiber terminals are closely associated with the taste cells; in fact, there

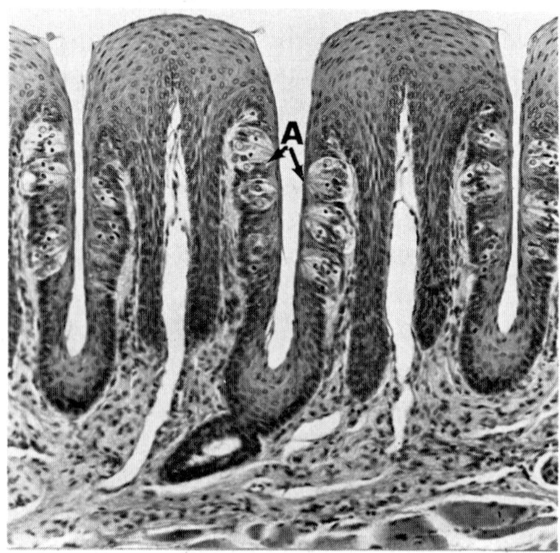

Fig. 10–10. *Tongue, rabbit. Foliate papillae with prominent taste buds (A). H & E. ×110.*

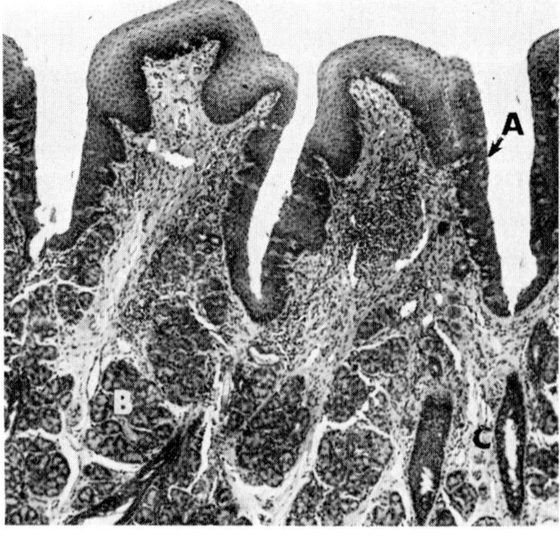

Fig. 10–11. *Tongue, dog. Foliate papillae (A), with less prominent taste buds than those of rabbits; serous glands (B) and duct (C) at the base of the papillae. H & E. ×48.*

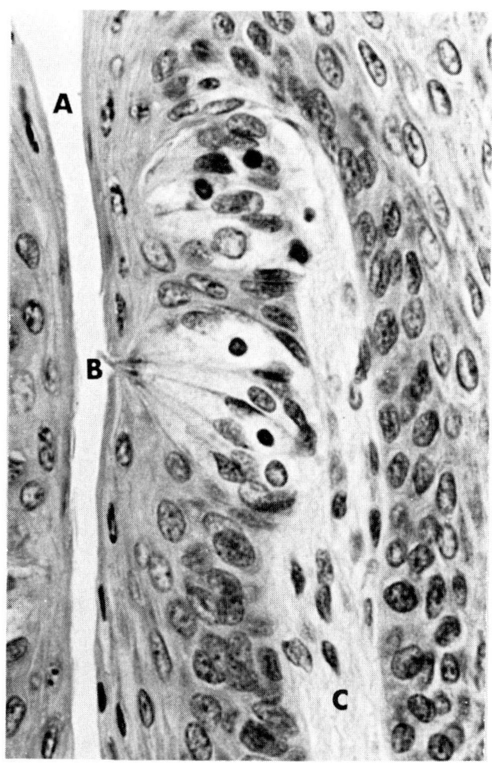

Fig. 10–12. *Taste buds, rabbit. Gustatory furrow (A); taste pore (B); nonmyelinated nerve fiber bundle (C). H & E. ×615.*

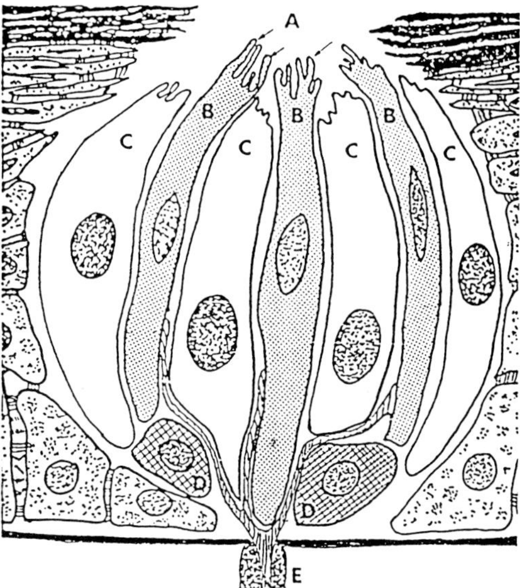

Fig. 10–13. *Taste bud. Taste pore (A); neuroepithelial taste cell (B) with microvilli (taste hairs) at arrows; sustentacular cells (C); basal cells (D); and nerve fiber (E).*

is evidence that they are enveloped by these cells.

The intrinsic *lingual muscle* mass is composed of longitudinally, transversely, and vertically arranged bundles of striated muscle (Figs. 10–6 and 10–7). The well-developed dorsal longitudinal fibers lie directly under the mucosa, whereas the ventral longitudinal fibers consist of a few strands below prominent horizontal and transverse bundles. Because of the diverse arrangement of the lingual muscle fibers, the tongue has extensive mobility in the movement of food into and within the oral cavity.

The *ventral surface* of the tongue is covered by nonkeratinized stratified squamous epithelium. The mucosa contains an abundance of capillaries, arteriovenous anastomoses, and branches of the lingual artery and vein. They are thought to play a part in the elimination of heat.

Scattered among the muscle fibers and in the submucosa of the tongue are clusters of seromucous glands, collectively called the *lingual glands,* which are part of the minor salivary glands discussed later.

SPECIAL STRUCTURES OF THE TONGUE

The *lyssa* of the carnivore tongue is a cordlike structure enclosed in a dense collagenous sheath and extends lengthwise near the ventral surface of the center of the tongue. The lyssa of the dog is filled with adipose tissue, striated muscle, blood vessels, and nerves, but that of the cat contains mainly fat (Fig. 10–14). The tongue of the pig contains a similar structure. A middorsal *fibroelastic cord* with hyaline cartilage, striated muscle, and fat is present in the horse.

The ruminant tongue has a *dorsal prominence* characterized by a thickened mucosa. Connective tissue papillae extend almost to the surface of the epithelium, which is thicker than that on the other re-

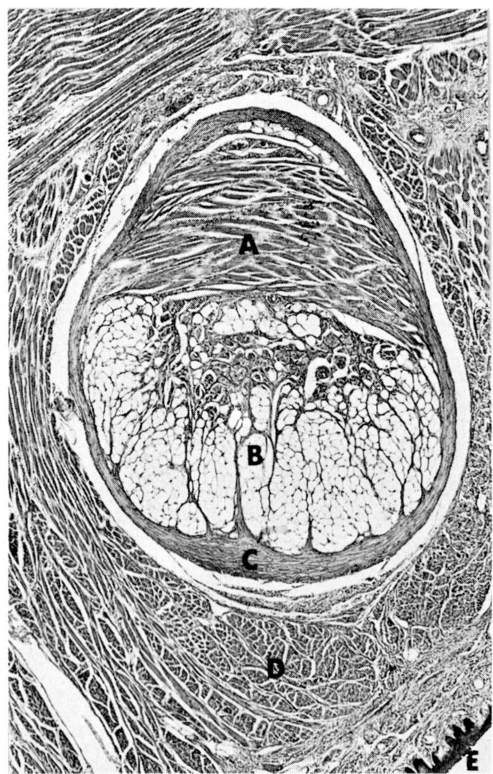

Fig. 10–14. *Lyssa, dog. Striated muscle (A); adipose tissue (B); collagen sheath (C); intrinsic lingual muscles (D); ventral surface of tongue (E). H & E. ×28.*

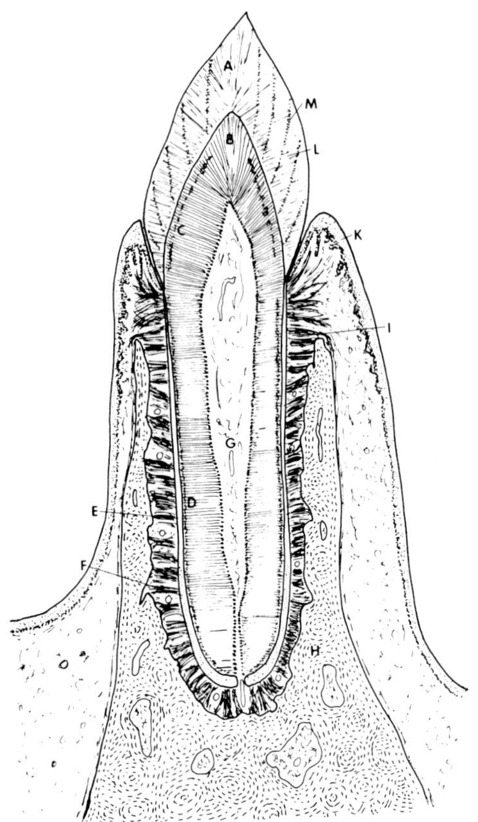

Fig. 10–15. *Schematic drawing of a section through an incisor tooth. Enamel (A); dentin (B) with interglobular dentin (C) and the granulosa layer of the root (D); acellular (E) and cellular (F) cementum; pulp cavity with peripherally located odontoblasts (G); alveolar bone (H); periodontal membrane (I); gingiva (K); lines of Hunter-Schreger (L); incremental lines (M). (From Dellmann, H.-D.: Veterinary Histology: An Outline Text-Atlas. Philadelphia, Lea & Febiger, 1971.)*

gions of the tongue. Flattened lenticular papillae are scattered over the surface of this area.

Teeth

Teeth are highly mineralized structures in the oral cavity that serve the domestic mammals in procuring, cutting, and crushing food and as weapons of offense and defense. The tooth consists of a highly mineralized outer part surrounding the pulp cavity, which contains a core of connective tissue, blood vessels, and nerves (Fig. 10–15).

HYPSODONT AND BRACHYDONT TEETH

Two types of teeth occur in the domestic animals: *brachydont* and *hypsodont.* These teeth differ in their rates of growth and in the arrangement of the layers of mineralized tissue.

Brachydont teeth are short and cease to grow after eruption is completed (Fig. 10–15). They have a *crown,* the portion above the gingiva; a *neck,* the constricted region just below the gingival line; and one or more *roots* embedded in a bony socket of the maxilla or mandible called the *alveolus.* The crown is covered by a cap of enamel that extends down to the neck region. The root is covered by a layer of cementum that may slightly overlap the enamel at their junction on the neck. Beneath both the enamel and cementum is a thick

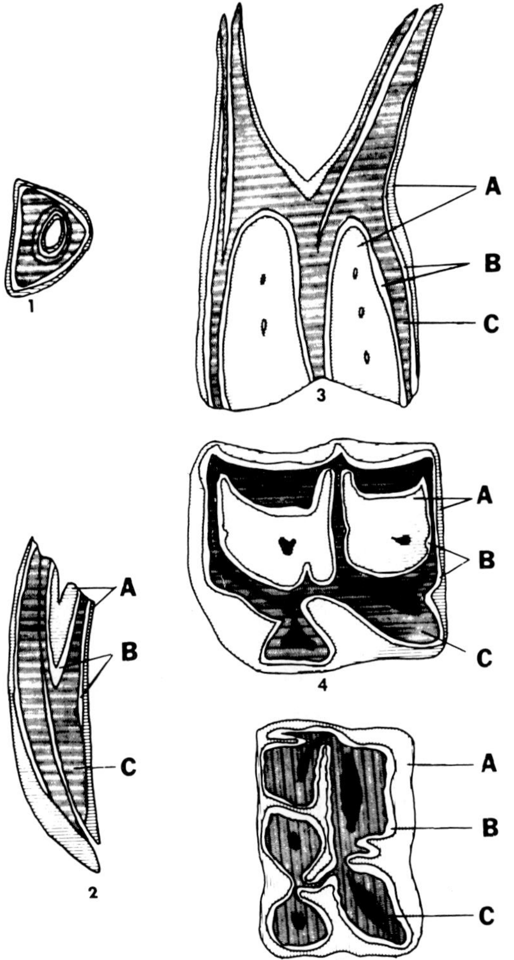

Fig. 10–16. *Hypsodont teeth, horse. 1, Cross section of incisor. 2, Longitudinal section of incisor. 3, Longitudinal section of upper molar. 4, Cross section of upper molar. 5, Cross section of lower molar. Cementum (A); enamel (B); dentin (C).*

layer of dentin. Brachydont teeth include all those of carnivores and man, the incisor teeth of ruminants, and the teeth of the pig except for the canine teeth of the boar.

Hypsodont teeth are much longer than brachydont teeth and continue their growth throughout a portion, if not all, of the adult life of the animal (Fig. 10–16). They do not have a crown and neck but, rather, an elongated *body,* with the roots and neck forming, in some species, only after a delayed period. The tusks of the boar continue to grow throughout its life and never develop roots. Cementum covers the outside of the tooth both above and below the gingiva. Beneath the cementum is a layer of enamel extending throughout the length of the body and almost to the apex of the root. The enamel, in turn, lies on a thick layer of dentin. Hypsodont teeth differ from brachydont teeth in that the hypsodont cementum and enamel invaginate into the dentin. Where these invaginations occur from the occlusal surface down into the tooth, they form the *infundibula,* whereas those infolding along the sides form the *enamel plicae,* characteristic of the molars. The occlusal aspect of the molars has a corrugated surface that results from the irregular wearing of the mineralized tissues. Because enamel is the hardest of the mineralized tissues, it is most resistant to wear and projects above the surface as *enamel crests.* Dentin and cementum are less resistant than enamel and wear away more readily. This irregular contour makes the occlusal surface very effective for grinding food. Hypsodont teeth include all those of the horse, the cheek teeth of ruminants, and the tusks of the boar.

STRUCTURE

The mineralized tissues of the teeth are *enamel, dentin,* and *cementum.* Each of these has a separate origin and differs morphologically and in degree of mineralization.

Enamel covers the crown of brachydont teeth but lies beneath a layer of cementum in the hypsodont teeth. It is the hardest substance in the body, composed of 99% mineral (hydroxyapatite) and 1% organic matrix by weight. Histologically, enamel is composed of long, slender enamel rods held together by mineralized interrod enamel. Parallel bundles of rods pursue a wavy or oblique course from the inner to the outer surface of the enamel layer (Fig. 10–17). Where these bundles change directions, curved lines appear; these are known as the *lines of Hunter-Schreger.* En-

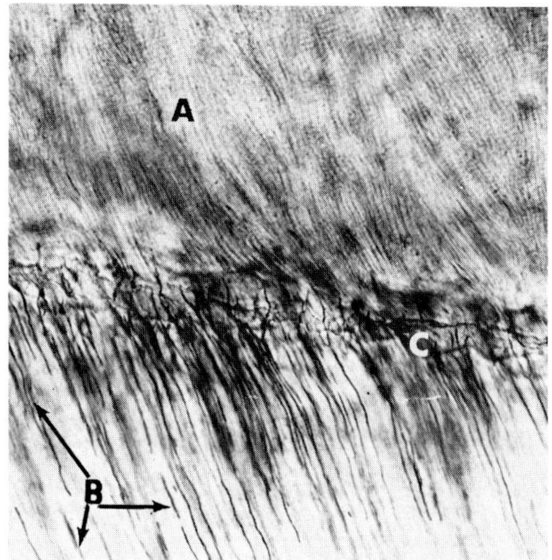

Fig. 10–17. *Ground tooth, man. Junction of enamel (A) (notice the cross striations of the enamel prisms) and dentin (B) with the odontoblastic processes penetrating the tubules; interglobular dentin (C). Unstained.* ×*235.*

amel is produced by ameloblasts that differentiate from the inner enamel epithelium of the enamel organ (see tooth development below).

Dentin is a highly mineralized tissue that constitutes the major part of the tooth. It underlies the enamel of the crown and the cementum of the root and forms the wall of the pulp cavity. It consists of a matrix of organic material, mainly collagen and glycoprotein, upon which is deposited crystallites and hydroxyapatite, the composition being about 70% mineral and 30% organic matter. The dentin is perforated by parallel dentinal tubules that extend from the inner to the outer surface of the dentin. The dentinal tubules contain the *dentinal processes* of the odontoblasts. The *peritubular dentin* immediately surrounds the dentinal processes and is more highly mineralized than the intertubular dentin, which constitutes the remainder of the dentin. The odontoblasts form a layer of columnar cells beneath the dentin and produce the organic matrix of dentin. This unmineralized organic material constitutes the *predentin,* which lies between the distal end of the odontoblasts and the mineralized dentin. *Globular dentin* is composed of small, unmineralized areas within the dentin immediately adjacent to the enamel. These areas are more numerous in the root of the tooth and form the granulosa layer of the dental root at the dentinocementum junction (Fig. 10–18). The odontoblasts continue to produce dentin throughout the life of the tooth, although at a somewhat slower rate after the tooth erupts.

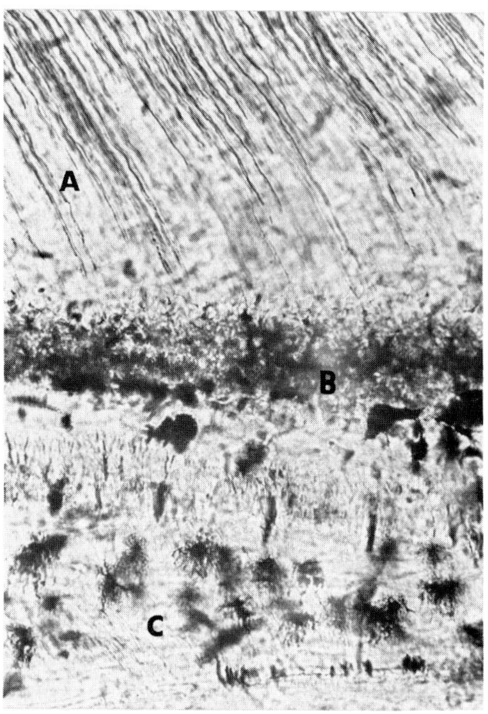

Fig. 10–18. *Ground tooth, man. Dentinocemental junction. Dentin (A) containing dentinal tubules (the dark lines); granulosa layer of the root (B); cementum (C) with lacunae. Unstained.* ×*185.*

Cementum is a yellowish, mineralized layer of slightly modified bone. It is composed of lamellae oriented parallel to the surface of the tooth, with cementocytes occupying the lacunae (Fig. 10–19). Cytoplasmic processes of the cementocytes extend into anastomosing canaliculi similar to those of bone. The cementum covering the upper part of the root may be devoid of cells, forming the acellular cement layer. Bundles of collagen fibers, called *perforating cementum fibers,* are embedded in the

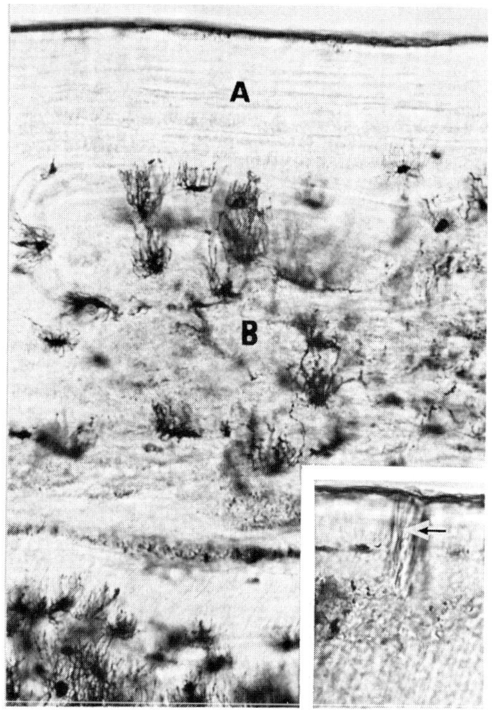

Fig. 10–19. *Ground tooth, man. Lamellae of acellular cementum (A) oriented parallel to the surface of the tooth. Cellular cementum with cementocytes (B). ×185. Insert, perforating fibers (arrow) embedded in the cementum. Unstained. ×185.*

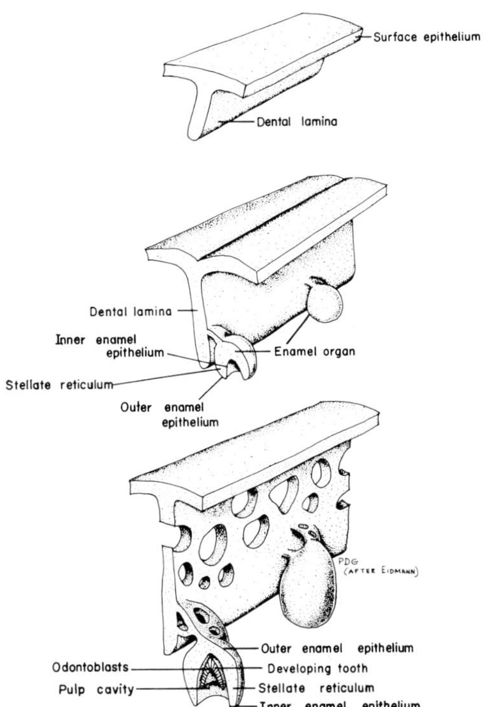

Fig. 10–20. *Stages in the development of the tooth.*

cementum of the tooth and extend into the bony socket (Fig. 10–19). These fibers form the *periodontal membrane,* which anchors the tooth in the socket.

Dental pulp is composed of connective tissue cells and fibers, matrix, numerous blood vessels, and nerves. It resembles embryonic connective tissue in texture, with delicate collagen fibers coursing through the matrix. The most peripheral part is the layer of odontoblasts, from which the odontoblastic processes extend into the dentinal canaliculi. Basal processes from the odontoblasts extend into the matrix or unite with similar processes from neighboring cells. Because dentin is continuously being deposited on the inside of the tooth, the pulp cavity is gradually reduced in older animals.

DEVELOPMENT

In the embryo, there is an invagination of the oral ectoderm into the underlying mesenchyme, forming the *dental lamina* (Fig. 10–20), a continuous, arch-shaped sheet of epithelial cells extending along the future site of the gingiva. Isolated thickenings arise on the labial side of the dental lamina at the site where each deciduous tooth develops. These thickenings are the primordia of the enamel organ, which eventually gives rise to the enamel.

The shape of the enamel organ suggests an inverted cup attached to the dental lamina by a thin stem (Fig. 10–20). The epithelial cells lining the inside of the cup form the *inner enamel epithelium,* and those covering the outside form the *outer enamel epithelium.* The epithelial cells between these two layers become stellate shaped and take on the appearance of connective tissue, thus forming the *stellate reticulum* of the enamel organ. The mesenchyme enclosed

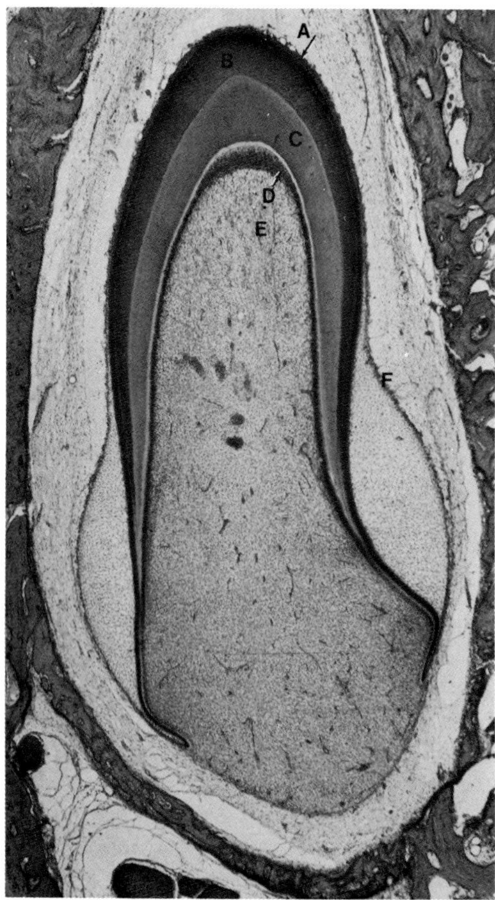

Fig. 10–21. *Developing permanent tooth, dog. (A) Ameloblasts; (B) enamel; (C) dentin; (D) odontoblasts; (E) dental papilla; (F) outer enamel cells. H & E. ×25. (Courtesy of A. Hansen.)*

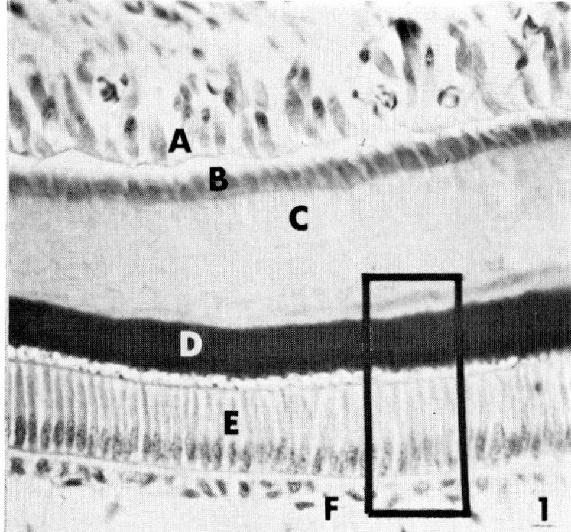

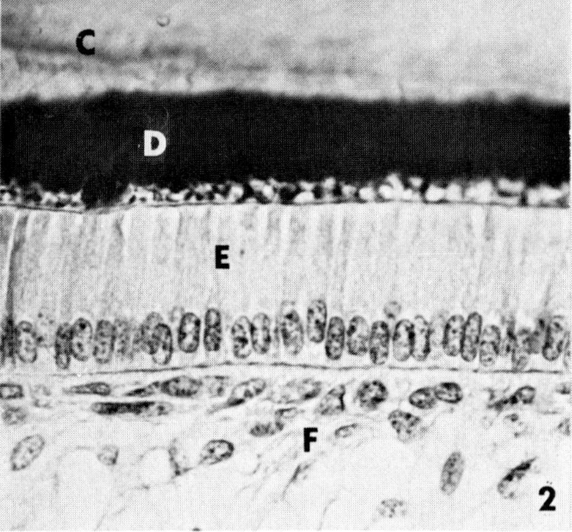

Fig. 10–22. *Developing tooth, dog. 1, Odontoblasts (A); recently deposited dentin (B); older dentin (C); enamel (D); ameloblasts (E); stellate reticulum (F). ×200. 2, Area marked in Figure 10–22-1. Trichrome. ×300.*

by the cup of the enamel organ condenses to form the dental pulp or dental papilla. The internal contour of the cup is a replica of the shape of the tooth crown to be produced (Fig. 10–21).

As the enamel organ enlarges, the cells of the inner enamel epithelium take on a distinct columnar shape and differentiate into *ameloblasts,* which will later produce the enamel. The mesenchymal cells of the dental pulp immediately adjacent to the ameloblasts differentiate into odontoblasts, which produce dentin. Dentin is deposited as sheaths of mineralized material around the odontoblastic processes that are anchored to the basal lamina of the enamel epithelium. As more dentin is produced, the cell body recedes toward the pulp cavity and the layer of dentin becomes thicker. Shortly after the first dentin is deposited, the ameloblasts begin to produce the enamel matrix (Fig. 10–22). The deposition of the dentin and enamel begins at the apex of the crown and continues down the sides of the crown to the neck region.

The formation of the root begins shortly before the eruption of the tooth. The root is formed by a downward growth of a sheet of cells originating from the enamel organ at the junction of the inner and outer enamel epithelium. This downward-growing sheet of cells, the *epithelial sheath of Hertwig,* surrounds the connective tissue of the pulp cavity and induces the formation of odontoblasts. The dentin of the root is produced by these odontoblasts.

The entire enamel organ and developing tooth are enclosed by the *dental sac,* a thickened connective tissue layer that completely surrounds the developing tooth. In brachydont teeth, the crown erupts through the dental sac while the root is still covered by it. The dental sac then collapses against the root dentin and gives rise to the cementocytes that deposit a covering of cementum over the roots. In hypsodont teeth, the dental sac collapses before the tooth erupts, and cementum therefore covers the entire tooth surface.

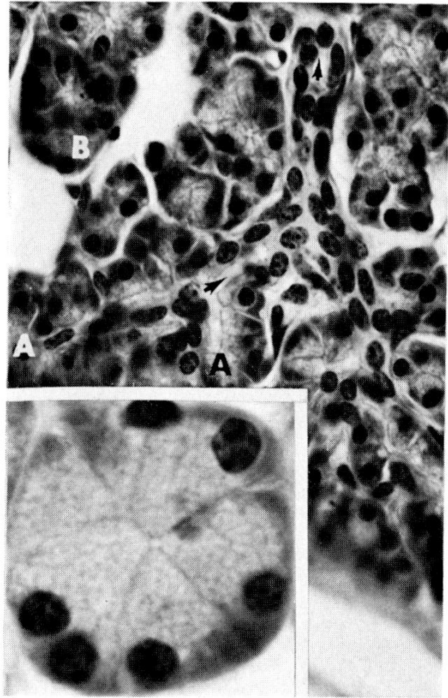

Fig. 10–23. *Parotid salivary gland, horse. Serous acini (A) opening into intercalated ducts (arrow); serous acinus (B). H & E. ×440. Insert, serous acinus. H & E. ×1382.*

SALIVARY GLANDS

The salivary glands comprise a series of secretory units that originate from the oral ectoderm and grow into the underlying mesoderm as large aggregates of compound tubuloacinar glands. The *major salivary glands* include the parotid, mandibular, and sublingual glands of all domestic species, the zygomatic gland of carnivores, and the molar gland of the cat. The *minor salivary glands* are small clusters of seromucous secretory units in the submucosa of the oral cavity and are named according to their location, e.g., labial, lingual, buccal, and palatine.

Saliva is a mixture of both serous and mucous secretory products of salivary glands. It is important in the moistening of the ingested food and lubrication of the surface of the upper digestive organs and thus enhances the flow of the ingesta into the stomach. Saliva dissolves water-soluble components of food, which facilitates access to the taste buds, making the sense of taste somewhat dependent on the saliva. Saliva in domestic animals is considered to play only a minor role in the digestion of food before it reaches the stomach. Ruminants, however, produce a large volume of saliva, which is an important source of fluids in the rumen.

Parotid Salivary Gland

The *parotid salivary gland* in domestic animals is predominantly serous, although occasional isolated mucous secretory units may occur in the dog and cat. Structurally, it is a compound gland composed of numerous lobular units separated by thin connective tissue septa. The lobule consists of acinar secretory units formed by pyramid-shaped cells with basal nuclei and surrounded by a well-developed basophilic granular endoplasmic reticulum (Fig. 10–23). The apex of each cell is filled with secretory granules containing digestive enzymes. The granules are commonly referred to as zymogen granules because they initiate the digestion of carbohydrates. Stellate-shaped myoepithelial cells *(basket cells)* located between the secretory cells and the basement membrane can be dem-

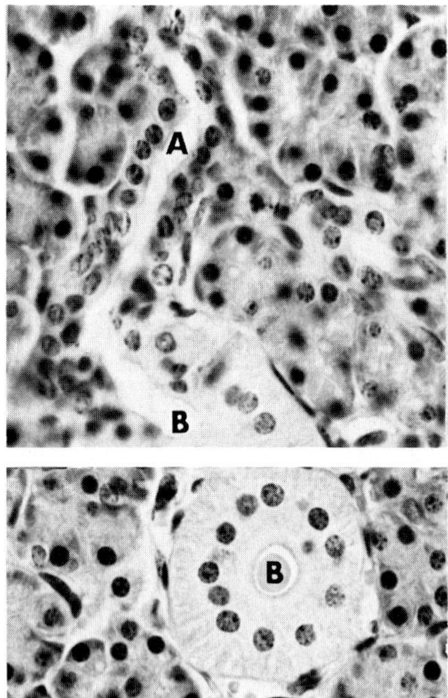

Fig. 10–24. *Parotid salivary gland, horse. Intercalated duct (A) joining striated duct (B). H & E. ×425. Lower portion, striated duct (B). H & E. ×480.*

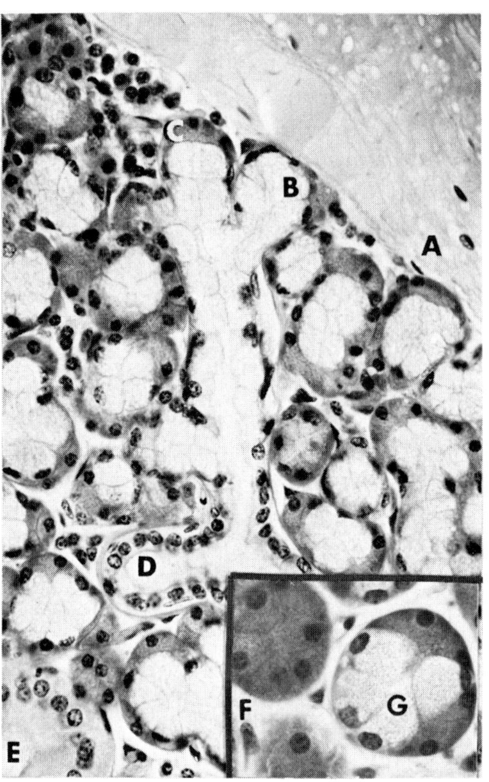

Fig. 10–25. *Mandibular salivary gland, horse. Capsule (A); tubuloacinar gland with mucous acini (B) and serous demilunes (C); intercalated duct (D); striated duct (E). H & E. ×384. Insert, serous acinus (F); mixed acinus (G). H & E. ×530.*

onstrated by special techniques. Their processes form a network around the acinus. The narrow lumen of the acinus opens into a short *intercalated duct* lined by low cuboidal epithelium. The intercalated duct joins a large *striated* or *salivary duct* lined by cuboidal or columnar epithelium. These ducts are distinguished by striations in the basal portion of the tall columnar cells (Fig. 10–24). This appearance is due to perpendicularly oriented mitochondria within numerous cytoplasmic compartments formed by deep infoldings of the basal cell membrane. This specialization creates a vast basal surface area with energy-producing mitochondria and participates in the active transport of ions and water between cells and underlying tissue fluids. The intralobular or striated ducts are easily recognized as the largest structures within the lobule and participate in the secretory process by the transport of ions and water and possibly the excretion of salt. The striated ducts extend to the edge of the lobule, where they join *interlobular ducts* located in the connective tissue septa between lobules. These ducts are lined by simple columnar epithelium, which changes to stratified columnar epithelium as the ducts become larger and fuse with similar ducts draining other lobules. The interlobular ducts converge to form the *main parotid duct,* and where it opens into the oral cavity, the epithelium changes from stratified columnar to stratified squamous epithelium.

Mandibular Salivary Gland

The mandibular salivary gland is a compound branched tubuloacinar gland composed of both mucous and serous acini. The morphologic structure of the secretory unit is somewhat variable from one species to another but generally consists of a tubular unit with an enlarged end-piece. Mucus-secreting cells border the lumen, and serous demilunes occur at the periphery (Fig. 10–25). The serous secretion reaches the lumen through small canaliculi located between the mucous acinar cells. Variations of this basic pattern may include separate serous and mucous units or mucous tubular units with enlarged, serous, acinar end-pieces. In the dog and cat, the mucous elements predominate, and even demilune cells may react faintly to histochemical tests for mucus. Myoepithelial cells occur between the base of the epithelial cells and the basal lamina. The tubuloacinar secretory units are connected to short intercalated ducts that in turn give rise to the striated ducts. The striated ducts have characteristics similar to those of the parotid gland. The columnar epithelium of the interlobular ducts gradually changes to two-layered cuboidal epithelium and finally becomes stratified squamous epithelium before it enters the oral cavity. Goblet cells may occur in the epithelium of the main duct.

The gland is innervated by both sympathetic and parasympathetic nerve fibers, and the nature of the secretion depends somewhat on the degree of stimulation of each system. It has been suggested that the sympathetic stimulation may affect the demilune cells, whereas the parasympathetic stimulation may act on the acinar cells.

Sublingual Salivary Gland

The sublingual salivary gland is a compound branched tubuloacinar gland (Fig. 10–26). The number of mucous acini and serous demilunes and the seromucous nature of their secretory product vary among species. Sublingual glands of the cow, sheep, and pig are almost entirely mucous, with relatively few demilunes. In addition to the typical mucous acini and demilunes, in the dog and cat these glands contain clusters of serous acini with well-developed intercellular canaliculi (Fig. 10–27). The basal portion of the cells bordering the canaliculi contains PAS-positive granules. The mucous cells form tubular structures that connect the serous acini with the intercalated ducts. Striated and intercalated ducts are present but not well developed in the cat and dog. However, in the horse, ruminants, and pig, they are well developed, but the intercalated ducts are much shorter compared to those of the parotid gland. The interlobular ducts have at their origin a low columnar epithelium that increases in height and becomes two-layered in larger ducts. The main duct is lined with stratified cuboidal epithelium, with goblet cells occurring in the cow and pig.

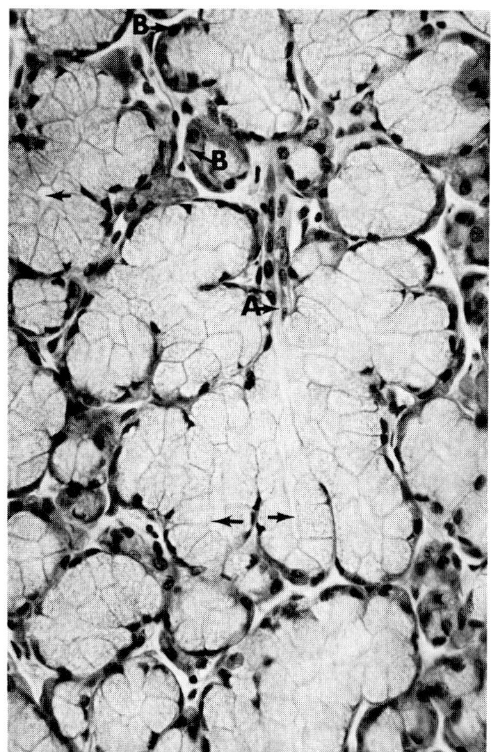

Fig. 10–26. *Sublingual salivary gland, dog. Mucous acini with lumina (arrows) emptying into intercalated duct (A); serous demilunes (B). H & E. ×280.*

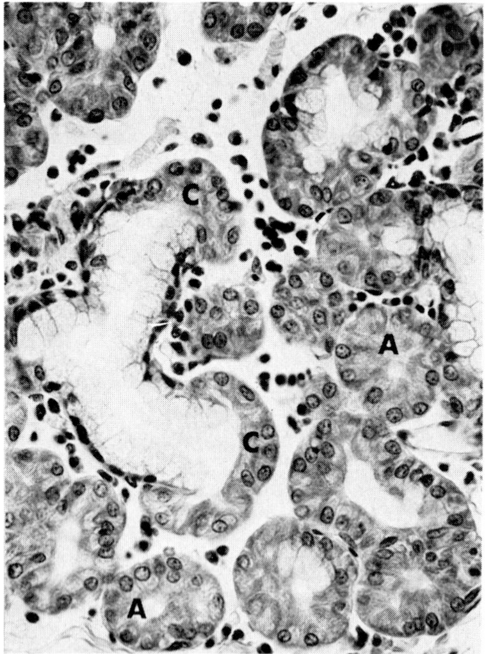

Fig. 10–27. *Sublingual salivary gland, dog. Serous acini (A). Serous demilunes (C) on tubular mucous structure. H & E. ×275.*

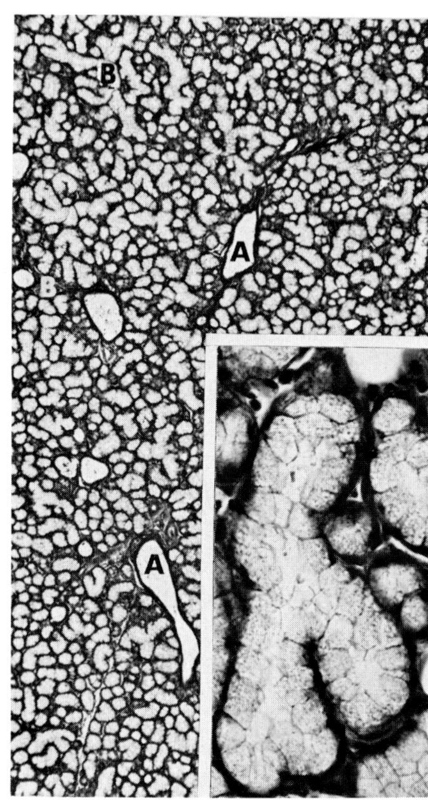

Fig. 10–28. *Zygomatic salivary gland, dog. Interlobular excretory ducts (A); tubuloacinar glands (B). H & E. ×38. Insert, detail of gland. H & E. ×300.*

Zygomatic Salivary Gland

Among the domestic species, the zygomatic salivary gland is present only in carnivores. It is named from its location beneath the zygomatic arch of the temporal bone. The parenchyma is composed of long, branched tubuloacinar secretory units that are predominantly mucus secreting (Fig. 10–28). Small, flattened serous demilunes occur at the periphery of the mucous cells, but their secretory product is considered to form only a small portion of the gland product. Intercalated and striated ducts are almost nonexistent, but isolated patches of tall, striated cells are present within the low cuboidal epithelium of the intralobular ducts. The interlobular and main ducts are similar to those of the other glands.

Molar Salivary Gland

The *molar salivary gland* of the cat, located in the fascia beneath the mucosa of the lower lip near the commissure, is histologically similar to the zygomatic salivary gland. It is a compound tubuloacinar gland that is predominately mucus secreting (Fig. 10–29). There are occasional serous demilunes both on the acinar end-pieces and along the tubular portion. Intercalated and striated ducts are not present, and the interlobular ducts have a two-layered cuboidal epithelium. Several main ducts empty into the oral cavity opposite the molar teeth.

Minor Salivary Glands

Clusters of serous, seromucous, or mucous minor salivary glands, occurring throughout the oral cavity, are generally named according to their location. The lin-

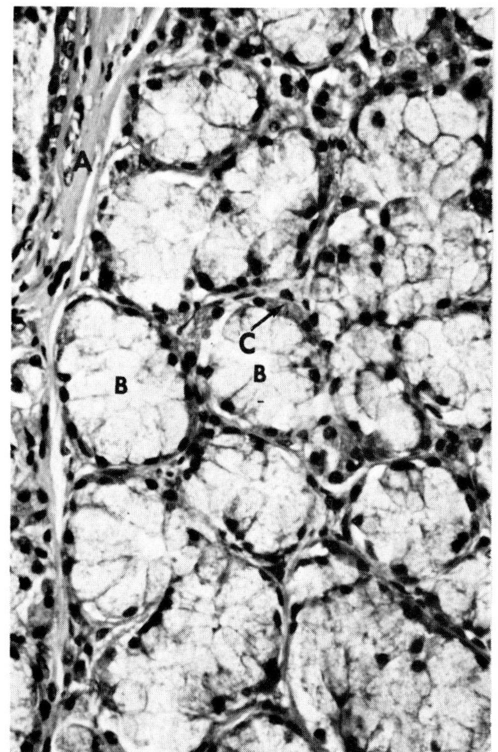

Fig. 10–29. *Molar salivary gland, cat. Interlobular connective tissue (A); mucous acini (B); serous demilune (C). H & E. ×257.*

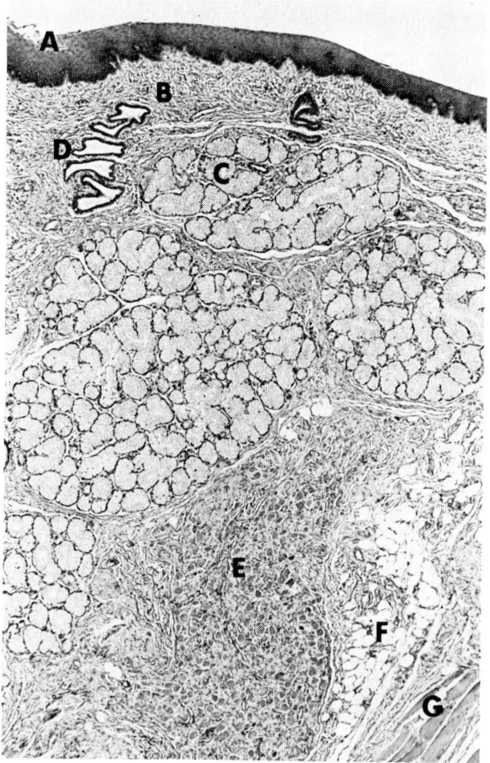

Fig. 10–30. *Pharynx, dog. Stratified squamous epithelium (A); lamina propria (B); mucous glands (C); excretory ducts (D); ganglion (E); adipose connective tissue (F); striated muscle (G). H & E. ×37.*

gual glands are located in the submucosa and between the intrinsic muscle bundles of the tongue. The gustatory glands, associated with the vallate and foliate papillae (Fig. 10–11), are entirely serous and their ducts open into the furrow at the base of the papillae. The labial, buccal, palatine, and pharyngeal glands also contribute mucous and serous secretory products to the saliva. Histologically, the secretory units resemble those of the major salivary glands and occur in a variety of forms, i.e., acinar, tubuloacinar, or tubular. Mucous tubular and acinar units frequently have serous demilunes associated with them; however, striated ducts are not characteristic of the minor salivary glands. The duct system consists of simple cuboidal epithelium within the lobules and two-layered cuboidal epithelium in the larger interlobular ducts. The stratification of the duct epithelium increases as it reaches the oral cavity, where it changes to a stratified squamous type.

PHARYNX

The pharynx connects the oral cavity to the esophagus and contains openings to the nasal cavity (nasopharynx), larynx, and auditory tubes. A mucous membrane, a striated tunica muscularis, and an adventitia make up the wall (Fig. 10–30). The mucosa is composed of a stratified squamous epithelium and a lamina propria containing fibroelastic tissue intermingled with lymphatic tissue and mucous glands. The pharynx lacks a lamina muscularis. The adventitia is a fibroelastic layer that attaches the pharynx to the surrounding tissue.

Table 10–1.
Esophageal Wall

	Horse	*Pig*	*Cow*	*Goat*	*Sheep*	*Dog*	*Cat*
Stratified squamous epithelium*	Keratinized	Keratinized	Keratinized	Keratinized	Keratinized	Non-keratinized	Non-keratinized
Lamina propria papillae	+	+	+	‡	+	−	−
Lamina muscularis smooth muscle	†	Absent in cranial part. Highly developed in lower end.	†	†	†	Absent in cranial part. Interrupted in middle part.	†
Submucosal glands compound tubuloalveolar seromucous	‡	More abundant in cranial than in caudal half.	‡	‡	‡	Present throughout and extend into stomach.	‡
Tunica muscularis§	Cranial two thirds are striated. Caudal one third is smooth.	Cranial is striated. Middle is mixed. Caudal is smooth.	Striated throughout and extends onto the reticular sulcus.			Striated throughout.	Cranial is striated. Caudal one third to one fifth is smooth.
Tunica adventitia	Loose connective tissue cells and fibers with blood and lymph vessels and nerves surround the esophagus. A serous membrane (mediastinum) may be present in the thoracic cavity or near the stomach. In the abdominal cavity, the parietal peritoneum may reflect on the abdominal esophagus when present.						

*Related to character of food: coarse food, highly keratinized; soft food, slightly keratinized to nonkeratinized.
†Longitudinal only: Isolated bundles of smooth muscle near pharynx, increases in thickness near stomach.
‡Present only at the pharyngoesophageal junction.
§Inner circular muscle layer becomes thicker toward the stomach in all animals, especially in the horse.

ESOPHAGUS

The esophagus (Table 10–1) joins the pharynx with the stomach and contains all the layers of a typical tubular organ of the digestive system (Fig. 10–31). An internal annular fold, most prominent ventrally, marks the junction of the pharynx and esophagus in carnivores.

TUNICA MUCOSA

The mucosa is composed of three layers: a stratified squamous epithelium, a lamina propria, and a lamina muscularis. The degree of keratinization of the stratified squamous epithelium varies with the species. It is usually nonkeratinized in carnivores, slightly keratinized in the pig, more so in the horse, and keratinized to a high degree in ruminants (Fig. 10–32). The *lamina propria* is made up of a feltwork of fine collagen fibers with an abundance of evenly distributed elastic fibers. The *lamina muscularis* contains only longitudinally oriented smooth muscle bundles. It is absent in the cranial end of the esophagus of the pig and the dog (Fig. 10–33-1,2), but the cat, horse, and ruminants have isolated smooth muscle bundles near the pharynx that increase in number and become confluent toward the caudal region (Fig. 10–33-3). In the pig, the lamina muscularis is especially well developed in the caudal end, where it is as thick as the outer layer of the tunica muscularis.

TELA SUBMUCOSA

The *submucosa* is loose connective tissue containing large, longitudinally oriented arteries, veins, large lymphatic vessels, and nerve trunks. Seromucous glands containing mucous acini with serous demilunes

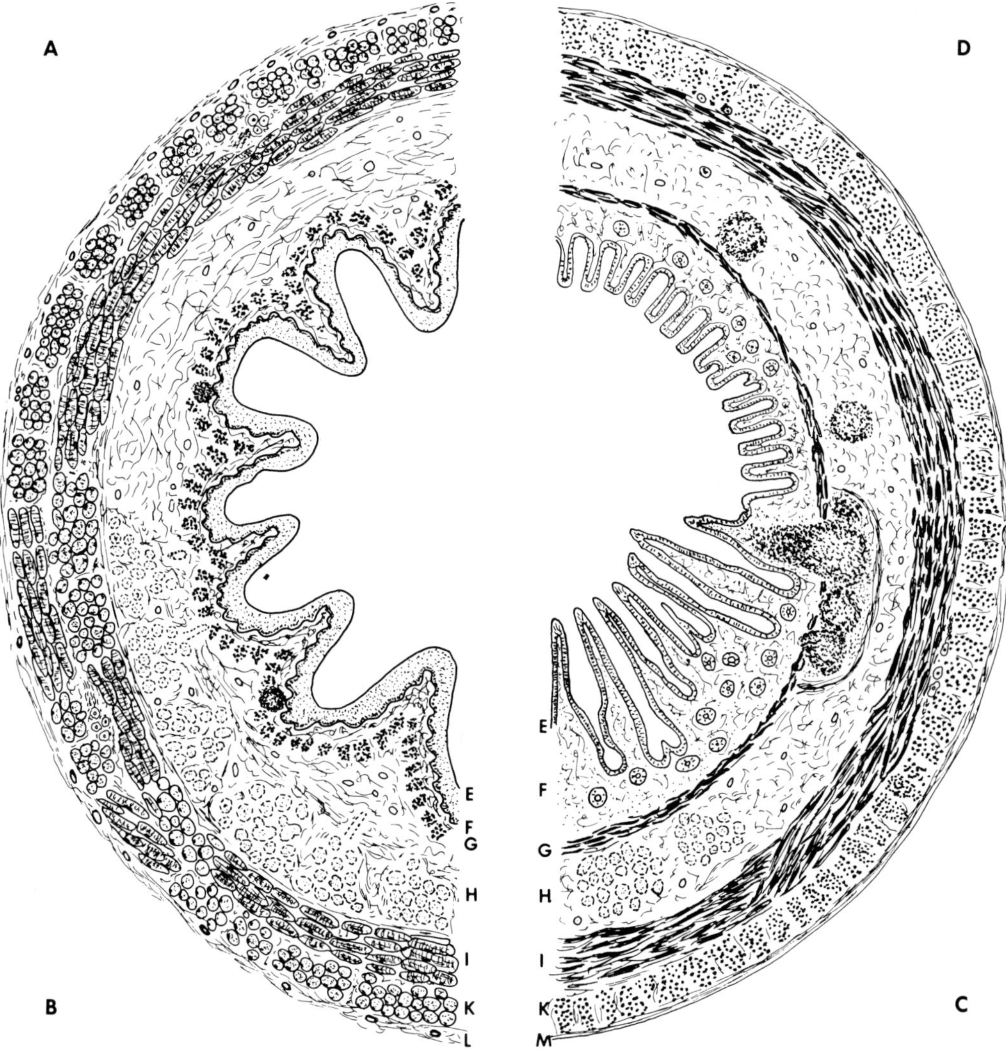

Fig. 10–31. *Schematic drawing of cross sections through various portions of the digestive tract. A, Esophagus without submucosal glands. B, Esophagus with submucosal glands. C, Small intestine with and without submucosal glands and with aggregated lymphatic nodules. D, Large intestine. Tunica mucosa: E, epithelium; F, lamina propria; G, lamina muscularis. H, Tela submucosa. Tunica muscularis: I, circular; K, longitudinal. L, Tunica adventitia. M, Tunica serosa. (From Dellmann, H.-D.: Veterinary Histology: An Outline Text-Atlas. Philadelphia, Lea & Febiger, 1971.)*

characterize this layer in the pig and dog (Fig. 10–33-2). In the pig, the glands are abundant in the cranial half but do not extend into the caudal half, whereas in the dog they are present throughout, extending into the cardiac region of the stomach (Fig. 10–34). The number of esophageal glands in the dog varies from 14,100 in dwarf breeds to 49,300 in the large breeds. Density of the glands may be as much as four times greater near the stomach (caudally) than at the beginning of the organ (cranially). Glands are present only at the pharyngoesophageal junction in the horse, cat, and ruminants. Mixed acini and demilunes occur in cattle. The loose nature of

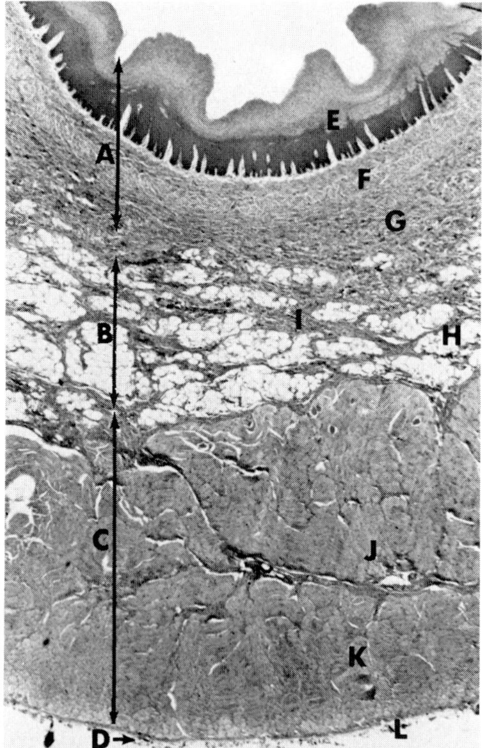

Fig. 10–32. *Esophagus, sheep. Typical layers of the digestive tube: mucosa (A); submucosa (B); tunica muscularis (C); tunica adventitia (D). Components of the esophagus: keratinized stratified squamous epithelium (E); dense irregular connective tissue of the lamina propria (F); lamina muscularis with longitudinal smooth muscle bundles (G); adipose tissue (H); collagen and elastic tissue in the submucosa (I); inner circular (J) and outer longitudinal (K) spiraling striated muscle; loose connective tissue (L). H & E. ×18.*

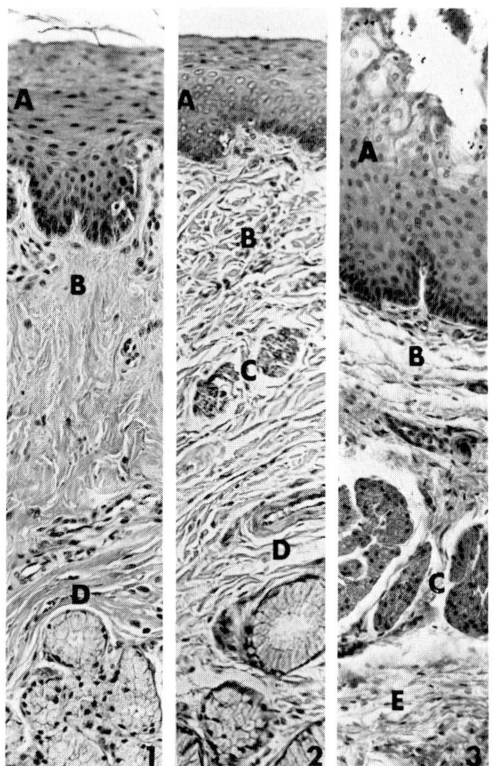

Fig. 10–33. *Esophagus: The variation of the structural components at three levels of three different species. 1, cranial level of pig; 2, middle level of dog; 3, caudal level of cat. Stratified squamous epithelium (A), lamina propria (B), lamina muscularis (C) absent in 1, scant and intermittent in 2, and well developed and continuous in 3. Submucosa with glands (D) and without glands (E). H & E. ×154.*

the submucosa allows the mucosa of the relaxed esophagus to form longitudinal folds.

TUNICA MUSCULARIS

The *tunica muscularis* of the esophagus of ruminants and dogs is entirely striated. In the horse, striated muscle makes up the rostral two thirds of the tunica muscularis but gradually changes to smooth muscle in the caudal third. The tunica muscularis of the pig is similar to that of the horse except that the middle third has mixed smooth and striated muscle. In the cat, the striated muscle may extend four fifths of the length of the esophagus before changing to smooth muscle. At the rostral end, there is some interdigitation and spiraling of the two layers of muscle comprising the tunica muscularis, but more caudally, these change to inner circular and outer longitudinal layers. The inner circular muscle layer thickens toward the stomach in all animals, but especially in the horse, where it is 10 to 15 mm thick. In ruminants, striated muscle extends from the esophagus into the wall of the *reticular sulcus.*

TUNICA ADVENTITIA

In the cervical region, the tunica muscularis is surrounded by the *tunica adven-*

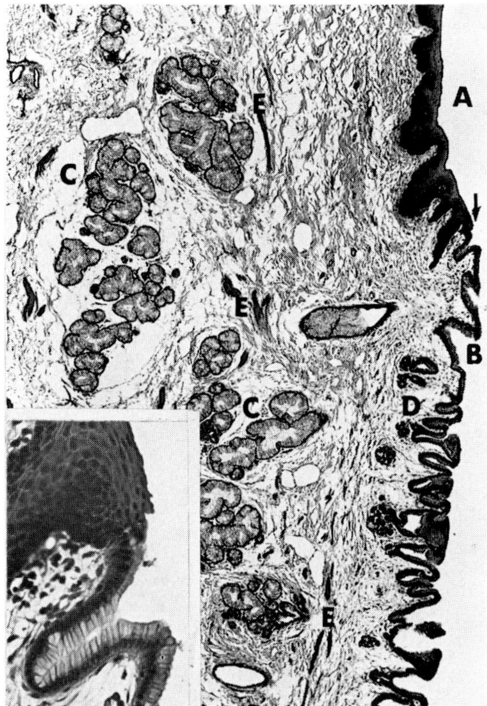

Fig. 10–34. *Esophagus-cardiac stomach junction, dog. Caudal esophagus (A); cardiac stomach (B). Notice the esophageal glands (C) extending into the cardiac gland region (D). Lamina muscularis (E). H & E. ×30. Insert, Junction of stratified squamous epithelium with simple columnar epithelium of the stomach (see arrow on large illustration). H & E. ×192.*

titia, a loose connective tissue containing blood and lymph vessels and nerves. The thoracic esophagus is largely invested by the mediastinal pleura in most species. The abdominal esophagus is most prominent in the horse, where it is about 2.5 cm in length and covered by a peritoneum giving rise to a serosa. In carnivores, a short, wedge-shaped, peritoneum-covered terminal portion makes up the abdominal esophagus. In other species the esophagus-stomach junction is at or near the diaphragm, and there is no mesothelial covering.

Esophagus-Cardiac Stomach Junction

The morphologic characteristics of this junction vary considerably because the junctions of the several layers do not take place at the same level. The skeletal muscle of the tunica muscularis changes gradually to smooth muscle. The glands of the esophagus may extend a short distance into the submucosa of the stomach, whereas the stratified squamous-simple columnar epithelial junction is very abrupt (Fig. 10–34). In the cat, the junction is 3 to 5 mm rostral to the cardia, whereas in the dog it is 1 to 2 cm rostral to the cardia. Only the pig has a well-developed internal sphincter muscle. A widening internal circular muscle at the esophagus-stomach junction in carnivores suggests a sphincterlike mechanism. In ruminants, the stratified squamous epithelium continues caudally to line the forestomach, and in the horse and pig, it extends throughout the nonglandular region of the stomach.

STOMACH

The stomach is an enlarged part of the digestive tube specialized for the enzymatic and hydrolytic breakdown of food into digestible nutrients (see Fig. 10–43). The muscular wall aids in mixing the ingesta. The stomach is lined exclusively by a glandular mucosa in carnivores, whereas herbivorous animals have, in addition to a glandular region, a nonglandular region lined with stratified squamous epithelium.

The wall of the stomach has all the layers of a typical tubular organ (Fig. 10–35-1). The tunica mucosa is composed of epithelium, a lamina propria (of collagen, elastic, and reticular fibers), and a lamina muscularis. The submucosa contains collagen fibers, fat, and the submucosal nerve plexuses. The tunica muscularis has three layers: an inner oblique, a middle circular, and an outer longitudinal layer. The myenteric plexuses are located between the middle and outer muscle layers. The tunica serosa is composed of mesothelium overlying a layer of loose connective tissue.

Nonglandular Region

The nonglandular region is absent in carnivores and small in the pig. In the

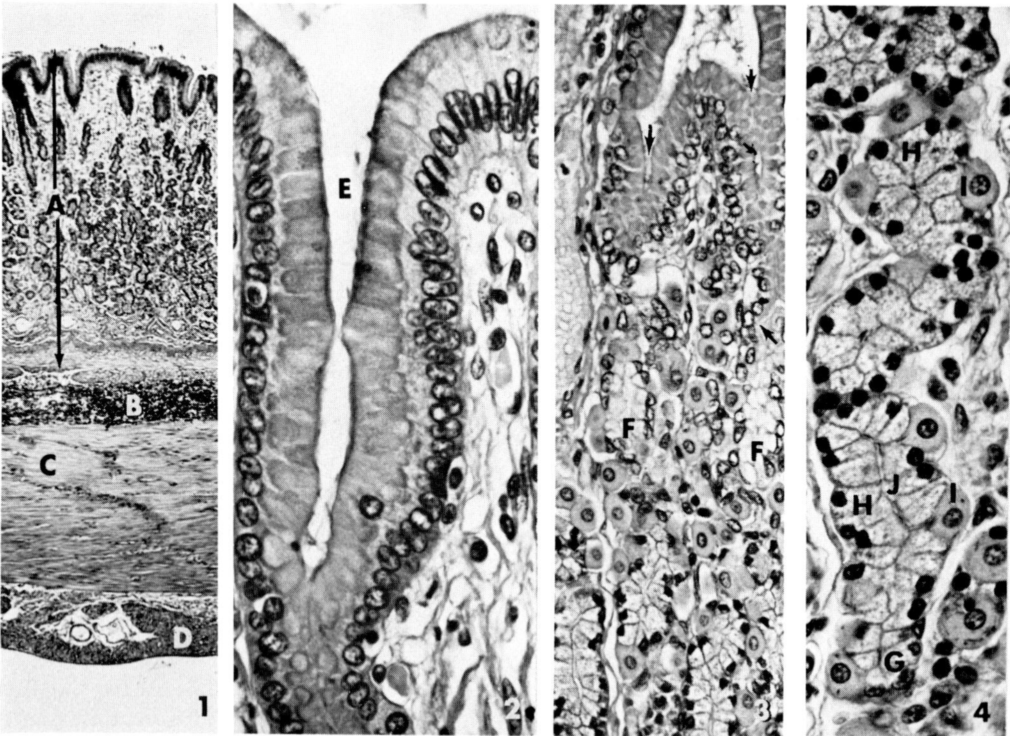

Fig. 10–35. *Fundic stomach, dog. 1, Section through fundic gland region. Trichrome. ×48. 2, Gastric pit. H & E. ×450. 3, Neck of fundic gland with mucous neck cells. H & E. ×210. 4, Base of fundic gland with chief and parietal cells. H & E. ×480. Mucosa (A); submucosa (B); circular (C) and longitudinal (D) layers of tunica muscularis; gastric pit (E); gastric gland lumen opening into gastric pit (arrows); mucous neck cells (F); base of gastric gland (G); chief cells (H); parietal cells (I); gland lumen (J).*

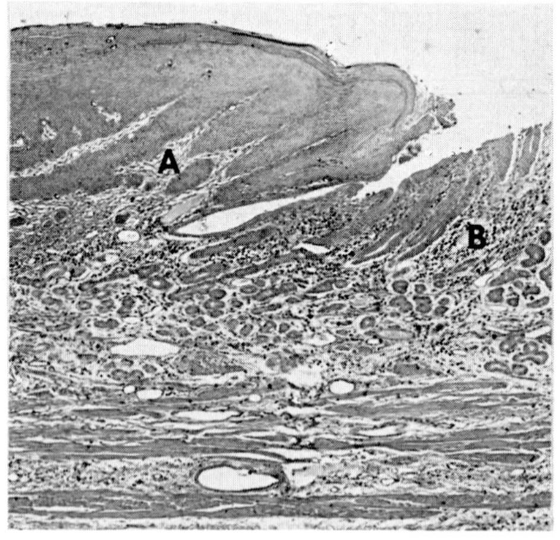

Fig. 10–36. *Junction of nonglandular and glandular regions of the stomach (margo plicatus), horse. Nonglandular region with stratified squamous epithelium (A); cardiac region with cardiac glands (B). H & E. ×48.*

horse, the nonglandular region extends a considerable distance and ends abruptly at the margo plicatus (Fig. 10–36). The nonglandular portion reaches its greatest development in ruminants and is subdivided into the rumen, reticulum, and omasum. These will be described in detail later in this chapter.

The lining epithelium of the nonglandular region is nonsecretory and may be keratinized, depending on species and diet. The lamina propria is composed of irregularly arranged collagen, elastic, and reticular fibers. There is a distinct lamina muscularis. The junction between the nonglandular and glandular portions of the stomach is abrupt, with the epithelium changing to a tall columnar type.

Glandular Region

The structure of the glandular region conforms to the general pattern described earlier (see Fig. 10–43). The glandular mucosa has extensive folds called *rugae,* which flatten as the stomach fills (see Fig. 10–39). Permanent elevations, called *gastric areas,* subdivide the mucosa and bulge into the lumen. The surface is studded with small depressions or invaginations called *gastric pits,* which are continuous with the gastric glands and receive their secretory products (Fig. 10–35-2). The mucosal surface is lined with tall columnar cells whose mucous secretory product is released continuously and serves as a protective coat that prevents autolysis of the mucosa. The surface epithelial cells have a rapid turnover rate; within approximately three to four days, they are replaced by lining cells from the gastric pit. The gastric glands occupy most of the lamina propria, so that only a few connective tissue fibers and cells are seen between them (Fig. 10–35-3). Indeed, the glands are so extensive that it is often difficult to visualize the lamina propria in this area.

The lamina muscularis is relatively thick, usually comprising three layers: an inner and outer circular layer and a middle longitudinal layer (Fig. 10–37). Small bundles of smooth muscle fibers extend into the mucosa, coursing through the connective tissue fibers between the gastric glands (Fig. 10–37).

In carnivores, a *subglandular layer* (lamina subglandularis) is interposed between the base of the glands and the lamina muscularis (Fig. 10–37). It is composed of the *stratum granulosum,* an inner layer containing many fibroblasts, and the *stratum compactum,* an outer layer that is a sheet of collagen fibers. The presence of this subglandular layer seems to be somewhat inconsistent, and its function is speculative; however, it is thought to provide some protection against perforations.

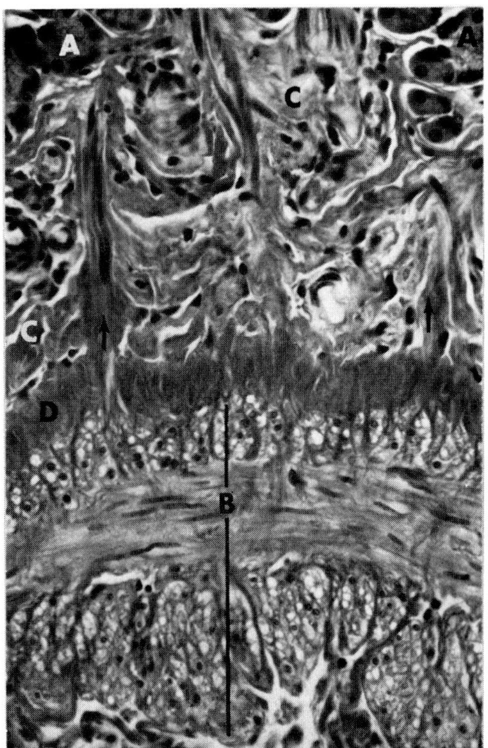

Fig. 10–37. *Fundic stomach, dog. Base of fundic glands (A); three-layered lamina muscularis (B) with muscle strands (arrows) penetrating the stratum compactum (D) and the lamina propria (C). Trichrome.* ×*428.*

The mucosa of the glandular stomach has three distinct regions named according to the various glandular types present: cardiac, fundic, and pyloric. The extent of the various glandular regions in the domestic animals is illustrated in Figure 10–43.

CARDIAC GLAND REGION

The *cardiac gland region* occupies a narrow strip at the junction of the glandular and nonglandular mucosae in all domestic mammals except the pig, where it covers nearly half of the stomach, including the diverticulum ventriculi (see Fig. 10–43). The cardiac glands are branched coiled tubular glands that open into the gastric pits. The body of the gland is relatively short and has a wider lumen than those of the fundic or pyloric glands. The mucous secretory epithelium is cuboidal with the nu-

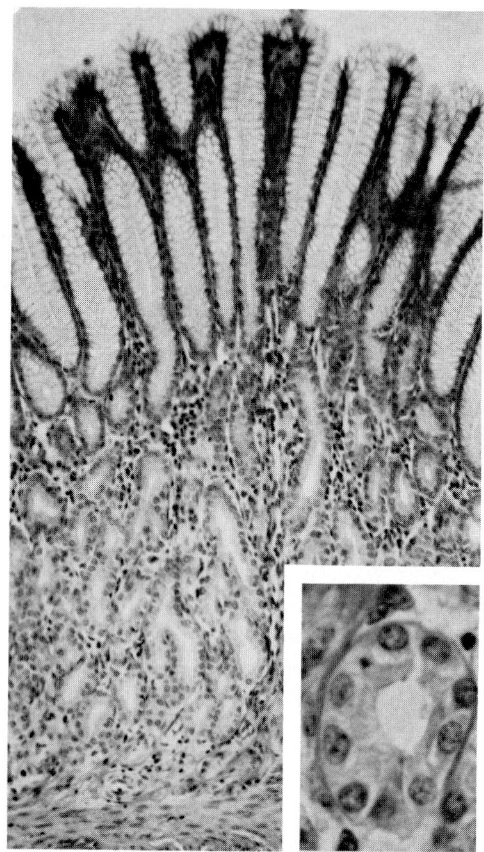

Fig. 10–38. *Cardiac stomach mucosa, pig. The mucous cells cover the surface and line the gastric pits. The cardiac mucosal glands are all mucous. Trichrome. ×50. Insert: Cross section of cardiac mucosal gland. Trichrome. ×535.*

clei located in the basal portion of the cells (Fig. 10–38). Parietal cells may occur at the junction of the cardiac and fundic regions.

FUNDIC GLAND REGION

The fundic gland region is well developed in all domestic species (see Fig. 10–43). In carnivores it occupies over half of the stomach, in the horse, over one third, and in the pig, approximately one quarter. Two thirds of the abomasum in ruminants contain fundic glands.

Fundic glands are straight, branched tubular glands that extend to the lamina muscularis (Fig. 10–35-3). The gland consists of a neck portion, a long body, and a slightly dilated blind end, also called the fundus of the gland. Four structurally and functionally distinct cell types comprise the secretory epithelium of the fundic gland: mucous neck cells, chief cells, parietal cells, and endocrine cells.

The *mucous neck cells* occupy the neck of the gland and are found among the parietal and chief cells (Fig. 10–35-3). They are typical mucous cells, with the flat nucleus located toward the cell base. They appear similar to the surface cells but have cytoplasm that is more basophilic. In addition, when treated with PAS, the mucous neck cells give an intensely positive reaction throughout, whereas the surface cells have PAS-positive material only in the upper two thirds of the cell.

The *chief cells* are the most numerous of the gastric gland cells (Fig. 10–35-4). They are cuboidal or pyramidal, with the spherical nucleus near the base of the cell. The area between the nucleus and the free surface appears lacy owing to the clear spaces that remain after fixation. In the living state, zymogen granules occupy these vacuoles and are demonstrable with special fixation and staining. It is for this reason that chief cells are also referred to as zymogen cells. The basal area of the chief cell has a well-developed rER, resulting in a basophilic staining reaction. Chief cells secrete pepsinogen, which is transformed into pepsin by hydrochloric acid.

The *parietal cells* are larger and less numerous than the chief cells. They have a tendency to occur singly, are pyramid-shaped, and are peripheral to the chief cells (Fig. 10–35-4). Usually only the apex of the cell borders on the gland lumen. Frequently, the base of the cell bulges outward from the external surface of the gland. The parietal cell has a spherical nucleus and the cytoplasm stains deeply with eosin. The cytoplasm contains a large number of mitochondria but no secretory granules. At the apex, the cell membrane invaginates to form a branching intracellular canaliculus that extends toward the center of the cell.

Numerous microvilli of varying length project into the intracellular canaliculus, thereby providing an extensive surface area associated with the active transport system necessary in the production of free hydrochloric acid. In addition to intracellular canaliculi, there are intercellular canaliculi between adjacent parietal cells. Because parietal cells contain an abundance of carbonic anhydrase, it is believed that carbonic acid is formed, the hydrogen ions from which are transported across the cell membrane and combine with chloride ions. Thus, free hydrochloric acid is formed in the canaliculi.

Throughout the glandular regions of the stomach and continuing into the intestines are a series of cells responsible for the production of gastrointestinal hormones such as secretin, gastrin, cholecystokinin, and gastric inhibitory peptides. In each case, the hormone is released from the endocrine cells into the bloodstream, where it circulates throughout the body, or the endocrine cells may release paracrine substances that diffuse locally to their target cells. These cells are difficult to identify in routine H & E sections and generally appear clear or poorly stained. Most frequently they are wedged between the basement membrane and the chief cells and do not reach the surface of the epithelium. Some of these cells do, however, extend to the lumen and are thought to monitor the luminal contents and respond with the release of hormones. At least 12 different endocrine cell types have been identified by electron microscopy in the gastrointestinal tract. They all possess numerous small membrane-bounded granules, mostly within the basal cytoplasm, and contain relatively little rough endoplasmic reticulum and small Golgi profiles. Those cells that have an affinity for silver stains are known as endocrine or argyophilic cells (see Fig. 10–65-4), and those that can be demonstrated with bichromate solutions are known as enterochromaffin cells. The endocrine cells of the gastrointestinal tract are part of a larger group of cells designated as APUD cells (see Chapter 15).

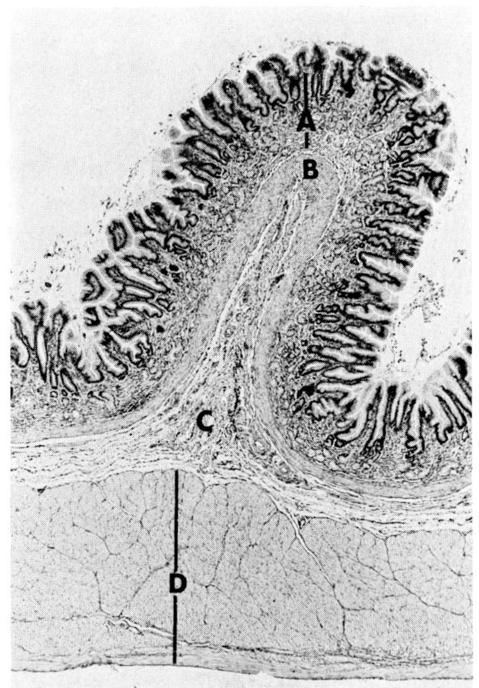

Fig. 10–39. *Pyloric stomach, cat. Longitudinal section through one mucosal fold or ruga. Lamina propria (A) covered by simple columnar epithelium; lamina muscularis (B); submucosa (C); tunica muscularis (D). Trichrome. ×30.*

PYLORIC GLAND REGION

The pyloric gland region occupies approximately half of the stomach in carnivores but only one third in the horse stomach and in the ruminant abomasum. In the pig the pyloric region is small, representing about one fourth of the stomach (see Fig. 10–43).

Pyloric glands are branched, coiled, and relatively short compared to the other gastric glands (Figs. 10–39 and 10–40). The gastric pits are considerably deeper than those in the cardiac and fundic gland regions. The cells are mucous and stain slightly basophilic, and the flat nuclei are located at the base of the cells.

At the pyloric-duodenal junction, the submucosal intestinal glands are found in

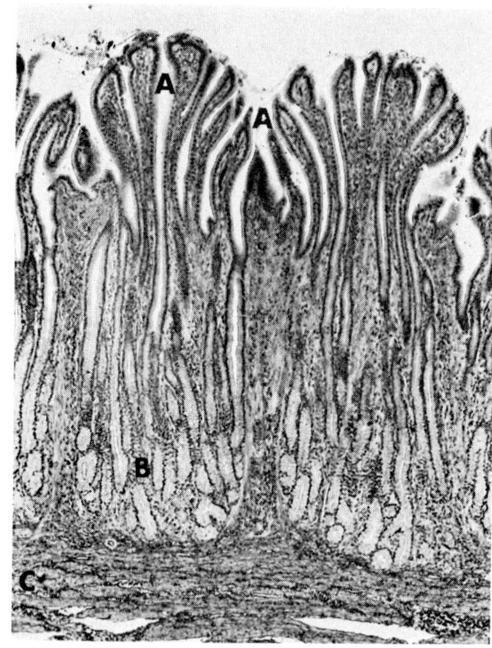

Fig. 10–40. *Pyloric stomach, pig. Gastric pits (A); pyloric glands (B); lamina muscularis (C). Trichrome. ×47.*

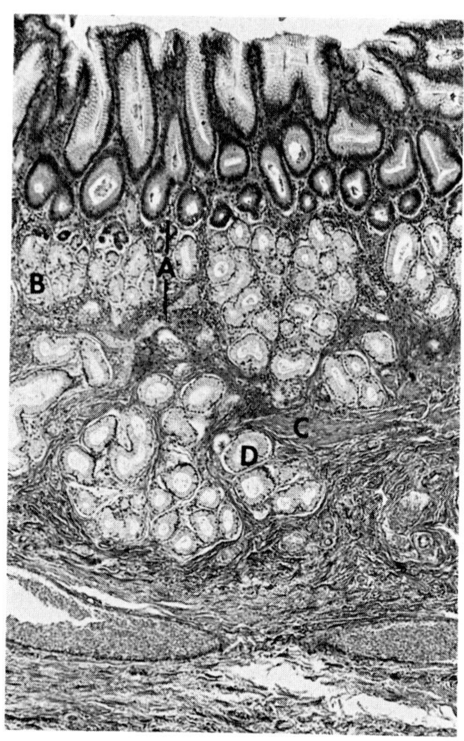

Fig. 10–41. *Caudal region of pyloric stomach, pig. Lamina propria (A); pyloric glands (B); lamina muscularis (C); submucosal glands (D); an extension of the submucosal intestinal glands. H & E. ×47.*

the submucosa of the pyloric region (Fig. 10–41). In addition, the middle circular muscle layer thickens, forming the pyloric sphincter. This encircles the caudal portion of the stomach and causes the submucosa and mucosa to bulge into the lumen. In ruminants and the pig this protuberance, called the pyloric torus, is especially prominent (Fig. 10–42).

Species Differences

In carnivores, the cardiac zone is a relatively narrow area, with the fundic and pyloric regions occupying the remainder of the stomach. In the dog, the fundic region is divided into two zones. The light zone has a thinner mucosa with deep gastric pits and short tortuous glands that appear in groups and do not reach the muscularis mucosae. The dark zone is adjacent to the pyloric region and has a thicker mucosa, shallow gastric pits, and fundic glands that more closely resemble those of the other species (Fig. 10–43).

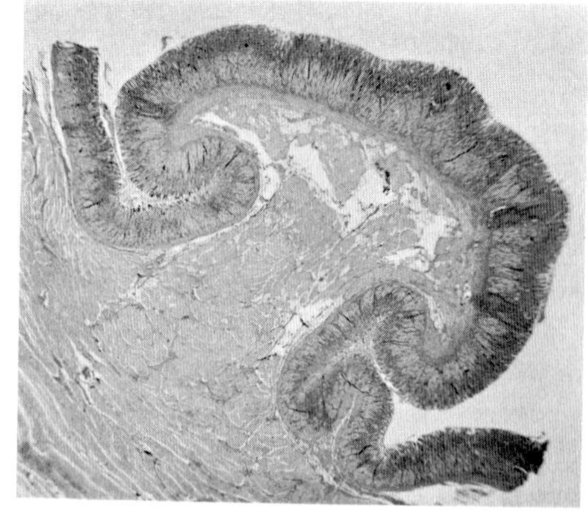

Fig. 10–42. *Pyloric torus, stomach, pig. H & E. ×3.7. (From: Dellmann, H.-D.: Veterinary Histology: An Outline Text-Atlas. Philadelphia, Lea & Febiger, 1971.)*

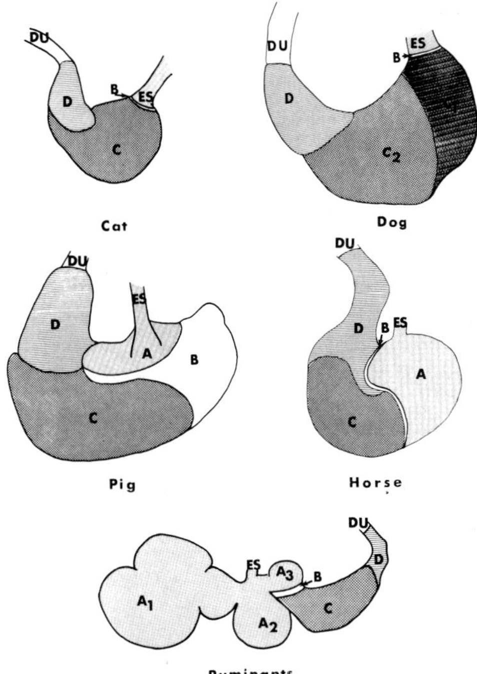

Fig. 10–43. *Drawing illustrating the simple and compound stomachs (originally drawn from fresh specimens). Nonglandular region lined by stratified squamous epithelium (A); rumen (A_1); reticulum (A_2); omasum (A_3); cardiac region (B); fundic gland zone, dog, with light (C_1) and dark (C_2) zones; pyloric gland region (D); esophagus (ES); duodenum (DU).*

The pig stomach has a large cardiac zone, and the parietal cells in the fundic region tend to occur in clusters.

The horse stomach has an extensive nonglandular region that terminates abruptly, forming the margo plicatus (Fig. 10–36). The cardiac region is almost nonexistent, whereas the fundic and pyloric zones follow the normal pattern.

Ruminant Stomach

The stomach of ruminants is composed of four structurally distinct parts. The first three parts, the *rumen, reticulum,* and *omasum,* are collectively called the *forestomach* (Fig. 10–43) and are lined with a nonglandular mucous membrane having a stratified squamous epithelium. The fourth part, the *abomasum,* is the glandular portion similar to the simple stomach of other species. The forestomach is effective in breaking down the coarse fibrous ingesta into absorbable nutrients by both mechanical and chemical action. The rumen acts as a fermentation vat where the large population of microorganisms acts on the ingesta, producing short-chain, volatile fatty acids, which are then absorbed through the mucosa into the blood. The reticulum and omasum exert a mechanical action on the ingesta, reducing the mass to fine particles. The wall of the omasum is especially well adapted for this function. In addition to fermentation and mechanical activities, there is considerable absorption through the mucosae of all three portions of the forestomach. The enzymatic digestive processes in the abomasum further degrade the ingesta to such substances as glucose and amino acids in a manner similar to that of the glandular portion of the simple stomach.

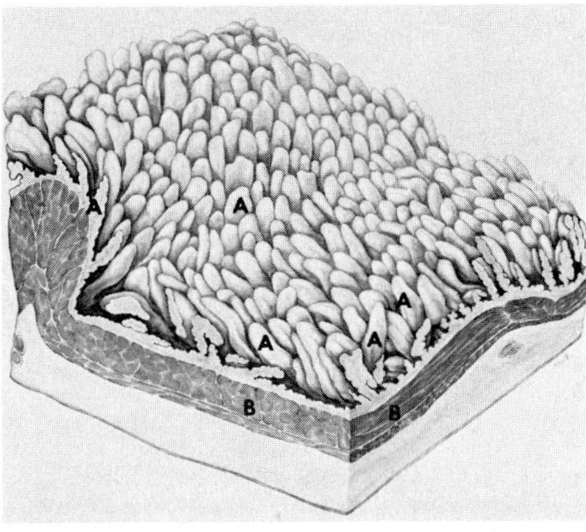

Fig. 10–44. *Three-dimensional drawing of a portion of the wall of the rumen. Papillae (A); tunica muscularis (B). (From Stinson, A.W., and Brown, E.M.: Veterinary Histology Slide Sets. East Lansing, Mich., Michigan State University, Instructional Media Center, 1970.)*

RUMEN

The rumen is characterized by small tongue-shaped papillae that may attain a length of 1.5 cm in adult cattle (Figs. 10–44 and 10–45). The size and shape of the pa-

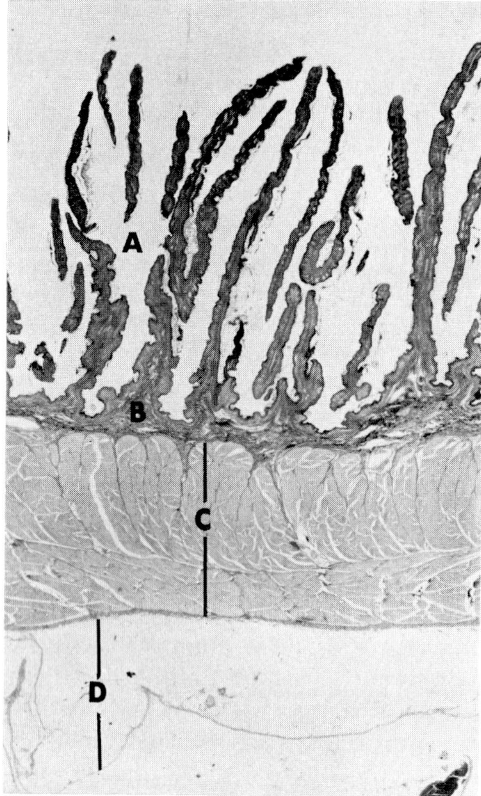

Fig. 10–45. *Rumen, cow. Papillae covered with stratified squamous epithelium (A); propria-submucosa (B); tunica muscularis (C); tunica serosa (D). H & E. ×7. (From Stinson, A.W., and Brown, E.M.: Veterinary Histology Slide Sets. East Lansing, Mich., Michigan State University, Instructional Media Center, 1970.)*

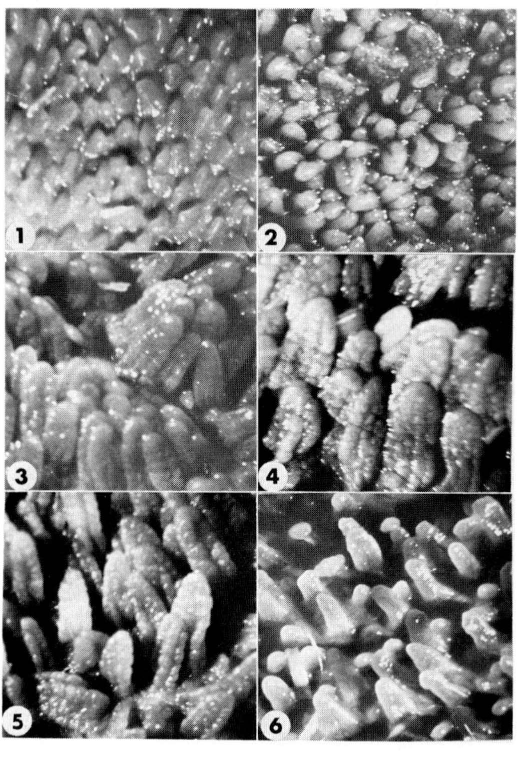

Fig. 10–46. *Changes in surface of rumen due to age and diet, same steer. ×2. 1, Six months of age, milk since birth. Papillae are rudimentary. 2, Hay and grain for three weeks. Papillae are enlarged. 3, Hay and grain for two months. 4, Hay and grain for three months. Papillae have reached maximal length. 5, After return to milk diet for three days. Papillae are smaller. 6, After return to milk diet for 10 days. Papillae are strikingly reduced. (From Stinson, A.W., and Brown, E.M.: Veterinary Histology Slide Sets. East Lansing, Mich., Michigan State University, Instructional Media Center, 1970.)*

pillae vary considerably from one region of the rumen to another. They first appear in the rumen of the bovine embryo when it measures 46 cm from the crown to rump, and at the time of birth they are about 1 mm long. They remain fairly underdeveloped as long as the animal remains on a milk diet. When roughage is included in the diet and fermentation begins in the rumen, the papillae increase rapidly in size (Fig. 10–46).

The ruminal epithelium is the stratified squamous type and performs at least three important functions: protection, metabolism, and absorption (Figs. 10–47 and 10–48). The upper keratinized layer forms a protective shield against the rough, fibrous ingesta, whereas the deeper layers metabolize the short-chain, volatile fatty acids particularly butyric, acetic, and propionic acids, the chief products of fermentation. Sodium, potassium, ammonia, urea, and many other products are also absorbed from the ruminal contents.

The stratum corneum varies in thickness from 1 to 2 cells to as many as 10 to 20 cells (Fig. 10–49). The cells are squamous shaped, and stainable nuclei may or may not be present. The stratum granulosum is usually 1 to 3 cells thick. The cells are distinctly flattened, and keratohyaline granules are present in the cytoplasm. The cells

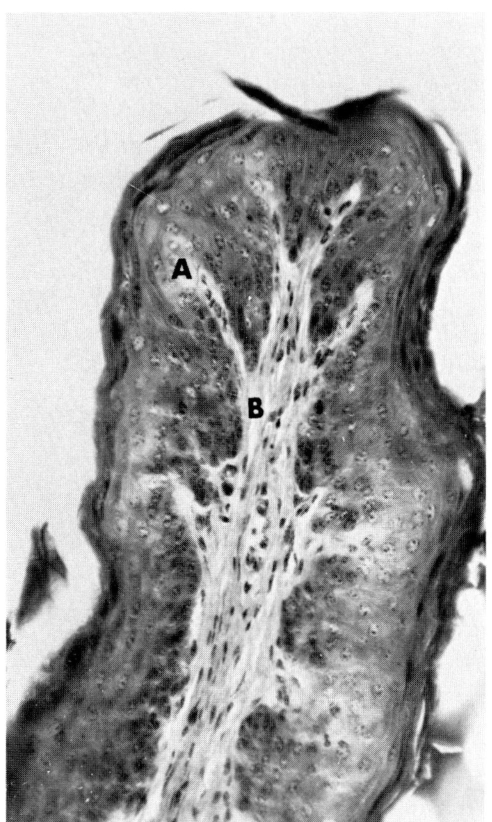

Fig. 10–47. *Tip of ruminal papilla, cow. Stratified squamous epithelium (A); lamina propria containing strands of connective tissue (B). H & E. ×250. (From Stinson, A.W., and Brown, E.M.: Veterinary Histology Slide Sets. East Lansing, Mich., Michigan State University, Instructional Media Center, 1970.)*

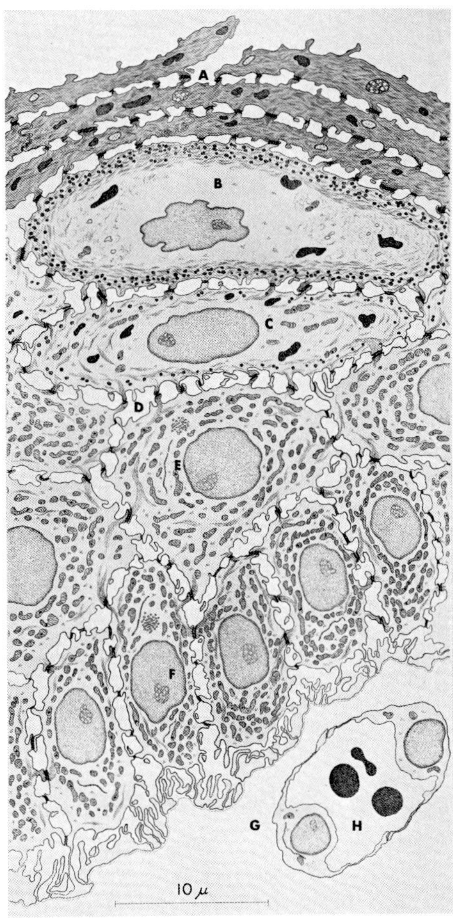

Fig. 10–48. *Drawing from an electron micrograph of ruminal epithelium. Stratum corneum (A); swollen cells of the stratum granulosum (B); flat cells of the stratum granulosum (C); intercellular canaliculi (D); stratum spinosum with desmosomal attachments between cells (E); stratum basale (F); lamina propria (G); capillaries in lamina propria (H). (From Stinson, A.W., and Brown, E.M.: Veterinary Histology Slide Sets. East Lansing, Mich., Michigan State Univerity, Instructional Media Center, 1970.)*

between the stratum granulosum and the stratum corneum are frequently swollen and are characterized by a shrunken nucleus surrounded by clear, electron-lucent cytoplasm. The peripheral cytoplasm of these cells contains keratohyaline granules, tonofilaments, and numerous membrane-bounded, electron-dense granules (Fig. 10–48). The stratum spinosum consists of polyhedral-shaped cells that are slightly larger than the basal cells (Fig. 10–50). The thickness of this layer varies considerably from 1 to 10 cells. The cytologic features of these cells include numerous mitochondria and ribosomes distributed throughout the cytoplasm (Figs. 10–51 and 10–52). A Golgi complex is not particularly well developed and membranes of the endoplasmic reticulum are scarce. Adjacent cells are connected through numerous desmosomes (Fig. 10–48). The stratum basale contains columnar cells located on a basement membrane (Fig. 10–53). Numerous processes extend to the basement membrane (Fig. 10–53) and greatly increase the cell surface at the junction with the lamina propria. The cytologic features of the basal

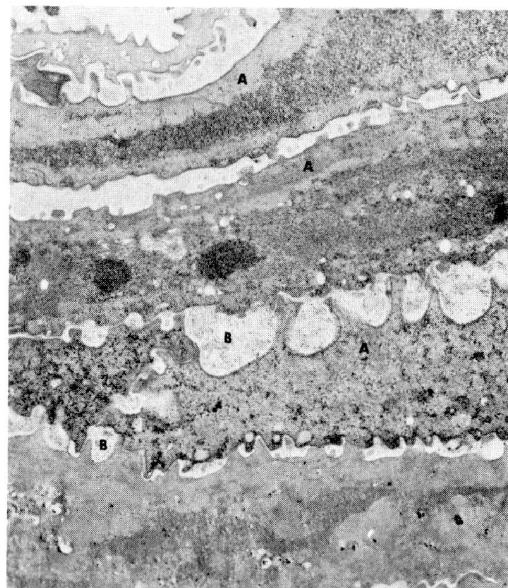

Fig. 10–49. *Electron micrograph of stratum corneum, rumen. Keratinized cell (A); intercellular canaliculi between cells (B). Notice the flocculent material within the canaliculi. ×6720. (From Stinson, A.W., and Brown, E.M.: Veterinary Histology Slide Sets. East Lansing, Mich., Michigan State University, Instructional Media Center, 1970.)*

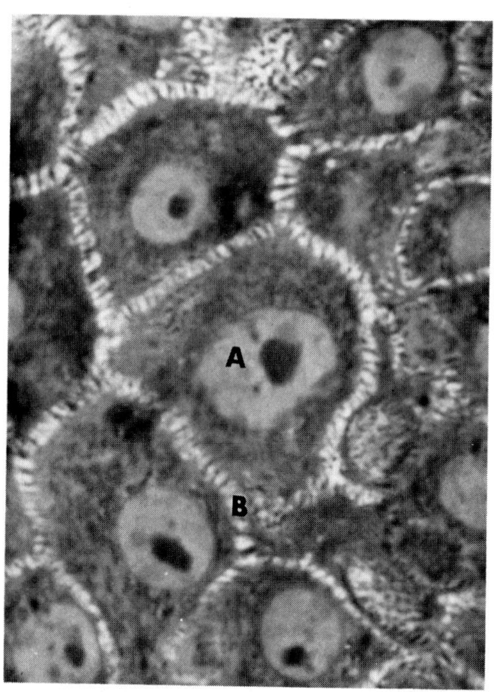

Fig. 10–50. *Stratum spinosum, rumen. Nucleus (A); intercellular space bridged by cytoplasmic processes of adjacent cells (B). Epon. Methylene blue. ×1000. (From Stinson, A.W., and Brown, E.M.: Veterinary Histology Slide Sets. East Lansing, Mich., Michigan State University, Instructional Media Center, 1970.)*

cells are similar to those of the stratum spinosum.

The intercellular spaces throughout the entire epithelium are distended to varying degrees. In some areas the space is wide and contains flocculent material that is being absorbed through the epithelium (Fig. 10–51). In other areas the spaces are collapsed and no flocculent material is present in the intercellular space, reflecting a period of little or no absorption (Fig. 10–52).

The lamina propria beneath the epithelium extends into the center of each papilla and consists of a dense feltwork of collagen, elastic, and reticular fibers. A dense network of fenestrated capillaries lies just beneath the basement membrane of the epithelium. Glands, as well as the lamina muscularis, are absent.

The tela submucosa is composed of loose connective tissue and blends into the lamina propria without any distinct line of demarcation. A network of blood vessels and the submucosal plexuses are located within this layer.

The tunica muscularis is composed of two layers of smooth muscle. The fibers of the inner layer have a circular arrangement, whereas those of the outer layer are longitudinally oriented. The myenteric plexuses are located between the longitudinal and circular muscle layers.

The tunica serosa of the rumen is composed of collagen and elastic connective tissue and is covered by a mesothelium. Varying amounts of fat, as well as blood and lymph vessels and nerves, are located in the serosa.

RETICULUM AND RETICULAR SULCUS

The *reticulum* has a mucosa with permanent anastomosing folds, giving it the appearance of a honeycomb (Fig. 10–54).

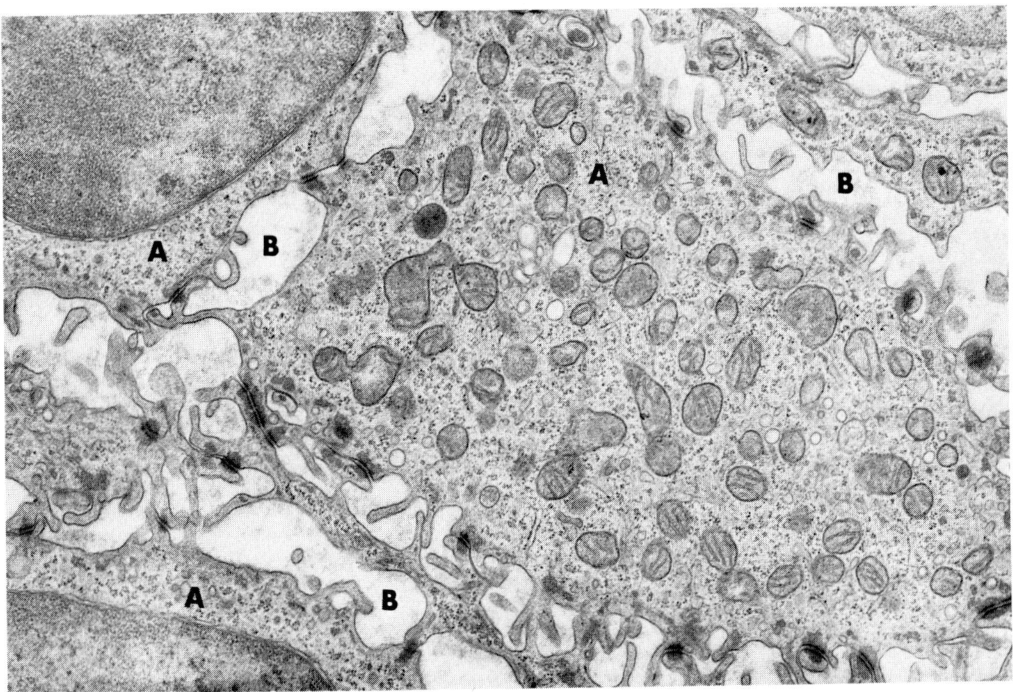

Fig. 10–51. *Electron micrograph of stratum spinosum, rumen. Epithelial cells with a large number of mitochondria and ribosomes (A); intercellular space with flocculent material (B). ×13,440. (From Stinson, A.W., and Brown, E.M.: Veterinary Histology Slide Sets. East Lansing, Mich., Michigan State University, Instructional Media Center, 1970.)*

There are two different heights of these folds. The taller folds separate the mucosal surface into shallow compartments that are further divided into smaller areas by shorter folds. The sides of the folds have vertical ridges, and the mucosa between the folds is covered by conical papillae that project into the lumen.

The keratinized stratified squamous epithlium resembles that of the rumen. The lamina propria is formed by a feltwork of collagen and elastic fibers. A well-developed band of smooth muscle is located in the upper part of the reticular folds and it is continuous with the lamina muscularis of the esophagus (Fig. 10–55). Where the reticular folds intersect, the muscle bundles pass from one fold into another, forming a continuous network of smooth muscle throughout the reticular mucosa.

The thin tela submucosa is composed of collagen and elastic fibers that blend into the lamina propria without any distinct junction. The tunica muscularis consists of two layers of smooth muscle fibers that follow an oblique course and cross at right angles. The myenteric and submucosal plexuses of nerve fibers and ganglia are present. The tunica serosa is composed of collagen and elastic fibers and is covered by a mesothelium.

The *reticular* or *esophageal sulcus* begins at the cardia and passes ventrally on the medial wall of the reticulum to end at the reticulo-omasal orifice. Contraction of the muscular wall of this sulcus closes off a channel that directs ingested fluids from the esophagus to the abomasum, thus bypassing the rumen and reticulum.

The entire sulcus is lined by stratified squamous epithelium (Fig. 10–56). The lamina propria is composed of collagen and elastic fibers. The lamina muscularis, an extension of the esophageal lamina

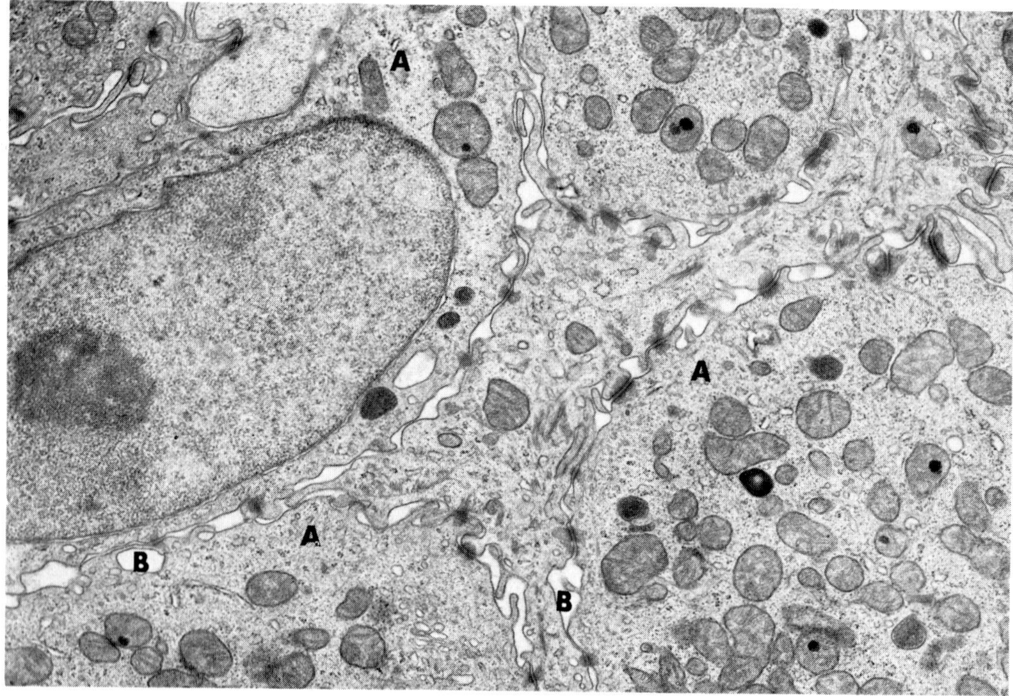

Fig. 10–52. *Electron micrograph of stratum spinosum, rumen. The intercellular space has collapsed. Compare to Figure 10–51. Epithelial cells (A); intercellular space (B). × 13,440. (From Stinson, A.W., and Brown, E.M.: Veterinary Histology Slide Sets. East Lansing, Mich., Michigan State University, Instructional Media Center, 1970.)*

muscularis, is incomplete and is most conspicuous in the lips of the sulcus. It forms a complete layer near the omasum. There are no glands in the mucosa.

The tela submucosa is made up of collagen and elastic fibers and blends with the lamina propria.

The internal layer of the tunica muscularis of the floor of the reticular sulcus is composed of transversely arranged smooth muscle fibers. Most of these fibers pass into the wall of the reticulum, where they blend with the external layer of the tunica muscularis, but a thin sheet curves around into the lips of the sulcus and inserts on the longitudinal muscle. A thin outer longitudinal layer contains both smooth and skeletal muscle fibers. The skeletal muscle fibers are a continuation of the esophageal musculature. They predominate over the smooth muscle at the cardia but fade out toward the termination of the sulcus. The tunica muscularis of the lips of the sulcus consists of smooth muscle fibers coursing parallel with the lips. These muscle fibers form a loop around the cardia corresponding to the cardiac loop of animals with simple stomachs. At the ventral end of the reticular sulcus, the muscle fibers pass into the sphincter of the reticulo-omasal orifice. At the side of the sulcus, the fibers spread out into the inner layer of the reticulum. The serosa is similar to other parts of the forestomach.

OMASUM

The *omasum* is organized into about 100 longitudinal laminae that arise on the greater curvature and sides of the organ (Fig. 10–57). The largest laminae, about 12 in number, have a thick, concave, free edge that reaches to within a short distance of the lesser curvature. There is a second

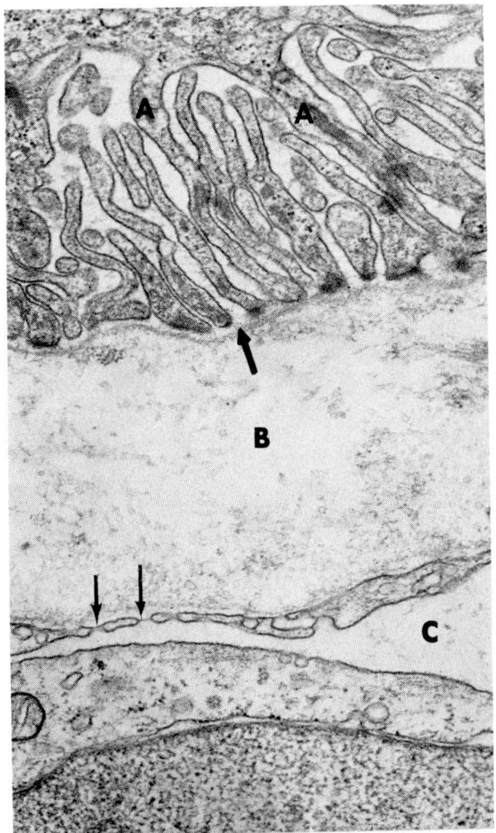

Fig. 10–53. *Electron micrograph of stratum basale and lamina propria, rumen. Cytoplasmic processes of the stratum basale cells (A) resting on basal lamina (thick arrow); lamina propria with collagen fibrils (B); capillary lumen (C) with fenestrations at thin arrows. ×20,000. (From Stinson, A.W., and Brown, E.M.: Veterinary Histology Slide Sets. East Lansing, Mich., Michigan State University, Instructional Media Center, 1970.)*

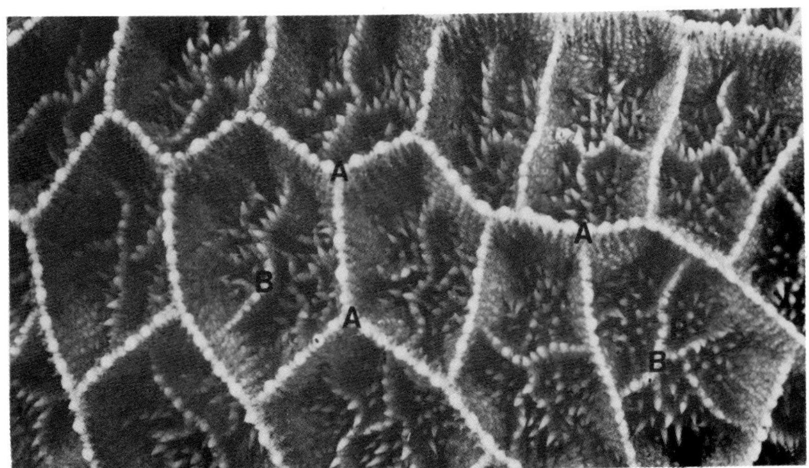

Fig. 10–54. *Surface view of the reticulum mucosa. (A) Primary folds; (B) secondary folds. (Courtesy of A. Hansen.)*

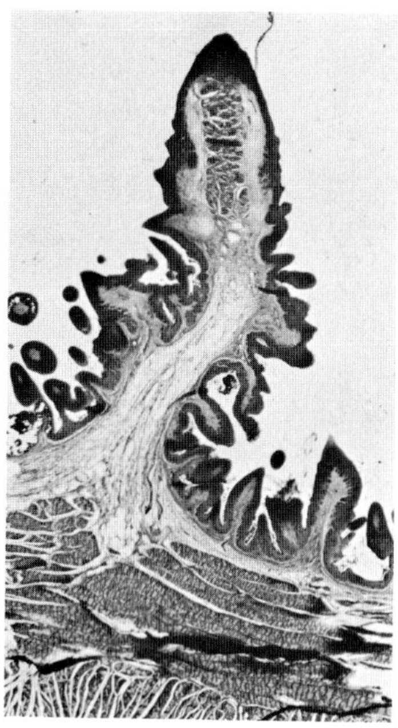

Fig. 10–55. *Reticulum, large ruminant. Cross section through a primary fold with condensed lamina muscularis in upper portion. H & E. ×9.5. (From Dellmann, H.-D.: Veterinary Histology: An Outline Text-Atlas. Philadelphia, Lea & Febiger, 1971.)*

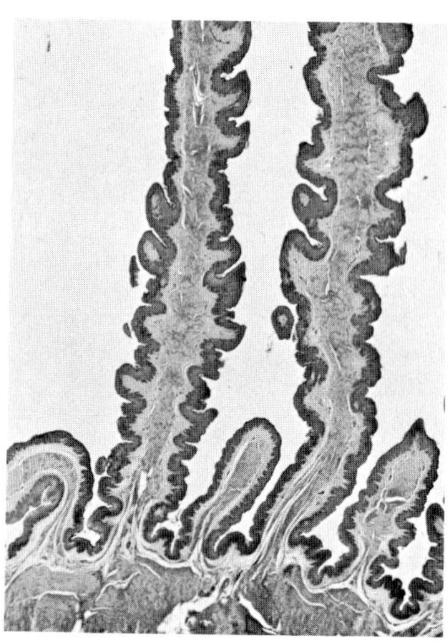

Fig. 10–57. *Omasum, large ruminant. Portion of the wall including the origin of laminae of different sizes. Large laminae are penetrated by an extension of the tunica muscularis, whereas the smaller laminae have muscle originating from the lamina muscularis only. H & E. ×10.7. (From Dellmann, H.-D.: Veterinary Histology: An Outline Text-Atlas. Philadelphia, Lea & Febiger, 1971.)*

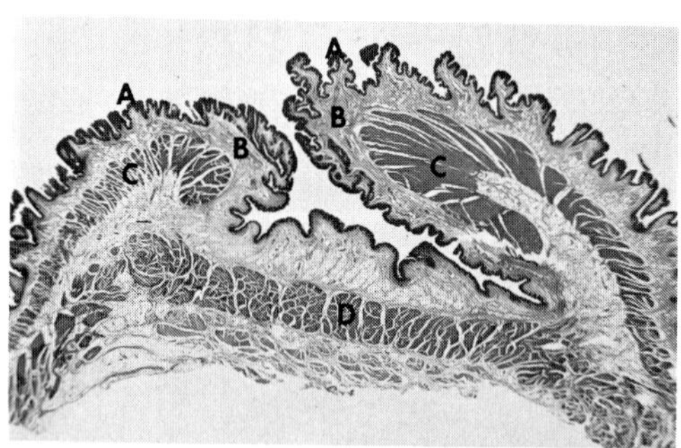

Fig. 10–56. *Reticular sulcus, cow. Stratified squamous epithelium covering the reticular papillae (A); lamina propria blending with the submucosa between scattered small bundles of the lamina muscularis (B); longitudinal musculature of the lips (C); transverse musculature of the floor (D). H & E. ×12. (From Dellmann, H.-D.: Veterinary Histology; An Outline Text-Atlas. Philadelphia, Lea & Febiger, 1971.)*

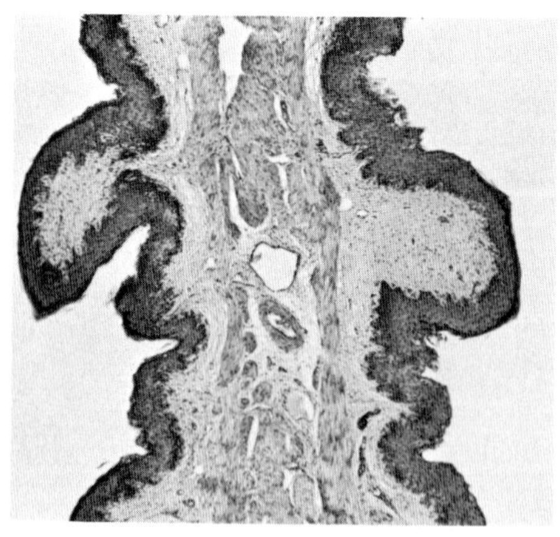

Fig. 10–58. *Omasum, large ruminant. Portion of a large lamina containing three layers of muscle. H & E. ×34.5. (From Dellmann, H.-D.: Veterinary Histology: An Outline Text-Atlas. Philadelphia, Lea & Febiger, 1971.)*

order of shorter laminae as well as third, fourth, and fifth orders, each decreasing in length. The food is pressed into thin layers in the narrow spaces between the laminae and reduced to a fine pulp by the numerous rounded, horny papillae that stud the surface of the mucosa. The papillae are directed so that the movement of the laminae works the solid food from the reticulo-omasal orifice into the interlaminar spaces and out at the abomasal end.

The lining is keratinized stratified squamous epithelium and the aglandular lamina propria is characterized by a dense subepithelial capillary network. A lamina muscularis forms a thick layer just beneath the lamina propria on both sides of the laminae. The tela submucosa is composed of collagen and elastic fibers, with blood and lymph vessels throughout. Nerve plexuses with ganglia may be present also.

The tunica muscularis is composed of an outer, thin longitudinal layer and an inner, thicker circular layer of smooth muscle whose innermost layer is continued into the large omasal laminae (first through third orders) as the intermediate muscle sheet (Fig. 10–58). The muscular pattern of a cross section of one of the larger laminae is characteristic. A thick inner layer of smooth muscle fibers, extending from the inner layer of the tunica muscularis to the free end of the lamina, forms the central part of the muscle. Smooth muscle fibers of the lamina muscularis are perpendicular to these fibers and lie on either side of it. Thus, in examining a cross section, three layers of smooth muscle will be seen. The tunica serosa is similar in structure to those described for the other parts of the forestomach.

ABOMASUM

The junction of the omasum with the abomasum is marked by a mucosal fold, the omaso-abomasal fold, where the epithelium changes abruptly from stratified squamous to simple columnar epithelium. In large ruminants, this change is on the apex of the fold, whereas in small ruminants it appears on the omasal side. The lamina propria becomes less dense on the abomasal side of the fold, and frequently there is a lymphatic nodule beneath the epithelial junction. The mucosa of the abomasum has all the characteristic glandular regions of the stomach described previously.

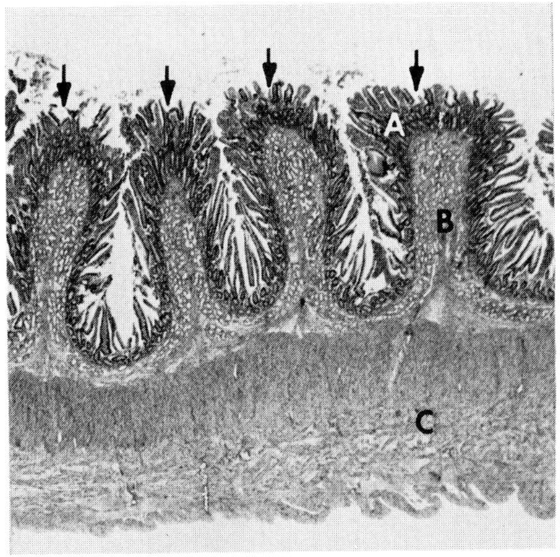

Fig. 10–59. *Longitudinal section of duodenum, cow. Circular folds (plicae circulares) (arrows). Mucosa (A); submucosal glands (B); tunica muscularis (C). H & E. ×42.*

SMALL INTESTINE

The small intestine is composed of the duodenum, jejunum, and ileum. Intestinal digestion, or reduction of food to an absorbable form, begins when the contents from the stomach are acted on by the pancreatic juice, bile, and intestinal secretions, and it continues throughout the length of the small intestine.

The digestive and absorptive functions of the small intestine are facilitated by several specialized structures. The efficiency of the absorptive function is enhanced by three structural features that increase the surface area exposed to the intestinal contents. (1) The upper two thirds of the small intestine have circularly disposed mucosal folds (plicae circulares) extending approximately two thirds of the way around the lumen. In the ruminants, these folds are permanent, but in all other domestic animals they are seen only in the relaxed mucous membrane and disappear when the organ is distended (Fig. 10–59). (2) The surface of the mucosa is studded with fingerlike projections, the intestinal *villi* (Figs. 10–60 and 10–61). The villi vary in length (0.5 to 1.0 μm), depending on the region and the species. They are long and slender in carnivores and short and wide in cattle. (3) Finally, the absorptive surface is further increased by the *microvilli* on the free surface of the simple columnar epithelial cells of the villi (Fig. 10–62).

The digestive functions require voluminous amounts of digestive enzymes, along with a copious supply of mucus to protect the lining cells from mechanical injury and irritating compounds. The enzymes are provided by special cells in the mucosa and submucosa, as well as by glands that lie outside the intestine and are connected to it by ducts, i.e., liver and pancreas. Mucus is produced by submucosal glands in the small intestine (Figs. 10–59, 10–63, and 10–64) and by goblet cells, which are intermingled with the absorptive surface cells throughout the entire intestine (Figs. 10–61, 10–62, and 10–65). The morphology of the small intestine varies to some extent among the domestic animals; the important differences are discussed throughout this section.

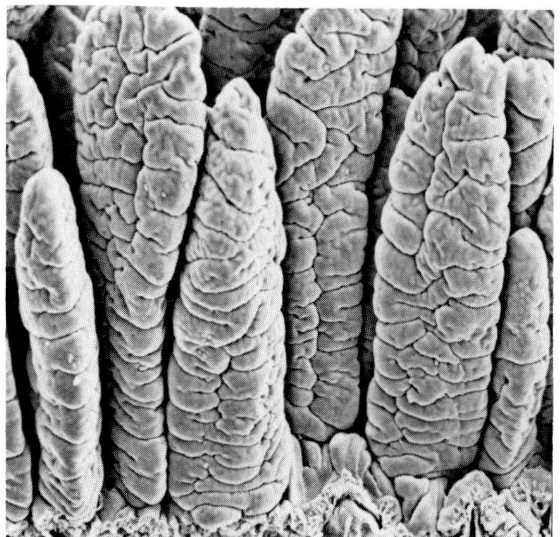

Fig. 10–60. *Scanning electron micrograph of intestinal villi, ileum, calf. These villi are in a contracted state. ×85. (Courtesy of J.F. Pohlenz.)*

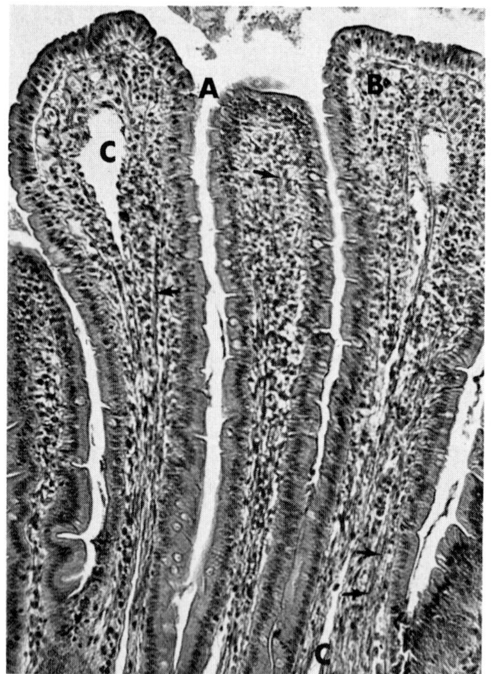

Fig. 10–61. *Villi of the small intestine, dog. Simple columnar epithelium with goblet cells (A); lamina propria (B); lymphatic vessel (lacteal) (C); smooth muscle (arrows). H & E. ×115. (From Titkemeyer, C.W., and Calhoun, M.L.: A comparative study of the structure of the small intestine of domestic animals. Am J Vet Res 16:152, 1955.)*

TUNICA MUCOSA

The mucosa includes the lining epithelium, lamina propria with glands, and a lamina muscularis. The villi are mucosal projections and are the most characteristic feature of the small intestine. The *intestinal glands (crypts)*, which open into pits between the bases of the villi, penetrate the mucosa as far as the lamina muscularis. These simple tubular glands are sometimes referred to as mucosal glands (Fig. 10–64).

EPITHELIUM. The lumen of the intestine

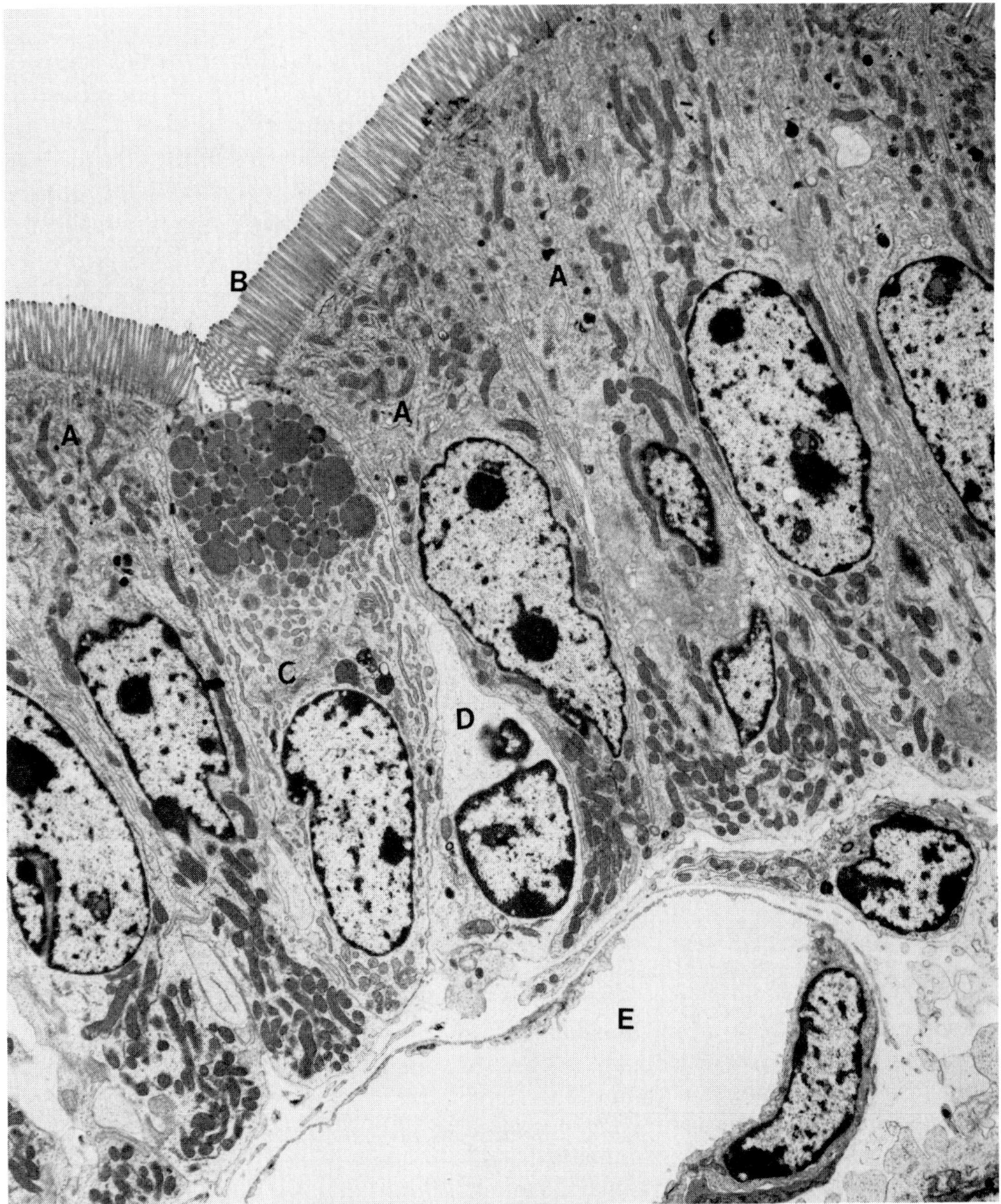

Fig. 10–62. *Electron micrograph of jejunum surface, epithelium, calf. Simple columnar epithelial cells (A) with microvilli (B). One goblet cell (C) and a migrating lymphocyte (D) are also present. Immediately below the epithelium is a capillary (E). ×5000. (Courtesy of J.F. Pohlenz.)*

is lined by simple columnar epithelium with numerous goblet cells interspersed among the columnar cells (Fig. 10–62). Well-developed junctional complexes, located between the epithelial cells at the luminal surface, prevent the fluid of the intestinal contents from diffusing into the lamina propria without going through the cells. The columnar absorbing cells have oval nuclei situated near the cell base and have prominent microvilli (striated border). In electron micrographs, rod-shaped

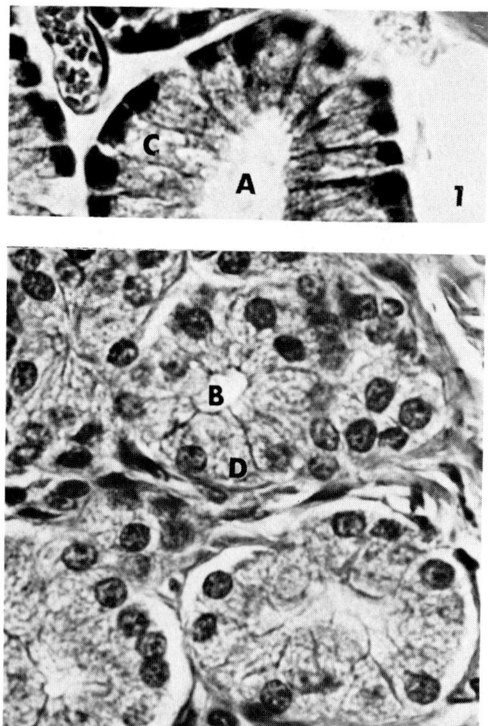

Fig. 10–63. *Submucosal glands, duodenum: 1, goat; 2, cat. Large lumen of goat submucosal gland (A); columnar cells of goat (C). H & E. ×600. Small lumen of cat submucosal gland (B); pyramidal cells of cat (D). H & E. ×580. (From Titkemeyer, C.W., and Calhoun, M.L.: A comparative study of the structure of the small intestine of domestic animals. Am J Vet Res 16:152, 1955.)*

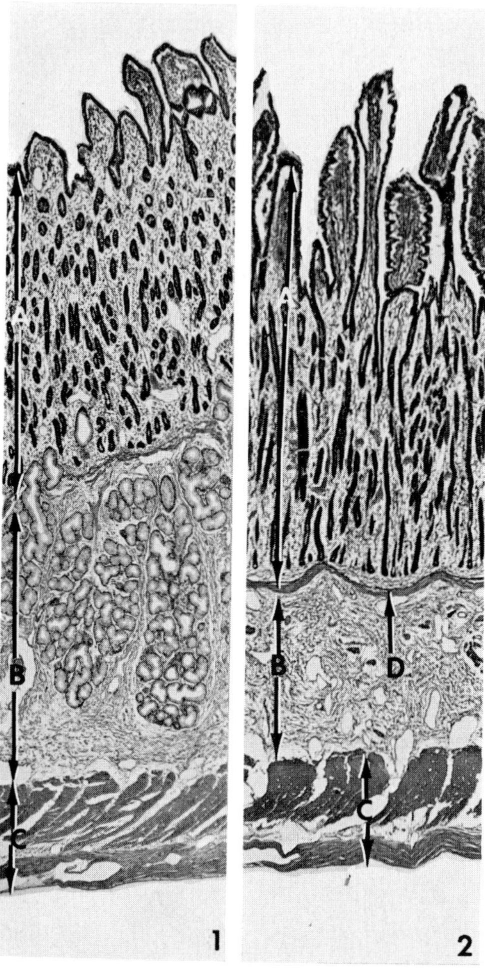

Fig. 10–64. *Duodenum, dog. 1, Area near pylorus with submucosal glands. 2, More caudal area without glands. Tunica mucosa (A); tela submucosa (B); tunica muscularis (C); lamina muscularis (D). H & E. ×28. (From Adam, W.S., Calhoun, M.L., Smith, E.M., and Stinson, A.W.: Microscopic Anatomy of the Dog: a Photoghraphic Atlas. Springfield, Ill., Charles C Thomas, 1970.)*

mitochondria are seen near the nucleus and in the basal region (Fig. 10–62). The apical cytoplasm contains a terminal web and extensive smooth ER necessary for the synthesis of triglycerides. A prominent supranuclear Golgi complex also functions in chylomicron formation, in addition to having secretory activity. Rough ER and free ribosomes are located in the basal part of the cell.

Goblet cells are dispersed among the columnar cells (Fig. 10–65-1). As mucin is produced within the cell, the apical portion of the cell becomes distended, mucigen droplets accumulate, and the nucleus and remaining cytoplasm are pushed into the narrow cell base that rests on the basal lamina (Fig. 10–62). (For more details, refer to Chapter 2.) The number of goblet cells decreases at the tip of the villi, and the density of the goblet cells is two to three times greater in the caudal part of the small intestine than in the cranial portion.

The simple tubular intestinal glands are lined by a variety of cell types. Undifferentiated, low columnar (cuboidal) cells in the glandular crypts multiply, differentiate, and migrate onto the villus, giving

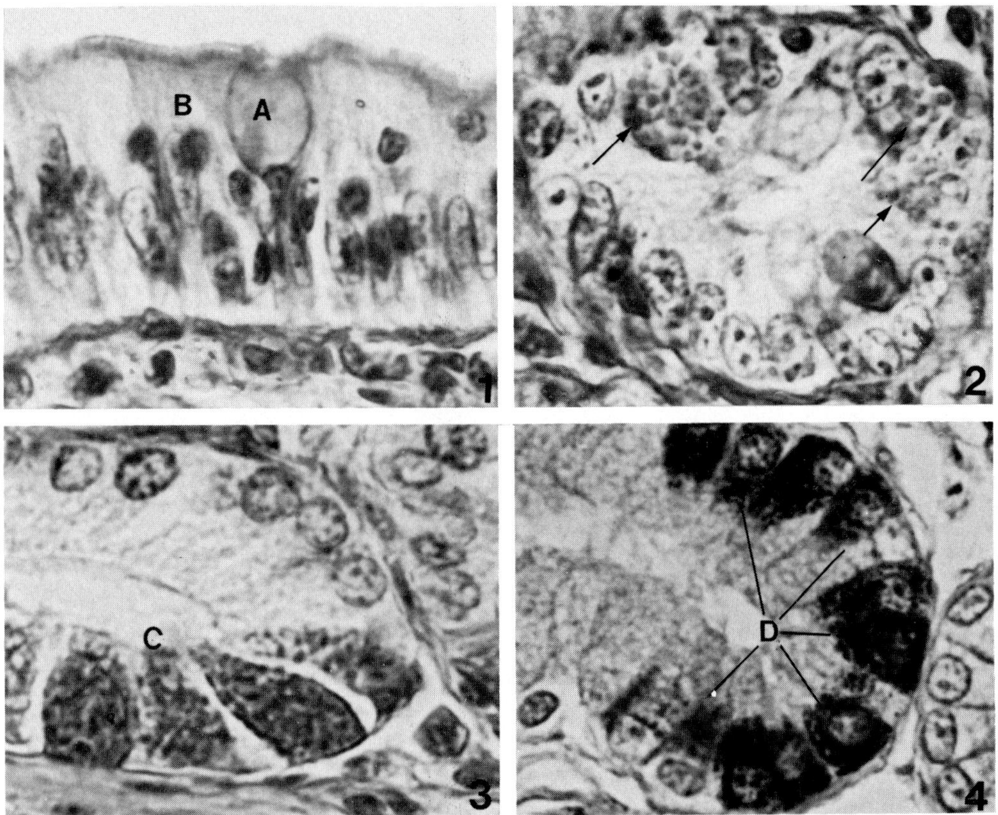

Fig. 10–65. *Intestinal mucosal cells. 1. Goblet cells (A); Simple columnar epithelium with microvilli (B), cat. Trichrome. ×1100. 2. Globular leukocytes (arrows), cat. Trichrome. ×1100. 3. Paneth cells (C), horse. Trichrome. ×1100. 4. Endocrine cells (D), dog. Fontana-Masson silver stain. ×1100.*

rise to the absorptive columnar cells and the goblet cells. They are pushed toward the tip of the villus by succeeding cells, where they slough off into the lumen. Because of this continuous cell renewal, many mitotic figures occur among the cells lining the glands. The mitotic activity is constant and bears no relation to the amount of ingesta or enzyme activity. It has been estimated that the epithelium is renewed every two to three days.

Near the base of the intestinal crypts, granular cells of Paneth are present in ruminants, the horse, and man (Fig. 10–65-3). They are pyramid-shaped cells with prominent spherical, acidophilic granules located between the nucleus and the cell apex. They have all the characteristics of enzyme-producing cells, and there is substantial evidence that they produce peptidase and lysozyme, an antibacterial compound. These cells also contain zinc, which has been reported to be important in the activation of peptidase. Endocrine cells, characteristic of both intestine and stomach, were discussed with cells of the fundic glands (Fig. 10–65-4).

LAMINA PROPRIA. The lamina propria is the loose connective tissue that forms the core of the villi and surrounds the intestinal glands. It is composed of collagen and elastic fibers enmeshed in a reticular fiber framework. Within this extensive fiber network are blood and lymph vessels, leukocytes, fibrocytes, smooth muscle cells, plasma cells, and mast cells. Globular leukocytes are found in the intestinal mucosa of most domestic species. They contain large eosinophilic globular material surrounding a small nucleus (Fig. 10–65-2). Their function is unknown. Diffuse lymphatic tissue or solitary lymphatic nodules are scattered throughout the small intestine. The number of nodules increases toward the distal portion. Between the base of the intestinal glands and the lamina muscularis of carnivores, there may be a subglandular layer similar to that found in the stomach.

A single lymphatic capillary, the *lacteal,* is located in the center of the lamina propria of the villus (Fig. 10–61). This vessel has a blind terminal end at the tip of the villus and is the origin of the lymph vessels that form a plexus at the base of the villi. This basal plexus gives rise to a larger one surrounding the intestinal glands and the lymphatic nodules. Longitudinally oriented smooth muscle fibers that originate from the lamina muscularis extend to the tip of the villus (Fig. 10–61). Contraction of these muscle cells causes the villus to shorten and undoubtedly is responsible for lateral movements as well. Usually, this smooth muscle aids in pumping the lymph out of the lacteal into the plexus below. A single arteriole from the submucosa penetrates the lamina muscularis and courses into the villus, where it forms an arteriovenous loop and a capillary network immediately beneath the surface epithelium. As a result of digestive activity, the vascular network becomes engorged with blood, causing the villus to lengthen. During muscular contraction, the blood is pumped out as the villus shortens. Thus, the villi act as pumping stations for moving food-laden blood and lymph into the general circulation.

LAMINA MUSCULARIS. The lamina muscularis is composed of inner circular and outer longitudinal layers of smooth muscle. With the exception of those of the dog, they tend to be thin and incomplete. The lamina muscularis of the dog is much thicker, the inner circular layer alone averaging 27 μm in thickness and the outer longitudinal layer 44 μm. However, the lamina muscularis may vary with the species, the individual animal, and the region (Fig. 10–66).

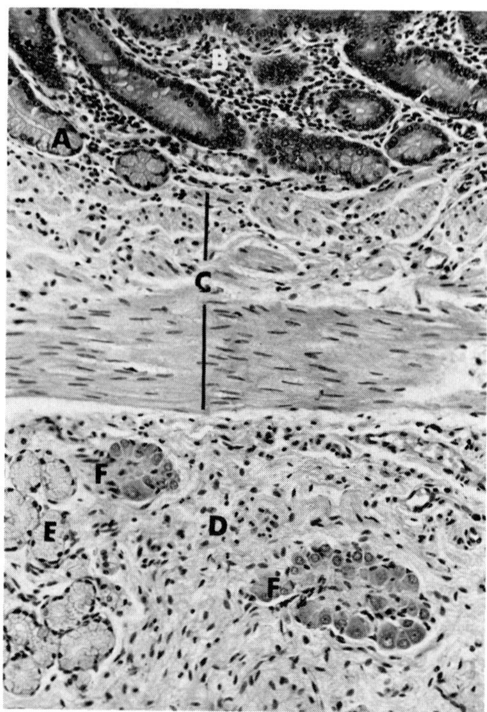

Fig. 10–66. *Duodenum, horse. Intestinal glands (A); lamina propria (B); lamina muscularis (C); submucosa (D); submucosal glands (E); submucosal plexuses (F), H & E. ×95.*

TELA SUBMUCOSA

The tela submucosa is a connective tissue layer of collagen and elastic fiber bundles located between the lamina muscularis and the tunica muscularis. The tubuloalveolar submucosal glands, located within this connective tissue network, open into the base of the intestinal mucosal glands. They are mucous in the dog and ruminants, serous in the pig and horse, and seromucous in the cat (Figs. 10–63 and 10–64). The lumina of the glands are largest in the goat and smallest in the pig. The serous (proteinaceous) or mucous secretory product

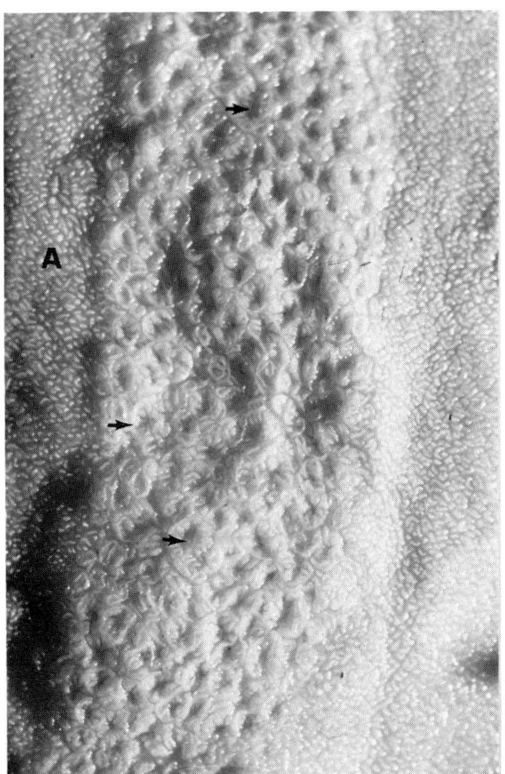

Fig. 10–67. *Mucosa of small intestine with aggregated lymphatic nodules, pig. Villi (A); surface depressions over lymphatic nodules (arrows). H & E. ×6. (From Titkemeyer, C.W., and Calhoun, M.L.: A comparative study of the structure of the small intestine of domestic animals. Am J Vet Res 16:152, 1955.)*

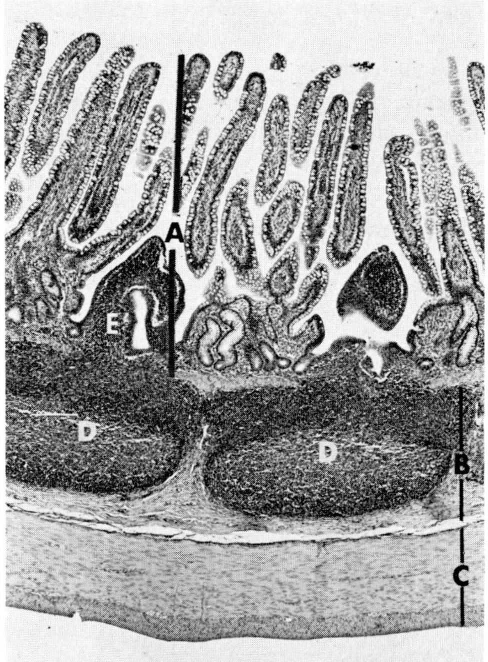

Fig. 10–68. *Ileum, cat. Tunica mucosa (A); submucosa (B); muscularis (C); aggregated lymphatic nodules (D). Notice the lymphatic tissue in the mucosa (E). H & E. ×48.*

from these glands lubricates the surface epithelium and provides protection from the acid gastric chyme. The glands are present in all domestic animals, but their distribution varies with the different species. For example, they are confined to the cranial portion of the duodenum in the dog, whereas in the horse they extend well beyond the gross anatomic limits of the duodenum. It is for this reason that in veterinary histology the term "submucosal glands" is far more descriptive than "duodenal glands," a term common in human histology.

Solitary lymphatic nodules are present in the submucosa throughout the small intestine. Large masses of aggregated lymphatic nodules occur in all three segments of the small intestine, but they are usually considered to be more characteristic of the ileum (Figs. 10–67 and 10–68). With the exception of the cat, they are visible grossly and are usually located in the submucosa on the side opposite the mesenteric attachment. However, they are discernible from the serosal surface of the dog intestine and tend to be located on either side of the mesentery. The nodules are largest in cattle and most numerous in the horse. The intestinal glands may extend into the submucosa in areas of the small intestine where the lamina muscularis is disrupted by the aggregated lymphatic nodules. (See Chapter 8 for details on this gut-associated lymphatic tissue.)

The submucosal nerve plexuses are scattered throughout the submucosa (Fig. 10–66). The nerve fibers from these plexuses extend into the villi.

TUNICA MUSCULARIS

In all species, the *tunica muscularis* consists of inner circular and outer longitudinal smooth muscle layers. The tunica muscularis is thickest in the horse, in which the two layers are nearly equal in thickness. The connective tissue between the two muscle layers contains the myenteric plexus.

TUNICA SEROSA

The tunica serosa of the small intestine, similar to that of the stomach, is a loose connective tissue continuous with that of the mesentery. Both are invested by the mesothelium of the peritoneum.

Blood Supply

Branches of the mesenteric artery penetrate the tunica muscularis, give off branches to supply this layer, and continue into the submucosa, where they form a plexus. Short arterioles supply the lamina muscularis and mucosal gland area, whereas long arterioles extend to the tip of the villi before forming a capillary network within the villus. At the tip of the villus, the arteriole is continuous with the venule, forming an arteriovenular loop. Veins from the villi and the periglandular capillary bed combine to form a submucosal venous plexus. This plexus gives rise to veins that traverse the tunica muscularis parallel to the arterial supply. The circulation in the small intestine of the horse, carnivores, and the pig differs from the above-described pattern in that these animals lack arteriovenous loops but have arteriovenous (A-V) anastomoses in the submucosa preceding the villous circulation. These occlusive structures shunt the blood to the villi during digestion. When the digestive process is inactive, these A-V anastomoses are open and there is a partial bypass of the villus circulation.

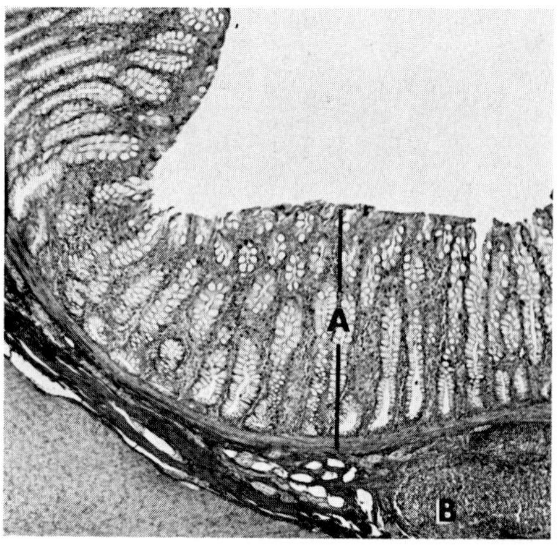

Fig. 10–69. *Cecum, cat. Mucosa (A); lymphatic tissue in submucosa (B). Trichrome. ×45.*

General Identifying Features

The various regions of the small intestine in the domestic animals are not clearly defined microscopically, as they are in man. For example, the submucosal glands do not extend the full length of the gross anatomical limits of the duodenum in most animals; however, in the horse these glands are often seen as far as the rostral part of the jejunum. Likewise, the mucosal aggregated lymphatic nodules, often considered an identifying feature of the ileum, may be seen anywhere along the small intestine of our domestic animals.

Because the length of the villi varies with physiologic activities and with species, it is not a reliable characteristic for the identification of the various segments.

The *ileocecal junction* is marked by lymph nodules in the pig and ruminants. In the cat and horse, the lymph nodules are near the blind end of the cecum. All domestic animals except the horse have a single sphincter at the ileocecocolic junction. The horse has both ileocecal and cecocolic sphincters.

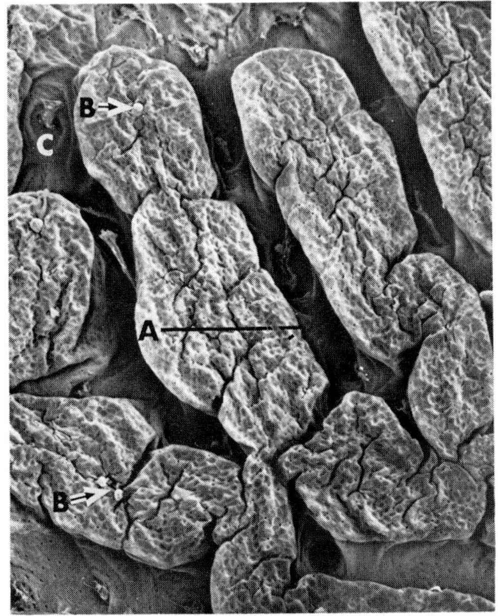

Fig. 10–70. *Scanning electron micrograph of colon, calf. Surface view of longitudinal folds of the mucosa (A); droplets of mucus (B); opening of crypt (C). ×200. (Courtesy of C.A. Mebus and L.E. Newman.)*

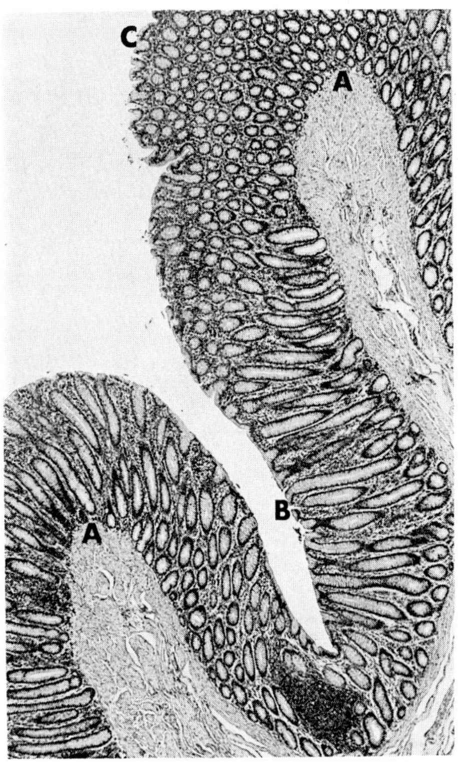

Fig. 10–71. *Colon, cow. Longitudinal folds of the mucosa (A), with intestinal glands cut longitudinally (B) and cross sectionally (C). H & E. ×27.*

LARGE INTESTINE

The large intestine is composed of the *cecum, colon, rectum,* and *anus.* It is a site for microbial action on the ingesta, absorption of water, vitamins, and electrolytes, and secretion of mucus. There are many gross and functional variations in the large intestine related to the necessity of breaking down the large masses of cellulose-containing materials consumed by the herbivores and ruminants. However, it is difficult to distinguish the various portions in histologic sections. Characteristics common to all segments of the large intestine are the absence of villi, the longer, straighter, more compact intestinal glands with large numbers of goblet cells (Fig. 10–69), the absence of Paneth cells, and the increase in the number of lymphatic nodules. Plicae circulares are absent in the large intestine, but longitudinal folds are present (Figs. 10–70 and 10–71). Animals fattened for slaughter tend to accumulate adipose tissue in the submucosa (Fig. 10–72).

Cecum

The cecum varies in size among the different species. In herbivores with simple stomachs, e.g., the horse, the relatively large cecum is an important bacterial fermentation reservoir, but in carnivores it is small. In all domestic animals, the cecum has a substantial number of lymphatic nodules scattered throughout its length (Fig. 10–69). In the dog, pig, and ruminants, lymphatic nodules are located around the ileocecal opening, and in the horse and cat they are concentrated to some extent near the blind end of the cecal sac. With the exception of the absence of villi in the cecum, the remaining structures are similar to those in the small intestine.

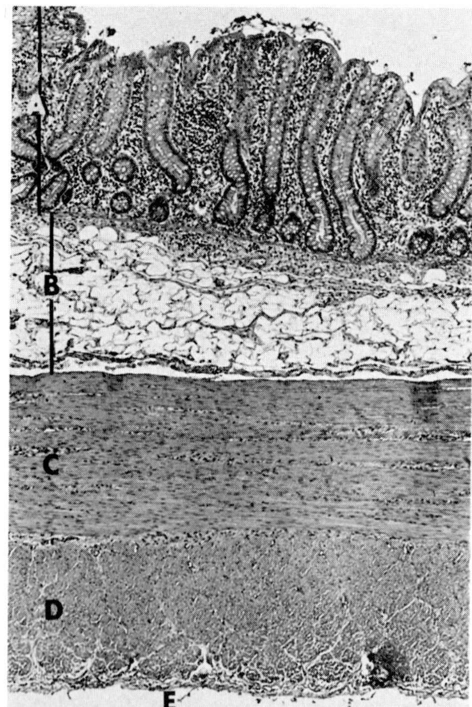

Fig. 10–72. *Cecum, pig. Mucosa (A); submucosa filled with adipose tissue (B); inner circular (C) and outer longitudinal (D) layers of the tunica muscularis; serosa (E). H & E. ×48.*

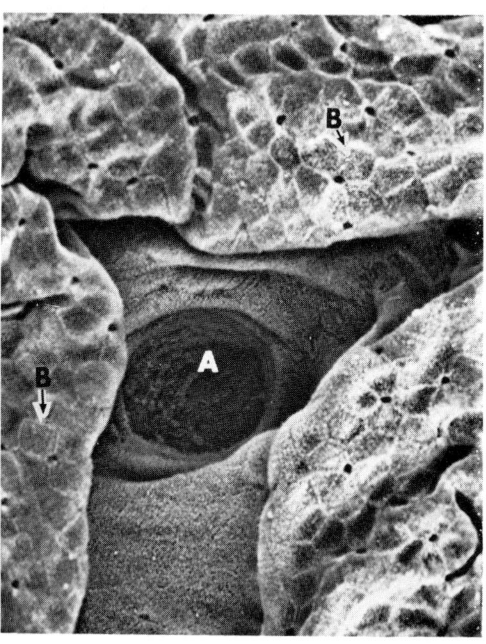

Fig. 10–73. *Scanning electron micrograph of colon, two-day-old calf. Surface view of an intestinal gland opening (A); individual epithelial cells with microvilli (stippling) (B); ×1000. (Courtesy of C.A. Mebus and L.E. Newman.)*

Colon

The tunica mucosa of the colon is substantially thicker, owing to the increased length of the intestinal glands, as compared to that of the small intestine. Because there are no villi, the mucosal surface is smooth (Figs. 10–73 and 10–74). There is an increase in the number of goblet cells. The submucosa often becomes distended by the lymphatic tissue and the lamina muscularis is interrupted. In such instances, intestinal glands may extend into the submucosa. Histochemical and ultrastructural studies indicate that these glands originate from the mucosa and are not true submucosal glands.

In the pig and horse, the outer longitudinal layer of the tunica muscularis of the cecum and colon forms large, flat muscle bands containing numerous elastic fibers, the *taenia coli* (Fig. 10–75), and *taenia ceci.* Those of the cecum and ventral large colon of the horse have more elastic fibers than smooth muscle cells.

Rectum

Like that of the colon and cecum, the mucosa of the rectum is smooth, and except for the increased number of goblet cells, the basic structures are similar as well. In the horse and cow, the rectal wall is thicker than the wall of the colon. In carnivores, there is a thickening of the outer longitudinal muscular layer. Elastic tissue is most prominent in the rectum of the horse and cow and least prominent in the sheep and goat. The outer muscle layer contains more elastic tissue than the inner layer. The retroperitoneal portion of the rectum lacks a serosa.

Near its junction with the anus, the rectal mucosa in ruminants is thrown into longitudinal folds, the *rectal columns* (columnae rectales). All domestic animals have a

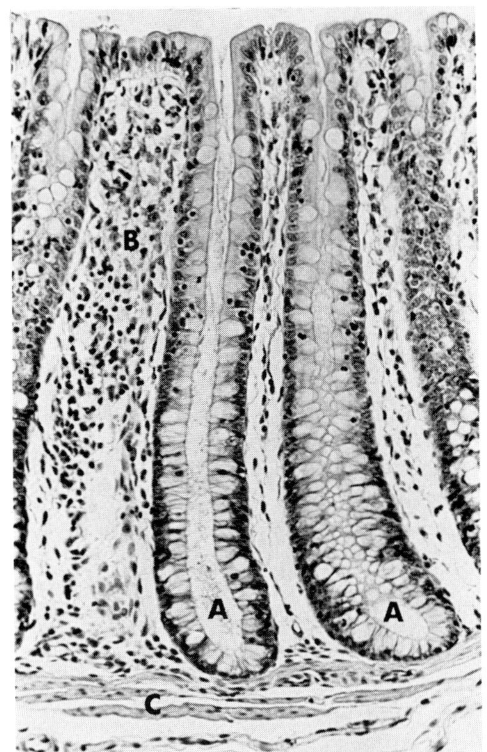

Fig. 10–74. *Colon, pig. Mucous membrane with intestinal glands and goblet cells (A); lamina propria (B); lamina muscularis (C). H & E. ×200.*

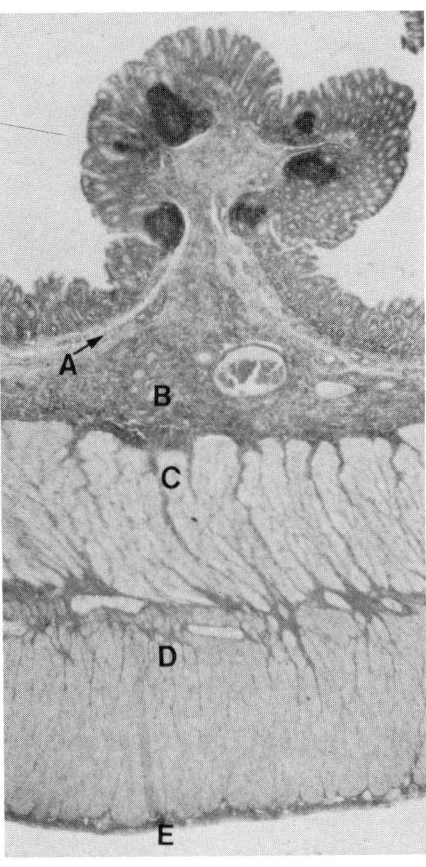

Fig. 10–75. *Descending colon, horse. Lamina muscularis (A); submucosa (B); tunica muscularis, circular layer (C); tunica muscularis, longitudinal layer, taenia (D); serosa (E). Notice the lymphatic nodules in the mucosa. H & E. ×22.*

rather large venous plexus in the lamina propria of this region of the rectum. In the dog, about 100 solitary lymphatic nodules are a prominent feature of the rectum. They are visible grossly because of pitlike depressions, *rectal pits,* in the mucosa overlying these lymphatic nodules.

Anus

The anus is the terminal segment of the digestive tract, and at the anorectal line the simple columnar epithelium of the rectum changes abruptly to stratified squamous nonkeratinized epithelium (Fig. 10–76). In ruminants, the short gland-free anal canal is continuous proximally with the rectal columns and ends distally at the anocutaneous line. In the horse, the anal mucosa is nonglandular, and at the anocutaneous line it joins the skin that covers the anal protuberance.

In the pig and carnivores, the anal canal has three distinct zones: (1) columnar zone (zona columnaris ani); (2) intermediate zone (zona intermedia); and (3) cutaneous zone (zona cutanea). The *columnar zone* contains longitudinal columns, or *anal columns,* between which are the *anal sinuses.* Modified tubuloalveolar sweat glands (anal glands) in the submucosa produce a lipid secretion in dogs (Fig. 10–76) and cats and a mucous secretion in pigs. They may extend into the columnar zone, which is less distinct in the cat than in the dog and pig. The *intermediate zone* is relatively narrow. The mucosa is lined with stratified squa-

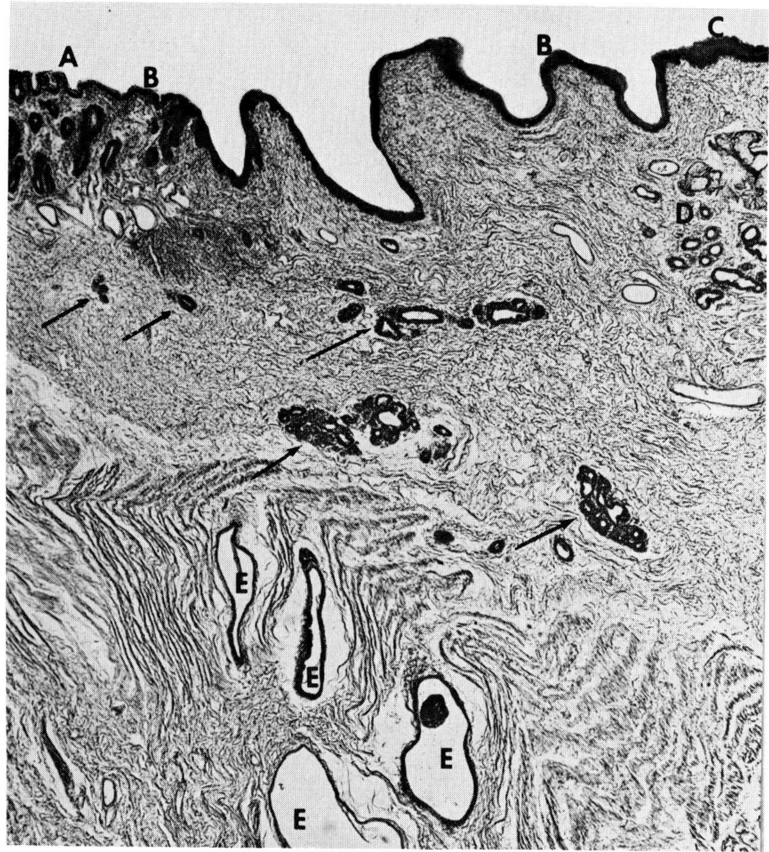

Fig. 10–76. *Rectum and anus, dog. Rectum (A); anus (B); skin with sweat and sebaceous glands (C); skin glands (D); deep veins (E); anal glands (arrows). H & E. ×66. (From Adam, W.S., Calhoun, M.L., Smith, E.M., and Stinson, A.W.: Microscopic Anatomy of the Dog: a Photographic Atlas. Springfield, Ill., Charles C Thomas, 1970.)*

mous epithelium, and anal glands occupy the submucosa. The *cutaneous zone* is lined by keratinized stratified squamous epithelium. In carnivores, the ducts from the *anal sacs* open at the junction of the intermediate and cutaneous zones. The anal sacs and ducts are bilateral evaginations of the anal mucosa. In the outermost part of the cutaneous zone, near the junction with the skin, the mucosa of the dog contains large modified sebaceous glands, the *circumanal glands*. The anal sacs, their associated glands, and the circumanal glands are discussed with the integument (Chapter 16).

The lamina muscularis and the outer longitudinal layer of the tunica muscularis terminate at the *anorectal junction*. The inner circular layer forms the internal anal sphincter and extends into the cutaneous zone, whereas the external anal sphincter, which is circularly disposed striated muscle, extends from the anorectal line to the perineal region.

LIVER

The liver is the largest gland in the body and is characterized by a multiplicity of complex functions: excretion (waste products), secretion (bile), storage (lipids, vitamins A and B, glycogen), synthesis (fibrinogen, globulins, albumin, prothrombin), phagocytosis (foreign particulate matter), detoxification (lipid-soluble drugs), conju-

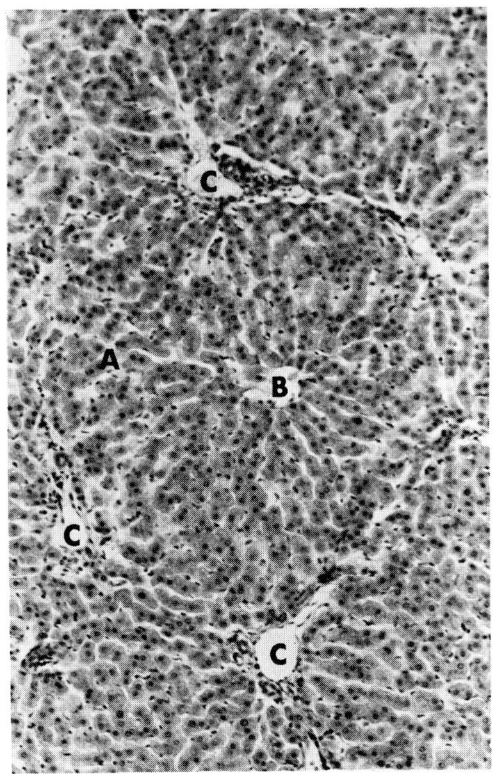

Fig. 10–77. *Liver, calf. Lobule (A) with central vein (B) is not separated from adjacent lobules by connective tissue as is that of the pig, in Figure 10–78. Interlobular portal veins (C) in portal areas. H & E. ×80.*

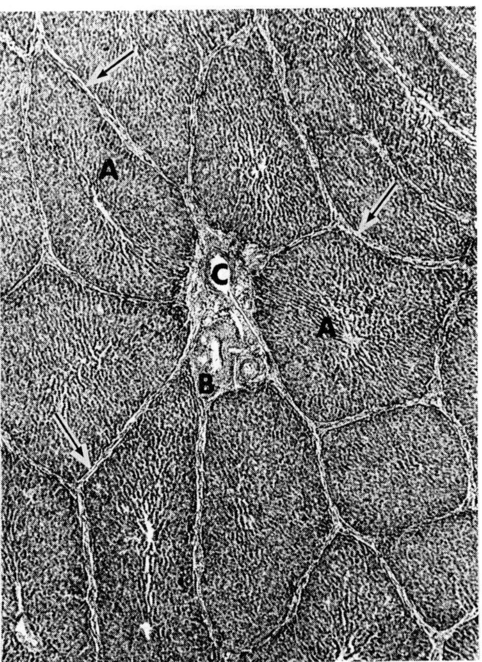

Fig. 10–78. *Liver, pig. Liver lobules (A); portal canal (B); branch of the portal vein (C); interlobular connective tissue (arrows). Trichrome. ×30. (From Stinson, A.W., and Brown, E.M.: Veterinary Histology Slide Sets. East Lansing, Mich., Michigan State University, Instructional Media Center, 1970.)*

gation (toxic substances, steroid hormones), esterification (free fatty acids to triglycerides), metabolism (protein, carbohydrates, fats, hemoglobin, drugs), and hemopoiesis (in the embryo and potentially in the adult). An understanding of the structure of the liver is vital to the interpretation of these processes.

Recall that the liver has a dual blood supply. The portal vein brings food-laden blood from the intestine and associated organs, and the hepatic artery supplies the liver cells with oxygenated blood. Branches of these two vessels follow the interlobular connective tissue of the portal areas; this extensive network of vessels ensures that the liver cells are never more than a few millimeters from a rich blood supply.

Capsule and Trabeculae

Each lobe of the liver is covered by visceral peritoneal mesothelial cells overlying a thin connective tissue capsule. Connective tissue from the capsule extends into the interlobular spaces and supports the vascular system and bile ducts. A fine network of reticular fibers surrounds the cells and sinusoids. The collagen content increases from 0.05% in immature animals to 0.7% in adults. Smooth muscle cells may be present in the capsule and interlobular tissue. Interlobular tissue and trabeculae are scant and difficult to see (Fig. 10–77), except in the pig, which has distinct fibrous connective tissue septa surrounding each liver lobule (Fig. 10–78). This accounts for the tougher nature of pork liver as a food, as opposed to beef liver.

The connective tissue supporting a lymph vessel and the branches of the he-

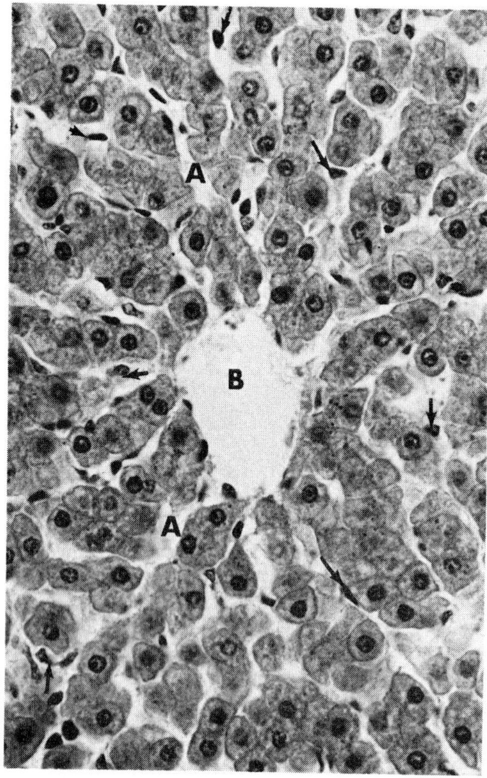

Fig. 10–79. *Liver, calf. Hepatic sinusoids (A); central vein (B); phagocytic cells (arrows). H & E. ×384.*

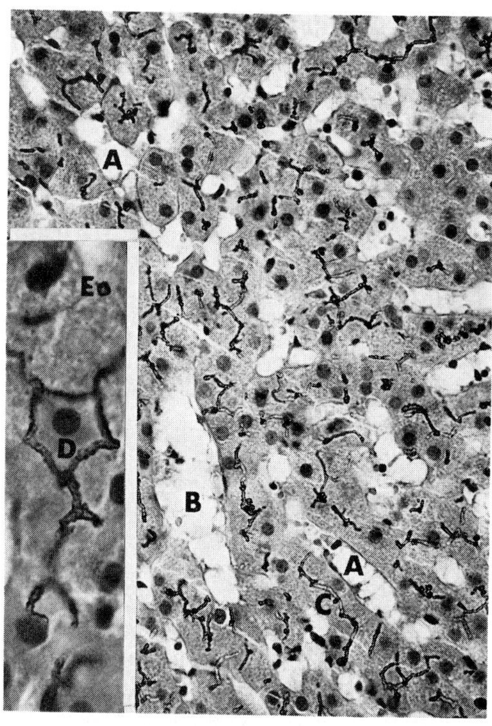

Fig. 10–80. *Liver, pig. Sinusoids (A), central vein (B), liver plates with bile canaliculi between the cells (C). Silver stain. ×300. Insert, bile canaliculi surrounding a liver cell (D) and a cross section of a bile canaliculus (E). Silver stain. ×768.*

patic artery and portal vein and the bile ductule appears throughout any section of liver. These groups of vessels and ducts, together with the supportive connective tissue, are called *portal canals* or *areas.* Blood from the portal canal reaches the central vein by way of the thin-walled sinusoids. Therefore, blood from branches of the hepatic artery and portal vein eventually mix within the sinusoids. Conversely, bile flow is opposite to that of the blood. All the parenchyma between the portal canal and the central vein consists of cells arranged in branching plates or laminae (Fig. 10–79). These laminae are one cell thick, with the free surface of the cells facing the sinusoids. Between adjacent cells, the bile canaliculi are formed by the apposing cell membranes of the hepatocytes. The canaliculi form an anastomosing network throughout the laminae (Fig. 10–80).

Liver Lobule Concepts

The lobular structure can be interpreted in three different ways, depending on which functional relationships are considered. The *hepatic lobule,* sometimes called the classic lobule, is a structural unit organized around the central vein (Figs. 10–77 and 10–78). Cross-sectional profiles of this lobule are roughly hexagon-shaped, with the sinusoids radiating from the periphery to the central vein into which they empty. *Portal canals* are present at approximately three of the six angles of the hepatic lobule. The hepatic lobule is especially well delineated in the pig because it is surrounded completely by connective tissue septa. In the other species, the septa are less conspicuous, and the parenchyma of one lobule appears to blend into adja-

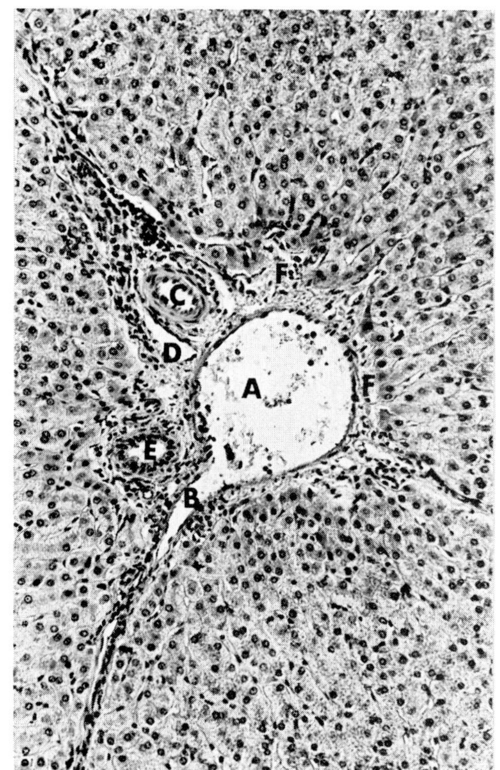

Fig. 10–81. *Liver, pig. Portal area composed of a branch of the portal vein (A); terminal branch (B); branch of the hepatic artery (C); lymph vessel (D); bile duct (E); interlobular connective tissue (F). H & E. ×154.*

cent lobules without a clear line of demarcation.

The *portal lobule* is a functional unit centered around the bile ductule in the portal area. It is defined as a triangular area consisting of the parenchyma of three adjacent hepatic lobules that are drained by the bile ductule in the portal canal. Thus the axis of the portal lobule is the interlobular bile ductule in the portal canal (Figs. 10–81 and 10–82), and the periphery is delineated by three central veins. This concept emphasizes the exocrine activities of the liver, since the bile flows from the periphery of the lobule toward the bile ductule of the portal canal, whereas blood flows from the center of the lobule to the periphery.

A third functional unit, the *liver acinus,* has received wide acceptance because it is based on the differences in the dynamics of blood flow, pressure, and oxygen tension and best explains a gradient in metabolic activity. The liver acinus is roughly a diamond-shaped area made up of parts of two hepatic lobules supplied by terminal branches of the interlobular portal vein and hepatic artery. The blood vessels course at right angles from a portal canal between two hepatic lobules to form the backbone of the acinus, and the two central veins are at the two opposing points of the diamond (Fig. 10–82). Because of the relationship of the vascular backbone to the central veins, there is a direct correlation between blood supply and metabolism. Thus, the liver acinus has three ill-defined zones. Zone 1 is the area nearest the vascular backbone; the hepatocytes are the first to receive blood and nutrients, are the last to die after exposure to noxious substances, and are the first to regenerate. Zone 3 is the region nearest the central vein; the liver cells are the most compromised, the most susceptible, and the first to die because they receive blood of inferior quality. Zone 2 is the area between the other two; hence, the cells receive blood of moderate quality.

Parenchyma

The polyhedron-shaped *liver cells* or hepatocytes have a centrally located spherical nucleus with one or more prominent nucleoli and scattered clumps of chromatin. Occasionally are seen binucleated cells that result from the incomplete division of the cytoplasm following normal mitotic nuclear division. The cytoplasm of hepatocytes is usually somewhat granular but may vary depending on nutritional and functional cellular changes. Mitochondria are abundant and the Golgi complex is usually near the bile canaliculus but may be juxtanuclear. There are numerous lysosomes, clusters of free ribosomes, and well-developed rER and sER, which are often contiguous with each other. At the fine-structural level, glycogen is seen as dense

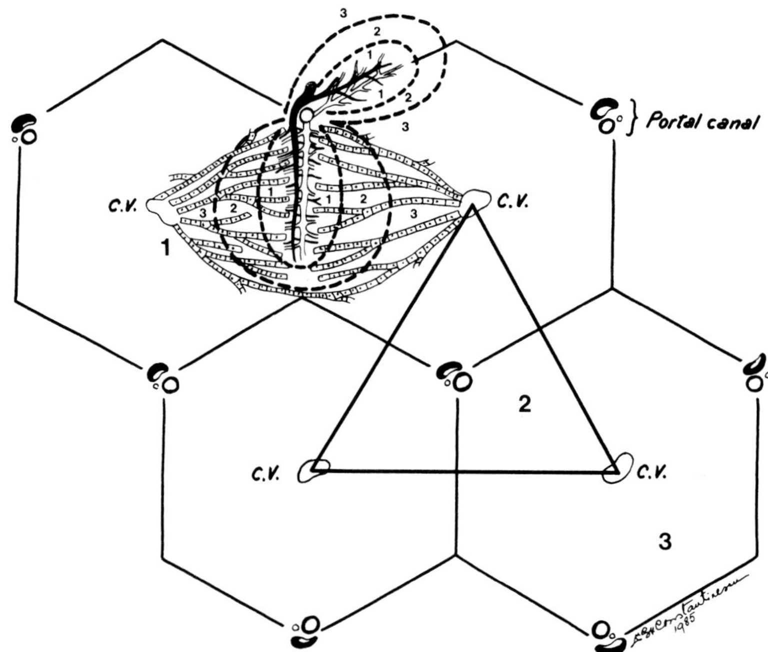

Fig. 10–82. *Schematic drawing of the various hepatic functional units. 1. Liver acinus with 3 zones on each side of the vascular backbone. 2. Portal lobule with a portal area as the axis and one central vein at each point of the triangle. 3. Hepatic lobule with the central vein as its axis. (Modified and redrawn from Rappaport, A.M., Borowy, Z.J., Laugheed, W.M., and Lotto, W.N. Anat Rec 119:11, 1954. Fig. 1.)*

granules in a rosette configuration. In ordinary histologic preparation glycogen-rich areas appear grainy or as irregularly shaped empty spaces, whereas sites occupied by fat appear as empty round vacuoles. It is not unusual to see bile pigments in normal hepatocytes.

There is considerable evidence that all hepatocytes may not be functionally identical, but rather certain enzyme patterns and metabolic systems may be related to the position of the cell within the lobule or acinus. While it is generally accepted that liver cell metabolic activity is closely associated with blood supply, the extent to which hepatocytes are similar or dissimilar with respect to metabolic systems, susceptibility to insults, and nutritional needs remains to be resolved.

The liver cell has six or more surfaces that are of three different types: 1) those surfaces that face the perisinusoidal space where the free surface has well-developed microvilli; 2) those surfaces that border the bile canaliculi; and 3) the contact surfaces between adjacent hepatocytes where apposed cell membranes may have gap junctions and desmosomes.

Bile Canaliculi and Bile Ducts

The minute canals (0.5 to 1.0 μm in diameter) between apposing hepatocytes are the bile canaliculi (Fig. 10–80). They are simply areas where the membranes of adjacent cells diverge, forming expanded intercellular spaces. The cell membranes bordering these spaces have short microvilli, and the upper and lower margins have tight junctions (zonulae occludentes) that prevent bile from filling the narrow intercellular space adjacent to the canaliculus.

Hepatocytes absorb bilirubin (bile pigment) from the blood, conjugate it, and secrete it as one component of bile. The bile salts, protein, and cholesterol are the other components. Bile is secreted into the bile canaliculi and reaches the portal areas by way of the ductule. The ductules join larger intrahepatic ducts and finally leave the liver through the main hepatic ducts. The extrahepatic bile passages are composed of the hepatic ducts, cystic duct, the common bile duct, and the gallbladder.

Bile ductules are lined with cuboidal epithelium, and as the ducts enlarge, the epithelium gradually increases in height and finally becomes columnar in the larger hepatic ducts. The lining epithelial cells have an abundance of mitochondria and a well-developed Golgi complex.

Blood Vessels and Sinusoids

The vascularity of the liver is directly related to its multitudinous functions. On entering the liver, the portal vein and hepatic artery immediately send branches to the lobes, the *interlobar vessels,* which in turn branch to form the *interlobular vessels* that are found in the portal areas.

The interlobular portal veins have small branches, sometimes referred to as distributing veins, which form the axis of the liver acinus. Short venules arise from the distributing veins and end directly in the sinusoids.

Most of the blood from the interlobular hepatic artery enters a capillary plexus within the portal areas that is drained by small branches of the portal vein. Only a small portion of the blood reaches the sinusoids directly by way of arteriolar branches of the interlobular artery.

Sinusoids are blood capillaries that course through the lobule carrying blood from the interlobular hepatic artery and portal vein to the central vein. They often communicate with each other via interruptions in the hepatic laminae. This ramifying arrangement ensures that hepatocytes have at least one surface adjacent to the sinusoids separated only by the perisinusoidal space. Sinusoids are lined by a discontinuous and porous endothelium and large stellate, active macrophages (Kupffer cells) of monocytic origin (Fig. 10–83). They occur at various places along the sinusoids, often sending long pseudopodia through the endothelial pores or between the endothelial cells.

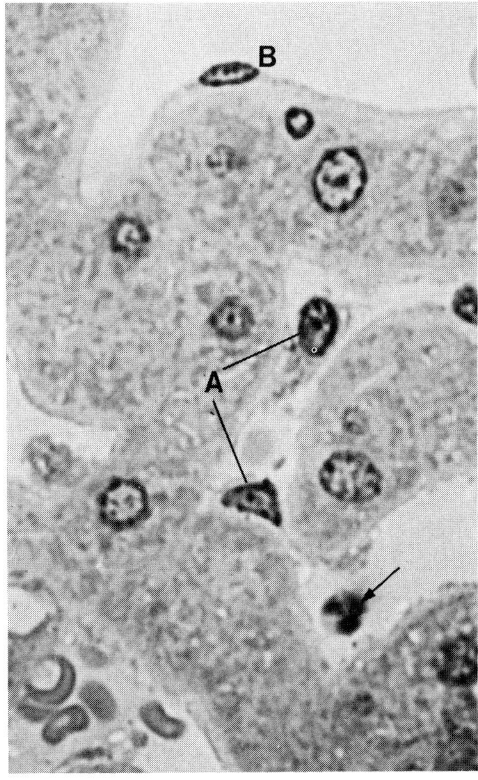

Fig. 10–83. *Liver laminae and sinusoids, cat. Two sinusoidal phagocytes (A) with abundant cytoplasm and one endothelial cell (B) comprise the sinusoidal living cells. Notice the erythrocytes (lower left) and one neutrophil (arrow). Epon. Toluidine blue.* ×*1600.*

The sinusoidal endothelium lacks a basal lamina and rests directly on the tips of the hepatocyte microvilli. Thus a perisinusoidal space exists between liver cells and the endothelium within which the microvilli are bathed in blood plasma, allowing a direct exchange of substances between blood and liver cells. However, in cattle the endothelium is continuous, and a distinct basal lamina is present in all ruminants.

In addition to the hepatocyte microvilli, the perisinusoidal space contains reticular fibers as well as *perisinusoidal stellate* cells, or *adipocytes.* These cells store vitamin A and are involved in fibrinogenesis by synthesizing type III collagen following liver injury.

Blood leaves the lobule by way of the *central veins* or *terminal hepatic venules.* They are lined by endothelium resting on a thin adventitia and communicate directly with the sinusoids. The central veins connect with the *sublobular veins* or intercalated veins at the periphery of the hepatic lobules. These two veins course along the base of the lobules where several join to form collecting veins that eventually join as the hepatic vein.

Lymph and Lymph Vessels

The origin and flow of lymph in the liver have been subjects of great controversy. Although lymph vessels are seen in the capsule and in portal areas, lymph capillaries have not been demonstrated among the parenchymal cells. At present, it is thought that liver lymph is formed in the perisinusoidal space, flows beside the interlobular blood vessels, and enters a space between the connective tissue of the portal area and the parenchyma. Here it diffuses through the connective tissue into the lymph vessels within the portal area. The lymph is carried from the portal areas by larger lymph vessels and ultimately leaves the liver with the efferent blood vessels.

GALLBLADDER

The gallbladder, a small sac attached to the liver of most domestic animals (though absent in the horse), is the storage site of bile produced by the liver. While bile is stored in the gallbladder, it is concentrated by the reabsorption of water and inorganic salts. There is some evidence that the epithelium also has a secretory function. In the contracted (empty) state the gallbladder mucosa is thrown into numerous anastomosing folds. As it fills and expands, these folds have a tendency to flatten, giving a smoother surface to the mucosa. The epithelium is a single layer of columnar

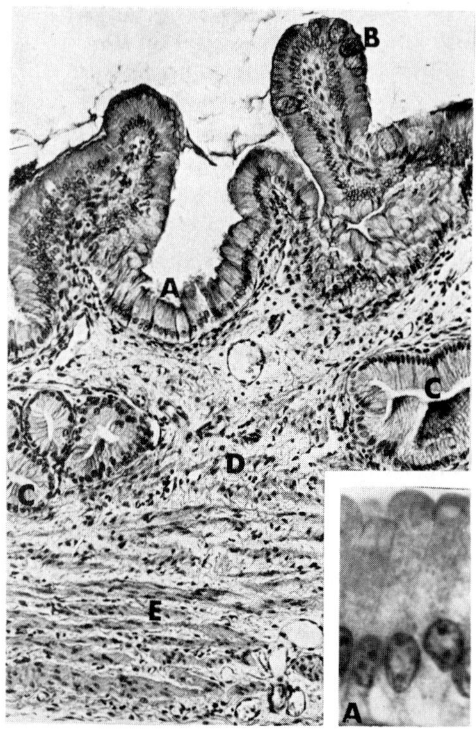

Fig. 10–84. *Gallbladder, dog. Simple columnar epithelium (A); goblet cells (B); cross sections of mucosal crypts (C); lamina propria (D); tunica muscularis (E). H & E. ×120. Insert, simple columnar epithelial lining. H & E. ×768.*

cells that covers the surface as well as the *mucosal crypts,* which are small epithelial diverticuli that sometimes give the impression of being glands (Fig. 10–84). Two types of columnar cells are located in the epithelium. The most numerous type is the "light" cell, which has a pale cytoplasm of uniform density. The cytoplasm of the apical region contains vesicles but is devoid of organelles. Electron-dense bodies with smooth outlines occur in the subapical and supranuclear cytoplasm. The less numerous "dark" cells are seen among the light cells. They have a narrow profile and contain a dark, dense cytoplasm with few organelles and a nucleus that is more heterochromatic than that of the light cells. The epithelial cell surface is covered with microvilli, and tight junctions between adjacent cells prevent the intercellular passage

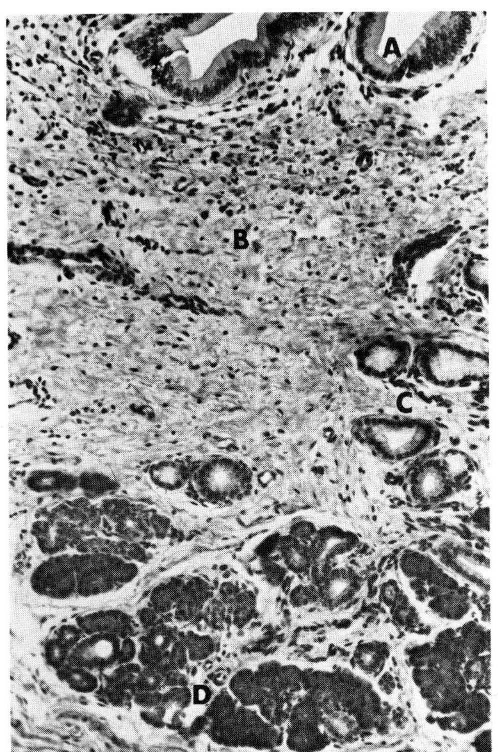

Fig. 10–85. *Gallbladder, cow. Simple columnar epithelium (A); lamina propria (B); mucous glands (C); serous glands (D). H & E. ×120.*

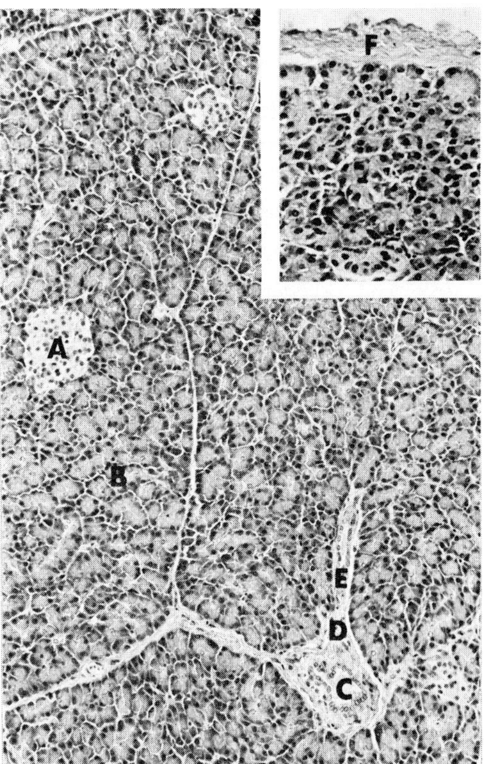

Fig. 10–86. *Pancreas, pig. Pancreatic islet (A); pancreatic acini (B); interlobular duct (C) in interstitial tissue (D); intralobular duct (E). H & E. ×120. Insert, capsule of sheep pancreas (F). H & E. ×192.*

of fluids from the lumen of the organ. Goblet cells are characteristic of the epithelium of some species, such as cattle, and globular leukocytes may be found in the epithelium of cats. Endocrine cells, possibly of the APUD system, have been described in the epithelium of the gallbladder of cattle.

The lamina propria is composed of loose connective tissue. Because there is no lamina muscularis, the lamina propria blends with the submucosa without a clear line of junction. Lymphatic tissue, either diffuse or nodular, may be present in the connective tissue. In some species, particularly the ruminants, glands are present in the mucosa. They may be serous or mucous depending on the species, individual, or location in the mucosa (Fig. 10–85). The smooth muscle fibers of the tunica muscularis generally course in a circular direction. The muscles are supplied by both sympathetic and parasympathetic nerves.

The hepatic and common bile ducts are similar in structure to that of the gallbladder. Both circular and longitudinal muscle layers are present. The muscle is thickest in the bovine species and thinnest in carnivores. In the other domestic animals, the muscle layer is discontinuous.

In the horse, the hepatic duct, which carries unconcentrated bile, and the major pancreatic duct open into the diverticulum duodeni. No sphincter is present, thus permitting a continuous flow of bile into the intestine.

The bile duct of the pig opens onto a duodenal papilla. In the dog, the bile duct has a 2.5- to 3-cm intramural section in the duodenal wall before opening with a minor pancreatic duct at the major duodenal pa-

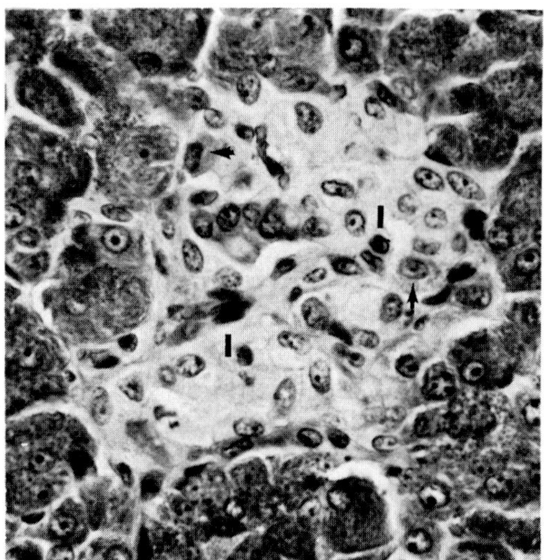

Fig. 10–87. *Pancreatic islet surrounded by pancreatic acini, dog. A cells (arrows); B cells (I). Trichrome. ×450.*

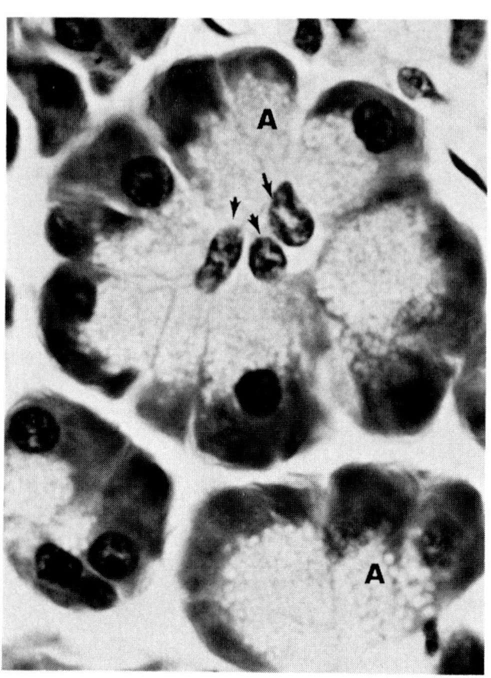

Fig. 10–89. *Pancreatic acinus with three centroacinar cells at arrows. Zymogen granules (A). H & E. ×1200.*

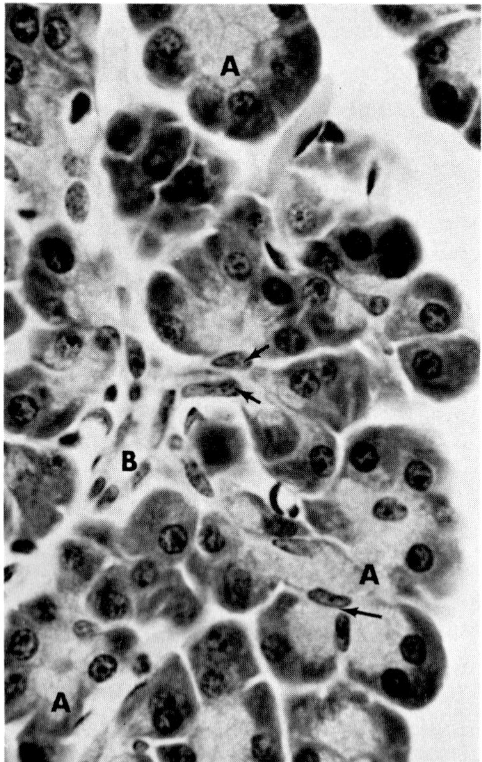

Fig. 10–88. *Pancreas, dog. Pancreatic acini (A); intercalated duct (B); centroacinar cells (arrows). H & E. ×768.*

pilla. In the cat, the bile duct opens into the duodenum similarly but is accompanied by the major pancreatic duct.

PANCREAS

The pancreas is an encapsulated, lobulated, compound tubuloacinar gland containing both exocrine and endocrine secretory units (Fig. 10–86). The function of the exocrine portion is to produce a variety of enzymes, including amylase, lipase, and trypsin, which act on the products of gastric digestion as they reach the duodenum. The endocrine portion (pancreatic islets [Fig. 10–87] produces mainly insulin and glucagon. The histologic structure of the islets is discussed in Chapter 15.

The stroma of the pancreas consists of a thin capsule that gives rise to delicate connective tissue septa separating the parenchyma into distinct lobules. The lobule is composed of secretory units and intralobular ducts. The secretory units are tubu-

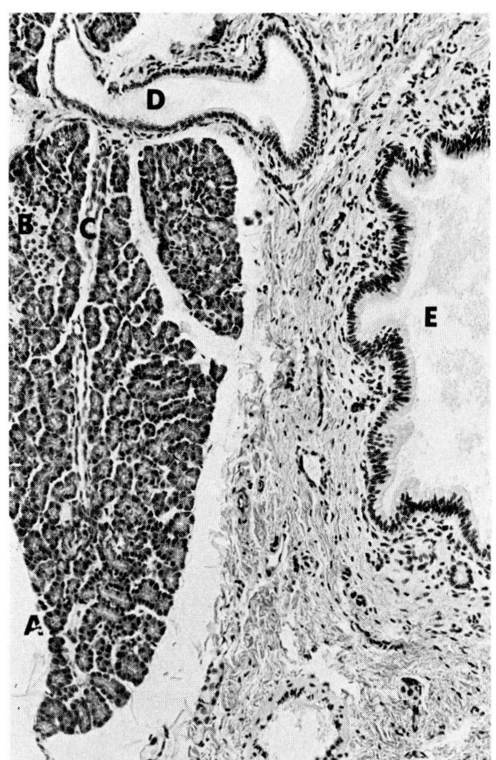

Fig. 10–90. *Pancreas, goat, Pancreatic lobule (A); pancreatic islet (B); intralobular duct (C); interlobular duct (D); main pancreatic duct (E). H & E. ×145.*

loacinar, with the tubular portion more prominent in ruminants. The secretory epithelial cells are generally pyramid-shaped, with a spherical nucleus near the base of the cells (Figs. 10–88 and 10–89). The basal portion of the cells rests on a basement membrane, and there are no myoepithelial or basket cells surrounding the secretory units. The cytoplasm surrounding the nuclear region contains a well-developed ER and numerous mitochondria. The apical region of the cells contains eosinophilic membrane-bounded zymogen granules, which are filled with the enzymes produced in the endoplasmic reticulum. Special staining reveals a well-developed Golgi complex between the nucleus and the zymogen granules. The tubuloacinar secretory unit has a small lumen, and the duct system begins as flattened centroacinar cells in the lumen (Fig. 10–89). These cells begin in the acinar portion and continue throughout the tubular part of the secretory unit. Intercalated ducts are continuous with the centroacinar cells. They join the secretory units to the intralobular ducts, which are lined by low cuboidal epithelium. The ductal epithelium changes from cuboidal in the intralobular ducts to columnar in the interlobular and collecting ducts (Fig. 10–90). Goblet cells may be present in the larger ducts. Frequently, pacinian corpuscles are present in the interlobular connective tissue of the pancreas of the cat.

The pancreas is very similar to the parotid salivary gland in histologic structure. However, it can be distinguished by the presence of pancreatic islets and centroacinar cells and by the absence of striated intralobular ducts.

REFERENCES

Adam, W.S., Calhoun, M.L., Smith, E.M., and Stinson, A.W.: Microscopic Anatomy of the Dog: A Photographic Atlas. Springfield, Ill., Charles C Thomas, 1970, pp. 102–157.

Boshell, J.L., and Wilborn, W.H.: Histology and ultrastructure of the pig parotid gland. Am J Anat *152*:447, 1978.

Chu, R.M., Glock, R.D., and Ross, R.F.: Gut-associated lymphoid tissue of young swine with emphasis on some epithelium of aggreated lymph nodules (Peyer's Patches) of the small intestine. Am J Vet Res *40*:1720, 1979.

Elias, H., and Sherrick, J.C.: Morphology of the Liver. New York, Academic Press, 1969.

Gemmell, R.T., and Heath, T.: Fine structure of sinusoids and portal capillaries in the liver of adult sheep and the newborn lamb. Anat Rec *172*:57, 1972.

Lindberg, L.-A., and Gröhn, Y.: Sinusoidal fat-storing cells in bovine liver. Anat Histol Embryol *11*:374, 1982.

Rappaport, A.M., Borowy, Z.J., Loughheed, W.M., and Looto, W.N.: Subdivision of hexagonal liver lobules into a structural and functional unit. Role in hepatic physiology and pathology. Anat Rec *119*:11, 1954.

Wünsche, A.: Anatomy of the liver lobule of pig. Anat Histol Embryol *10*:342, 1981.

11

Urinary System

ESTHER M. BROWN

The urinary system includes the paired kidneys and ureters, and the urinary bladder and urethra. The kidneys have a major role in fluid and electrolyte balance and in the control of blood pressure. Waste products are eliminated from the kidneys as urine, which is carried by the ureters to the urinary bladder, where it is stored until evacuated through the urethra.

KIDNEY

The numerous functions performed by the kidneys require an intricate array of tubules closely associated with blood vessels. Knowledge of the definitive anatomic relationships among the secretory tubules, excretory ducts, and capillaries helps to clarify kidney structure and function.

The *uriniferous tubule* of the adult kidney is composed of two portions, the collecting tubule and the nephron, each of which has separate embryologic primordia. The collecting tubule or duct develops from that portion of the embryonic *mesonephric duct* that forms the ureteric bud. The proximal part of this bud develops into the ureter; the distal portion dilates into the renal pelvis, forming the calyces, papillary ducts, and collecting ducts. Concurrently, *metanephrogenic* cells form a cap over the developing collecting ducts so that the future nephrons develop along with each order of developing collecting ducts.

While the collecting tubules and nephrons are developing, the blood supply to the metanephron begins to evolve. Branches from the renal artery form capillary tufts at the blind end of each future nephron and establish the final intimate association of the capillaries with the nephron.

Macroscopic Structure

A kidney cut in a longitudinal plane has two distinct zones. The peripheral dark area is the *cortex* and the remaining, lighter portion is the *medulla,* shaped like an inverted pyramid. The broadest aspect or base fits against the innermost border of the cortex, and the apex or *papilla* faces the pelvis. Each medullary pyramid and the cortical tissue that forms a cap over the base and covers the sides constitute a *lobe,* the gross anatomic unit of the kidney. The cortical and medullary portions of the kidney lobes in the domestic animals are fused to varying degrees. In kidneys of large ruminants, the fusion of the cortex is incomplete and the outside surface has fissures outlining the lobes. The kidney of the pig has a fused cortex with separate medullary papillae. These two animals have *multilobar* or *multipyramidal* kidneys (Fig. 11–1). Carnivores, small ruminants, and the horse all have *unilobar* or *unipyramidal* kidneys, owing to the nearly complete fusion of the lobes so that the apices of the pyramids form a ridgelike common papilla, the *renal crest,* where the papillary ducts drain into the renal pelvis. In the horse, the papillary ducts open into a long (6- to 10-cm) cavity called the *terminal recess* that courses from the pelvis to each pole of the kidney. The terminal recess is lined with transitional epithelium.

The papilla of unipyramidal kidneys projects into the expanded end of the ureter, the *renal pelvis,* situated on the medial border in an indentation called the *hilus.* In multipyramidal kidneys, major and minor calyces are formed as a result of the repeated branching of the ureteric bud during its development. The minor calyces fit against the apex of each papilla, and the major calyces join the renal pelvis. In the kidneys of large ruminants, the major calyces make a direct junction with the ureter, and there is no renal pelvis (Fig. 11–1).

Microscopic Structure

In a low-power view of a kidney section, the dark cortex is seen to be interrupted at intervals by projections of lighter-staining medullary tissue, called *medullary rays,* which contain branched collecting ducts, together with the descending and ascending limbs of the nephron loop. The cortical substance surrounding each medullary ray is the *cortical labyrinth.* A medullary ray and the renal corpuscles and associated nephrons that empty into the branched collect-

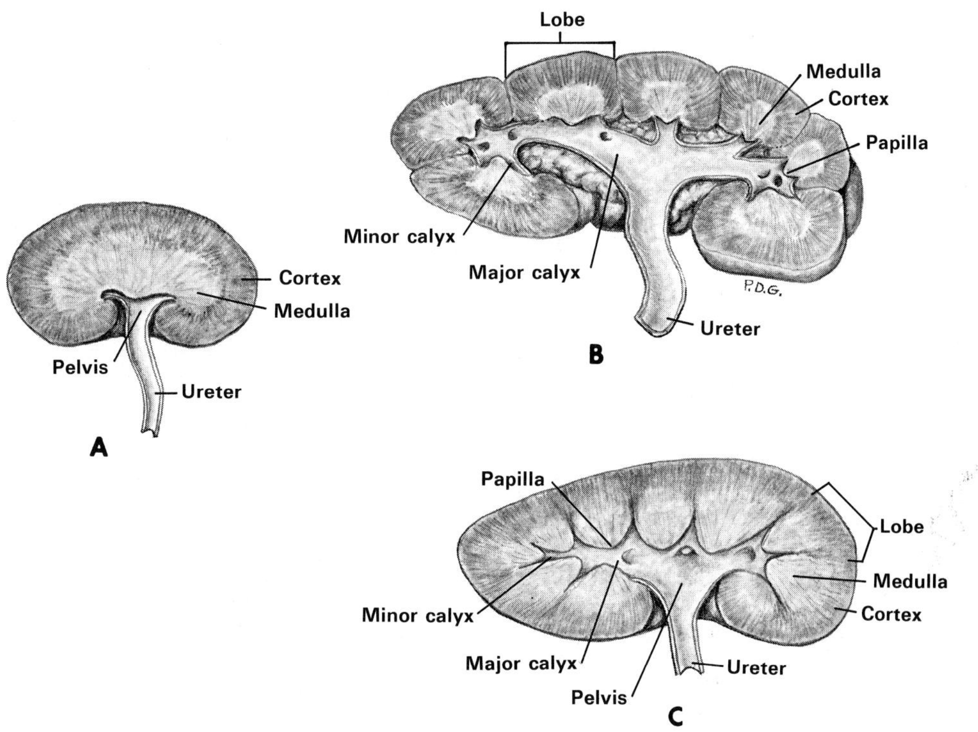

Fig. 11–1. *Schematic drawing illustrating the different types of kidneys. True unipyramidal kidney (A), typical of the cat; multipyramidal kidney (B), typical of large ruminants with external demarcation of the lobes (notice absence of a renal pelvis); multipyramidal kidney of the pig (C).*

ing ducts of that ray constitute a *kidney lobule.* The limits of each lobule, although not clearly defined, are indicated by the interlobular arteries that course into the cortex from the corticomedullary junction. The dark cortical tissue extending into the medulla outlines the lateral boundaries of the pyramids. These cortical striations are the *renal columns.*

The medulla appears lighter than the cortex and presents a striated pattern because of the alignment of the straight portions of the uriniferous tubules and their associated blood vessels. The medulla has a distinguishable zonation that reflects regional specialization of the tubules (Fig. 11–2).

CAPSULE AND CONNECTIVE TISSUE STROMA

The capsule surrounding the kidney has a dense outer layer of collagen and elastic fibers, and an inner layer composed of loose connective tissue that in the dog, horse, and pig has some smooth muscle fibers (Fig. 11–3). Kidney capsules in the ruminants have a distinct smooth muscle layer, which is thickest in the sheep and goat. There is no smooth muscle in the kidney capsule of the cat.

The renal stroma is sparse and consists essentially of loose connective tissue surrounding blood vessels, lymph vessels, and nerves.

NEPHRON

The nephron is the functional unit of the kidney and has six morphologically distinct segments: (1) the glomerular capsule (expanded blind end of the nephron), (2) the convoluted and (3) straight portions of the proximal tubule, (4) a thin segment, and (5) the straight and (6) convoluted portions

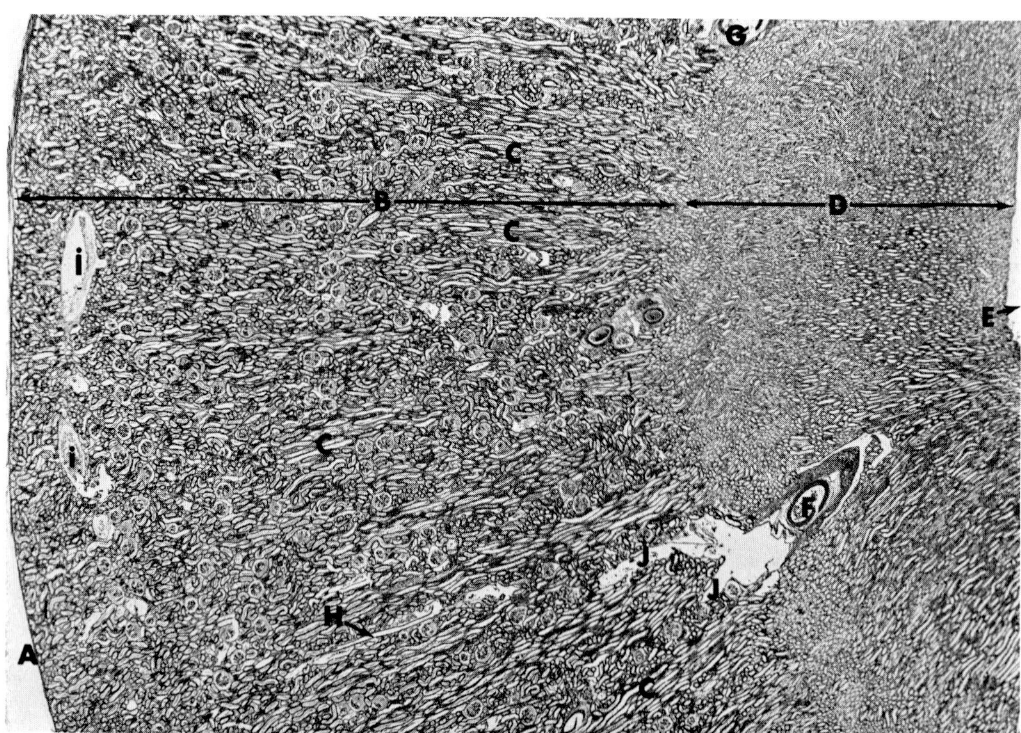

Fig. 11–2. *Kidney, dog. Capsule (A); cortex (B) containing medullary rays (C); medulla (D); pelvis (E); arteries: interlobar (F), arcuate (G), interlobular (H); veins: stellate (i), interlobular (J). H & E. ×10. (From Adam, W.S., Calhoun, M.L., Smith, E.M., and Stinson, A.W.: Microscopic Anatomy of the Dog: A Photographic Atlas. Springfield, Ill., Charles C Thomas, 1970.)*

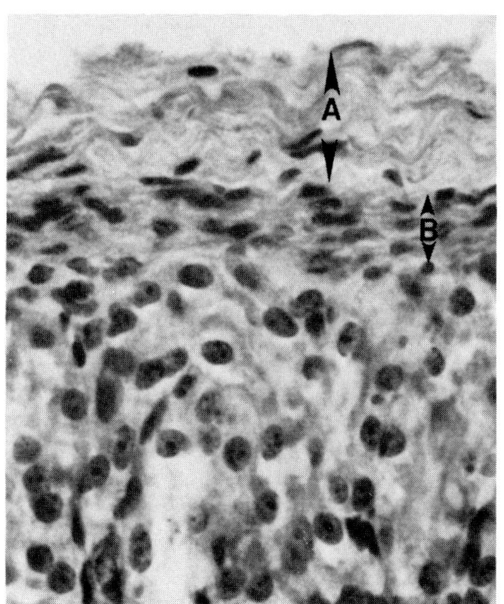

Fig. 11–3. *Kidney, pig. The capsule is composed of a connective tissue layer (A) and layer of smooth muscle beneath it (B). H & E. ×600.*

of the distal tubule. The proximal and distal convoluted tubules are located in the cortex surrounding the renal corpuscle. The straight portions of the proximal and distal tubules and the thin segment make a loop that extends into the medulla, called the *loop of the nephron (Henle)*. The *thick descending limb* is the straight portion of the proximal tubule, the *thin descending* and *ascending limbs* make up the thin segment of the nephron, and the *thick ascending limb* is the straight portion of the distal tubule (Fig. 11–4).

In unipyramidal kidneys, the segments of the nephron loop are so regularly arranged that a separation of the medulla into definite outer and inner zones is visible with the naked eye. The junction of the ascending thin and thick limbs marks the boundary between the *outer* and *inner zones* of the medulla. The *outer zone* is further subdivided into *inner* and *outer bands,* and the boundary between these bands is marked by the junction of the straight portion of the proximal tubule with the thin descending limb of the nephron loop (Fig. 11–4).

Zonation is less distinct in multipyramidal kidneys because the loops of the nephron have different lengths. The short loops originate from the renal corpuscles located near the surface of the kidney and are the most numerous type. These are referred to as *superficial nephrons.* The bend of the loop is formed by the thick ascending limb and is located in the outer zone of the medulla. The long loops come from the renal corpuscles nearer the medulla and are called *juxtamedullary nephrons.* The bend is formed by the thin segment. Occasionally the loops are very long, extending nearly to the apex of the papilla.

RENAL CORPUSCLE. The renal corpuscle is formed when the capillary tuft, or *glomerulus,* invaginates the epithelium-lined, dilated end of the nephron called the *glomerular capsule.* As a result, a double-walled capsule invests the capillary loops, which project into the lumen of the expanded blind end of the tubule. This intimate association of capillaries and tubule epithelium forms a complex structure known as the *renal corpuscle.* The epithelium covering the capillaries is the *glomerular epithelium* or the *visceral layer,* and that lining the opposing wall is known as the *capsular epithelium* or the *parietal layer.* The space between the glomerular epithelium and the capsular epithelium is the *capsular space.* That region of the renal corpuscle where the afferent and efferent arterioles are located is known as the *vascular pole.* Opposite the vascular pole is the *urinary pole,* where the capsular epithelium is continuous with the cuboidal epithelium of the proximal convoluted tubule (Fig. 11–5).

Because the capillary tuft is situated between two arterioles, the glomerular filtration efficiency is enhanced tremendously. On entering the renal corpuscle, the afferent arteriole forms four to six primary branches, from which hang lobules of capillary loops (Fig. 11–5). These drain into one of the few primary branches of the

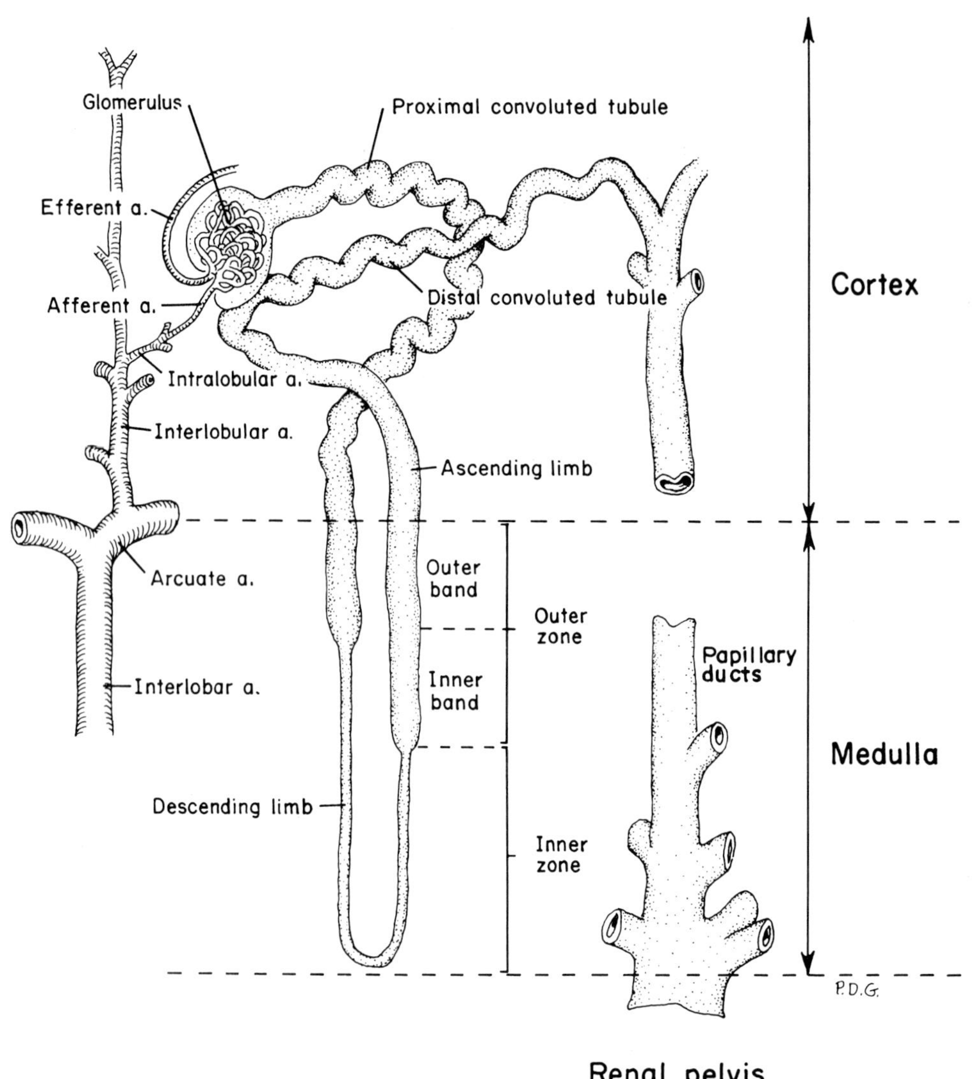

Fig. 11–4. *Schematic diagram illustrating the various segments of the uriniferous tubule, their locations within the cortex and medulla, and their relationship to the major arteries.*

efferent arteriole. Capillaries from each lobule spiral around a common axis that serves as a point of fixation. On section, the axis appears like a stalk radiating from the vascular pole to the glomerular periphery (Fig. 11–5).

The filtration barrier of the renal corpuscle is composed of three layers: (1) glomerular endothelium, (2) basal lamina, and (3) glomerular epithelium (visceral layer). The basal lamina is common to both epithelial layers (Fig. 11–6A).

The cytoplasm of the glomerular endothelium is porous (Fig. 11–6B). Because the pores range in size from 50 to 100 nm, this part of the filtration barrier merely acts as a prefilter by holding back large particulate matter and blood cells.

The basal lamina of the renal corpuscle is more than three times thicker (325 to 340 nm) than those found elsewhere in the body and, when stained with PAS, is readily visualized with the light microscope (Fig. 11–7). Three layers are detectable with the

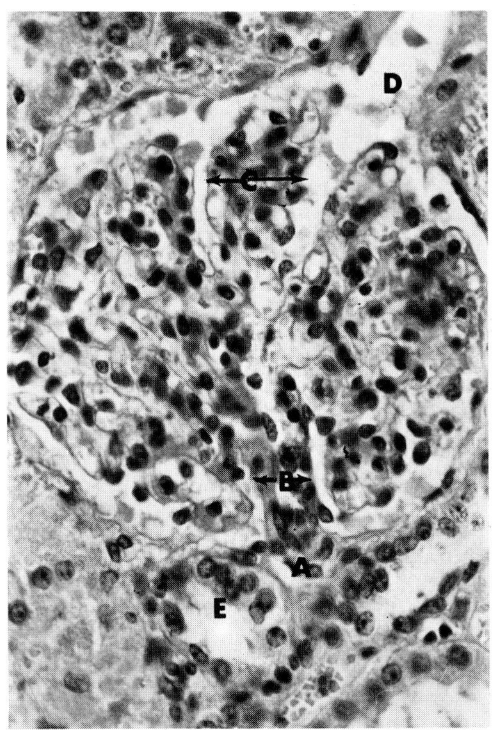

Fig. 11–5. *Renal corpuscle, horse. Afferent arteriole (A); vascular stalk (B); capillary lobule in glomerulus (C); urinary pole (D); macula densa (E). H & E. ×425.*

electron microscope: (1) the *lamina densa,* a thick central layer; (2) the *lamina rara externa,* located next to the visceral epithelium; and (3) the *lamina rara interna,* adjacent to the capillary endothelium. This unusually thick basal lamina is produced continuously by the glomerular epithelium. The basal lamina is a major part of the filtration barrier, capable of holding back macromolecules with molecular weights of approximately 160,000. In sites where the loops of capillary lobules are suspended from the arteriolar branches, the capillaries are close together and the glomerular epithelium does not penetrate far enough to cover each capillary. Located in this centrolobular axis are cells referred to as *mesangial* or *intercapillary cells* (Fig. 11–7). These cells secrete a matrix, similar to the basal lamina, that covers the endothelium, and thus have a supportive role. The mesangial cells may become phagocytic and remove fragments of old basal lamina to prevent it from becoming excessively thick.

The third layer is the glomerular epithelium. The large cells, called *podocytes,* have numerous long processes that radiate from the cell body and course parallel to the long axis of the capillary. These *major processes* in turn break up into *minor processes* or pedicels (end feet) that terminate on the basal lamina. The cell body and the major processes are separated from the basal lamina by spaces filled with glomerular filtrate. The pedicels from one podocyte interdigitate with one another and with the pedicels from other podocytes. Between these interdigitations are slits, the *filtration slits,* covered with a thin diaphragm, the *filtration-slit membrane* (Fig. 11–6A and B). Filtration-slit membranes have a pore size somewhere between 6 and 9 nm and constitute the final filtration site capable of stopping substances with a molecular weight slightly less than 60,000. The size of the macromolecules is important in considering the efficiency of the filtration barrier, but it is also necessary to consider the numbers and kinds of electrostatic charges the macromolecules carry, as well as whether they are associated with larger molecules. Glomerular permeability is also affected by the fixed negative charges associated with the glycosaminoglycan portion of the filtration barrier.

The capsular epithelium of the renal corpuscle is typical simple squamous epithelium. It becomes cuboidal at the urinary pole and continues as such into the proximal convoluted tubule.

PROXIMAL TUBULE. The proximal tubule of the nephron has two major segments: a convoluted part, which makes several loops in the cortex near the renal corpuscle, and a straight portion, extending into the outer zone of the medulla. The convoluted portion is the longest segment of the nephron and makes up the bulk of the cortex. The cells are more acidophilic than those in other parts of the nephron; therefore, it is

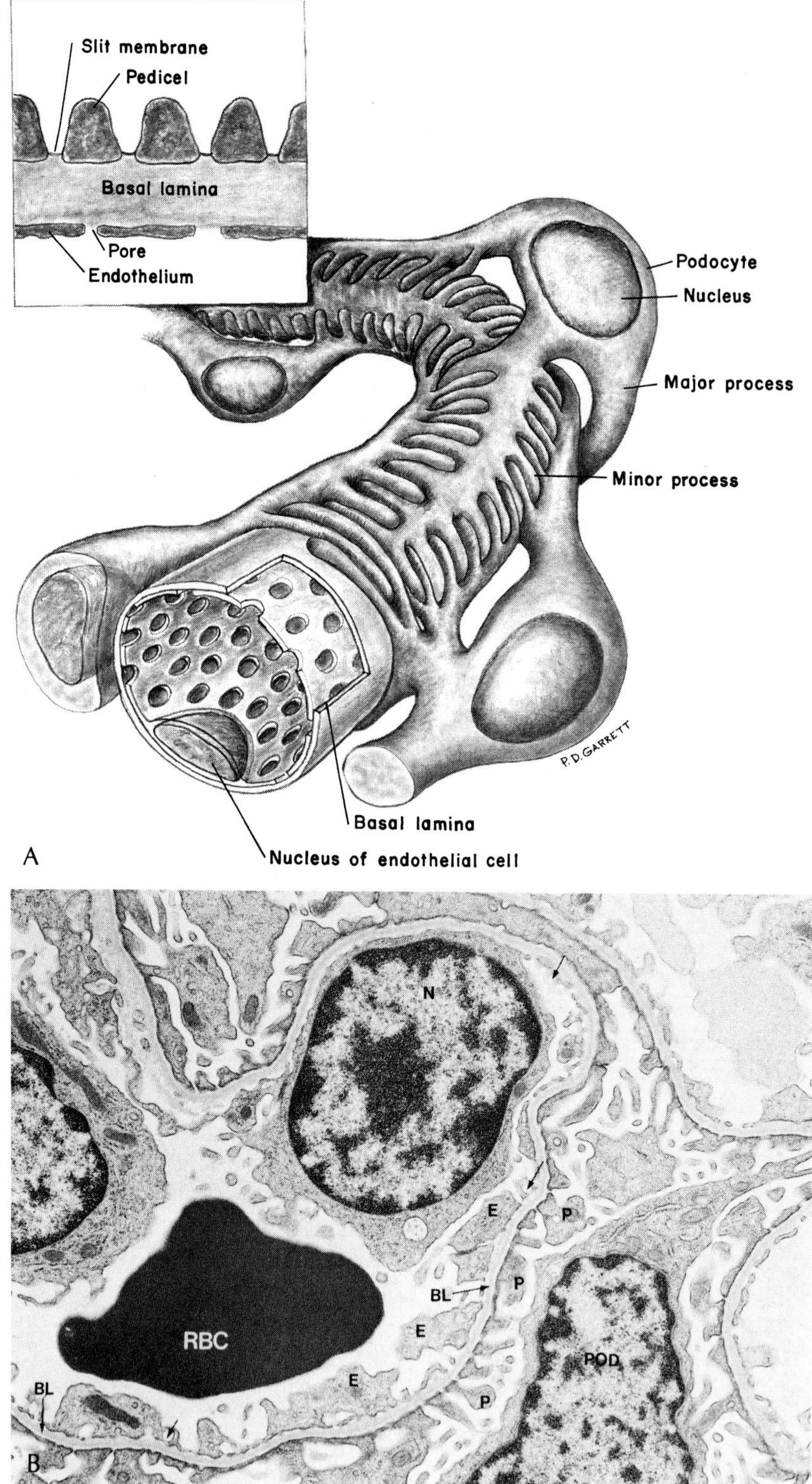

Fig. 11–6. *A, Schematic drawing illustrating the ultrastructure of the glomerular filtration apparatus. The major cytoplasmic processes branch to form the minor processes or pedicels, which make intimate contact with the basal lamina. Between the pedicels are the slit membranes seen in the inset. B, Renal corpuscle, cat. Electron micrograph illustrating the filtration apparatus. Erythrocyte (RBC) in the capillary lumen; endothelial cell nucleus (N) and cytoplasm (E) with pores (arrows); basal lamina (BL); podocyte nucleus (POD) and the interdigitating pedicels (P).* ×*16,000 (Courtesy E.J. King and D.A. Kinden.)*

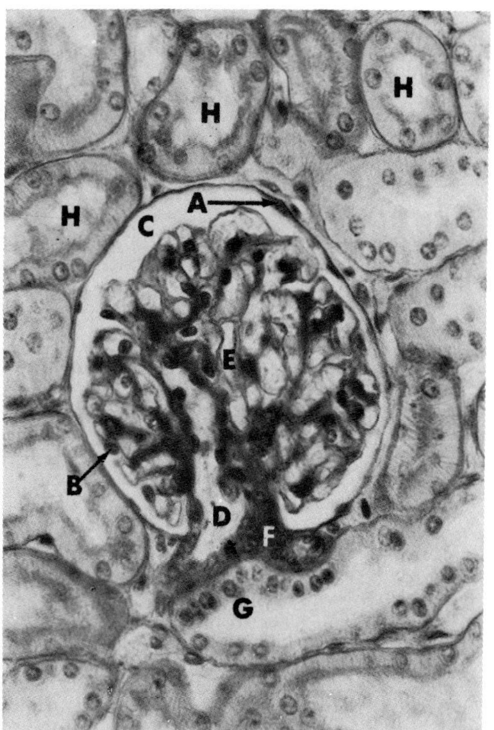

Fig. 11–7. *Renal corpuscle, cat. Capsular epithelium (A); glomerular epithelium (B); capsular space (C); afferent arteriole (D); glomerulus (E); mesangial cells (F); macula densa (G); proximal tubules (H). Basement membranes are dark-stained. PAS. ×425.*

possible to identify proximal tubules on the basis of their stainability. In a cross section of a tubule, the epithelial cells are pyramidal. The spherical nucleus is located near the base, and the free surface has long microvilli, the brush border, which sometimes appear to fill the lumen. The numerous narrow basal interdigitating cell processes and their associated mitochondria (Fig. 11–8) are visible in the light microscope as vertical striations (see Fig. 11–13).

Electron micrographs reveal that the long microvilli have an abundant glycocalyx. Between the bases of the microvilli, invaginations that extend into the cytoplasm expand and give rise to pinocytotic vesicles (Fig. 11–8). At the cell base, narrow lateral and basal processes interdigitate to form complex ridges and grooves. Likewise, the basal infoldings of adjacent cells interdigitate, so that a basal process in a single section may actually belong to a contiguous cell. These extensive infoldings and interdigitations are functionally important in the operation of the sodium pump described later in this chapter.

The straight portion of the proximal tubule has essentially the same histologic characteristics as the convoluted portion. It is located in the medullary rays and the medulla and is the first portion of the nephron loop. The proximal tubular epithelia of carnivores, and especially the cat, contain numerous lipid droplets that give the cells a foamy appearance in paraffin sections. While this lipid is more prevalent in the convoluted portion of the tubule in cats, it is present throughout the nephron. On the basis of histochemical and ultrastructural studies it appears that the lipids are triglycerides and phospholipids.

THIN SEGMENT. The thin segment is the thin descending and ascending portion of the nephron loop. It is lined with simple squamous epithelium whose nuclei tend to bulge into the lumen. The surface has a few short microvilli and less-numerous cell organelles, and the lateral and basal infoldings and interdigitations are less complex than those in the proximal portion of the nephron (Fig. 11–8).

DISTAL TUBULE. The straight portion of the distal tubule is the thick ascending limb of the nephron loop, which rises through the outer zone of the medulla into the cortex, where it comes into juxtaposition with the renal corpuscle. Here it loops between the afferent and efferent arterioles, so that the wall of the distal tubule is in close contact with the wall of the afferent arteriole. At this point, the tubular epithelium is taller; consequently, the nuclei are closer together and the epithelium appears denser than it does in other areas. This is the *macula densa,* the significance of which will be discussed later (Fig. 11–7). In the horse, the cells of the macula densa often appear stratified, with nuclei at two or three different levels (Fig. 11–5). The

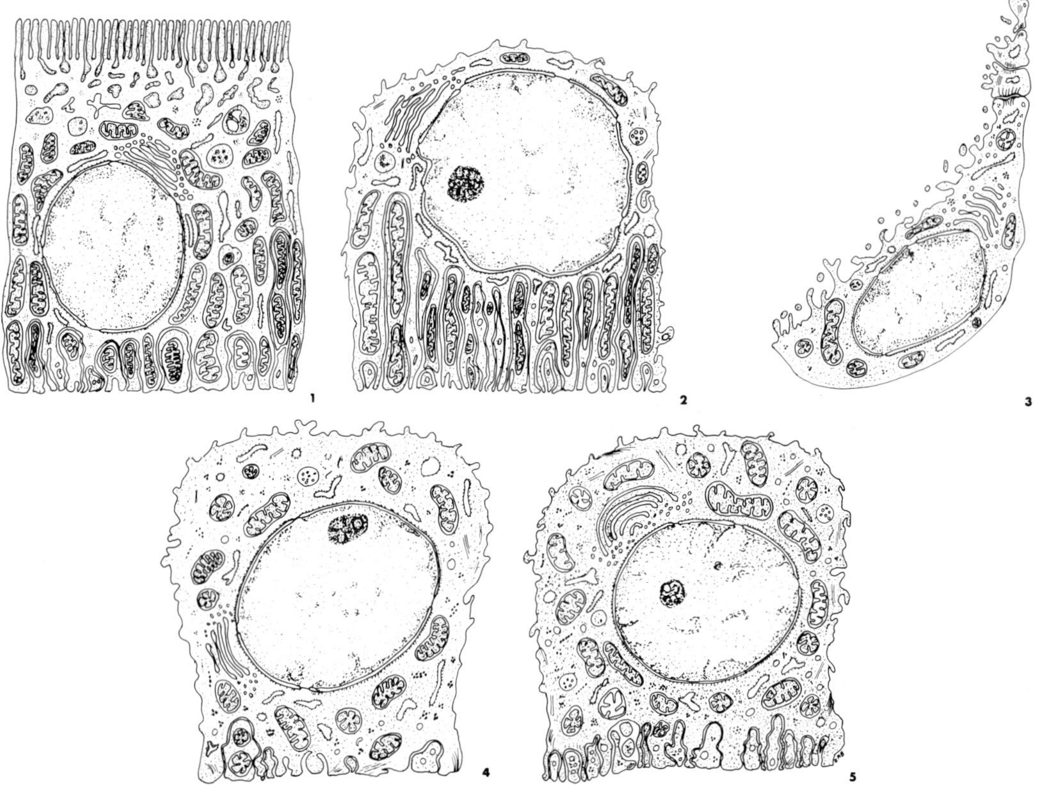

Fig. 11–8. *Schematic drawing of cell types in the various portions of the uriniferous tubule. (1) Proximal convoluted tubule; (2) distal convoluted tubule; (3) thin limb of nephron loop; (4) light and (5) dark cells of collecting duct.*

epithelium of the distal tubule is higher than that in the thin segment, and distinct vertical striations are seen in the basal region (Fig. 11–9). A few short microvilli extend from the cell apex and occasionally one long cilium projects into the lumen. Electron micrographs reveal a well-developed rER and many free ribosomes. Deep basal cell membrane infoldings are associated with vertically oriented mitochondria (Fig. 11–8).

The convoluted portion of the distal segment forms a loop toward the kidney surface and then joins an arched collecting tubule near a medullary ray. Although the convoluted distal and proximal tubules are intermingled within the cortex, some histologic characteristics make it possible to differentiate the two segments (Fig. 11–7). There are fewer cross and oblique sections of the distal segment because it is not as long as the proximal portion. The lumen of the distal tubule tends to be larger because the epithelium is lower, and because the cells are narrow there are more nuclei than in cross sections of the proximal segments. Unlike the proximal tubules, there are no brush borders on the free surfaces of the cells in the distal tubule, and the pale cytoplasm is usually less acidophilic.

In electron micrographs, the basal infoldings and compartmentalization appear more elaborate than those in the cells of the proximal tubule. Large, long mitochondria lie between the basal cytoplasmic infoldings. The surface cytoplasm is free of invaginations, and a few short microvilli extend from the cell apex (Fig. 11–8).

COLLECTING TUBULES

The nephrons join the collecting tubules in the cortex, and although they do absorb

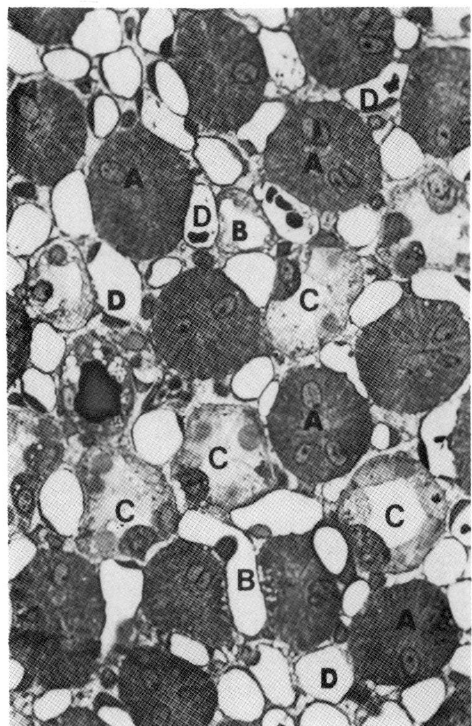

Fig. 11–9. *Kidney medulla, outer zone, dog. Descending thick limb of the nephron (A); thin limb (B); collecting ducts (C) and capillaries of vasa recta (D). Epon. Toluidine blue. ×425.*

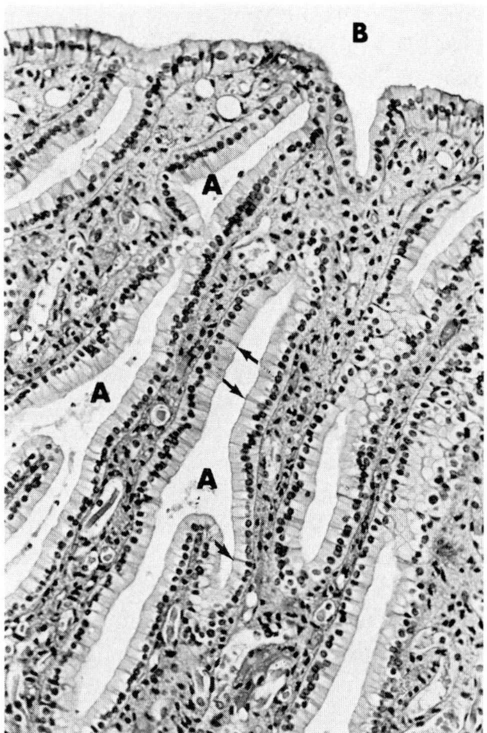

Fig. 11–10. *Renal papilla, dog. Papillary ducts (A), lined with simple columnar epithelium; a few dark cells (arrows) interspersed with clear cells; area cribrosa (B). H & E. ×80. (From Adam, W.S., Calhoun, M.L., Smith, E.M., and Stinson, A.W.: Microscopic Anatomy of the Dog: A Photographic Atlas. Springfield, Ill., Charles C Thomas, 1970.)*

some substances, e.g., bicarbonates, they are not a part of the nephron itself. Collecting tubules are the terminal segments of the uriniferous tubules; they enter the medullary rays and course into the inner zone of the medulla where they join other tubules, and finally converge into large straight collecting ducts called *papillary ducts.* These ducts open into the renal pelvis at the apex of the papilla; this region is called the *area cribrosa.*

ARCHED COLLECTING TUBULES. These tubules are the direct continuation of the collecting tubules from several nephrons of one lobule. The cuboidal epithelial cytoplasm is pale and has a dark, spherical nucleus. The arched collecting tubules open directly into the straight collecting tubules.

STRAIGHT COLLECTING TUBULES. The straight tubules, located in the medullary ray, course through the outer zone of the medulla and, on reaching the inner zone, join other straight tubules. The cuboidal epithelium lining these tubules is somewhat taller than that in the arched portion, and their lateral cell margins are usually clearly defined. There are two epithelial cell types: clear cells, predominant in the more distal segment and less numerous in the proximal portion, and dark cells, more numerous in the proximal tubule and fewer toward the papilla. The clear cells contain few organelles; the dark cells have a dense cytoplasm containing numerous mitochondria and polyribosomes. The apical surface has many short microvilli and occasionally a single cilium (Fig. 11–8).

PAPILLARY DUCTS. Several straight collecting tubules join at acute angles to form the large collecting or papillary ducts, which open at the apex of the papilla (Fig. 11–10). The epithelium is columnar and may become transitional toward the duct opening. However, in the dog it is columnar throughout the entire length. In the horse and ruminants, the transitional epithelium extends farther along the papillary ducts than in the other domestic animals. The other cytologic features are similar to those of the straight collecting tubules.

BLOOD VESSELS

Waste products in the blood are removed most effectively by the kidney. Such efficiency depends on the kidney's receiving a large volume of blood delivered under high pressure. Likewise, the regulation of fluid and electrolyte balance is enhanced by the intricate association of blood vessels with the various segments of the uriniferous segments of the uriniferous tubule (Figs. 11–9, 11–10, 11–11 and 11–12).

The renal artery enters the hilus and divides into several *interlobar arteries* that course within the renal columns between the pyramids. At the base of the pyramids, these arteries form branches that arch over the pyramids at the corticomedullary junction as the *arcuate arteries.* The arcuate arteries send branches into the cortex at the lateral margins of the lobules. These are the *interlobular arteries,* which give rise to the numerous *afferent arterioles* supplying the glomeruli forming several capillary lobules. The glomerular capillaries converge at the vascular pole as the *efferent arteriole.* Upon leaving the glomeruli, the efferent arterioles supply different capillary beds, depending on their location within the cortex. Those from the glomeruli in the outer part of the cortex form the *peritubular plexus* surrounding the proximal and distal convoluted tubules. Efferent arterioles from the deep or juxtamedullary cortex contribute to the adjacent peritubular plexus and also send long bundles of vessels, the *vasa recta,* deep into the medulla. Because some blood is supplied to the medulla by arter-

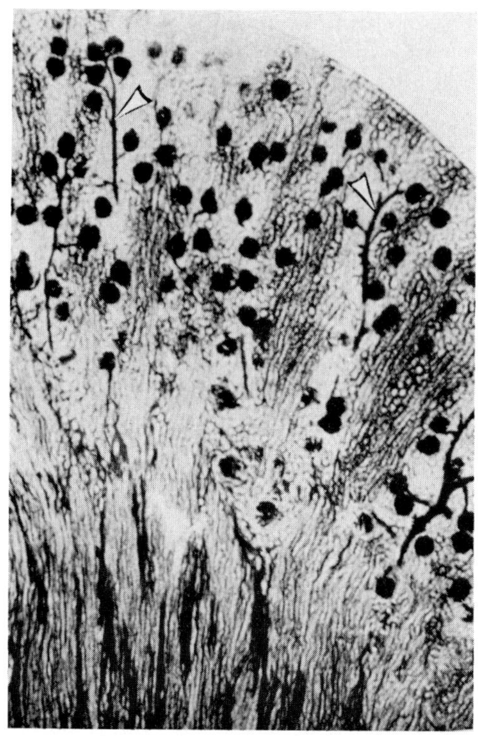

Fig. 11–11. *Kidney, dog. This section of india ink–injected kidney illustrates the interlobular arteries (arrowheads), afferent and efferent arterioles, the cortical peritubular plexuses, and the vasa recta in the medulla. ×25. (Courtesy E.J. King.)*

ioles that arise directly from the arcuate arteries, the vasa recta are divided into two groups: those originating directly from the arcuate arteries are the true straight arterioles, the *arteriolae rectae verae,* and those arising from the efferent arterioles are the false straight arterioles, the *arteriolae rectae spuriae.* These descending arterioles give rise to capillaries with an arterial descending limb and a venous ascending limb, functioning as countercurrent exchangers (Figs. 11–11 and 11–12). The arterial vasa recta are lined with a relatively thick endothelium, while the endothelium in the venous vasa recta is much thinner. The capillaries that form the plexuses at various levels throughout the medulla are fenestrated.

The capillary beds in the outer portion of the cortex drain toward the surface by

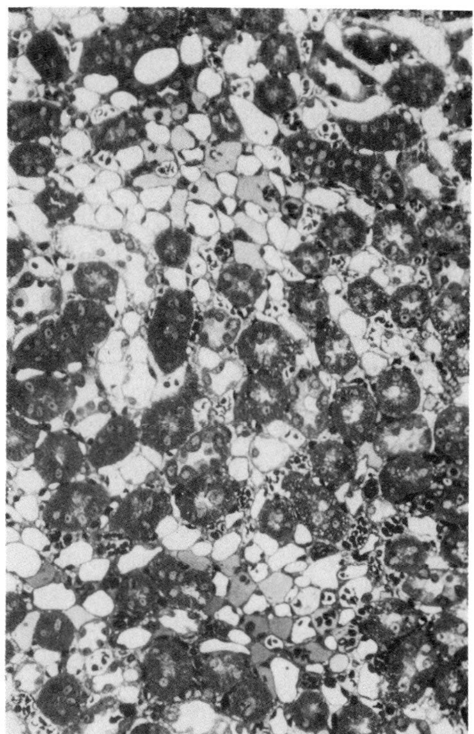

Fig. 11–12. *Subcortical zone of the outer medulla, dog. This illustrates the vessel bundles and associated tubules. The venous vasa recta appear gray due to stained plasma. Epon. Toluidine blue. ×175.*

the *superficial cortical veins,* which eventually join the *stellate veins* beneath the capsule. Dog and cat kidneys are distinguished by exceptionally large stellate veins, located immediately beneath and partly within the capsule in the cat, and a short distance away from the capsule in the dog (Fig. 11–2). *Interlobular veins* drain the stellate veins, which meet with the arcuate veins at the corticomedullary junction. The deeper cortical capillaries join the *deep cortical veins,* which course parallel to the interlobular arteries and unite with the *arcuate veins.* The arcuate veins continue as *interlobar veins* in the renal columns and empty into the *renal vein* at the hilus.

INTERSTITIAL TISSUE

Because the tubules and blood vessels dominate the appearance of the renal parenchyma, little attention has been given to the interstitial tissues until recently. This is particularly true for the cortex, where the capillaries occupy most of the area between the tubules, particularly when seen with the light microscope. However, several ultrastructural studies of the cortex have clearly demonstrated the presence of mononuclear cells with phagocytic properties as well as the presence of fibroblasts. The exact function of the mononuclear cells is as yet unknown.

The morphology and function of the medullary interstitial tissue have been investigated far more extensively than the morphology and function of the cortex. At the light-microscopic level, the cells are seen to be oriented with their long axes perpendicular to the long axis of the tubules and vasa recta. These cells produce prostaglandins, particularly PGA_2 and PGE_2, whose actions have an antihypertensive effect by increasing urine and blood flow along with the intensified sodium excretion. In addition, the medullary interstitial cells apparently synthesize an intercellular matrix rich in glycosaminoglycans and hyaluronic acid. These substances slow electrolyte transport, owing to their water-binding ability.

LYMPHATIC VESSELS

Lymphatic vessels accompany the interlobar arcuate and interlobular arteries. They converge at the renal pelvis, where they form large trunks, and then leave at the hilus with the renal vein. Those renal corpuscles near the interlobular arteries often have branches of the lymphatic vessels either completely or partially surrounding them, as seen in the horse and dog, respectively. Recent studies of the dog kidney revealed small lymphatic channels in close association with the proximal and distal tubules. In addition, kidneys of the dog and cat have rather prominent subcapsular lymphatic vessels. There is as yet no conclusive evidence of lymphatic vessels in the kidney medulla. These interlobular lymphatics are lined by an endothelium surrounded by a basement membrane, and the interlobar and hilar vessels of dogs and calves have valves.

NERVES

Branches of the celiac ganglion and the splanchnic nerves accompany the arteries at the hilus and follow their course into the kidney. Sympathetic and parasympathetic fibers supply the muscular walls of the arteries. They penetrate to the level of the afferent glomerular arterioles, but there are no nerve terminals within the glomerulus or on the epithelial cells of the uriniferous tubules.

JUXTAGLOMERULAR COMPLEX

Three structures are included in the juxtaglomerular complex: (1) the juxtaglomerular cells of the afferent arteriole, (2) the macula densa in the distal tubule, and (3) a cluster of cells adjacent to both the afferent arteriole and the macula densa, called mesangial cells. All these structures are located in a triangular area at the vascular pole of the renal corpuscle (Fig. 11–13). The afferent and efferent arterioles form the sides of the triangle; the macula densa is the base and the vascular pole itself is the apex.

At the point where the afferent arteriole enters the renal corpuscle, the muscle cells in the tunica media are modified. The nuclei are spherical, rather than spindle-shaped as they are in normal smooth muscle cells, and the cytoplasm contains many secretory granules and a few myofilaments. These modified muscle cells are the *juxtaglomerular (JG) cells.* The granules are not visible with most stains but can be demonstrated with the PAS reaction and are seen in Epon sections stained for light microscopy (Fig. 11–13). In addition to the cytoplasmic granules, another modification is significant. The internal elastic lamina is absent; therefore, the cells are in close con-

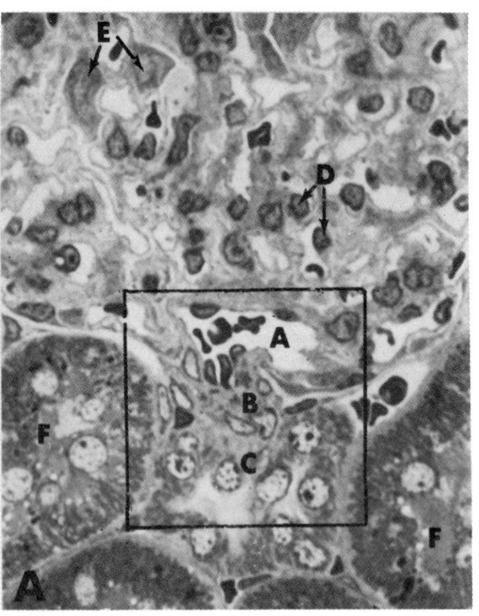

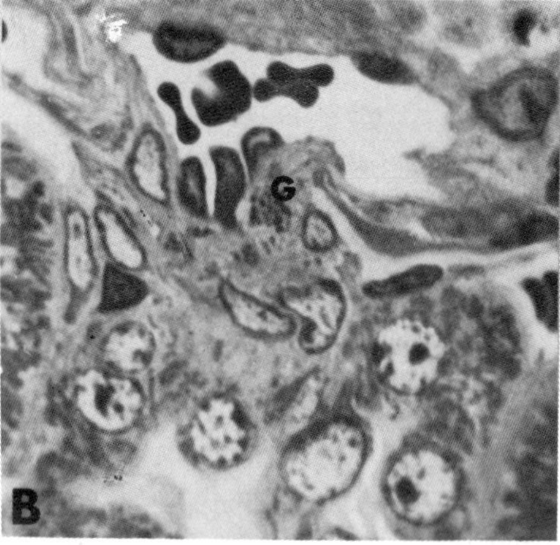

Fig. 11–13. *Kidney, cat. A, Afferent arteriole (A) containing erythrocytes (black) and modified smooth muscle cell nuclei (B) adjacent to macula densa (C); glomerular endothelial cell nuclei (D); glomerular epithelial nuclei (E); proximal tubules (F) with vertical striations. ×650. B, Area outlined in A; juxtaglomerular granules (G) in modified muscle cells. Notice the endothelial nuclei in afferent arteriole. Epon. Toluidine blue. ×880.*

tact with the endothelium and nearer to the blood in the lumen.

The epithelium of the macula densa of the distal tubule differs from that in other parts of the tubule. The mitochondria are short and scattered throughout the cytoplasm, and the granular ER is scanty. The Golgi complex is located between the nucleus and the base of the cell, which lies adjacent to the juxtaglomerular cells in the afferent arteriole. In addition, the basement membrane is frayed and discontinuous in some places, providing more intimate contact with the modified muscle cells.

The third element is composed of mesangial cells (also called Lacis cells, Polkissen, or polar cushion cells) located within the limits of the triangle and in close contact with the other two components of the juxtaglomerular complex. The cytoplasmic processes of these cells contain myosinlike filaments. They penetrate the glomerulus as part of the intercapillary cell population. The function of the juxtaglomerular complex is discussed in the next section of this chapter.

Functional Morphology

By eliminating waste products from the blood, the kidneys perform a significant excretory function. Of equal importance is their conservational function, by which electrolytes, proteins, carbohydrates, and other substances are retained. These two functions maintain body homeostasis by providing a constant internal environment for the entire animal. The elaboration of urine requires three processes: glomerular ultrafiltration, tubular resorption, and tubular secretion. The various components with their unique organization are ideally adapted to carry out these processes.

GLOMERULUS

The location of the glomerular capillaries between two arterioles is a unique arrangement and provides an extremely efficient mechanism for producing vast amounts of ultrafiltrate from the blood. This efficiency is the result of the relatively high filtration pressure maintained throughout the capillary network owing to the resistance produced by the efferent arteriole. This is in contrast to other capillary networks, located between arterioles and venules, where the pressure in the venules is much lower than the pressure in the arterioles.

NEPHRON

More than 99% of the glomerular filtrate is resorbed as the fluid flows through the various segments of the uriniferous tubule. The remaining portion, the urine, is modified by selective absorption, diffusion, and excretion of other substances as well.

PROXIMAL CONVOLUTED TUBULE. Structurally, the cells in the proximal convoluted tubules are well adapted for their functions. Approximately 85% of the sodium and water is resorbed into the blood by the action of a cellular sodium pump. The sodium moves from the tubule lumen into the cytoplasm and, together with the chloride ions, is pumped out of the cell base into the tissue fluid, where numerous capillaries are located. The chloride ions pull water from the cytoplasm, which sets up a concentration gradient between the fluid in the tubule lumen and the cell cytoplasm. This gradient is responsible for the movement of sodium and water into the cytoplasm. Therefore, the sodium pump operates at the base of the cell and is responsible for the movement of the sodium out of the cell into the tissue fluid.

The sodium pump requires an extensive surface area and a considerable amount of energy. The numerous basal infoldings of the cell membrane increase the available surface area, and the long and abundant mitochondria provide a vast source of energy.

Some blood protein passes the filtration

barrier in the glomerulus and is absorbed at the free surface of the proximal convoluted tubular cells. Small pinocytotic vesicles filled with protein form from the cell membrane between the microvilli and fuse with cytoplasmic lysosomes. The lysosomal enzymes digest the protein, and the respective amino acids leave by way of the cell base and enter the adjacent capillaries.

In addition to sodium and protein, all the glucose is resorbed in this segment along with free amino acids and urea.

LOOP OF THE NEPHRON. The loop of the nephron concentrates the filtrate to reduce the volume, and creates a hypertonic tissue fluid surrounding adjacent collecting tubules. This hypertonic environment pulls water from the collecting tubule lumen, thus reducing the volume of urine.

The descending limb is permeable to sodium and water, and because it is located near the ascending limb where sodium is pumped from the lumen into the interstitial fluid, it is in a hypertonic environment. This pulls water from the descending limb, and the tubular fluid becomes increasingly hypertonic as it approaches the bottom of the loop. In the ascending limb, sodium is pumped out, but the cells are impermeable to water and the tubule fluid becomes isotonic and gradually hypotonic as more sodium is lost to the interstitial fluid. The ascending and descending limbs of the blood vessels of the vasa recta are under low hydrostatic pressure, and much of the osmotic pressure is due to blood colloids; therefore, they can survive in a hypertonic tissue fluid and not upset the osmotic gradient necessary for urine concentration.

The arrangement of the vasa recta and the descending and ascending limbs of the nephron, along with the collecting ducts, takes on a definite pattern in the medulla to facilitate the countercurrent mechanisms involved in the movement of water and electrolytes described above. These blood vessels and tubules are seen in bundles scattered throughout the medulla (Fig. 11–12). In the subcortical zone of the outer medulla, the central core of the bundle is composed of arterial and venous vasa recta, surrounded by descending limbs of the nephron. Finally, the periphery of the bundle is made up of ascending thin limbs and collecting ducts. Thus, the organization of the bundle is such that groups of three pairs of tubes are juxtaposed to each other; the fluid flow in each pair is in opposite directions. The pairs are (1) the arterial and venous vasa recta, (2) the venous vasa recta and the descending limb and (3) the ascending limbs and the collecting ducts. This opposite-flow arrangement of the vessels and tubules maximizes the exchange of material between them and the interstitial tissue.

Although the bundles in the inner medulla are considerably smaller, the same opposite-flow relationships exist because the ascending thin limbs are next to the collecting ducts and the descending limbs are closely related to the venous vasa recta.

DISTAL CONVOLUTED TUBULE. On reaching the distal convoluted tubule of the nephron, the tubular fluid is hypotonic. Sodium and water continue to be pumped out, as evidenced by the extensive basal infoldings and interdigitations of the cell membrane. The sodium ions are replaced by potassium, hydrogen, and some ammonia, thereby acidifying the urine. Because more water is resorbed owing to the influence of the antidiuretic hormone, the urine becomes isotonic.

COLLECTING TUBULES. The final concentration of urine takes place in the collecting tubules. The withdrawal of water from the tubular fluid is regulated by the antidiuretic hormone and by the hypertonic environment created by the loop of the nephron. Therefore, the urine delivered into the kidney pelvis is hypertonic.

JUXTAGLOMERULAR COMPLEX. The JG cells respond to a fall in blood pressure by elaborating renin; this can be demonstrated within the granules of these cells by immunocytochemical methods. Renin acts upon angiotensinogen and splits off angiotensin I, a decapeptide that is enzymatically converted to angiotensin II, a powerful vasoconstrictor. Since JG cells are sensitive to stretching, they are *baroreceptors,* and whenever they are not stretched by normal blood pressure they secrete more renin. The resulting increase in the blood level of angiotensin II acts directly on the arteriolar muscle and also stimulates the synthesis and release of the hormone aldosterone from the adrenal cortex. Aldosterone further contributes to increased blood pressure by acting on the kidney tubules to increase sodium and water resorption. However, sustained high blood pressure is prevented because the baroreceptors in the arterioles stop releasing renin, and the *chemoreceptors* in the macula densa act as sodium sensors to regulate tissue hydration and blood volume.

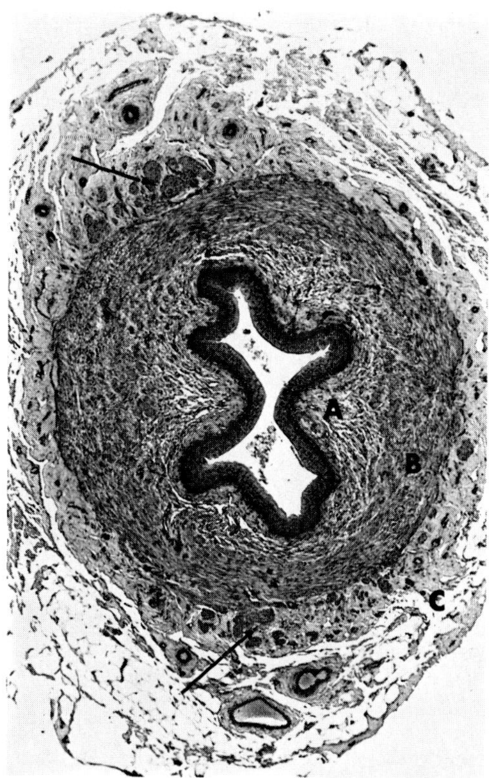

Fig. 11–14. *Section near kidney, ureter, dog. Mucosa (A); tunica muscularis (B); serosa (C). The lumen has a stellate shape. Notice that the outer longitudinal muscle bundles are scattered (arrows). H & E. ×40. (From Adam, W.S., Calhoun, M.L., Smith, E.M., and Stinson, A.W.: Microscopic Anatomy of the Dog., A Photographic Atlas. Springfield, Ill., Charles C Thomas, 1970.)*

URINARY PASSAGES

Renal Pelvis

The renal pelvis is the expanded proximal end of the ureter that faces the apex of the renal papilla.

The renal pelvis is lined with typical transitional epithelium. It rests on a propria-submucosa of loose connective tissue. In the horse, the propria-submucosa contains numerous tubuloalveolar mucous glands.

The tunica muscularis is usually composed of three layers: inner and outer longitudinal layers and a middle circular layer. The tunica adventitia is thin and composed of loose connective tissue, blood vessels, and fat.

Ureter

The ureter leaves the kidney at the hilus and enters the urinary bladder, coursing obliquely through the tunica muscularis. Where the ureter pierces the bladder lining, there is a valvelike mucosal flap, which closes off the ureteral opening as the bladder fills. This is part of a safety mechanism preventing urine reflux.

The wall of the ureter has three layers: (1) the mucous membrane, (2) a tunica muscularis, and (3) either an adventitia or a serosa. The mucosa is thrown into longitudinal folds, which may produce a stellate-shaped lumen seen in cross sections (Fig. 11–14). The mucous membrane is lined with five to six layers of transitional epithelial cells. The thickness varies with the species. The epithelium rests on a loose connective tissue stroma. Ureters of the horse, donkey, and mule have simple branched tubuloalveolar mucous glands in the propria-submucosa (Fig. 11–15). They extend from the renal pelvis through the

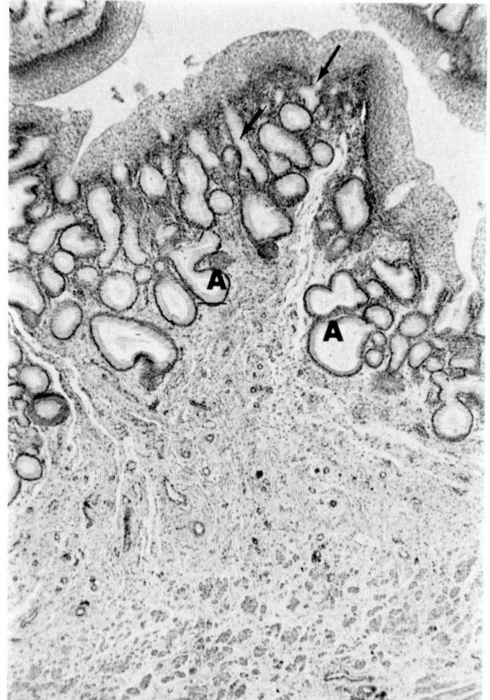

Fig. 11–15. *Ureter, horse. Mucous glands (A) in the mucosa. The secretion enters the lumen by ducts (arrows). H & E. ×40.*

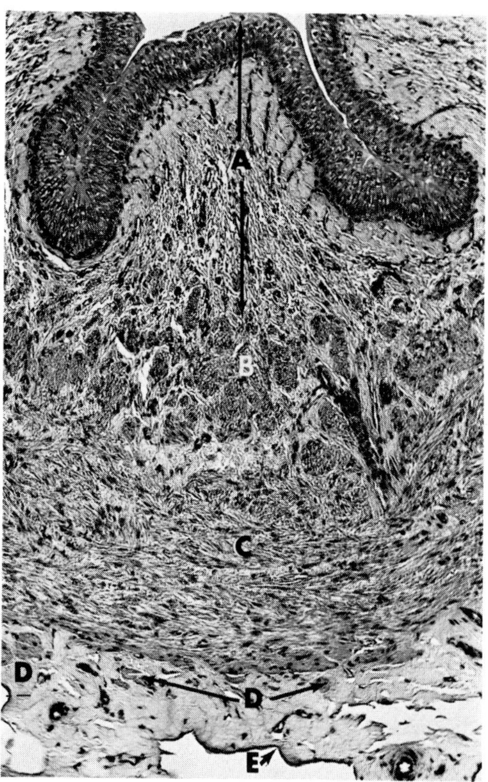

Fig. 11–16. *Ureter, dog. Cross section near bladder. The mucosa (A) and the three layers of the tunica muscularis, inner longitudinal (B), middle circular (C) and outer longitudinal (D), and the serosa (E) make up the wall. H & E. ×110. (From Adam, W.S., Calhoun, M.L., Smith, E.M., and Stinson, A.W.: Microscopic Anatomy of the Dog: A Photographic Atlas. Springfield, Ill., Charles C Thomas, 1970.)*

upper one third (10 cm) of the ureter. Their secretory products give the urine of these species the characteristic stringy, mucous consistency.

The muscularis has three ill-defined layers: inner and outer longitudinal layers and a middle circular layer (Fig. 11–16). Loose connective tissue often separates the smooth muscle bundles, particularly in the longitudinal layers. This arrangement results in a spiraling of the muscle and assists in the peristaltic action that sweeps distally toward the urinary bladder and propels urine into the bladder. The inner longitudinal muscle layer is absent in the cat ureter, except for a scant amount in the proximal portion. As the ureters course through the bladder wall, the middle circular layer disappears and the two longitudinal layers intermingle with those of the bladder (Fig. 11–17).

The outermost coat of the ureter may be either an adventitia or a serosa, depending on the extent of the peritoneal investments, the amount of periureteral fat, and the level of the section. The adventitia is composed of loose collagen and elastic fibers with varying amounts of adipose tissue around the periphery.

Urinary Bladder

The bladder is the reservoir for urine. Histologically it is an expanded ureter, because most of the layers present in the ureter are present in the bladder. The major differences are the relative increases in the thickness of the individual layers of the bladder tunica muscularis and the pres-

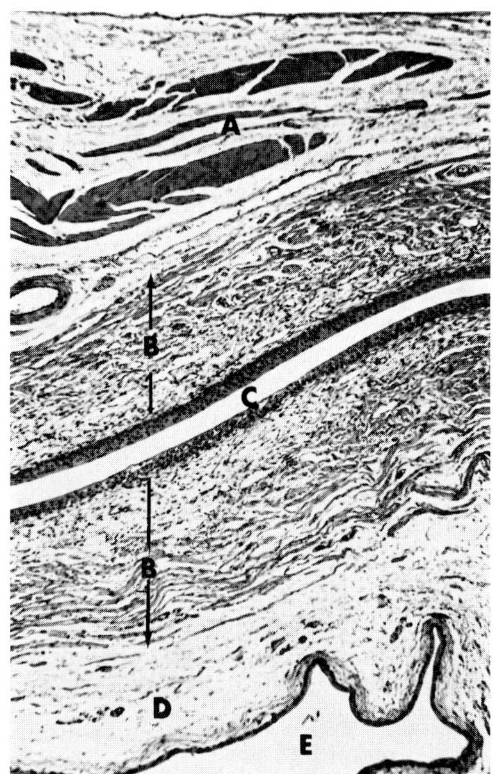

Fig. 11–17. *Ureter penetrating urinary bladder, dog. Muscle of bladder wall (A); ureter (B) with lumen (C); bladder mucosa (D) with scattered lamina muscularis fibers; lumen of urinary bladder (E). H & E. ×50. (From Adam, W.S., Calhoun, M.L., Smith, E.M., and Stinson, A.W.: Microscopic Anatomy of the Dog: A Photographic Atlas. Springfield, Ill., Charles C Thomas, 1970.)*

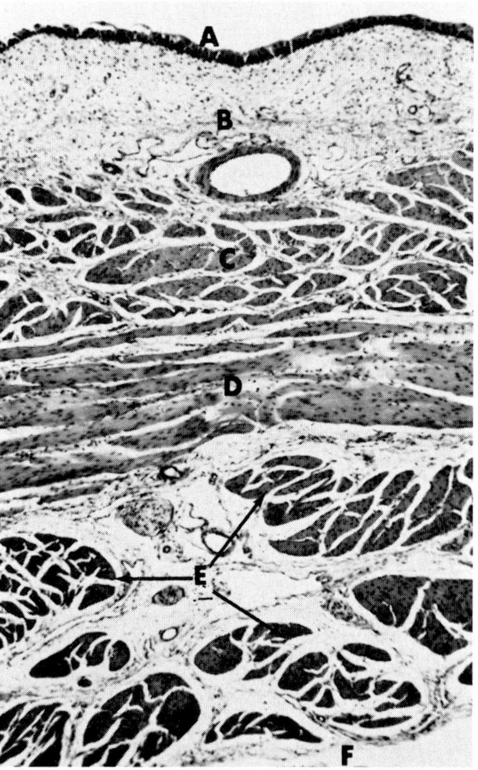

Fig. 11–18. *Urinary bladder, dog. Transitional epithelium (A) resting on the propria-submucosa (B), the inner longitudinal layer (C), middle circular layer (D) and outer longitudinal layer (E) of the tunica muscularis, surrounded by the serosa (F). H & E. ×12. (From Adam, W.S., Calhoun, M.L., Smith, E.M., and Stinson, A.W.: Microscopic Anatomy of the Dog: A Photographic Atlas. Springield, Ill., Charles C Thomas, 1970.)*

ence of a scanty lamina muscularis in bladders of some animals (Figs. 11–18 and 11–19).

The transitional epithelium varies in thickness from 3 to 14 cell layers, depending on the species and degree of distention. Lymphocytes migrate from the lamina propria and come to lie between the epithelial cells. They are particularly numerous in ruminants.

The epithelium rests on a lamina propria composed of loose connective tissue with a substantial amount of elastic fibers. The fibers become more abundant at the bladder neck, where they are arranged circularly. Lymphatic nodules in the lamina propria are a common finding in all domestic animals. Numerous capillaries are present near the epithelium, and in ruminants they tend to form a definite layer immediately beneath the basement membrane (Fig. 11–20).

The presence and amount of a lamina muscularis vary with the species. It is best-developed in the horse bladder, where the fiber bundles are separated by loose connective tissue (Fig. 11–21). They occur deep in the lamina propria near the muscularis externa. In ruminant, dog, and pig bladders, the lamina muscularis is extremely thin, and sometimes only isolated smooth muscle cells are seen. In the cat bladder, the lamina muscularis is absent al-

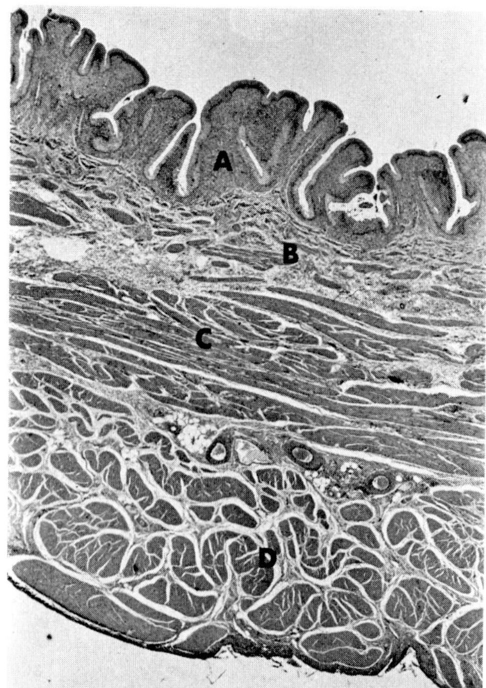

Fig. 11–19. *Urinary bladder, pig. Beneath the mucosa (A) is the tunica muscularis. The inner longitudinal layer (B) is scattered. The middle circular layer (C) and the outer longitudinal layer (D) are the thickest layers. H & E. ×9.*

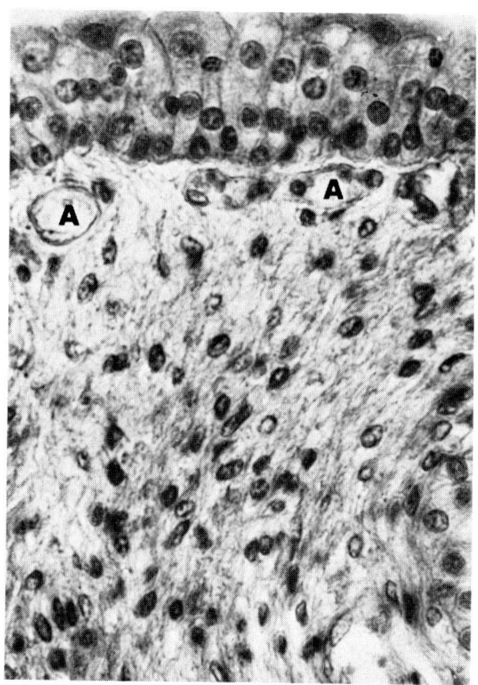

Fig. 11–20. *Urinary bladder, sheep. Capillaries (A) immediately beneath the epithelium, typical of ruminants. H & E. ×570.*

together. At the bladder neck, the lamina muscularis tends to diminish in all animals.

The connective tissue of the bladder submucosa is somewhat looser and contains more elastic fibers than that of the lamina propria. Large blood vessels are located here, along with small ganglia. At the bladder neck, the submucosa becomes extremely thin.

The bladder muscularis is composed of three rather ill-defined layers: an inner and outer longitudinal layer and a middle circular layer. The interweaving pattern of the muscle layers is a distinguishing feature of the bladder. In some regions, such as the vertex and lateral walls, the layers are more definite than in other areas.

The urinary bladder musculature is called the *detrusor muscle,* and at the ureterovesicular junction, the longitudinal ureteral muscle interdigitates with the same layer of the bladder. This forms a functional sphincter, preventing urine reflux. At the bladder neck, the detrusor muscle continues into the urethra and converges toward the urethral orifice. Contraction of the longitudinally oriented muscle bundles widens the urethral lumen and shortens the length. This mechanism initiates micturition. The circularly arranged elastic fibers in the bladder neck and proximal urethra assist in the closure of the urethra following micturition.

As it does in the ureter, the extent of the peritoneal investment of the urinary bladder varies with the different species. The bladders of the dog, cat, and pig are completely invested. The horse bladder has peritoneum over the entire dorsal surface and over half of the ventral aspect. In ruminant bladders, the peritoneum extends farther caudad than in the horse.

The mesothelium rests on a loose connective tissue layer, and in areas where it is absent, only a loose adventitia remains.

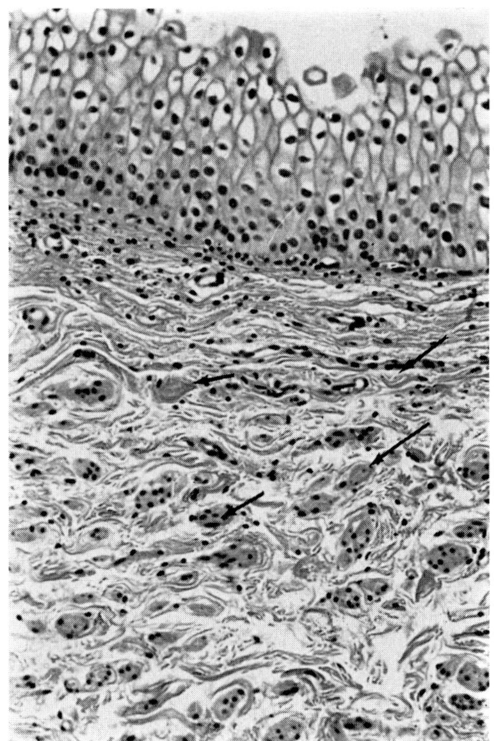

Fig. 11–21. *Urinary bladder, horse. Scattered smooth muscle fiber bundles of the lamina muscularis (arrows). H & E. ×175.*

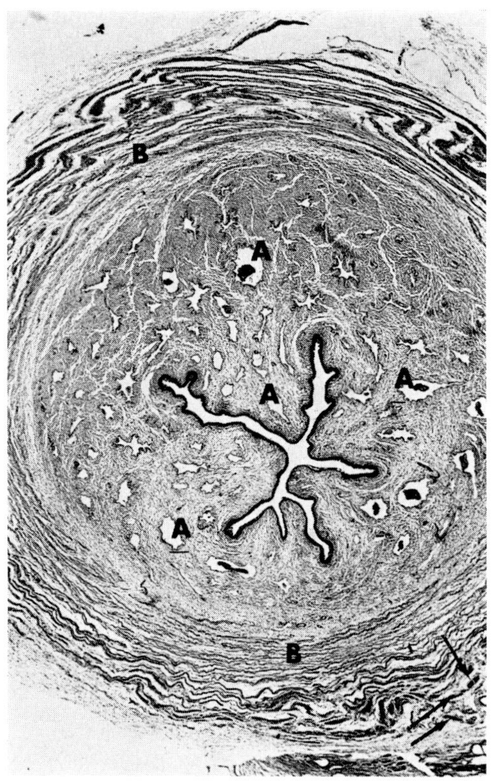

Fig. 11–22. *Urethra, bitch. Section through the middle portion has numerous venous plexuses (A) scattered throughout the lamina-submucosa. The urethral crest is at the nine o'clock position of the lumen. The tunica muscularis is made up primarily of a circular layer (B) with a few scattered longitudinal muscle fiber bundles (arrows). H & E. ×100. (From Adam, W.S., Calhoun, M.L., Smith, E.M., and Stinson, A.W.: Microscopic Anatomy of the Dog: A Photographic Atlas. Springfield, Ill., Charles C Thomas, 1970.)*

Ganglia, blood vessels, and nerves are in the subserosa.

Urethra (Female)

Only the female urethra will be discussed in this section; that of the male is discussed with the male reproductive organs (Chapter 12). The female urethra is a relatively short tube extending from the bladder to the external urinary orifice. The wall has four coats: (1) mucosa, (2) submucosa, (3) muscularis, and (4) adventitia.

The mucosal ridges, which form where the two ureters enter the bladder, converge at the median plane of the bladder neck and continue throughout the entire length of the urethra. The most prominent mucosal fold, the *urethral crest,* and adjacent shallow longitudinal folds tend to give the urethral lumen a stellate appearance (Fig. 11–22). Sections taken distally often have a crescent-shaped lumen owing to the urethral crest and a lack of the other longitudinal folds (Fig. 11–23).

In all domestic animals, the lining epithelium is transitional near the bladder neck and gradually changes to stratified squamous epithelium at the external orifice. Between these two sites are areas of stratified cuboidal or columnar epithelium, either as isolated patches intermixed with transitional epithelium or as a continual lining. The amount and location of these epithelial types are subject to species variations.

In all domestic animals except the doe

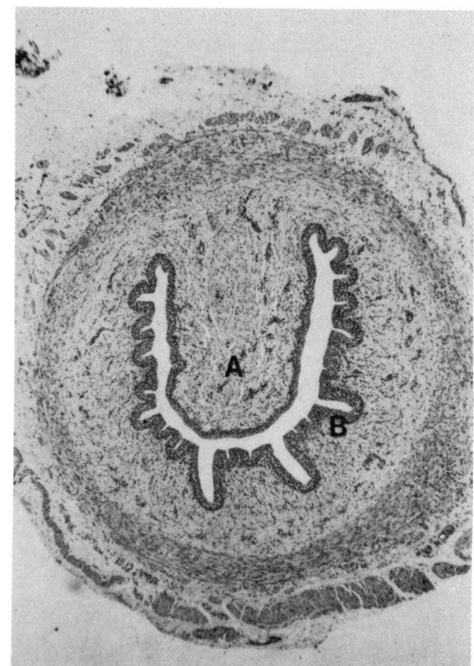

Fig. 11–23. *Urethra, queen. Prominent urethral crest (A) and lumen lined with transitional epithelium (B). H & E. ×37.*

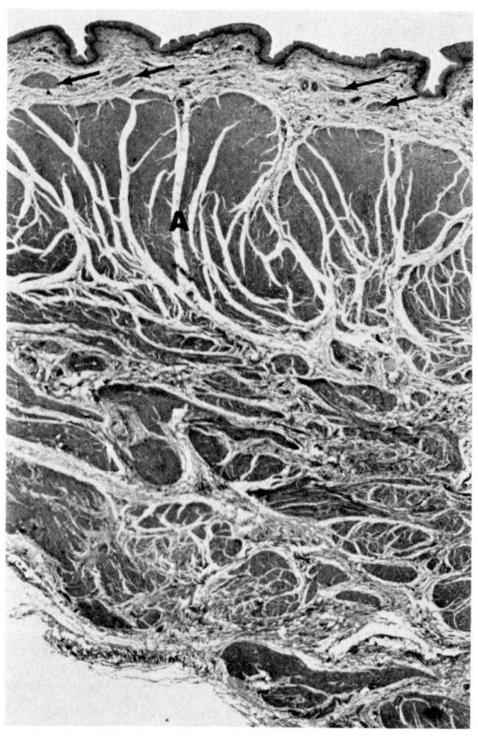

Fig. 11–24. *Urethra, cow. The tunica muscularis has a thick inner circular layer (A), whereas the remaining layers are less discrete. Scattered smooth muscle fiber bundles (arrows) form an incomplete lamina muscularis. H & E. ×9.*

and bitch, some surface cells give a positive reaction for mucous secretion, and in the sow and mare, goblet cells are present near the bladder neck. Only the mare, doe, and ewe have stratified squamous epithelium at the external orifice. In the other domestic animals, the stratified squamous epithelium of the vestibule changes immediately to stratified cuboidal or transitional (sow) epithelium at the external orifice. Frequently, cysts are seen in the epithelium, and in the cow, mare, and sow, there are occasional intraepithelial glands formed by epithelial tubular evaginations.

The fibroelastic propria-submucosa is more compact immediately beneath the epithelium than it is in the deeper portion. In the cow, there is a conspicuous capillary bed adjacent to the epithelial basement membrane. Diffuse lymphatic tissue and occasional lymphatic nodules are common in all domestic animals. Lymphocytes migrate into the epithelium and lie between the surface cells. The propria-submucosa is permeated by cavernous spaces, giving it the appearance of erectile tissue. There are species differences with respect to the distribution and the amount of cavernous tissue throughout the length of the urethra. In the cow, sow, bitch, and mare, cavernous spaces are present throughout the entire length, and they increase both in number and in size toward the urethral orifice. In the queen, ewe, and doe, no cavernous spaces are found in the proximal urethra, but they appear in the lower two thirds.

The existence of a true urethral lamina muscularis is somewhat questionable. Nonetheless, in all domestic animals, isolated longitudinal smooth muscle bundles are scattered in the deep portion of the mucosa, and some bundles extend into the longitudinal mucosal folds. The muscle bundles are more numerous and larger in the mare and cow than in carnivores (Fig. 11–24).

In the proximal urethra, the tunica muscularis contains a thick inner circular and a thin outer longitudinal layer. In the mare, the inner circular layer sometimes has a mixture of longitudinally and circularly oriented fibers, which may give the appearance of three layers.

Distally, where the urethra is related to the ventral vagina, the smooth muscle fibers become intermixed with striated muscle fibers; the amount and the distribution of each type are species-dependent. In carnivores, smooth muscle is replaced by circular striated muscle bundles with a few striated longitudinal fibers. A thin layer of circular smooth muscle lies on the inner side of the striated muscle bundles.

In the other domestic animals, the outer longitudinal layer gradually changes to striated muscle arranged circularly. The inner smooth muscle layer is a mixture of circular and longitudinal fiber bundles.

In ruminants and the pig, there is a suburethral diverticulum at the urethral orifice, lined with transitional epithelium that gradually changes to stratified squamous epithelium. The lamina propria is loose connective tissue infiltrated with lymphocytes and, occasionally, with well-defined lymphatic nodules.

REFERENCES

Bargmann, W., Krisch, B., and Leonhardt, H.: Lipids in the proximal convoluted tubule of the cat kidney and the reabsorption of cholesterol. Cell Tissue Res *177*:523, 1977.

Bharadwaj, M.B., and Calhoun, M.L.: Histology of the urethral epithelium of domestic animals. Am J Vet Res *20*:841, 1959.

Brenner, B.M., and Rector, F.C.: The Kidney. Vols. I and II. Philadelphia, W.B. Saunders Co., 1981.

Bulger, R.E., Siegel, F.L., and Pendergrass, R.: Scanning and transmission electron microscopy of the rat kidney. Am J Anat *139*:483, 1974.

Calhoun, M.L.: Comparative histology of the ureters of domestic animals. Anat Rec *133*:365, 1959.

Kris, W.: Structural organization of the renal medullary counterflow system. Fed Proc *42*:2379, 1983.

Lacy, E.R.: The mammalian renal pelvis: physiological implications from morphometric analyses. Anat Embryol *160*:131, 1980.

Michael, A.F., Keane, W.F., Raij, L., Vernier, R.L., and Mauer, S.M.: The glomerular mesangium. Kidney Int *17*:141, 1980.

Stephenson, J.L.: Renal concentrating mechanism. Fed Proc *42*:2377, 1983.

12

Male Reproductive System

H.-DIETER DELLMANN
KARL-HEINZ WROBEL

The male reproductive system consists of (1) the testes surrounded by the tunica vaginalis and the testicular envelopes, (2) the epididymides, (3) the ductus deferentes, (4) the accessory glands (vesicular, prostate, and bulbourethral), (5) the urethra, and (6) the penis surrounded by the prepuce.

TESTIS

Tunica Vaginalis

When the testis is removed from the scrotum, the parietal layer of the *tunica vaginalis* remains attached to the scrotum, whereas the visceral layer, the peritoneal covering of the testis (and epididymis) remains intimately associated with the underlying capsule of the testis, the *tunica albuginea.* The visceral layer of the tunica vaginalis consists of a mesothelium and a connective tissue layer that blends with the tunica albuginea.

Tunica Albuginea

The *tunica albuginea* is a solid capsule of dense irregular connective tissue (Fig. 12–1). It consists predominantly of collagen fibers and a few elastic fibers. In the stallion, boar, and ram occasional smooth muscle cells are present. Numerous branches of the testicular artery and vein are concentrated in the vascular layer. This layer is located in the deep portions of the tunica albuginea in the boar and stallion and superficially in the dog and ram.

Septula Testis and Intralobular Connective Tissue

The tunica albuginea is continuous with connective tissue trabeculae, the *septula testis,* which converge toward the mediastinum testis. These trabeculae are thick, complete septa in the dog and boar, whereas in ruminants and the cat (Fig. 12–1) they are thin, often inconspicuous, and incomplete. They are composed predominantly of collagen fibers, contain vessels and nerves and divide the testis into a varying number of testicular lobules, each containing one to four convoluted tubules. The septula are continuous with the intralobular connective tissue. Each convoluted seminiferous tubule is surrounded by a basal lamina, often with club-shaped projections into basal infoldings of sustentacular cells, followed by a layer of collagen

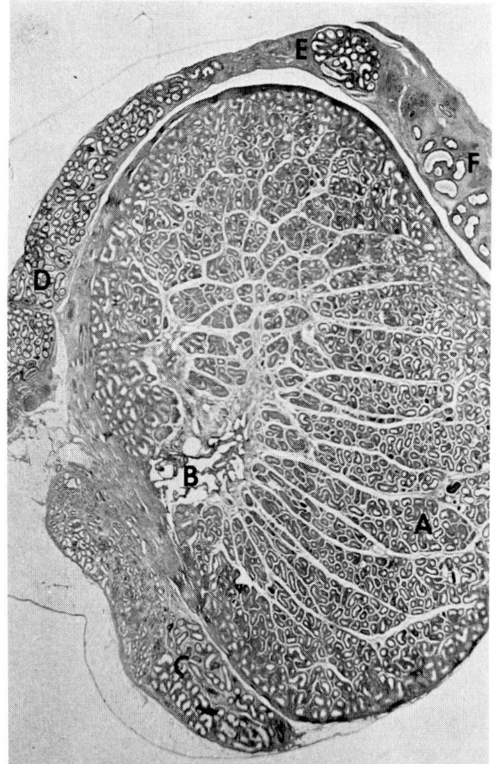

Fig. 12–1. *Testis, cat. The convoluted seminiferous tubules in the lobuli testis (A) are separated by thin septula testis and converge toward the rete testis (B); head (C), body (D) and tail (E) of the epididymis; initial portion of the ductus deferens (F). H & E. ×5.3.*

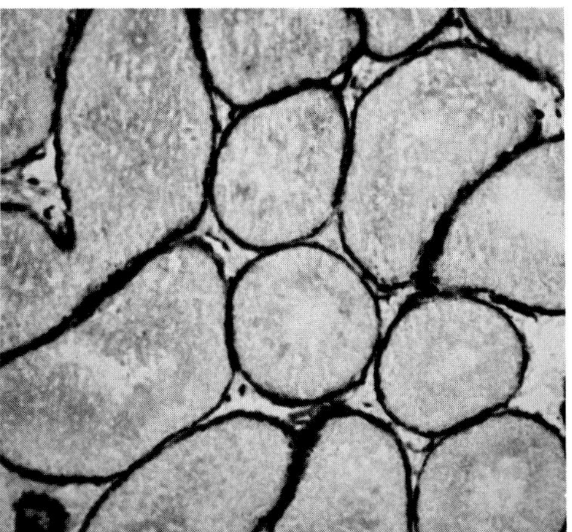

Fig. 12–2. *Testis, goat. Positive alkaline phosphatase reaction of the contractile elements surrounding the seminiferous tubules. ×50.*

fibrils and elastic fibers. In addition, peritubular cells that have a strong alkaline phosphatase activity surround the tubules in one or several layers (Fig. 12–2). They are ensheathed by a basal lamina that is complete in the boar and indistinct in the bull. In the prepubertal testis, the peritubular cells resemble fibroblasts that acquire characteristics of smooth muscle cells at puberty (micropinocytotic vesicles at the cell surface and numerous filaments, 6 to 7 nm thick, in the cytoplasm). These changes are induced by hypophyseal hormones and androgen. The peritubular cells are responsible for the contractions observed in isolated seminiferous tubules; they participate in spermiation and transport of tubular content. The outermost layer of the tubular propria consists of fibrocytes and irregularly arranged bundles of collagen fibrils.

Mediastinum Testis

Centrally, the septula are continuous with the loose connective tissue of the *mediastinum testis* (Fig. 12–1). In the stallion, the mediastinum testis is restricted to the cranial pole of the testis, but in most other domestic mammals it occupies a central position.

Interstitial Cells

The intertubular spaces contain blood and lymph vessels, fibrocytes, free mononuclear cells, and interstitial endocrine (Leydig) cells (Fig. 12–3). The latter produce testicular androgens and, in the boar, large amounts of estrogens as well. The number of interstitial cells varies considerably in the different species and is age-dependent. In the adult bull, interstitial cells constitute approximately 7% of the entire testicular volume. The interstitial cells are particularly abundant in the boar (20 to 30% of the testicular tissue in the adult boar) and stallion. Interstitial endocrine cells occur in cords or clusters, not

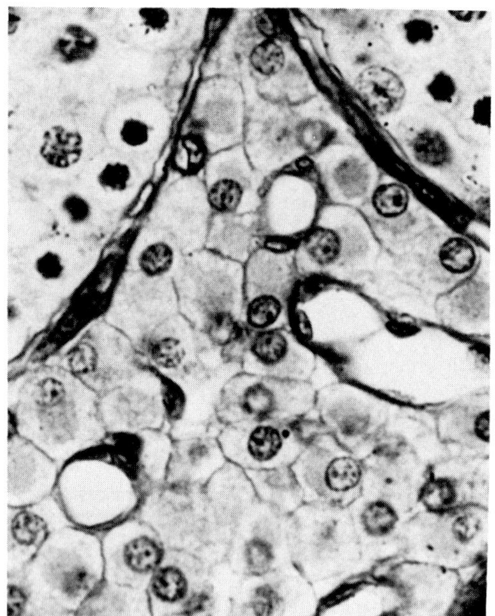

Fig. 12–3. *Testis, boar. Interstitial cells are particularly abundant in the intertubular connective tissue. PAS. ×700.*

every cell being in close contact to a capillary. Between adjacent cells are intercellular canaliculi and gap junctions. High concentrations of steroids are found in testicular tissue and lymph.

The interstitial endocrine cells are irregular, polyhedral cells with spherical nuclei containing peripherally concentrated chromatin (Fig. 12–3). Lipid inclusions are found in all species. In the stallion and cat, a varying amount of glycogen is present. The abundant smooth ER of the interstitial endocrine cells contains steroid dehydrogenases and increases considerably at puberty, as does the number of mitochondria. These possess tubular cristae and are involved in some of the steps in testosterone synthesis, e.g., the cleavage of the side chain of cholesterol in the transformation of cholesterol to pregnenolone. The function of the relatively small Golgi complex in hormone secretion is obscure. Storage of testosterone within the cell and its release from the cell are morphologically inconspicuous. Among the main functions of testosterone are (1) promotion of normal sexual behavior (libido), (2) triggering of the growth and maintenance of the function of the male accessory glands and secondary sex characteristics, (3) control of spermatogenesis (together with FSH), (4) negative feedback action on the hypophysis and hypothalamus, and (5) general anabolic effects.

Convoluted Seminiferous Tubules

The convoluted seminiferous tubules (tubuli seminiferi convoluti) (Fig. 12–1) are tortuous tubules with a diameter of 200 to 400 μm lined by a stratified epithelium consisting of two different basic cell types: sustentacular (supporting, Sertoli) cells and spermatogenic cells.

SUSTENTACULAR CELLS

Sustentacular cells are derived from undifferentiated supporting cells of the prepubertal gonad. These cells are mitotically active, contain large amounts of rough ER, and produce the anti-paramesonephric-hormone, a glycoprotein that suppresses development of uterine tubes, uterus, and vagina in the male.

During puberty, sustentacular cell differentiation is accompanied by a morphologic transformation and loss of mitotic capability.

The adult sustentacular cells are irregularly outlined, elongated cells. Their broad base rests on the basement membrane and the remaining cytoplasm extends upward to the tubular lumen (Fig. 12–4). They are rather evenly spaced; between 25 and 30 sustentacular cells are seen in a cross section of a seminiferous tubule. Lateral cytoplasmic processes of the sustentacular cells fill all the spaces between adjacent spermatogenic cells. The spherical, oval, or pear-shaped nucleus is generally located in the broad portion of the cell and often deeply infolded; furthermore, an exceptionally large nucleolus is present. The sustentacular cells of all do-

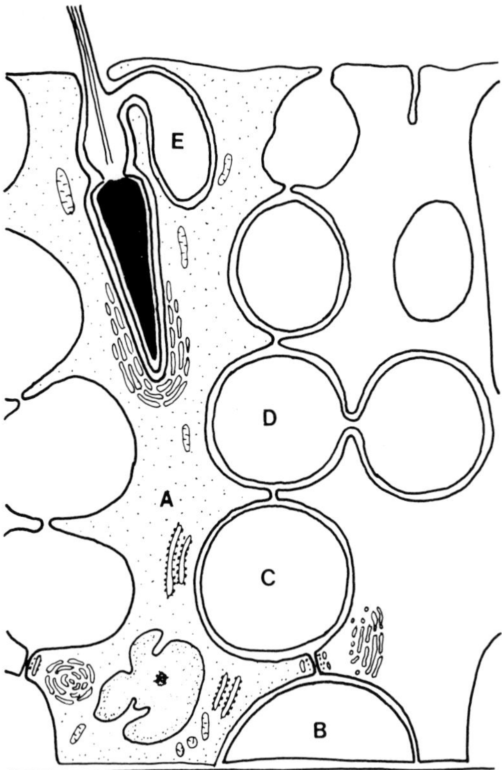

Fig. 12–4. *Diagrammatic representation of sustentacular cell-germ cell interrelationships. (A) sustentacular cell; (B) spermatogonium; (C) spermatocyte; (D) spermatid; (E) residual cytoplasm (body). (Modified from L. Plöen.)*

mestic mammals contain varying amounts of lipid inclusions and glycogen. Microfilaments, microtubules, and smooth ER are abundant, but little granular ER is found. Often, the apical cell surface is deeply indented by old spermatids, and at the level of their acrosomal region, superficially located cisternae of ER associated with microfilaments are a characteristic feature of the sustentacular cells. Similar structures are present in regions of close contact between adjacent sustentacular cells.

These regions are localized near the bases of adjacent sustentacular cells, above the level of the spermatogonia and early spermatocytes. Here the sustentacular cells are joined by special junctions that separate a basal from an adluminal (apical) compartment. The division of the spermatogonia and the renewal of the stem cells take place in the basal compartment, i.e., in an area that has access to tissue fluid. The tight junctions constitute a diffusion barrier, also referred to as the blood-testis barrier, that provides a microenvironment in the adluminal compartment within which the complicated processes of meiosis and spermiogenesis occur without major outside disturbance. Early spermatocytes have to pass through these junctions without interrupting the physiologic blood-testis barrier. This is probably accomplished by a zipperlike opening of these junctions, which close again below the spermatocytes before they reach the adluminal compartment. It is important to realize that all the descendants of one spermatogonium form a syncytium, i.e., they are interconnected by cytoplasmic bridges.

Sustentacular cells have nutritive, protective, and supportive functions for the spermatogenic cells. In addition, they phagocytize regressive spermatozoa and detached residual bodies of spermatids. They release the spermatozoa into the lumen of the seminiferous tubules (spermiation). They mediate the action of FSH on the germ cells, participate in the synchronization of spermatogenic events, produce an androgen-binding protein, and secrete the intratubular fluid, containing potassium, inositol, glutamate transferrin, and inhibin. Inhibin of Sertoli cell origin is reabsorbed from the lumen of the efferent ductules and the initial segment of epididymis. It then reaches the blood stream and exerts a negative feedback on hypophyseal FSH secretion. Although normal sustentacular cells have only a minimal proven steroidogenic function, sustentacular cell tumors may produce large amounts of estrogen, leading to feminization of the organism.

SPERMATOGENIC CELLS

Various *spermatogenic cells,* representing different phases in the development and differentiation of the spermatozoon, are located between and above the sustentacular cells. The sequence of events in the development of spermatozoa from spermatogonia is referred to as *spermatogenesis* and is subdivided into three phases: (1) spermatocytogenesis, the process during which spermatogonia develop into spermatocytes; (2) meiosis, the maturation division of spermatocytes that results in spermatids with a reduced (haploid) number of chromosomes; and (3) spermiogenesis, the process of transformation of spermatids into spermatozoa.

SPERMATOCYTOGENESIS. The spermatogenic stem cell is a diploid cell referred to as a spermatogonium. In all mammals, the spermatogonia undergo a phase of multiplication; however, the number of mitotic divisions is species-dependent. In the bull, ram, and boar, essentially three types of spermatogonia can be distinguished—A type, intermediate (I) type, and B type—but the morphologic differences are too subtle to be discussed here. In the bull, they undergo a total of six mitotic divisions: three A divisions, one I division, and two

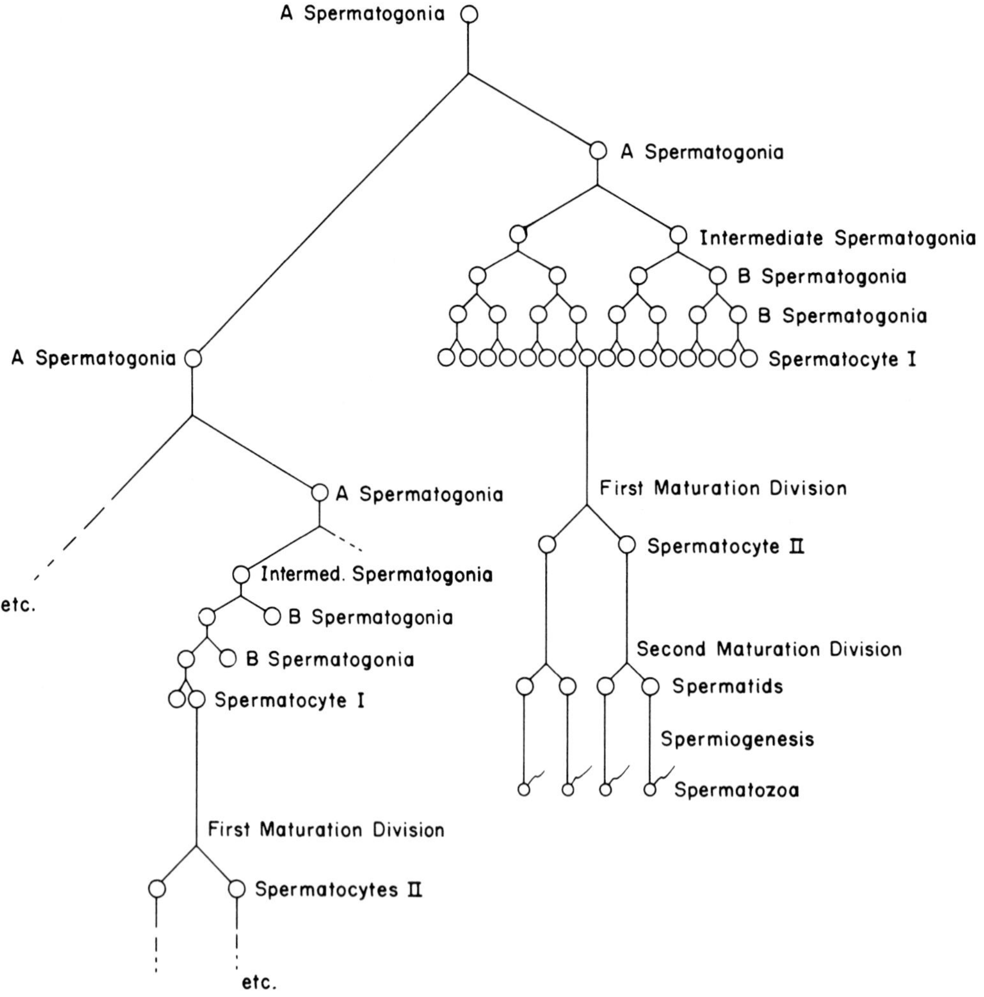

Fig. 12–5. *Schematic drawing of the sequential events during spermatogenesis, bull, boar, stallion. (Redrawn and slightly modified from Ortavant, R., Courot, M., and Hochereau, M.T.: Spermatogenesis and morphology of the spermatozoon.* In *Reproduction in Domestic Animals, 2nd Ed. Edited by H.H. Cole and P.T. Cupps. New York, Academic Press, 1969, pp. 251–276.)*

B divisions. The division of a stem spermatogonium (type A) results in one daughter cell that is the beginning of a spermatogenic series. The other daughter cell becomes a new stem cell (Fig. 12–5). It remains inactive until the descendants of the first daughter cell give rise to primary spermatocytes, at which time it divides and again gives origin to one new stem cell and one cell that begins a spermatogenic series. Thus, the continuity of stem cells and uninterrupted spermatogenesis are guaranteed. The diploid set of chromosomes (stallion, bull, buck, 60; ran, 54; boar, 38; dog, 78; cat, 38) is visible particularly during the long prophase.

Primary spermatocytes are the result of the last mitotic division of (and at the beginning of their development are similar to) B-type spermatogonia. Subsequently, the spermatocytes develop into the largest cells of the entire spermatogenic series. They are located in a more central position within the wall of the tubule than those of the previous stages (Fig. 12–6). Between 25 and 60% of the developing spermatogonia degenerate during spermatocytogenesis.

MEIOSIS. During meiosis, two successive nuclear divisions occur, resulting in a reduction of the number of chromosomes from diploid (2 n) to haploid (n). The primary spermatocytes go through the initial phase of meiosis, called the first maturation division. The results of this division are secondary spermatocytes.

The prophase of the first maturation division is subdivided into the leptotene, zygotene, pachytene, diplotene, and diakinesis stages. During the leptotene phase, the chromosomes replicate during interphase; consisting of two daughter chromatids, they become arranged in thin, threadlike strands. In the zygotene stage, homologous chromosomes begin to pair (synapse). Completion of pairing initiates the pachytene phase, during which crossover occurs between the two non-sister chromatids of the paired chromosomes (tetrads). In microscopic preparations, primary spermatocytes are best identified when they are in this phase of meiosis (Fig. 12–6). During the diplotene phase, the paired chromosomes pull away from each other, but sister chromatids remain attached through chiasmata, i.e., sites where crossover has occurred. During diakinesis, the chromosomes shorten and broaden and the four separate chromatids in each chromosome are clearly evident.

The metaphase, anaphase, and telophase occur rapidly. During these phases, the paired chromosomes are first arranged at the equatorial plate; subsequently homologous chromosomes are separated and individual chromosomes move to opposite poles of the cell to be distributed to the daughter cells, at which time they uncoil and lengthen. The small secondary spermatocytes resulting from this first maturation division are more centrally located than the primary spermatocytes (Fig. 12–6).

After a very short period of interphase, during which no duplication of genetic material occurs, the secondary spermatocytes undergo the second maturation division, with a short prophase followed by meta-, ana-, and telophases, which are essentially similar to those of mitotic divisions. During this division, the centromeres divide and the sister chromatids of the secondary spermatocytes separate and are distributed to each of the spermatids resulting from that division. Thus, these cells possess a haploid set of chromosomes. It is important to emphasize once more that germ cells of the same developmental stages, from spermatogonia through spermatids, are frequently and perhaps regularly interconnected by cytoplasmic bridges, which contributes to the synchronized maturation of the cells.

SPERMIOGENESIS. The process by which the spermatids differentiate into spermatozoa involves a certain number of nuclear and cytoplasmic transformations and is referred to as *spermiogenesis*. Early spermatids

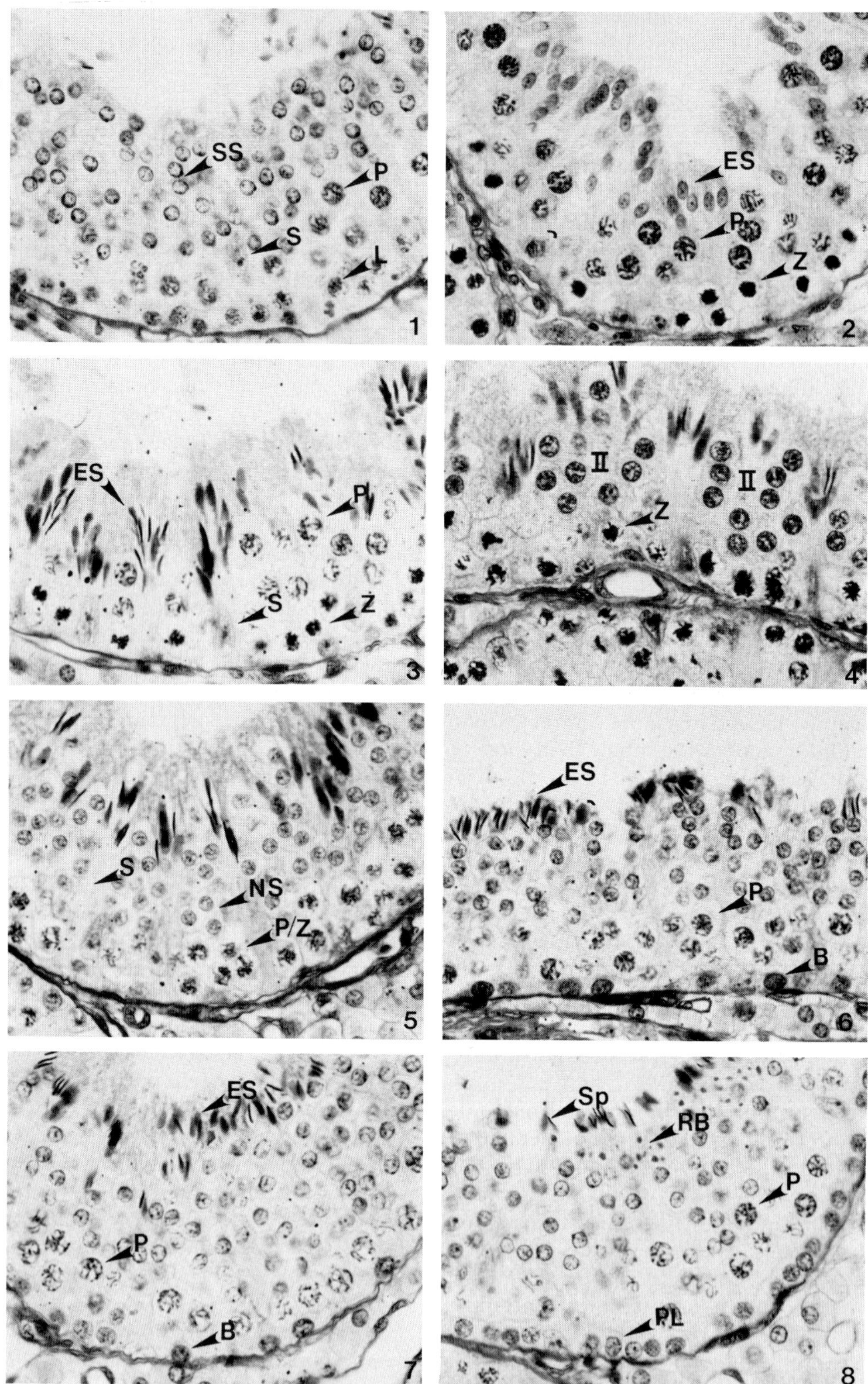

Fig. 12–6. *The eight stages of the spermatogenic cycle, boar. (B) B spermatogonia; (ES) elongated spermatids; (L) Leptotene primary spermatocytes; (NS) Newly formed spermatids; (P) pachytene primary spermatocytes; (PL) preleptotene primary spermatocytes; (P/Z) primary spermatocytes leaving zygotene and entering pachytene; (RB) Residual bodies; (S) Sustentacular cell; (Sp) Spermatozoa in spermiation; (SS) Spherical spermatids; (II) Secondary spermatocytes. PAS. ×500.*

are small, spherical cells with a central spherical nucleus (Fig. 12–6). They are smaller than the secondary spermatocytes and located in a more central position in the tubule. During their maturation, the spermatids are surrounded by the processes of the supporting cells.

The most important morphologic changes during spermiogenesis are the formation of the acrosome, the condensation, transformation, and shift of the nucleus to an eccentric location within the cell, and the formation of the motile tail. In the spermatid nucleus a shift occurs in the histone content from a lysine-rich to an arginine-rich variety, which helps to condense and stabilize the DNA of the spermatozoon.

Spermiogenesis is divided into Golgi phase, cap phase, acrosomal phase, and maturation phase.

During the *Golgi phase* of spermiogenesis, proacrosomal granules appear in the Golgi vesicles and eventually fuse to form a single acrosomal granule (Fig. 12–6) within the acrosomal vesicle. During the *cap phase,* both the acrosomal granule and vesicle move toward the anterior pole of the nucleus. Here the acrosomal granule flattens and is now called the acrosome. The acrosomal vesicle grows and covers approximately the anterior two thirds of the nucleus at the head cap. During the transition from the cap phase to the *acrosomal phase,* the nucleus elongates and becomes eccentrically located within the cell, directed toward the periphery of the tubule and the forming tail toward the lumen. During the *acrosomal phase,* most of the acrosome remains localized at the anterior pole of the nucleus, and the remainder of the acrosome spreads into the head cap. At this point the entire structure is referred to as the acrosomal cap. Both the spermatid nucleus and the spermatid become elongated. During the *maturation phase,* after the development of the tail is completed, the residual body, which consists of excess cytoplasm containing a few inclusions and organelles, is separated from the spermatozoon, and the intercellular bridges between the germ cells are now interrupted.

During early acrosome formation, the centrioles move toward the caudal pole of the cell where the distal centriole gives rise to the outgrowing flagellum, and subsequently move back to the caudal pole of the nucleus with the base of the flagellum. Microtubules project caudally from a ring-like specialization of the cell membrane at the caudal edge of the acrosomal cap to form the caudal sheath or manchette, a temporary structure whose significance is not fully understood. At the same time, elongation of the spermatid takes place. Concurrently, two rings, one small and dense and the other large and less dense, arise around the distal centriole. The distal centriole and the large ring disappear during further maturation, and the small ring (annulus) moves distad and marks the distal end of the middle piece of the mature spermatozoon. Concomitantly with the aforementioned changes, the caudal sheath disappears and mitochondria form a helix in the periphery of the middle piece. The connecting piece forms nine longitudinally oriented columns around the centrioles, connected distally to nine longitudinal fibers peripheral to the nine double fibrils of the flagellum. Finally, in some mysterious way, semicircular ribs form the fibrous sheath around the tail fibers in the principal piece of the spermatozoon.

In most species, all cells originating from a B-type spermatogonium (i.e., two primary spermatocytes, four secondary spermatocytes and finally eight spermatids) are linked together by cytoplasmic bridges. These bridges are interrupted when the individual spermatozoa are released into the lumen of the seminiferous tubule. At the same time, the residual body is disconnected from the spermatozoa.

SPERMATOZOON

With the light microscope, the spermatozoon appears to consist essentially of two

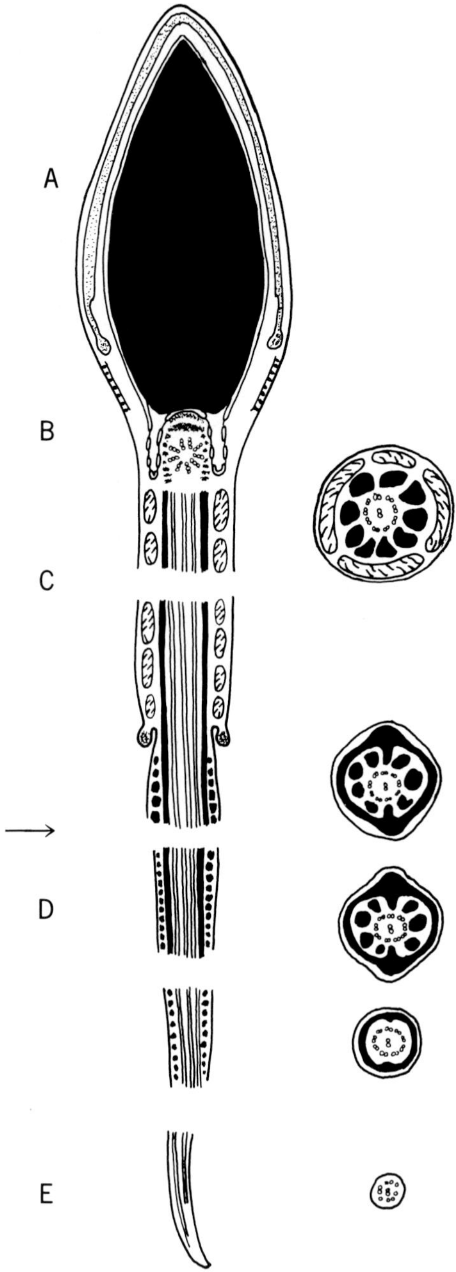

Fig. 12–7. *Schematic drawing of a spermatozoon. Left, longitudinal section; right, cross sections located at the levels from which they are taken. A, Head containing the nucleus covered by the acrosome. Notice equatorial segment of the acrosome and post-acrosomal sheath. B, Neck. C, Middle piece with central fibrils, nine outer dense fibers and the surrounding mitochondria. The middle piece terminates with the anulus (arrow). D, Principal piece in which the central fibrils continue to be surrounded by the fibrous sheath and terminate before the end of the principal piece. E, End piece made up of the irregularly arranged central fibrils terminating at various levels.*

portions: the head and the tail. With the electron microscope, the tail is seen to be further subdivided into neck, middle piece, principal piece, and end piece (Fig. 12–7).

HEAD. The shape of the nucleus determines the shape of the head of the spermatozoon, which is species-dependent and subject to great variations. The anterior pole of the nucleus is covered by the acrosomal cap, which contains a number of hydrolytic enzymes: hyaluronidase, aryl sulfatase, unspecific esterase, and acrosin. These are needed for the penetration of the cumulus oophorus and zona pellucida by the spermatozoa. The caudal region of the acrosome is characterized by a narrowing of the cap and condensation of its contents. This is the equatorial segment of the acrosome. The base of the nucleus is surrounded by the postacrosomal sheath, which consists of fibrous proteins rich in sulfur. In dead spermatozoa, it stains intensely with certain dyes, such as eosin or bromophenol blue. This reaction is used to evaluate the quality of an ejaculate. Both the equatorial segment and the postacrosomal sheath participate in the process of fertilization.

NECK. The neck is a relatively short and narrow structure between the head and middle piece. It consists of a centrally located centriole and nine peripheral, longitudinally oriented, coarse fibers continuous with the outer fibers of the middle piece.

MIDDLE PIECE. The core of the middle piece has the characteristic structure of a flagellum: two central microtubules and nine peripheral doublets (microtubules) making up the axial filament complex. They are surrounded by nine longitudinally oriented, tapered outer fibers that are connected to the fibers of the connecting piece. These in turn are surrounded by the mitochondria in a helicoidal arrangement. A ring-shaped thickening of the plasma membrane (anulus) of the middle piece marks the limit between middle piece and principal piece.

PRINCIPAL PIECE. The principal piece is the longest portion of the tail of the spermatozoon. The axial filament complex has a structure identical to that of the middle piece and is surrounded by the continuing outer fibers of the middle piece. The fibers are subject to variations in size and shape and gradually taper toward the end of the principal piece. Semicircular ribs of structural proteins in a helicoidal arrangement fuse to two of the outer fibers to form the characteristic peripheral fibrous sheath of the principal piece.

END PIECE. The termination of the fibrous sheath marks the beginning of the end piece, which contains only the axial filament complex. Proximally in the end piece, this complex has its characteristic nine-plus-two arrangement; distally, the peripheral doublets gradually become reduced to singlets and terminate at various levels.

CYCLIC EVENTS IN THE SEMINIFEROUS TUBULES

Before one spermatogenic series is completed, several new spermatogenic series are initiated at the same level within the seminiferous tubule. As all the descendants of each stem cell develop synchronously, successive cell generations follow each other with cyclic regularity, from the periphery toward the center of the seminiferous tubule.

Changes in the shape and stainability of the nuclei during cell division and the release of spermatozoa into the tubular lumen provide a basis for dividing the spermatogenic cycle into stages. In testes of the bull, ram, and boar, it is possible to identify eight stages.

Stage 1. Following spermiation, spherical spermatids lie nearest to the lumen, followed basally by two generations of primary spermatocytes, i.e., old pachytenes and young leptotenes (Fig. 12–6-1).

Stage 2. The spermatids and their dark-stained nuclei are elongated. There are two generations of primary spermatocytes: old pachytenes and young zygotenes (Fig. 12–6-2).

Stage 3. Elongated spermatids are arranged in bundles in close association with the apical portion of the sustentacular cells (Fig. 12–6-3).

Stage 4. The first and second maturation divisions take place. In addition to bundles of maturing spermatids and zygotene primary spermatocytes, either diplotene secondary spermatocytes or spherical spermatids are seen (Fig. 12–6-4).

Stage 5. Two generations of spermatids are present, older elongated spermatids and newly formed spherical spermatids. The zygotenes of stage 4 enter pachytene stage and leave their basal position (Fig. 12–6-5).

Stage 6. The bundles of older spermatids have moved away from the vicinity of the sustentacular cell nuclei. In addition to spherical spermatids, pachytenes and dark spermatogonia lie near the basal lamina.

Stage 7. The older spermatids continue to migrate centrally. Spermatogonia divide to form preleptotenes (Fig. 12–6-6).

Stage 8. Spermatozoa leave the tubular epithelium following separation from their residual bodies. Remaining within the epithelium are spherical spermatids and two generations of primary spermatocytes (older pachytenes and young preleptotenes).

In all domestic animals, not only are the descendants of one spermatogonium all at the same stage of development, but identical cellular associations are found over a certain distance in cross and longitudinal sections of seminiferous tubules. These spermatogenic segments, portions with synchronized development of germ cells, are usually arranged so that one specific segment is adjacent to the preceding and following stages of the spermatogenic cycle. If stages 1 through 8 succeed each other along the length of the seminiferous tubule, the sequence is referred to as a spermatogenic wave, which is about 10 mm long in the bull. However, it seems that variations such as repetition of wave fragments (1-2-3-4-1-2-3-4) or inversions (1-2-3-4-5-4-3-2) occur more frequently. Exactly what determines the spermatogenic cycles, segments, and waves is not known at this time.

Straight Testicular Tubules

In all domestic mammals, most of the convoluted seminiferous tubules terminate in the vicinity of the rete testis; they continue into the straight testicular tubules (tubuli recti), which connect them to the rete testis. Straight testicular tubules are short and have either a straight or tortuous course. In the stallion and boar, some of the convoluted seminiferous tubules terminate at the periphery of the testis and join the rete testis by long, straight *tubuli recti.* The terminal segment of the convoluted seminiferous tubule is lined by modified sustentacular cells that occlude the tubular lumen and project their apices into the cup-shaped initial portion of the straight testicular tubule (Fig. 12–8). All spermatozoa have to pass through the narrow intercellular slits between adjacent modified sustentacular cells on their way to the straight tubule. The terminal segment may further function as a valve preventing reflux of rete testis fluid into the seminiferous tubules.

The straight testicular tubules are lined with a simple squamous to columnar epithelium. In the bull a simple cuboidal epithelium lines the proximal portion of the straight tubules, and a simple columnar epithelium lines the distal portion (Fig. 12–9). This epithelium contains numerous macrophages and lymphocytes and is able to phagocytize spermatozoa.

Rete Testis

Irregularly anastomosing canals, surrounded by the loose connective tissue of the mediastinum testis, form the rete testis. It is lined by simple squamous or columnar epithelium. Elastic fibers and contractile cells are present underneath the epithelium. Most of the testicular fluid, which is reabsorbed in the head of the epididymis, is produced in the rete testis (in the ram, approximately 40 ml/day). Rete testis fluid differs in composition from tubular seminiferous fluid, testicular lymph, and blood plasma.

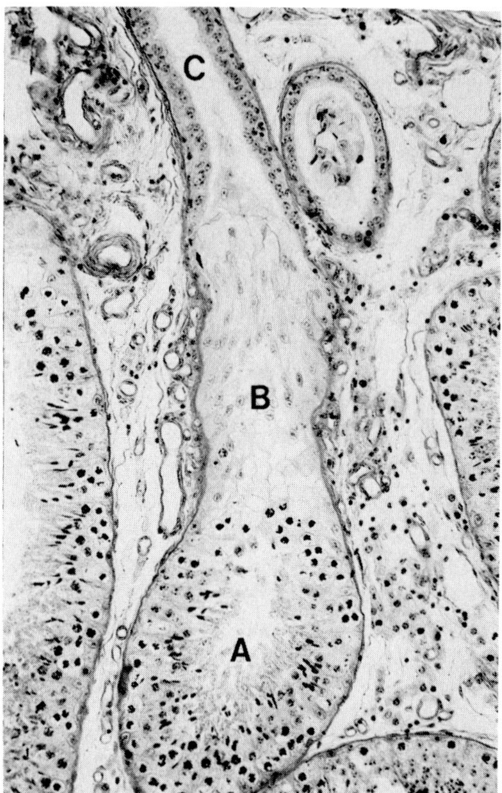

Fig. 12–8. *Convoluted seminiferous tubule (A), terminal segment (B) surrounded by a vascular plexus, and straight testicular tubule (C). Testis, bull. Ironhematoxylin. ×140.*

Testicular Blood Supply

The testicular artery has a straight abdominal portion and becomes highly coiled after reaching the spermatic cord. Very small nutritive twigs and the epididymal arteries branch from the coiled portion. As the artery enters the testis it courses parallel to the epididymis and is embedded in

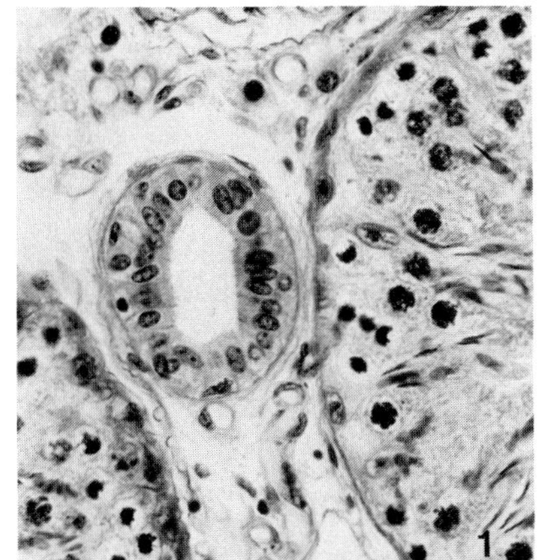

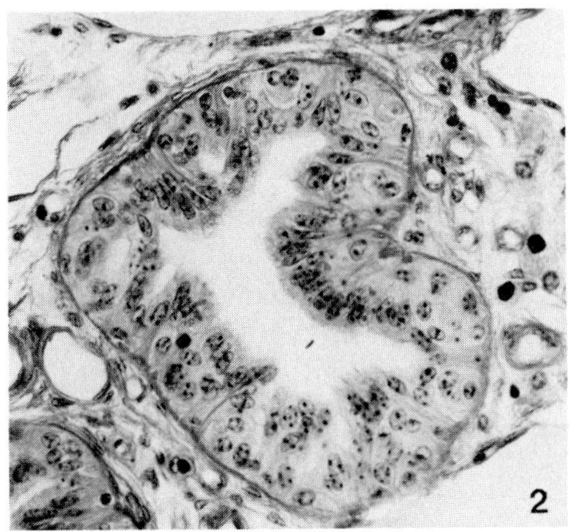

Fig. 12–9. *Proximal (1) and distal (2) portion of the straight testicular tubules, bull. Notice differences in tubule diameter and the lining epithelium. Masson-Goldner. ×350.*

the tunica albuginea. The testicular artery divides at the caudal testicular pole to form the arterial contributions to the vascular layer of the tunica albuginea. Within the septula testis, centripetal arteries course to the mediastinum testis. From here smaller centrifugal arteries return to supply the testicular parenchyma. Most of the testicular veins empty into superficial veins situated in the tunica albuginea. These converge at the base of the spermatic cord to form the pampiniform plexus, which is composed of three interconnected networks filling the available space in such a way that the windings of the testicular artery are completely surrounded by the valveless veins. This remarkable vascular topography in the mammalian spermatic cord is believed to function as a thermoregulator and venous-arterial steroid transfer.

EPIDIDYMIS

The mammalian epididymis is a dynamic accessory sex organ, dependent on testicular androgens for the maintenance of a differentiated state of its epithelium. It comprises several (8 to 25) ductuli efferentes and a long, coiled ductus epididymidis. Macroscopically, the epididymis is divided into a head, body, and tail. It is surrounded by a thick tunica albuginea of dense irregular connective tissue covered by the visceral layer of the tunica vaginalis. In the stallion, the tunica albuginea has a few smooth muscle cells scattered throughout the dense connective tissue.

Ductuli Efferentes

Between 8 and 25 ductuli efferentes connect the rete testis to the ductus epididymidis. The ductules are gathered in small lobules (coni vasculosi) with distinct boundaries of connective tissue. The epithelium of the efferent ductules is simple columnar and consists of ciliated and nonciliated cells (Figs. 12–10 and 12–11-1). Scattered lymphocytes in the basal epithelial area have been misinterpreted as a third genuine cell type. The ciliated cells (apical row of nuclei) help to move the spermatozoa toward the ductus epididymidis. The nonciliated cells (basal row of nuclei) have microvilli and a well-developed endocytotic apparatus consisting of coated micropinocytotic invaginations, coated vesicles, microcanaliculi, and resorptive vacuoles. The majority of the nonciliated cells are involved in resorptive processes; others may have a secretory activity. The nonciliated cells contain globular PAS-positive residual bodies following resorption and digestion of ductular fluid (Fig. 12–11-2). Intermediate forms between ciliated and nonciliated epithelial

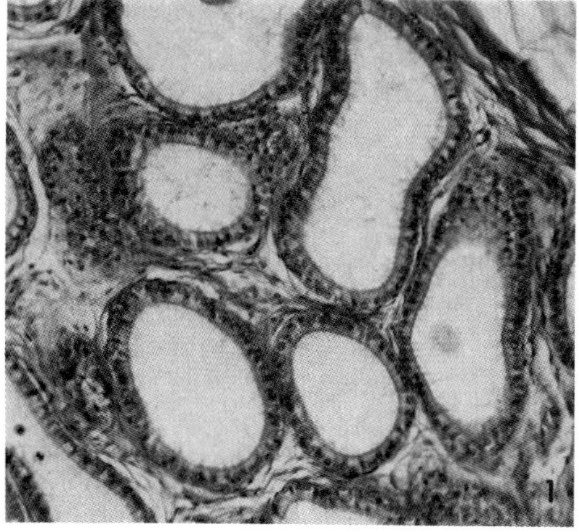

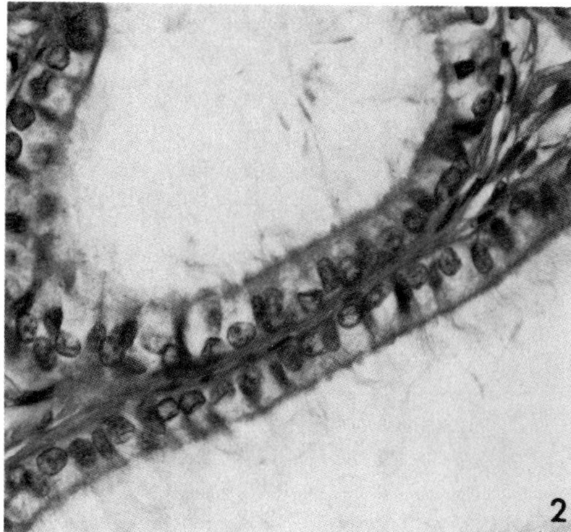

Fig. 12–10. *Testis, cat. 1, Ductuli efferentes surrounded by highly vascularized loose connective tissue. H & E. ×95. 2, Higher-power photomicrograph of the wall of two adjacent ductuli. H & E. ×133.*

cells are occasionally observed. The ductular epithelium is surrounded by 3 to 6 loosely arranged layers of modified smooth muscle cells and connective tissue. The ductuli efferentes and the initial portions of the ductus epididymidis constitute the head of the epididymis.

Ductus Epididymidis

The ductus epididymidis is extremely tortuous and coiled. The length of the duct varies considerably among species and has been estimated to be 40 m in the bull and boar and 70 m in the stallion. Despite these differences, sperm transport through the epididymis seems to require 10 to 15 days in most mammalian species.

The ductus epididymidis is lined by a pseudostratified epithelium, surrounded by a small amount of loose connective tissue and circular smooth muscle fibers, the number of which increases significantly toward the tail of the epididymis. Two cell

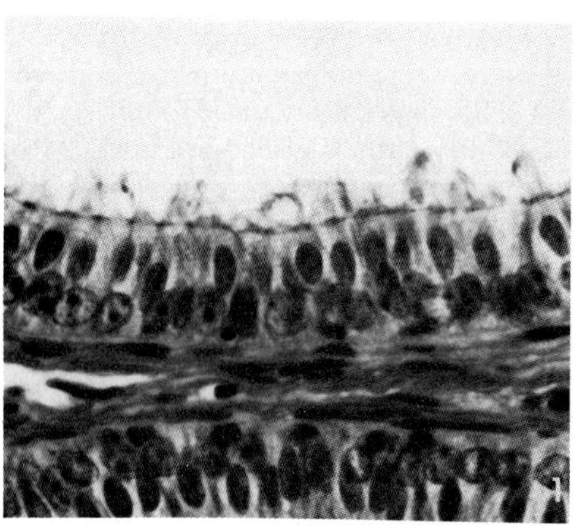

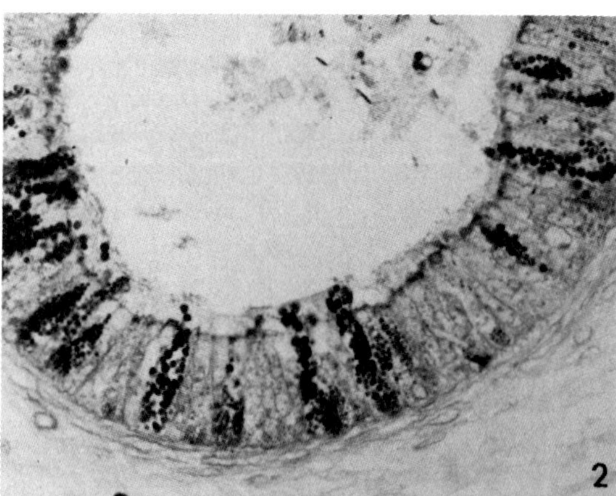

Fig. 12–11. *Efferent ductules, bull. 1, The pseudostratified columnar epithelium consists of basal cells (dense basal nuclei), secretory and resorptive cells (light spherical nuclei) and ciliated cells (dense ovoid nuclei). Masson-Goldner-Jerusalem trichrome. ×560. 2, Selective staining of nonciliated cells. PAS reaction following digestion by diastase. ×350.*

types are invariably present in the epithelium: columnar principal cells and small, polygonal basal cells (Fig. 12–12). In many species, additional cell types such as apical cells and clear cells are present. Macrophages and lymphocytes also occur within the epithelium.

The principal cells are generally taller in the head of the epididymis than in the remainder of the organ. The apical surfaces of the columnar cells bear long and sometimes branching microvilli (stereocilia), whose lengths decrease toward the tail. The occurrence of micropinocytotic invaginations at the bases of the microvilli and the presence of coated vesicles and multivesicular bodies in the apical cytoplasm indicate that the epididymal epithelium has a high resorptive capacity. Most of the fluid (over 90%) that leaves the testis is reabsorbed in the ductuli efferentes and the proximal part of the epididymal duct. Androgen-binding protein produced by the sustentacular cells of the seminiferous tubules is also reabsorbed in the initial segment of the ductus epididymidis. The secretion of various substances such as glycerophosphoryl choline, and glycoproteins, such as phosphatase and glycosidase, is also well established.

On the basis of histologic, histochemical, and ultrastructural criteria, the ductus epididymidis may be subdivided into several segments (six in the bull), the distribution and number of which are characteristic for each species (Fig. 12–12). Generally, the proximal parts of the duct (head and body) are involved in the maturation process of spermatozoa, whereas the cauda epididymidis serves as their main storage place. It is here that 45% of the bull's epididymal spermatozoa are stored. Spermatozoa leaving the testis are both immotile and infertile, whereas spermatozoa leaving the epididymis have gained motility and fertility. During their sojourn through the ductus epididymidis, spermatozoa undergo a series of morphologic and functional

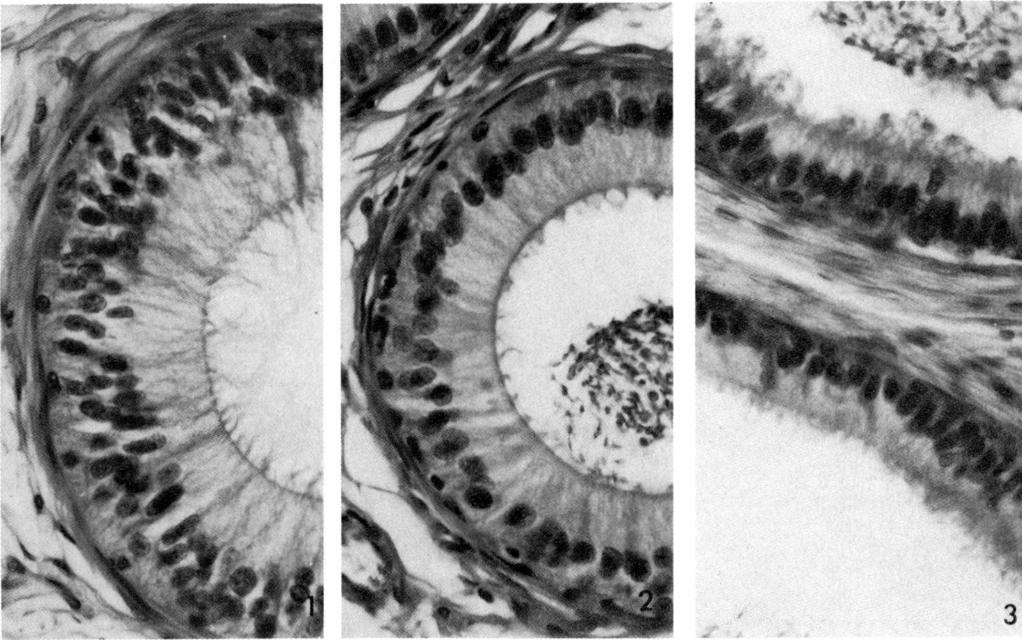

Fig. 12–12. *Epididymis, cat. Sections through the wall of the ductus epididymidis taken at the level of 1, head, 2, body, and 3, tail of the epididymis. Notice the variations in the position of the nuclei, in the height of the pseudostratified epithelium and in the length of the microvilli. H & E. ×435.*

changes that lead to the acquisition of full fertilizing capacity by the time they reach the cauda. The change in the functional status of the spermatozoa is reflected in (1) development of progressive motility, (2) modification of their metabolism, (3) alteration of the plasma membrane surface characteristics—activation of membrane-bound molecules necessary for recognition processes during fertilization, (4) stabilization of plasma membrane by oxidation of incorporated sulfhydryl groups, and (5) caudad movement and eventual loss of the cytoplasmic droplet, a remnant of the spermatid cytoplasm; spermatozoa with persisting droplets are probably infertile. Once fully mature, spermatozoa can be stored in the cauda epididymidis for a remarkably long period, much longer than if they were maintained at a similar temperature in vitro.

DUCTUS DEFERENS

The ductus deferens is the continuation of the ductus epididymidis, which after a sharp bend at the end of the tail gradually straightens and acquires the histologic characteristics of the ductus deferens. The initial portion of the ductus deferens is located within the spermatic cord. In its intra-abdominal course, it is located within a peritoneal fold (plica ductus deferentis). In the stallion and ruminants, the ductus deferens unites with the excretory duct of the vesicular gland to form a short ejaculatory duct, which opens at the colliculus seminalis into the urethra. In the boar, the ductus deferens and the excretory duct open separately into the urethra. In carnivores, the ductus deferens joins the urethra alone because the vesicular gland is absent.

The folded mucosa of the ductus deferens is lined by a pseudostratified columnar epithelium; toward the end of the duct it may become a simple columnar epithelium (Fig. 12–13). In the proximity of the epididymis, the columnar cells possess short, branched microvilli (Fig. 12–13-2). In the bull, small lipid droplets are present in the basal cells. The loose connective tissue of the propria-submucosa is highly vascularized and rich in fibroblasts and elastic fibers. In the stallion, bull, and boar, the tunica muscularis consists of intermingled circular, longitudinal, and oblique layers; in small ruminants and carnivores (Fig.

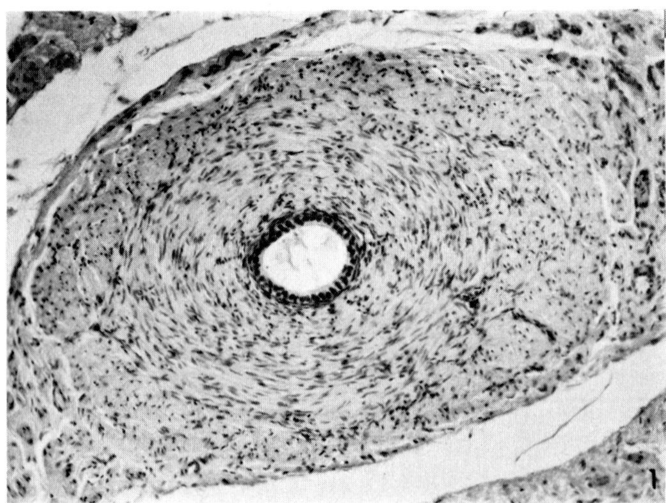

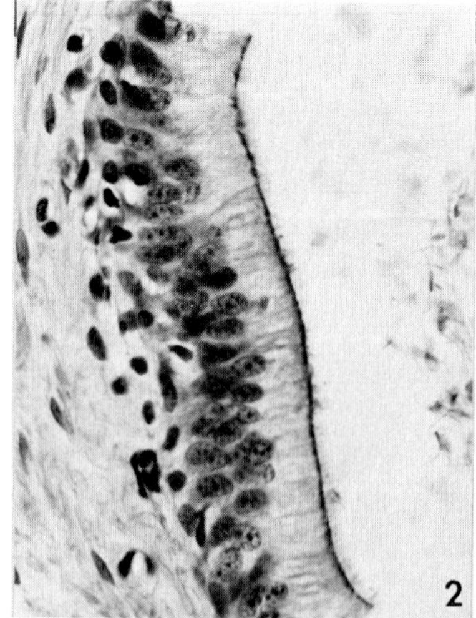

Fig. 12–13. *Ductus deferens. 1, Cross section through the intra-abdominal portion of the ductus deferens, cat. H & E. ×130. 2, Pseudostratified columnar epithelium of the ductus deferens of the dog taken at the same level. H & E. ×435.*

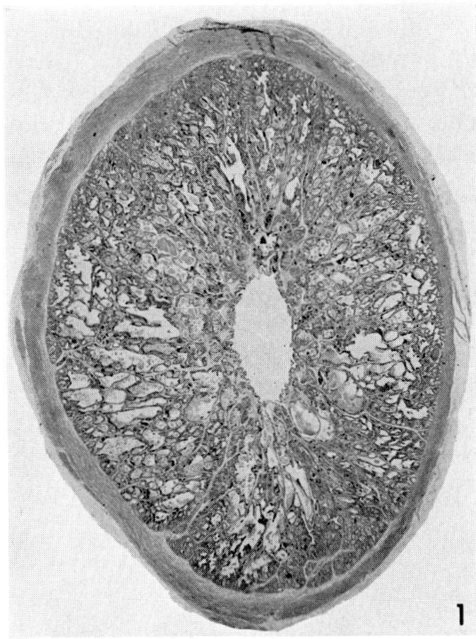

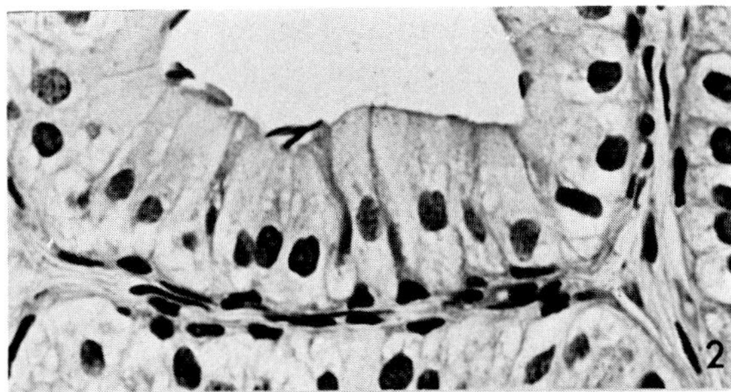

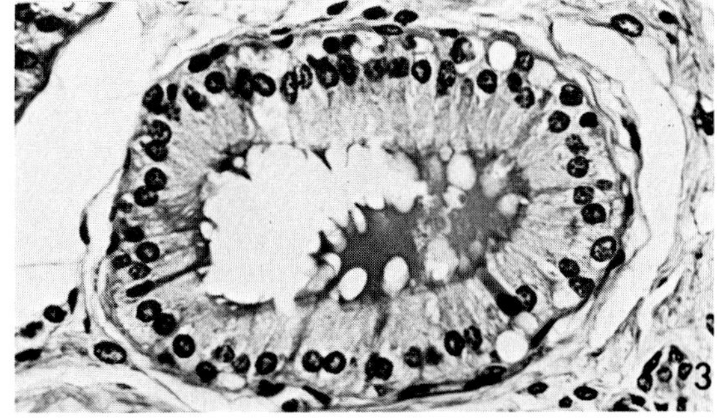

Fig. 12–14. *1, Cross section through the glandular portion of the ductus deferens, bull. Notice the abundance of glands in the propria-submucosa and the relatively thin tunica muscularis. H & E. ×4. 2, Secretory alveolus, goat. Basal and columnar cells and heads of spermatozoa in the lumen. Weigert's hematoxylin. ×560. 3, Secretory alveolus, bull. Some of the basal cells contain a huge lipid droplet (vacuole). Weigert's hematoxylin. ×350.*

12–13), an inner circular layer and an outer longitudinal layer are present. A tunica serosa with its usual components covers the organ.

The terminal portion of the ductus deferens, regardless of whether it forms an ampulla (stallion, ruminants, dog) or not (boar, cat), contains simple branched tubuloalveolar glands in the propria-submucosa. In the stallion, bull (Fig. 12–14-1), and ram, these glands occupy practically the entire propria-submucosa, which is rich in smooth muscle cells. In the dog and buck, the glands are surrounded by periglandular connective tissue devoid of smooth muscle cells. The glands are lined by cells that vary from tall columnar cells with ovoid nuclei to cuboidal cells with spherical nuclei (Fig. 12–14-2, 3). Apical, bleblike protrusions suggestive of secretory activity are often observed. Spherical or polyhedral basal cells are distributed irregularly between the columnar cells. In ruminants the glandular epithelium is rich in glycogen and the basal cells contain lipid droplets of variable size. Lipid droplets are also present in the columnar cells of the bull. The lipids in bovine basal cells may coalesce and give these cells the appearance of fat cells (Fig. 12–14-3). The tunica muscularis of the terminal portion of the ductus deferens consists of variably arranged smooth muscle bundles surrounded by the highly vascularized loose connective tissue of the tunica adventitia.

The lumen of the glandular portion of the ductus deferens and the wide openings of the glands into the lumen contain a considerable amount of spermatozoa in all domestic animals. In the bull, there are sufficient numbers for at least one normal ejaculate following recent castration or vasectomy.

ACCESSORY GLANDS

The ejaculate consists of spermatozoa and seminal plasm that is composed of secretions from epididymis and male accessory glands. These glands are (1) the glandular portion of the ductus deferens, (2) the vesicular gland, (3) the prostate, and (4) the bulbourethral gland. All accessory glands are present in the stallion, ruminants, and boar, the vesicular glands are absent in carnivores, and the bulbourethral gland is absent in the dog.

Vesicular Gland

The paired vesicular gland is a compound tubular or tubuloalveolar gland (Fig. 12–15). The glandular epithelium is pseudostratified columnar epithelium with tall columnar cells and small, spherical, often sparse basal cells. The intralobular and main secretory ducts are lined by a similar cuboidal epithelium, or by a stratified columnar epithelium in the horse.

The highly vascularized loose connective tissue of the propria-submucosa is continuous with the dense connective tissue trabeculae, which may subdivide the organ into lobes and lobules. A tunica muscularis of varying width and arrangement surrounds the organ, followed by a tunica serosa or a tunica adventitia.

SPECIES DIFFERENCES. In the stallion, the vesicular glands are true vesicles, with wide central lumina (ducts) into which open the short branched tubuloalveolar glands, separated by relatively thin connective tissue trabecular with irregularly arranged smooth muscle cells.

In the boar, the two vesicular glands possess a common connective tissue capsule; the tunica muscularis is thin. The interlobular septa consist predominantly of connective tissue and a few small muscle cells. The tubular lumina are wide; the secretory epithelium is folded (Fig. 12–16).

In the bull, the vesicular gland is a compact, lobulated organ (Fig. 12–15). Intralobular secretory ducts drain the slightly coiled tubular portions of the tubuloalveolar gland and in turn are drained by the main secretory duct. The secretory columnar cells have small lipid droplets and glycogen (Fig. 12–15) and give a positive alkaline phosphatase reaction. Some of the columnar cells possess light, bleblike apical projections. The basal cells are characterized by large lipid droplets, often in an in-

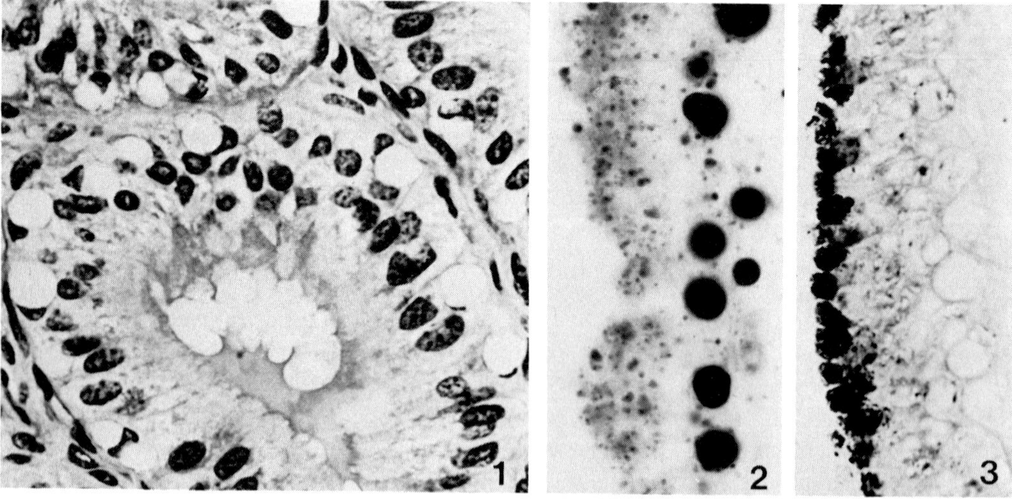

Fig. 12–15. *Vesicular gland, bull. 1. The basal cells in the pseudostratified columnar epithelial lining of the alveoli are characterized by large vacuoles containing lipid in vivo. Masson-Goldner. ×560. 2. Lipids were specifically stained with Sudan black B. Notice large lipid droplets in the basal cells and small lipid droplets in the secretory columnar cells. ×560. 3. The apices of the secretory columnar cells contain large amounts of glycogen. PAS. ×560.*

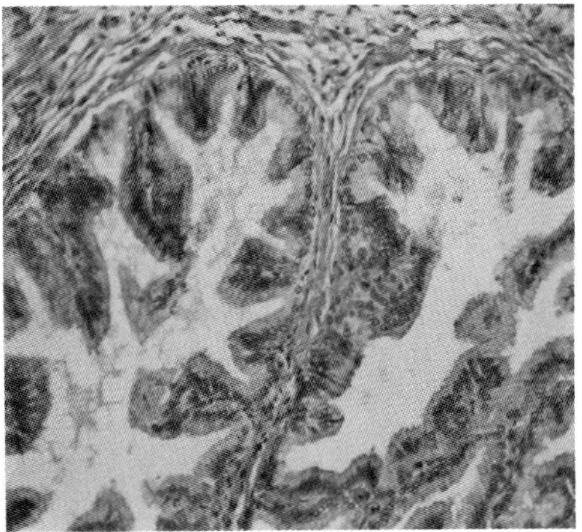

Fig. 12–16. *Vesicular gland, boar. Notice the folding of the epithelium in the secretory alveoli. H & E. ×130.*

franuclear position (Fig. 12–15). Approximately 50% of the lipid material is cholesterol and its esters; approximately 25% is triglycerides and approximately 10% is phospholipids. The interlobular septa are predominantly muscular, derived from the thick tunica muscularis, which is surrounded by a capsule of dense irregular connective tissue with a few smooth muscle cells.

The vesicular glands of the ram and buck are similar to that of the bull. Lipid droplets in the basal cells are absent in the ram but may be present in the buck. During the breeding season, the epithelium of the vesicular gland of the buck is considerably higher than during the nonbreeding season.

The gelatinous, white or yellowish white secretory product of the vesicular gland amounts to about 25 to 30% of the total ejaculate in the bull, 10 to 30% in the boar, and 7 to 8% in the ram and buck. It is rich in fructose, which serves as an energy source for ejaculated spermatozoa.

Prostate Gland

The prostate consists of a varying number of individual tubuloalveolar glands derived from the epithelium of the pelvic urethra. Two portions may be distinguished, according more to topographic than to histologic features: the compact or external portion (corpus prostatae), and the disseminate or internal portion (pars disseminata prostatae). The external portion either entirely surrounds part of the pelvic urethra at the level of the colliculus seminalis or covers part of its dorsal aspect. The disseminate portion is located in the propria-submucosa of the pelvic urethra (see Fig. 12–18).

The secretory tubules, alveoli, and intraglandular ducts of the prostate gland are lined by a simple cuboidal or columnar epithelium, with occasional basal cells (see Fig. 12–17-1). The simple epithelium changes to stratified columnar or transitional epithelium toward the terminal portions of the ducts. Some of the epithelial cells give a positive mucus reaction; the majority contains proteinaceous secretory granules. The tall columnar cells possess microvilli and sometimes bleb-like apical protrusions. Occasionally, concentrically laminated concretions of secretory material are found in the tubules and alveoli.

Secretory portions and ducts of the prostate gland are surrounded by loose connective tissue containing smooth muscle cells, which are particularly abundant in the external portion of the gland. Large trabeculae, which are predominantly muscular in the external portion of the gland, separate both the external and internal portions into individual lobules. These trabeculae originate from a capsule of dense irregular connective tissue with many smooth muscle cells around the internal portion (Fig. 12–17-2). The internal portion of the prostate is surrounded by the striated urethral muscle (Figs. 12–17-2 and 12–18).

SPECIES DIFFERENCES. In carnivores, the external portion of the prostate gland is particularly well developed and separated into two distinct bilateral lobes. In the dog, these lobes completely surround the proximal portion of the pelvic urethra. In the

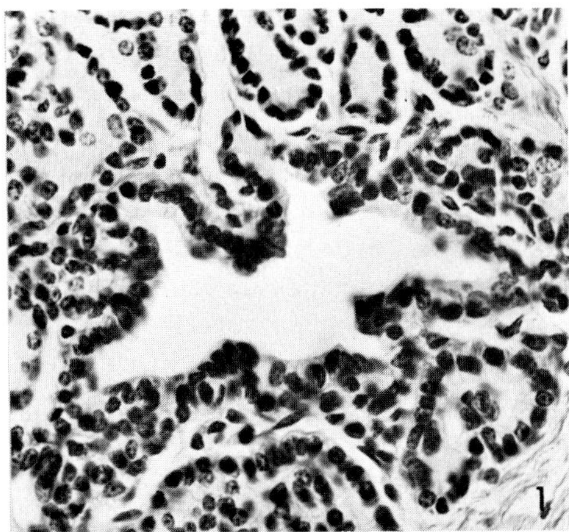

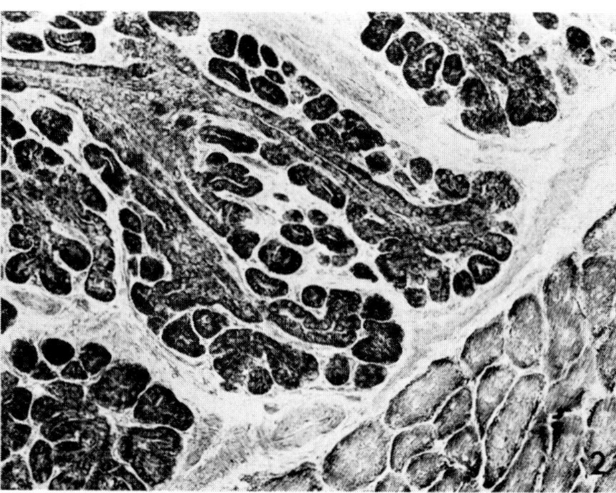

Fig. 12–17. *1, Prostate, buck. Parenchyma surrounds a small central duct partially lined by plasmodium-like cells on top of the folds. Van Gieson's stain.* ×*400. 2, Prostate (disseminate), boar. Notice the general organization of the gland; smooth muscle fibers (light gray) are seen in the capsule and the septa. β-D-galactosidase reaction.* ×*100.*

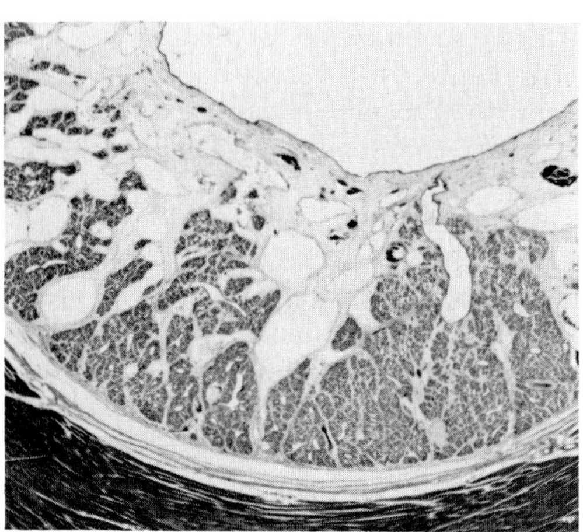

Fig. 12–18. *Pelvic urethra, bull. Large veins of the erectile tissue and the disseminate prostate in the propria-submucosa, surrounded by the urethral muscle. Crossmon's trichrome.* ×*11.*

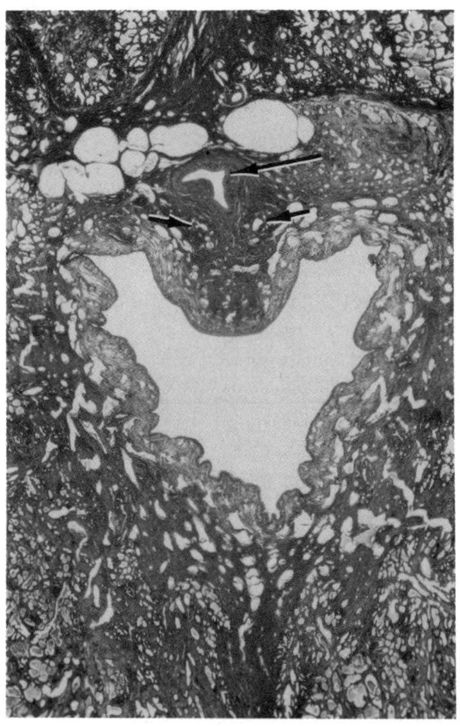

Fig. 12–19. *Prostatic urethra, dog. The urethral crest protrudes into the lumen and contains the terminal portions of the ductus deferentes (short arrows) and a rudimentary uterus masculinus (long arrow). Notice the thin-walled cavernous veins and the glandular tissue of the prostate around the urethra. Masson's trichrome.* ×*11.*

cat, they are located on the lateral and dorsal aspects of the urethra. The internal portion in the dog consists of a few glandular lobules (Fig. 12–19). In the cat, individual lobules of the internal portion are found scattered between the colliculus seminalis and the bulbourethral glands. Lamellar corpuscles may be observed in the interstitium.

In the stallion, only the external portion

of the prostate gland is present. The tubules are expanded with accumulations of secretory material. The capsule, trabeculae, and interstitial connective tissue are rich in smooth muscle.

The external portion of the prostate gland of the bull is relatively inconspicuous; it is absent in small ruminants. The particularly well-developed internal portion (Fig. 12–18) encircles the urethra in the bull and buck; in the ram it is U-shaped, the midline of the ventral aspect of the urethra being free of glandular tissue.

In the boar, the external portion of the prostate gland is a platelike organ; the internal portion (Fig. 12–17-2) is well developed and completely encircles the pelvic urethra.

The contribution of the prostatic secretions to the total volume of the ejaculate varies with the species. In ruminants it is 4 to 6%, in the stallion 25 to 30%, and in the boar 35 to 60%. One of the functions of the prostate is to neutralize the seminal plasma, made acid by accumulation of metabolic carbon dioxide and lactate, and to initiate active movements of the ejaculated spermatozoa.

Bulbourethral Gland

This paired gland is located dorsolaterally from the bulbar portion of the urethra. It is a compound tubular (boar, cat, buck) or tubuloalveolar (stallion, bull, ram) gland (Fig. 12–20). It is absent in the dog.

The secretory portions of the gland are lined with a tall simple columnar epithelium and occasional basal cells (Fig. 12–21). They open into collecting ducts either directly or through connecting pieces lined by a simple cuboidal epithelium characterized by a dark cytoplasm. The collecting ducts (Fig. 12–20), lined by a simple cuboidal or columnar epithelium, unite to form larger intraglandular ducts lined by a pseudostratified columnar epithelium (Fig. 12–20). These in turn open into a single (or multiple) bulbourethral duct with a lining of transitional epithelium.

The gland is ensheathed by a fibroelastic capsule containing a variable amount of striated muscle cells. Trabeculae, extending from the capsule, consist of dense irregular connective tissue and some smooth and striated muscle fibers. The interstitium consists of loose connective tissue and a few smooth muscle fibers.

SPECIES DIFFERENCES. In the cat, the gland consists of spacious, sinuslike intraglandular ducts and short, narrow, mostly unbranched tubular end-pieces. The secretory surface of the cells is increased by a

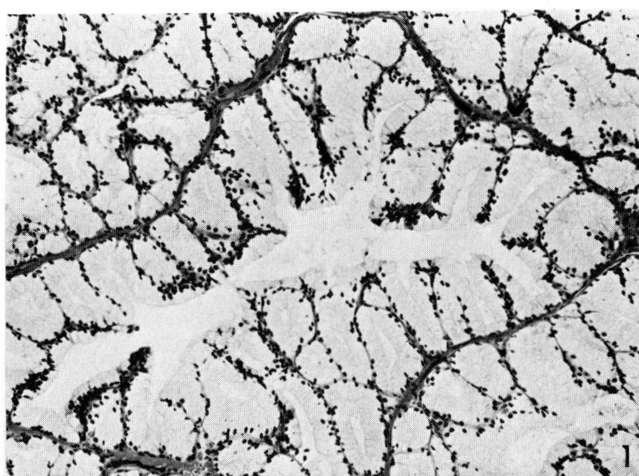

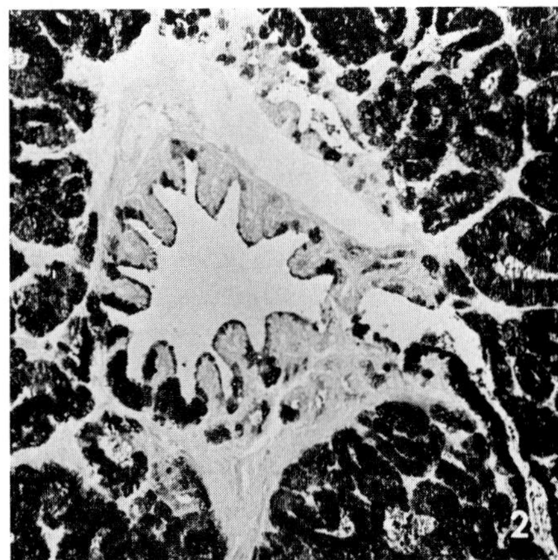

Fig. 12–20. *Bulbourethral gland, bull. 1, Notice the light tall columnar secretory epithelium and the dense basal nuclei, characteristic for intracellular accumulation of secretory product. Masson-Goldner-Jerusalem trichrome. ×100. 2, Positive PAS reaction in the parenchyma and some of the lining cells of the central duct. ×100.*

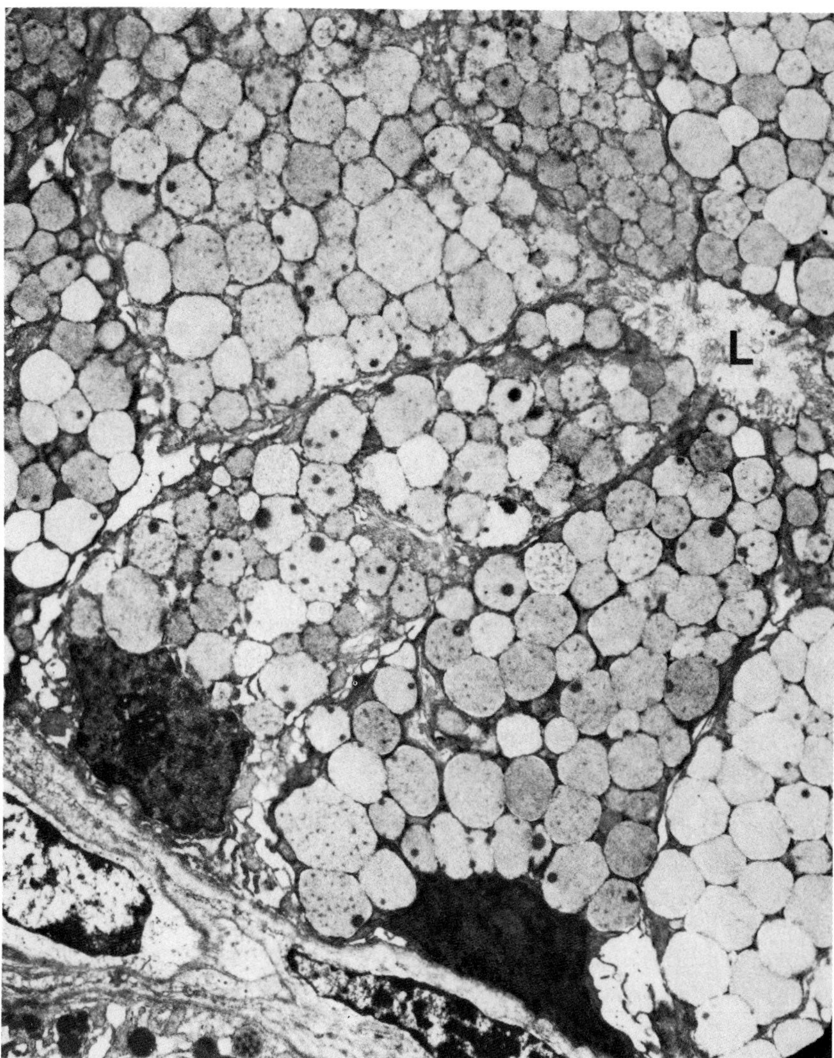

Fig. 12–21. *Bulbourethral gland, goat. Cross section through a secretory acinus. The secretory cells bordering the lumen (L) are filled with mucous secretory granules. ×5100.*

well-developed system of intercellular canaliculi.

In the stallion, the bulbourethral gland is completely surrounded by the bulbocavernous muscle. Three to four individual bulbourethral ducts are present.

The exceptionally large bulbourethral gland of the boar is surrounded by the ischioglandular muscle. Only a few smooth muscle cells are present in the interstitium. The collecting ducts are lined by a simple columnar epithelium.

In ruminants, the gland is also surrounded by the bulbocavernous muscle. In the bull and ram, short connecting pieces link the secretory portions to the collecting ducts, which are lined by a simple cuboidal epithelium (sometimes also secretory) (Fig. 12–20-2). In the buck, the secretory portions empty directly into these ducts. Smooth muscle cells are particularly abundant within the interstitium.

The mucous and proteinaceous secretory product of the bulbourethral gland is

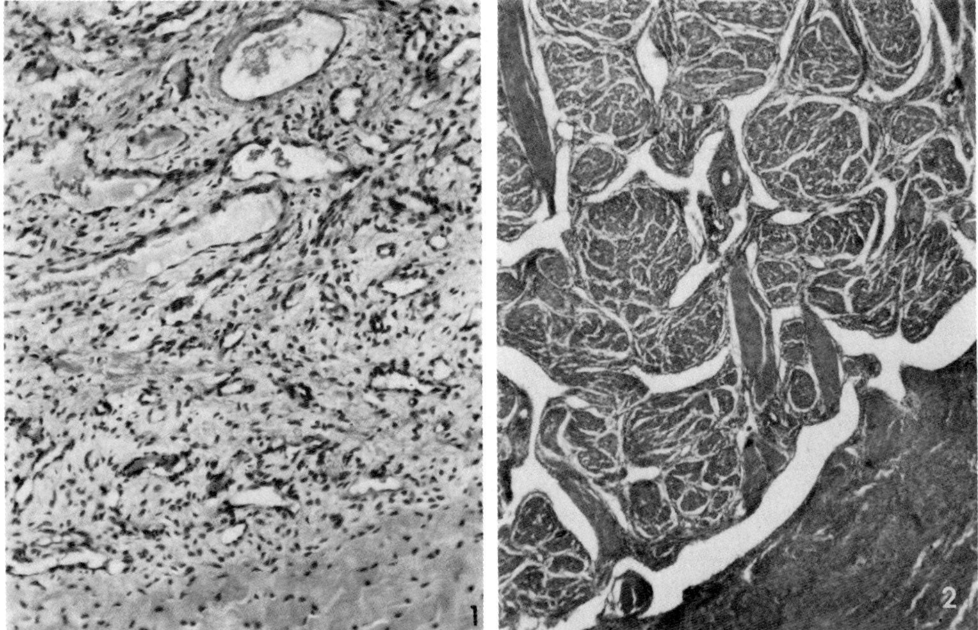

Fig. 12–22. *1, Penis, bull. Connective tissue predominates in the fibroelastic corpus cavernosum penis. H & E. ×130. 2, Penis, stallion. The collapsed cavernous spaces are surrounded by thick bundles of smooth muscle cells in the corpus cavernosum penis of the vascular type. H & E. ×40.*

discharged prior to ejaculation in ruminants, where it apparently serves to neutralize the urethral environment and to lubricate both the urethra and the vagina. In the boar, the exclusively mucous secretory product, rich in sialic acid, is part of the ejaculate (15 to 30%) and possibly involved in the occlusion of the cervix to prevent sperm loss. In the cat, the secretory product is mucus and also contains glycogen. In the absence of a vesicular gland, this bulbourethral glycogen may be the source of feline seminal fructose. It may provide energy for the metabolism of the spermatozoa.

URETHRA

The male urethra is divided into the prostatic, membranous, and spongiose portions. The prostatic portion extends from the urinary bladder to the caudal edge of the prostate. The membranous portion begins here and terminates at the point where the urethra enters the bulb of the penis, from which level the spongiose portion continues to the external urethral opening.

The entire urethral mucosa is thrown into longitudinal folds that flatten or disappear during erection and micturition. In the prostatic urethra, a prominent, permanent dorsomedian fold, the urethral crest, terminates as a slight enlargement, the *colliculus seminalis.* There, the ejaculatory ducts in ruminants and the stallion, the ductus deferentes and the ducts of the vesicular glands in the boar, and the deferent ducts in carnivores (Fig. 12–19) open into the urethra. Between these ducts, vestiges of the fused paramesonephric ducts, the uterus masculinus, may be found as either a solid epithelial cord or a short canal (Fig. 12–19).

The predominant lining of the urethra is a transitional epithelium with variably sized patches of simple columnar epithelium, stratified columnar epithelium, or cuboidal epithelium. The propria-submucosa consists of a dense irregular connective tissue with many elastic fibers and smooth muscle cells, and frequent diffuse lymphatic tissue or lymphatic nodules (dog). In the stallion and cat, simple tubular mucous (urethral) glands are present.

Throughout the entire length of the urethra, the propria-submucosa possesses erectile properties by virtue of endothelial-lined caverns of variable size that constitute the so-called vascular stratum in the prostatic and membranous urethra. Around the spongiose urethra the quantity and size of the cavernous spaces are greatly increased (see Fig. 12–25); here the vascular stratum is referred to as the corpus spongiosum, which begins at the ischiadic arch with a bilobed expansion, the bulb of the penis.

The tunica muscularis of the urethra consists of smooth muscle in the vicinity of the bladder or striated muscle in the remainder of the urethra. It is surrounded by a tunica adventitia of loose or dense irregular connective tissue.

In ruminants and the stallion, the terminal portion of the urethra protrudes incompletely (bull) or completely (stallion, ram, and buck) above the glans penis to form the processus urethrae. The transitional or squamous epithelial lining is surrounded by a corpus spongiosum containing many cavernous spaces in the stallion and fewer and smaller ones in ruminants. Two longitudinal fibrocartilaginous cords flank the urethra in the buck and ram. The urethral process is covered by a cutaneous mucous membrane.

PENIS

The penis consists of (1) two erectile structures, the corpora cavernosa penis, (2) the corpus spongiosum penis surrounding the spongiose urethra, and (3) the glans penis.

Corpora Cavernosa Penis

The paired corpora cavernosa penis arise from the ischiadic tuberosities and merge to form the body of the penis. They are surrounded by the tunica albuginea, a thick layer of dense irregular connective tissue containing variable numbers of elastic fibers and smooth muscle cells. A connective tissue septum completely (as in the dog) or partially divides the corpora cavernosa penis.

The spaces between the tunica albuginea and the trabecular network are filled with erectile tissue (Fig. 12–22). In the stallion (Fig. 12–22-2) and carnivores, this tissue consists of caverns lined by endothelium and surrounded by many smooth muscle cells and a small amount of connective tissue, the appearance of which varies between loose and dense irregular. In the stallion, these muscle bundles are oriented with the longitudinal axis of the corpus penis (Fig. 12–22-2), often causing a virtually complete obturation of the lumina of the cavernous spaces. Relaxation of these muscle cells causes the penis to elongate and emerge from the preputial sheath, which usually happens during micturition. In ruminants (Fig. 12–22-1) and the pig, the connective tissue surrounding the caverns contains few if any smooth muscle cells.

The cavernous spaces receive their main blood supply from arteries with a helical arrangement and referred to as helicine arteries (arteriae helicinae). Characteristically, they have epithelioid smooth muscle cells in the tunica intima. They protrude into the lumina of these vessels as ridges or pads, causing partial obliteration. As the smooth muscle cells relax, the blood flow into the caverns increases considerably and causes erection (see below). The cavernous spaces are drained by venules, several of which give origin to thick-walled veins.

The penis of the stallion is classified as a vascular penis because of the predominance of caverns in the corpus caver-

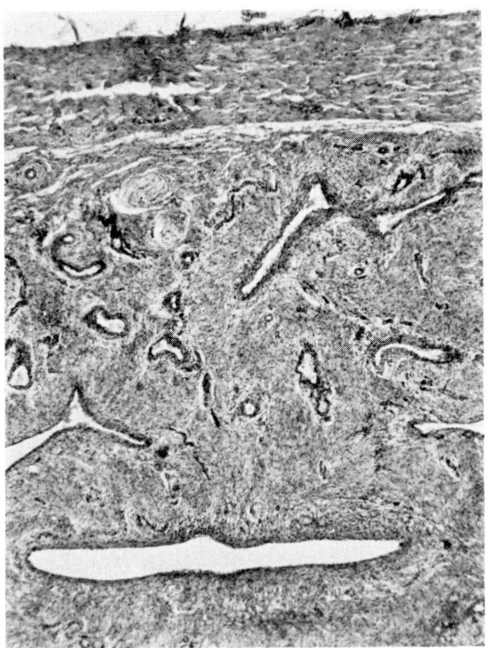

Fig. 12–23. *Corpus spongiosum glandis, stallion, H & E. ×39.*

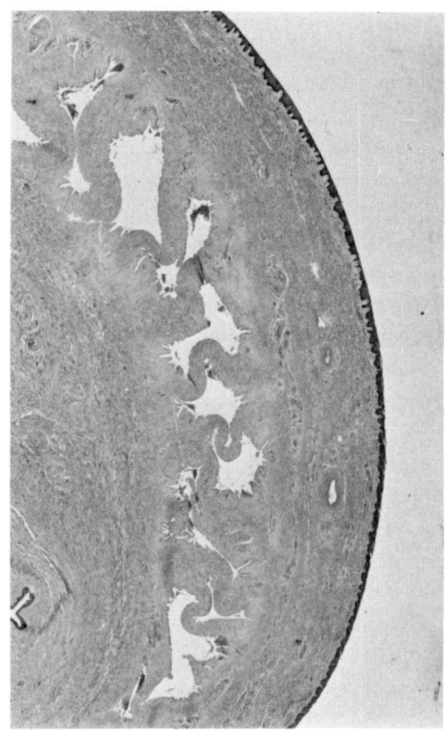

Fig. 12–24. *Glans penis, pars longa, dog. Large venous sinuses of the erectile tissue. H & E. ×11.*

nosum. In ruminants and the boar the caverns are less extensive and connective tissue prevails, thus the designation of the penes as fibroelastic. The dog and cat penes are best classified as an intermediate type.

Glans Penis

A well-developed glans penis is present only in the stallion and dog. It is surrounded by a tunica albuginea rich in elastic fibers. It continues into trabeculae that delineate spaces containing erectile tissue similar to that of the corpus spongiosum penis (horse) (Fig. 12–23), or a plexus of large caverns (dog) (Fig. 12–24). The glans penis is covered by the prepuce (see p. 311).

SPECIES DIFFERENCES

The corpora cavernosa penis of the dog are completely separated by a connective tissue septum and are continued cranially by the os penis, which terminates in a fibrocartilaginous tip. The glans penis consists of the bulbus glandis and the pars longa glandis. Both almost completely surround the os penis and the distal portion of the spongiose urethra and its associated corpus spongiosum. The *bulbus glandis* consists of large venous caverns separated by connective tissue trabeculae rich in elastic fibers. The *pars longa glandis* forms the rostral portion of the glans penis; its structure (Fig. 12–24) is identical to that of the bulbus.

In the cat, many adipose cells are present between the caverns of the corpus cavernosum penis. They increase in number toward the tip of the corpus cavernosum, which contains very little erectile tissue. A small os penis surrounded by the corpus cavernosum of the glans is present.

The connective tissue of the corpus cavernosum of the stallion contains many elastic fibers and smooth muscle cells. The glans covers the corpus cavernosum penis rostrally and possesses a long, caudally directed, dorsomedian process and an enlargement, the corona glandis, the epithelial covering of which bears cylindrical papillae. An indentation of the glans, the fossa glandis, contains the slightly protruding end of the urethra (processus urethae). At the level of the glans, the urethral muscle bundles are interrupted by the retractor penis muscle.

A corkscrew-like left turn characterizes approximately the cranial third of the penis of the boar. Its structure is similar to that of the penis of the bull.

The corpus penis of the bull contains a central connective tissue strand formed by the converging trabeculae. The tip of the penis (glans) (Fig. 12–25) consists of mesenchymal cells, adipose cells, and large intercellular spaces. An extensive erectile venous plexus (Fig. 12–25) is present. The penes of the buck and ram are similar to that of the bull. The glans is a large caplike enlargement similar to that of the bull. Two lateral outpocketings of the corpus spongiosum penis protrude from it laterally.

Mechanism of Erection

In animals with either a vascular or an intermediate-type penis, erection causes an increase in size and a stiffening of the organ. In animals with a fibroelastic penis, erection results essentially in an increase in the length of the penis that emerges from the prepuce.

Relaxation of the smooth muscle cells in the helicine arteries results in an increased blood flow into the spaces of the corpora cavernosa. The increased blood volume compresses the veins and subsequently decreases the outflow, eventually filling the erectile tissue spaces in the corpora cav-

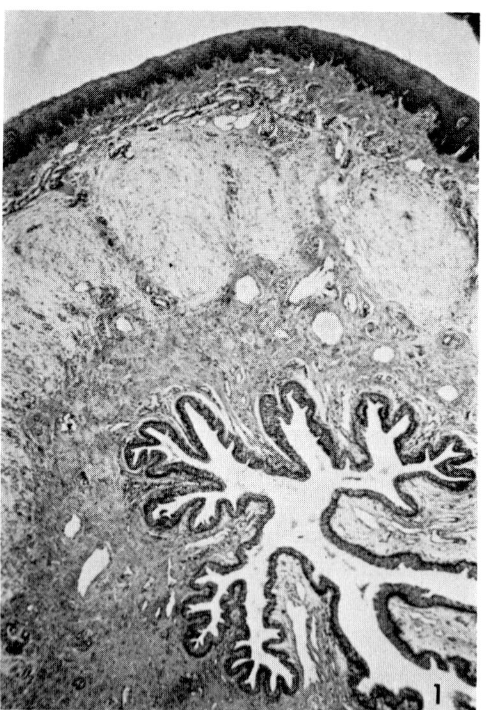

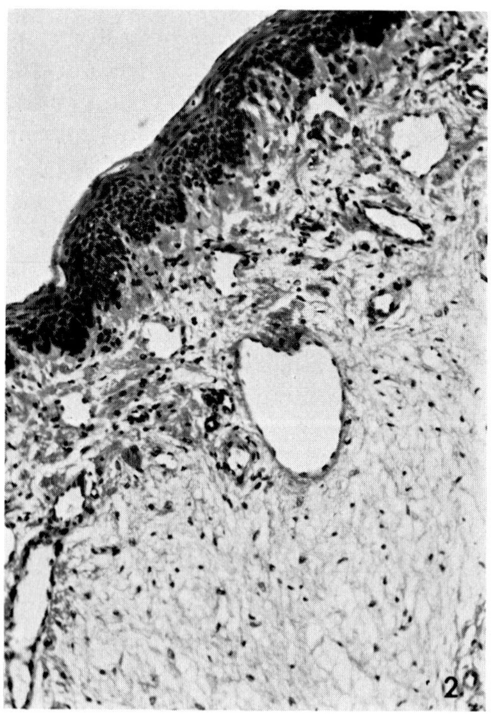

Fig. 12–25. *Glans penis, bull. 1, The urethra is surrounded by erectile tissue and a relatively thick connective tissue layer. H & E. ×40. 2, A higher-power photomicrograph of the surface of the glans with venous erectile tissue in, and especially underneath, the dense irregular connective tissue underlying the covering epithelium. Notice the peculiar appearance (see text) of the connective tissue of the glans. H & E. ×130.*

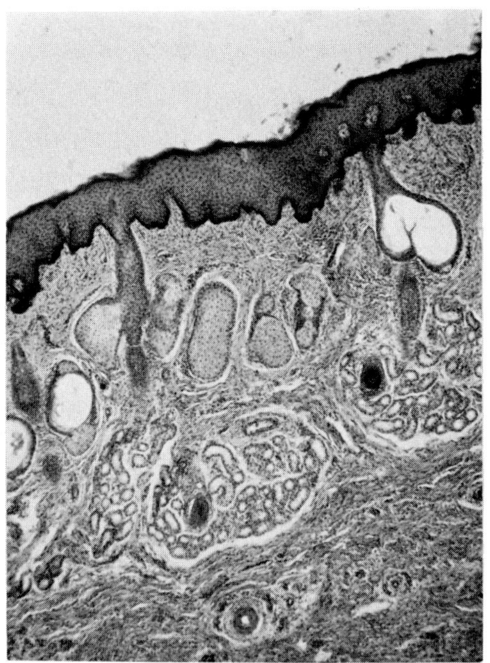

Fig. 12–26. *Skin with hairs and sebaceous and sweat glands covering the corpus penis, stallion. H & E. ×40.*

ernosa and spongiosa penis and in the glans penis.

Detumescence is initiated by contraction of the musculature of the helicine arteries and thus by a decrease in arterial inflow. The contraction of the smooth muscle cells of the tunica albuginea, the trabeculae, and the erectile tissue causes the penis to return to the flaccid state. In ruminants and the boar, the retractor penis muscle plays an essential role in retracting the penis into the prepuce.

During copulation, the constrictor vestibuli muscle of the bitch constricts the veins of the dog that drain the entire glans and especially the bulbus glandis. This causes the bulbus to enlarge to such a degree that immediate withdrawal of the penis from the vagina is impossible; consequently, coitus is prolonged.

Prepuce

The cranial portion of the penis and the glans penis are located in a tubelike reflection of the skin, the prepuce, composed of an external and an internal layer. The external layer reflects inward at the preputial opening to form the internal layer of the prepuce. It reflects on the cranial portion of the penis and is securely attached cranially to the glans penis.

The external layer is typical skin. Numerous sebaceous glands, not always related to hairs, are present at the preputial opening. In addition, long, bristlelike hairs are found in ruminants and the boar. In the stallion, ruminants, boar, and dog, fine hairs and sebaceous and sweat glands are located over a variable distance in the internal layer. In the stallion, occasional hairs occur, even in the penile skin (Fig. 12–26), which is also rich in sebaceous and sweat glands. In the dog and ruminants, both the internal layer of the prepuce and the skin covering the penis contain solitary lymphatic nodules; in the boar, they are present only in the internal layer. In the cat, the skin covering the glans has numerous keratinized papillae.

In the boar, a dorsal evagination of the prepuce is referred to as the preputial diverticulum. It is incompletely separated into two lateral portions by a median septum. Frequently, the keratinized cutaneous mucous membrane is folded. A mixture of desquamated epithelial cells and urine forms a substance with a most unpleasant odor.

REFERENCES

Aumüller, G.: Prostate gland and seminal vesicles. *In* Handbuch der Mikroskopischen Anatomie des Menschen. Vol. 7, Part 6. Berlin, Springer-Verlag, 1979.

Bedford, J.: Maturation, transport and fate of spermatozoa in the epididymis. *In* Handbook of Physiology. Sect. 7, Vol. V. Edited by R.O. Greep and E.B. Astwood, American Physiological Society. Baltimore, Williams & Wilkins, 1975, pp. 303–317.

Bishop, D.W.: Biology of spermatozoa. *In* Sex and Internal Secretions. Edited by W.C. Young. Baltimore, Williams & Wilkins, 1961, pp. 707–796.

Cole, H.H., and Cupps, P.T.: Reproduction in Domestic Animals. 3rd Ed. New York, Academic Press, 1977.

Fawcett, D.W., and Bedford, J.M. (eds.): The Spermatozoon. Maturation, Motility, Surface Properties and Comparative Aspects. Baltimore-Munich, Urban and Schwarzenberg, 1979.

Hamilton, D.W.: Structure and function of the epithelium lining the ductuli efferentes, ductus epididymidis and ductus deferens in the rat. *In* Handbook of Physiology. Sect. 7, Vol. V. Edited by R.O. Greep and E.B. Astwood, American Physiology Society. Baltimore, Williams & Wilkins, 1975, pp. 259–301.

Setchell, B.P.: The Mammalian Testis. London, Paul Elek, 1978.

Steinberger, A., and Steinberger, E.: Testicular Development, Structure and Function. New York, Raven Press, 1980.

Van Blerkom, J., and Motta, P. (eds.): Ultrastructure of reproduction. Boston, M. Nijhoff, 1984.

13

Female Reproductive System

JĀNIS PRIEDKALNS

The female reproductive system consists of bilateral ovaries and uterine tubes (oviducts), a usually bicornuate uterus, cervix, vagina, vestibule, vulva, and associated glands. It is concerned with the production and transport of ova, the transport of spermatozoa, fertilization, and the accommodation of the conceptus until birth.

EMBRYOLOGIC DEVELOPMENT

Gonads: Ovary

Initially, the gonads are longitudinal, ridgelike thickenings, called *gonadal ridges,* located on the ventromedial borders of the mesonephric kidneys. The ridges are covered by a cuboidal or squamous mesothelium known as the *surface epithelium.* Cells similar to those of the surface epithelium appear in the underlying gonadal mesenchyme to form cordlike *internal epithelial cell masses.* Large pale cells from the yolk sac entoderm, known as *primordial germ cells* (PGCs) migrate into the gonadal ridge at an early stage of development. Opinion is divided regarding whether the PGCs (1) represent progenitors of future sex cells, (2) induce the differentiation of sex cells from the surface epithelium or from the internal epithelial cell masses in the gonadal ridge, or (3) represent an ancestral germ cell that no longer participates in the formation of sex cells.

The internal epithelial cell masses proliferate centrally to form the *rete cords,* which cavitate to become the rete testis in the male and the rete ovarii in the female. A *medullary proliferation* of the internal epithelial cell masses follows the rete proliferation and forms the testis cords in the male and a rudimentary primary cortex in the female. In postnatal life, the testis cords cavitate to form the seminiferous tubules. In the female, a *cortical proliferation* of the internal epithelial cell masses follows the medullary proliferation, resulting in the formation of a secondary cortex with cordlike cell masses containing ova. These cell masses proliferate rapidly by mitotic activity and become separated into cell clusters.

The central cell of a cluster becomes the *oogonium,* or egg. The oogonia enlarge to form *primary oocytes.* As the primary oocyte forms, the surrounding cells form a single layer of flat *follicular cells.* Together the components constitute the *primordial follicle.* Prior to birth, the primary oocyte enters the first meiotic division, which is arrested in prophase. Celluar interaction of the oocytes with the rete ovarii is considered important for the initiation of meiosis. The first meiotic division of an oocyte is not completed until near the time of its ovulation, i.e., after puberty. The long duration of the first meiotic division may account in part for meiotic errors such as nondisjunction.

Development of the follicle is characterized by proliferation of the single layer of follicular cells, establishing a multilaminar stratum of *granulosa cells,* and by the formation of a vascularized multilaminar layer of *theca cells* around the granulosa cells.

Genital Ducts: Uterine Tubes, Uterus, and Vagina

Whereas the same embryonic gonadal ridge becomes either a testis or an ovary, two separate genital duct systems are formed in the sexually undifferentiated embryo. One of these duct systems, the *mesonephric (Wolffian) ducts and tubules,* develops in male fetuses, and the other, the *paramesonephric (Müllerian) ducts,* develops in female fetuses. Thus, both potential male and potential female genital duct systems are present in all embryos. Normally only the system determined by the genetic sex of the embryo develops, while the other system regresses (Fig. 13–1 and Table 13–1). The genetic sex, established at the time of conception, governs the development of gonadal sex, which regulates the development of phenotypic sex by genetic and endocrine mechanisms.

In the female, the mesonephric ducts and tubules regress and become vestigial ovarian appendages and the longitudinal duct of the epoophoron (Gärtner's duct). In the male they form the ductuli efferentes, epididymides, ductus deferentes, vesicular glands, ampullae, and ejaculatory ducts. The paramesonephric ducts, which arise parallel and lateral to the mesonephric ducts, form the *uterine tubes, uterus, cervix,* and part of the *vagina* in the female. They regress in the male, leaving a vestigial testicular appendage and the uterus masculinus (Fig. 13–1 and Table 13–1).

Genitalia: Vestibule and Vulva

The embryonic cloaca is divided by the urorectal septum into a dorsal rectum and a ventral urogenital sinus. The urogenital sinus forms the bladder, urethra, and associated glands, and, additionally in the female, the *vestibule, vestibular glands,* and in part the *vagina* (Table 13–1). Caudally, the entoderm-lined vestibule is completed by the ectoderm-lined *vulva,* and cranially, at the position of the hymen, it is continuous with the mesodermal vagina. In some species, however, entodermal cells of the urogenital sinus invade the vaginal and cervical mesodermal epithelia.

The external genitalia also pass through a stage occurring in both male or female. A *genital tubercle* develops ventrally to the cloacal membrane, and *urogenital folds* form on each side of the cloacal membrane. *Labioscrotal swellings* develop laterally to the urogenital folds.

In the male, closure of the urogenital folds establishes the urethral surface of the penis. The rest of the penis, including the glans, is formed from the genital tubercle. The labioscrotal swellings become the scrotum. In the female, the genital tubercle becomes the *clitoris,* the urogenital folds become the inner labia minora, and the labioscrotal swellings become the outer labia majora. The inner and outer labia fuse in domestic animals to form the *labia vulvae* (Table 13–1).

OVARY

The ovary is a combined exocrine and endocrine gland, i.e., it produces both ova (exocrine "secretion") and ovarian hormones, chiefly estrogens and progesterone (endocrine secretion). The structure of the normal ovary varies greatly with the species, age and phase of the sexual cycle. It is an ovoid structure divided into an outer cortex and an inner medulla (Fig. 13–2). In the mature mare, these areas are reversed, and the cortical tissue lies on the surface only in the ovulation fossa, which is the site of all ovulations.

The cortex is the broad peripheral zone containing follicles and corpora lutea. It is covered by a low cuboidal surface epithe-

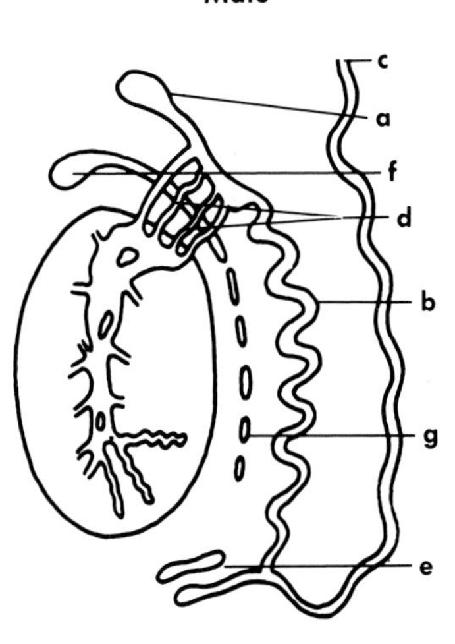

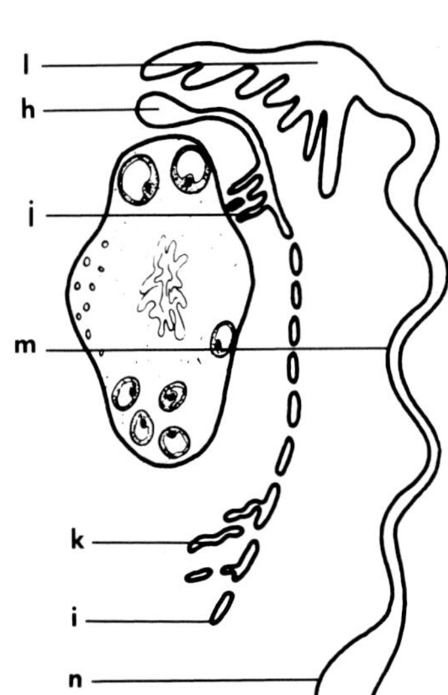

Fig. 13–1. *Diagrams illustrating the fates of the mesonephric duct and tubules and the paramesonephric duct in the adult male and female. Appendix epididymidis* (a); epididymis (b); ductus deferens (c); ductuli efferentes (d); paradidymis* (e); appendix testis* (f); uterus masculinus* (g); appendix ovarii* (h); longitudinal duct of epoophoron* (i); epoophoron* (j); paroophoron* (k); infundibulum (1); oviduct (m); uterus (n). *Vestigial structure.*

lium. The cortical stroma is loose connective tissue. The tunica albuginea is a thick connective tissue layer immediately beneath the surface epithelium. It is disrupted by the growth of ovarian follicles and corpora lutea and may be inconspicuous during increased ovarian activity. In rodent, bitch and queen ovaries, the cortical stroma contains cords of polyhedral interstitial gland cells. In the bitch ovary, 'cortical tubules' are also prominent. They are narrow channels lined by a cuboidal epithelium which in some sites are continuous with the surface epithelium.

The medulla is the inner area containing nerves, many large and coiled blood vessels and lymph vessels. It consists of loose connective tissue and strands of smooth muscle continuous with those in the mesovarium. Retia ovarii are located in the medulla; they are networks of irregular channels lined by a cuboidal epithelium or solid cellular cords. The rete may differentiate into follicular cells when in juxtaposition to an oocyte. They are prominent in carnivores and ruminants.

Ovarian Follicles

Primary (unilaminar) follicles are composed of a *primary oocyte,* approximately 20 μm in diameter in most species, surrounded by a single layer of squamous or cuboidal epithelial cells, the *follicular cells* (Fig. 13–3). The earliest primary follicles, surrounded by a simple squamous epithelium, are termed *primordial follicles.* The later stages have a simple cuboidal epithelium. The primary follicles, approximately 40 μm in diameter, are surrounded by a basement membrane and located mainly in the outer cortex close to the surface epithelium. Primary follicles are evenly distributed in ruminants and the sow and occur in clusters in carnivores.

In the oocyte, Golgi complexes and mitochondria occur near the nucleus. Microvilli may be present on parts of the oocyte surface. Several hundred thousand to one million potential oocytes may be present in a single ovary at birth in various species. Only several hundred of these ovulate during a lifetime. Most of them degenerate

Table 13–1.
Homologies of the Urogenital System

Embryologic (Indifferent) Structure		Adult Male (M) or Female (F) Structure
Mesonephric (Wolffian) duct	M	Appendix epididymidis,* epididymis, ductus deferens, vesicular glands, ampulla, ejaculatory duct
	F	Appendix ovarii,* longitudinal duct of epoophoron (Gärtner's duct)*
Mesonephric tubules	M	Ductuli efferentes, paradidymis*
	F	Epoophoron,* paroophoron*
Paramesonephric (Müllerian) duct	M	Appendix testis,* uterus masculinus*
	F	Uterine tube, uterus and cervix, vagina (in part)
Gonadal ridge and primordial germ cells	M	Testis — Three gonadal epithelial proliferations: 1, rete cord; 2, medullary; 3, cortical. Functional structures are produced by 1 and 2 in testis (rete testis, seminiferous tubules) and by 1 and 3 in ovary (follicles).
	F	Ovary
Labioscrotal swellings	M	Scrotum
	F	Labia majora of vulva
Genital tubercle	M	Penis except its urethral surface
	F	Clitoris
Urogenital folds	M	Urethral surface of penis
	F	Labia minora of vulva
Urogenital sinus	M	Bladder and urethra; prostate gland; bulbourethral glands; urethral glands
	F	Bladder, urethra, vestibule and vagina (in part); urethral glands; major vestibular (Bartholin's) glands; minor vestibular glands

*Vestigial structure.

before birth. The processes involved in the selection of follicles for growth, from a pool of nonproliferating primordial follicles, are poorly understood.

Secondary (multilaminar or *growing) follicles* consist of a stratified epithelium of polyhedral *granulosa cells* surrounding a *primary oocyte* (Fig. 13–4). A fluid-filled cavity is not yet present among the epithelial cells. In carnivores, the sow, and the ewe, follicles called polyovular follicles containing oocytes may develop (Fig. 13–5). In the cow, the late secondary follicle measures approximately 120 μm and contains an oocyte approximately 80 μm in diameter.

Secondary follicles are marked by the development of a 3- to 5-μm thick glycoprotein layer, the *zona pellucida,* around the plasma membrane of the oocyte. There is partial penetration of this zone by microvilli of the oocyte surface. The zona pellucida is secreted by the granulosa cells immediately surrounding the oocyte and in part by the oocyte itself. Cytoplasmic extensions of the granulosa cells around the oocyte penetrate the zona pellucida and associate closely with microvilli of the oocyte surface (Fig. 13–6).

As follicular development continues, small fluid-filled cavities (clefts) are formed among the granulosa cells. A vascularized layer of spindle-shaped cells, the *theca cells,* begins to form around the granulosa cell layer in late secondary follicles.

Tertiary (antral, vesicular, or *Graafian) follicles* are characterized by the development of a central cavity, the *antrum.* The antrum is formed when the fluid-filled clefts among the granulosa cells of secondary follicles coalesce to form a single large cavity

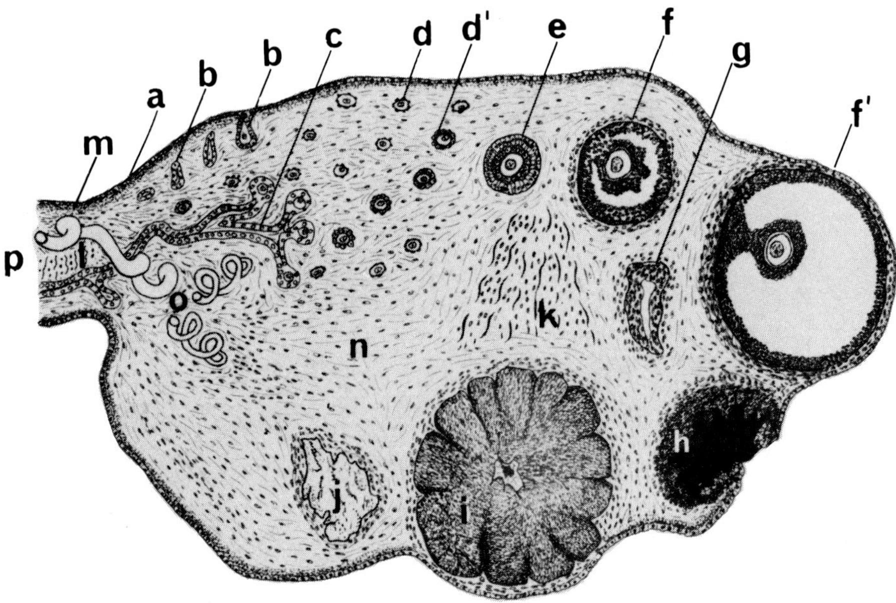

Fig. 13–2. *Diagram of the mammalian ovary illustrating the development and regression of follicles and corpus luteum and other ovarian structures. Surface epithelium (a); cortical tubules—bitch (b); rete ovarii—queen, rodents, cow (c); primordial (d) and late (d') primary follicles; secondary follicle (e); early (f) and mature (f') tertiary follicles; atretic follicle (g); corpus hemorrhagicum (h); corpus luteum (i); corpus albicans (j); interstitial gland—woman, bitch, queen, rodents (k); hilus cells—woman (l); tunica albuginea (m); stroma (n); blood vessels (o); mesovarium (p). (Part adapted from Patten, B.M.: Human Embryology. New York, Blakiston, 1953.)*

containing *liquor folliculi* (Fig. 13–7). Tertiary follicles just before ovulation are termed *mature follicles.*

The *primary oocyte* in tertiary follicles measures from 150 to 300 μm in diameter, depending on the species. It has a spherical, centrally located nucleus with a sparse chromatin network and a prominent nucleolus. The Golgi complexes, initially dispersed in the cytoplasm, become concentrated near the plasma membrane. Lipid granules and lipochrome pigment occur in the cytoplasm. As the antrum enlarges through the accumulation of liquor folliculi, the oocyte is displaced eccentrically, usually in a part of the follicle nearest to the center of the ovary. The oocyte then lies in an accumulation of granulosa cells, called the *cumulus oophorus.* In large tertiary follicles, the granulosa cells immediately surrounding the oocyte become columnar and radially disposed; they are then termed the *corona radiata.* The corona radiata cells are believed to provide nutrient support for the oocyte. They are lost at the time of ovulation in ruminants but persist until just before fertilization in other species.

In tertiary follicles, the granulosa cells form the parietal follicular lining, the *stratum granulosum,* which rests on a basement membrane. Most of the parietal granulosa cells are polyhedral but the basal layer may be columnar. Some of the granulosa cells may contain large PAS-positive inclusions, the Call-Exner bodies, which may represent intracellular precursors of liquid folliculi. In the large tertiary follicle, the granulosa cells have the ultrastructural characteristics of protein-secreting cells, notably a granular ER. Before ovulation, the granulosa cells of the mature follicle assume the characteristics of steroid-secreting cells, especially an agranular ER and mitochondria with tubular cristae.

The stratum granulosum is surrounded by the theca, which in tertiary follicles differentiates into two layers, an inner vas-

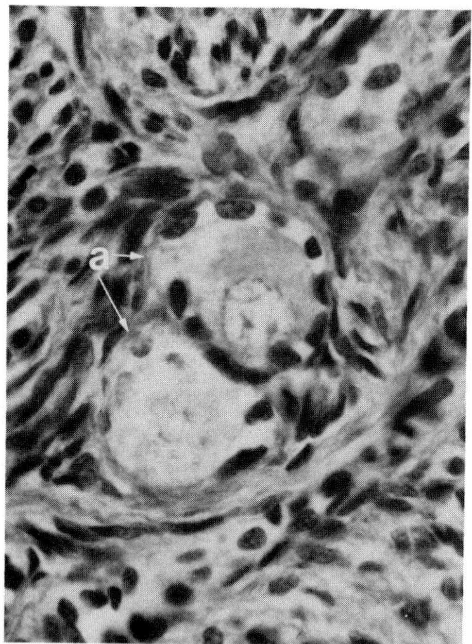

Fig. 13–3. *Primary follicles (a), mature bitch. (Early primary follicles, in which the primary oocyte is surrounded by simple squamous epithelium, are termed primordial follicles.) ×710. (From Adam, W.S., Calhoun, M.L., Smith, E.M., and Stinson, A.W.: Microscopic Anatomy of the Dog: A Photographic Atlas. Springfield, Ill., C.C Thomas, 1970, Plate 86, Fig. 1, with permission.)*

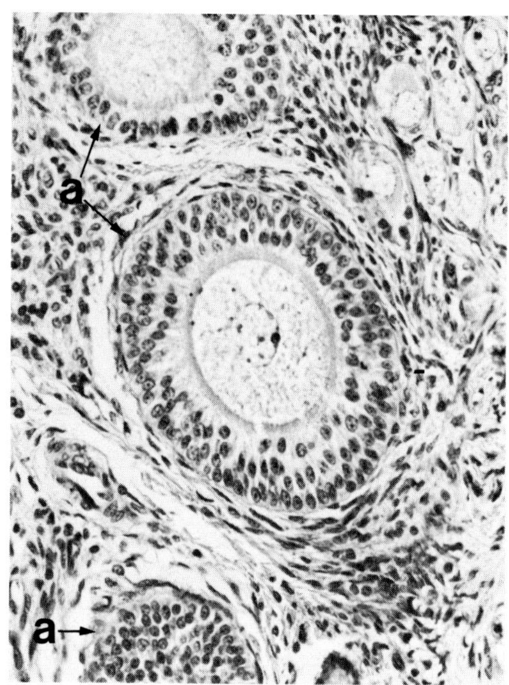

Fig. 13–4. *Secondary follicles (a), mature bitch. The primary oocyte is surrounded by a zona pellucida and a stratified epithelium of polyhedral cells. ×270. (From Adam, W.S., Calhoun, M.L., Smith, E.M., and Stinson, A.W.: Microscopic Anatomy of the Dog: A Photographic Atlas. Springfield, Ill., C.C Thomas, 1970, Plate 86, Fig. 2, with permission.)*

cular *theca interna* and an outer supportive *theca externa* (Fig. 13–8). The theca interna cells are spindle-shaped and located in a delicate reticular fiber network. An extensive blood and lymph capillary network is present in the theca interna, but it does not penetrate the stratum granulosum. In mature follicles, some of the *spindle-shaped* theca interna cells increase in size and assume polyhedral shapes and *epithelioid* characteristics. The nuclei of the epithelioid cells have a lighter chromatin pattern and more distinct nucleoli than the nuclei of the spindle-shaped cells. Cytoplasmic organelles in the epithelioid cells become typical of steroid-secreting cells: the mitochondria have tubular cristae, and agranular tubular ER, Golgi complexes, and lipid inclusions are abundant. The epithelioid cells are especially abundant in mature follicles during proestrus and estrus and during early regression. "Wedges" of epithelioid cells may protrude into the granulosa layer, giving a folding appearance to the wall of the mature follicle (Fig. 13–9). In rodent ovaries, the epithelioid theca interna cells of regressing follicles contribute to the formation of the ovarian interstitial gland.

The theca externa consists of a thin layer of loose connective tissue arranged concentrically around the theca interna. Blood vessels of the theca externa supply capillaries to the theca interna.

One or more mature follicles reach maximal development near the time of ovulation. The *primary oocyte* in these follicles completes the first meiotic division to become a *secondary oocyte.* During the first meiotic division, chromosome pairs are established and a mixture of parental genetic material occurs. This is followed by separation of the pairs and the production of

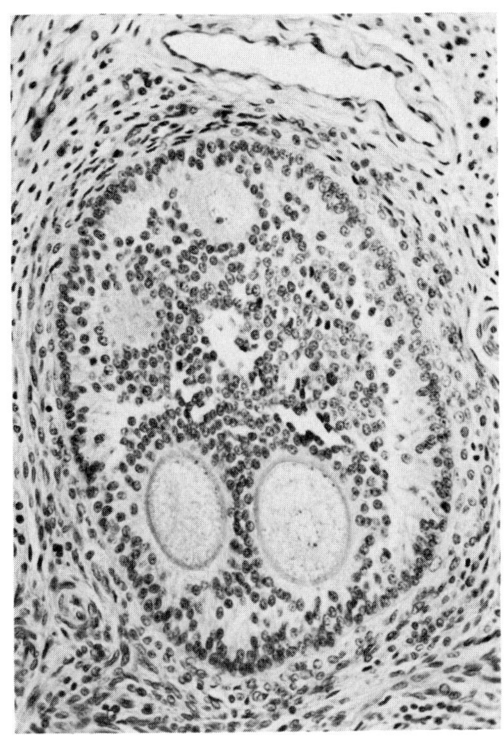

Fig. 13–5. *A polyovular secondary follicle, mature bitch. ×270. (From Adam, W.S., Calhoun, M.L., Smith, E.M., and Stinson, A.W.: Microscopic Anatomy of the Dog: A Photographic Atlas. Springfield, Ill., C.C Thomas, 1970, Plate 87, Fig. 3, with permission.)*

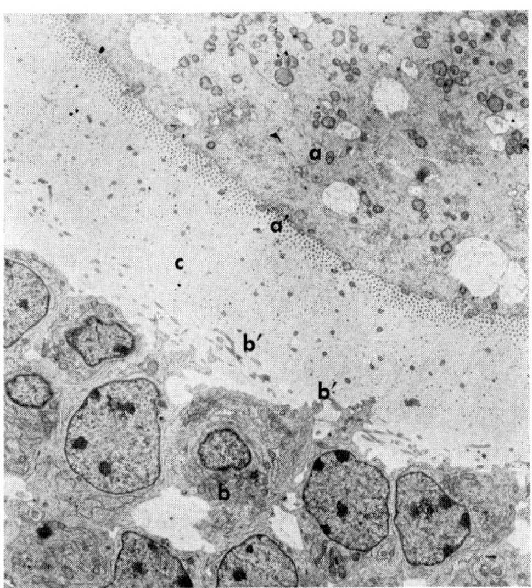

Fig. 13–6. *Electron micrograph of the oocyte (a) and cumulus granulosa cells (b) of a tertiary follicle, cow. Microvilli (a') of the oocyte extend into the zona pellucida (c) to the proximity of processes (b') of the cumulus granulosa cells. A distinct corona radiata has not yet developed. ×2,550. (From Priedkalns, J., and Weber, A.F.: Ultrastructural studies of the bovine Graafian follicle and corpus luteum. Z Zellforsch 91:554, 1968.)*

the first *polar body,* with little cytoplasm, at the completion of the division. In domestic animals, the first meiotic division is completed shortly before ovulation, except in the bitch and mare, in which both meiotic divisions are completed after ovulation. The second meiotic division begins immediately after the first meiotic division, but is arrested in metaphase; it is not completed unless fertilization occurs. At fertilization, the secondary oocyte becomes an *ovum* and the second polar body is given off. The ovum becomes a *zygote* when the male and female pronuclei in the ovum fuse.

Both the granulosa and theca cells of late secondary or early tertiary follicles become responsive to gonadotropic hormones. The granulosa cells develop follicle-stimulating hormone (FSH) receptors and the theca cells develop luteinizing hormone (LH) receptors. In mature tertiary follicles, the granulosa cells develop LH receptors.

In tertiary follicles, LH interacts with receptors on the theca interna cells to stimulate the production of androgens and small amounts of estradiol. The androgens either are secreted into capillaries or traverse the basement membrane to reach the granulosa cell layer. Receptors on the granulosa cells interact with FSH to activate the aromatase enzyme system, which converts the thecal androgens (testosterone, androstenedione) to estrogens (estradiol-17β, estrone). Granulosa cells themselves are unable to produce the androgens. The estrogens are secreted into the follicular fluid and capillaries. The antral concentration of estradiol-17β is some 1000 times greater than that of the bloodstream. The high local concentration of estrogens maintains a favorable environment for follicular maturation. In mature follicles, FSH induces LH receptors on granulosa cells. The action of FSH as well as LH on follicular cells is mediated by an increased produc-

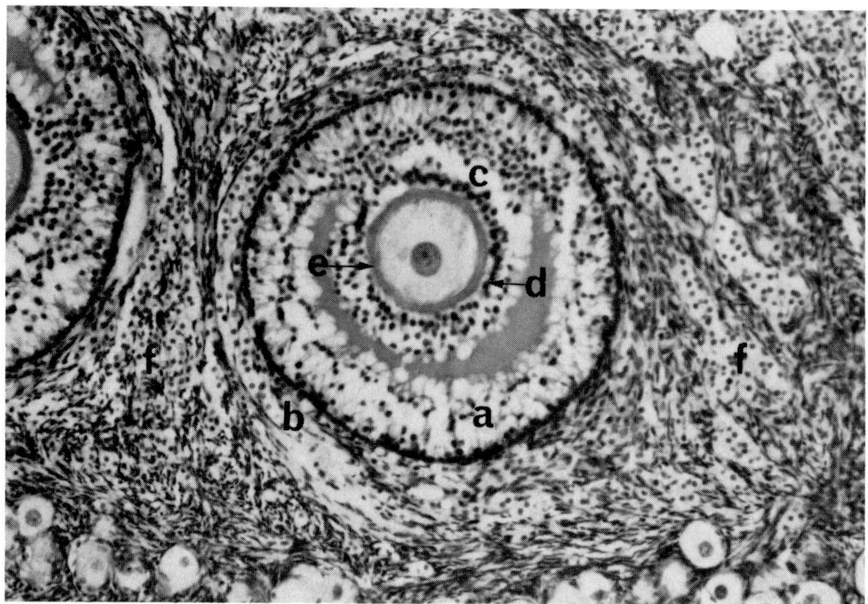

Fig. 13–7. *Early tertiary follicle in atresia, bitch. Pyknosis in the stratum granulosum (a), epithelioid reaction in the theca interna (b), cumulus oophorus (c), corona radiata (d), primary oocyte (e), interstitial gland (f).* ×*166.*

tion of cyclic adenosine-3′,5′-monophosphate (cyclic AMP), which acts as an intracellular "second messenger."

Immediately prior to ovulation, the ovulatory surge of LH interacts with the LH receptors on granulosa cells to induce events leading to ovulation. In addition, the LH surge appears to inhibit the aromatase activity of granulosa cells and thus to diminish estrogen secretion. In the preovulatory follicle, LH is also involved in the induction of oocyte maturation, i.e., the completion of the first meiotic division. A number of other physiologically active substances accumulate in the preovulatory follicular fluid, including "inhibin," a large protein that selectively suppresses pituitary FSH secretion.

Ovulation

When the follicle is maximally developed, it protrudes from the surface of the ovary. The blood and lymph vessel networks surrounding the follicle promote an increased rate of secretion of a thin liquor folliculi. The increased secretion rate is influenced by increases in the follicular blood capillary pressure and permeability during proestrus and estrus. The increased accumulation of liquor folliculi causes the follicles to swell, but intrafollicular pressure does not increase. Small hemorrhages occur in the follicular wall. The follicular wall becomes very thin and transparent at the peripheral site of ovulation, the *stigma.* The mature ovulatory follicles attain a size of 15 to 20 mm in the cow, 50 to 70 mm in the mare, approximately 10 mm in the ewe, goat, and sow, and approximately 2 mm in the bitch and queen.

Changes in the wall of the follicle preceding rupture are due to the release of collagenase enzymes. LH stimulates the production of prostaglandins $PGF_{2\alpha}$ and PGE_2. $PGF_{2\alpha}$ is believed to release collagenase enzymes from follicular cells, causing digestion of the follicular wall and its distension at the stigma. The process of digestion also releases proteins that provoke an inflammatory response with leukocytic infiltration and the release of histamine. All these processes degrade the connective tissue of the follicular wall and

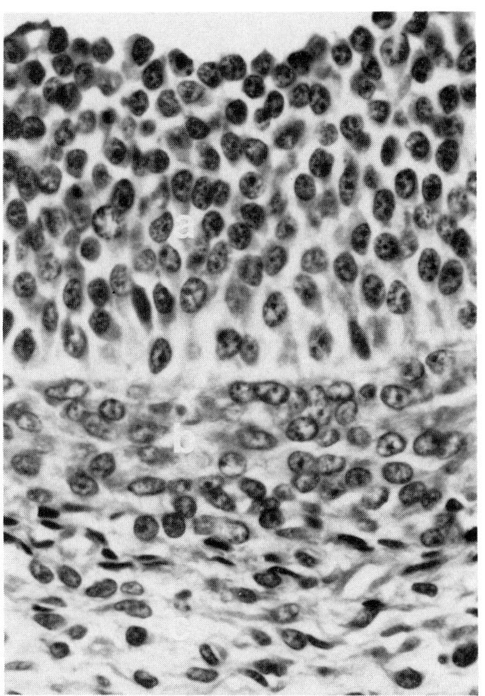

Fig. 13–8. *Stratum granulosum (a), theca interna (b), and theca externa (c) of a tertiary ovarian follicle, mature bitch. ×710. (From Adam, W.S., Calhoun, M.L., Smith, E.M., and Stinson, A.W.: Microscopic Anatomy of the Dog: A Photographic Atlas. Springfield, Ill., C.C Thomas, 1970, Plate 87, Fig. 2, with permission.)*

the ground substance of the cumulus oophorus, so that the follicle ultimately ruptures at the stigma and the oocyte is released. The oocyte, usually surrounded by the corona radiata, escapes into the peritoneal cavity, from which it is swept into the infundibulum of the uterine tube. On rare occasions, an oocyte may fail to enter the uterine tube and, if fertilized, may establish ectopic pregnancy. In most species, corona radiata cells disperse in the uterine tube in the presence of spermatozoa; however, they are lost at the time of ovulation in ruminants. The ovum probably remains fertilizable for less than one day; when not fertilized, it degenerates and is resorbed. In some species, one ovary ovulates more frequently than the other. Thus in the mare, the left ovary ovulates about 60% of the ova, whereas in the cow 60 to 65% of the ova come from the right ovary. Most domestic animals ovulate spontaneously, but ovulation in the queen is induced by a copulatory stimulus.

Atresia

Because only a small percentage of the potential oocytes is released from the ovary at ovulation, most follicles regress at some time during their development. This regression is called *atresia;* many more follicles become atretic than ever attain maturity. In atresia of primary and secondary follicles in the cow, the egg cell appears to degenerate before the follicular wall, whereas in tertiary follicles, the reverse is true. Atretic changes in tertiary follicles may result in the formation of two different morphologic types of atretic follicles: obliterative and cystic. In obliterative atresia, the granulosa and theca layers both infold, hypertrophy, and extend inward to occupy the antrum. In cystic atresia, both the granulosa and theca layers may atrophy, or only the granulosa layer may atrophy and the theca layer may either luteinize, fibrose, or hyalinize around the antrum (Figs. 13–10 and 13–11). In cases of hormonal (especially LH) insufficiency, large cystic atretic follicles may not regress, and ovulated follicles may not luteinize adequately to form a functional corpus luteum. In cystic atretic follicles, the theca interna cells containing LH receptors may continue to synthesize androgens following regression of the granulosa cells (that converted the androgens to estrogens.)

Prominent signs of atresia in follicular wall cells are nuclear pyknosis and chromatolysis. During atresia, the basement membrane of the granulosa layer may fold, thicken, and hyalinize, and is then called the *glassy membrane.*

Interstitial Gland Cells

Ovarian interstitial gland cells arise chiefly from the epithelioid theca interna cells of atretic antral follicles (i.e., follicles containing an antrum), or from hypertro-

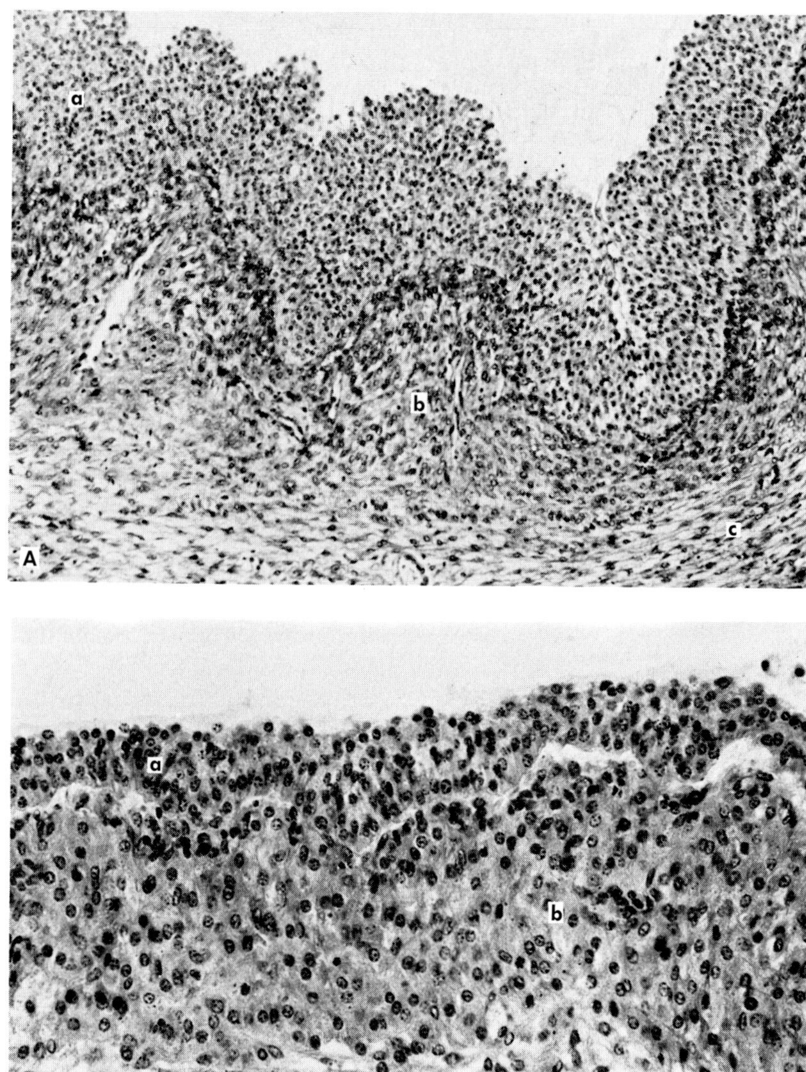

Fig. 13–9. *Large, developed tertiary ovarian follicles, cow. A, Folded wall of a mature proestrous follicle with hypertrophy of stratum granulosum (a) and theca interna (b). Theca externa (c). ×55. B, Follicle in early atresia with regression of stratum granulosum (a), whereas theca interna (b) is hypertrophied and contains epithelioid cells. ×110. (From Priedkalns, J.: Effect of melengestrol acetate on the bovine ovary. Z Zellforsch 122:85, 1971.)*

phied granulosa cells of atretic preantral follicles (Fig. 13–12). The interstitial gland is prominent in rodent ovaries, as well as in the ovaries of the bitch and queen. It is usually absent from the ovaries of other adult domestic animals. The interstitial gland cells are polyhedral and epithelioid and contain lipid inclusions. In species such as the rabbit and hare, they secrete large amounts of steroid hormones. The interstitial gland cells are to be distinguished from ovarian stromal cells, which are spindle-shaped and embedded in networks of reticular fibers.

In humans and certain other mammals, groups of epithelioid cells with structural

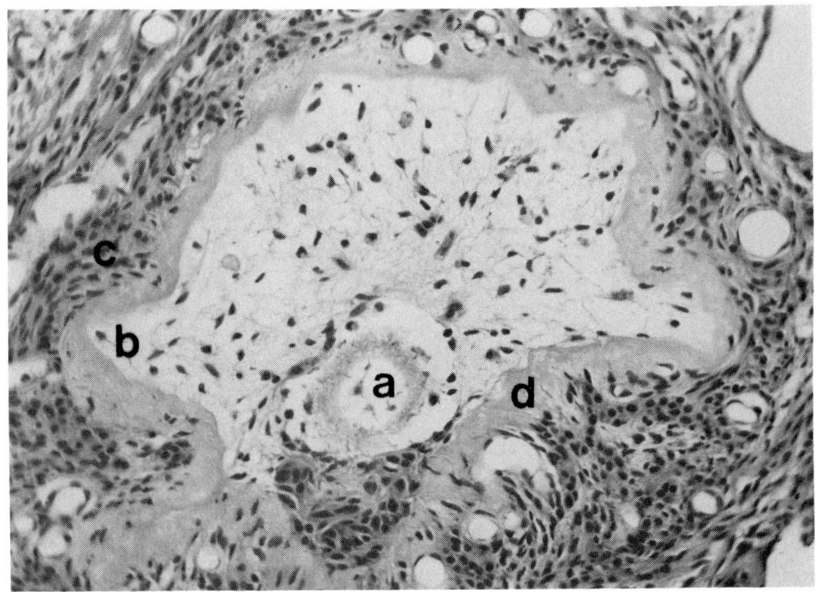

Fig. 13–10. *An atretic tertiary follicle, mature bitch. The oocyte (a) and granulosa layer (b) have degenerated, and the theca layer (c) has fibrosed. 'Glassy membrane' (d).* ×*170. (From Adam, W.S., Calhoun, M.L., Smith, E.M., and Stinson, A.W.: Microscopic Anatomy of the Dog: A Photographic Atlas. Springfield, Ill., C.C Thomas, 1970, Plate 87, Fig. 4, with permission.)*

features similar to those of ovarian interstitial gland cells occur in the hilus of the ovary near rete ovarii and in the adjacent mesovarium. They are called *hilus cells*. Cytochemically, they resemble testicular interstitial cells, and their tumors or hyperplasia are accompanied by masculinization in women.

Corpus Luteum

At ovulation, the follicle ruptures, collapses, and shrinks as the pressure is reduced. Folding of the follicular wall is extensive. The ruptured follicle is referred to as a *corpus hemorrhagicum* because of the blood that may fill the antrum. In the mare, cow, and sow there is more blood following rupture than in carnivores and small ruminants. Immediately before ovulation, some cells of the stratum granulosum exhibit signs of pyknosis. After ovulation, however, it becomes vascularized by vessels from the theca interna. The granulosa cells then enlarge, luteinize, and contribute to the *large luteal (lutein) cell* population of the corpus luteum. In most species, the theca interna cells also contribute to the formation of the corpus luteum. After ovulation, folding of the follicular wall results in the incorporation of parts of the theca layer into the corpus luteum. The theca cells appear to contribute to the *small luteal cell* population of the corpus luteum.

Luteinization is the process by which the granulosa and theca cells transform into luteal cells. It includes hypertrophy and hyperplasia of both cell types. A yellow pigment, lutein, appears in the luteal cells in the cow, mare, and carnivores; it is absent in the ewe, goat, and sow. A black pigment has been observed in the luteal cells of the mare. In the cow, postovulatory mitosis continues for about 40 hours in the granulosa (large) luteal cells, and for about 80 hours in the theca (small) luteal cells. The increase in size of the corpus luteum, after the period of mitotic activity, is mainly due to hypertrophy of the large luteal cells. The small luteal cells make up a minor part of the corpus luteum and occupy mainly trabecular and peripheral areas. However, the two luteal cell types may become mixed in the corpus luteum and are then difficult

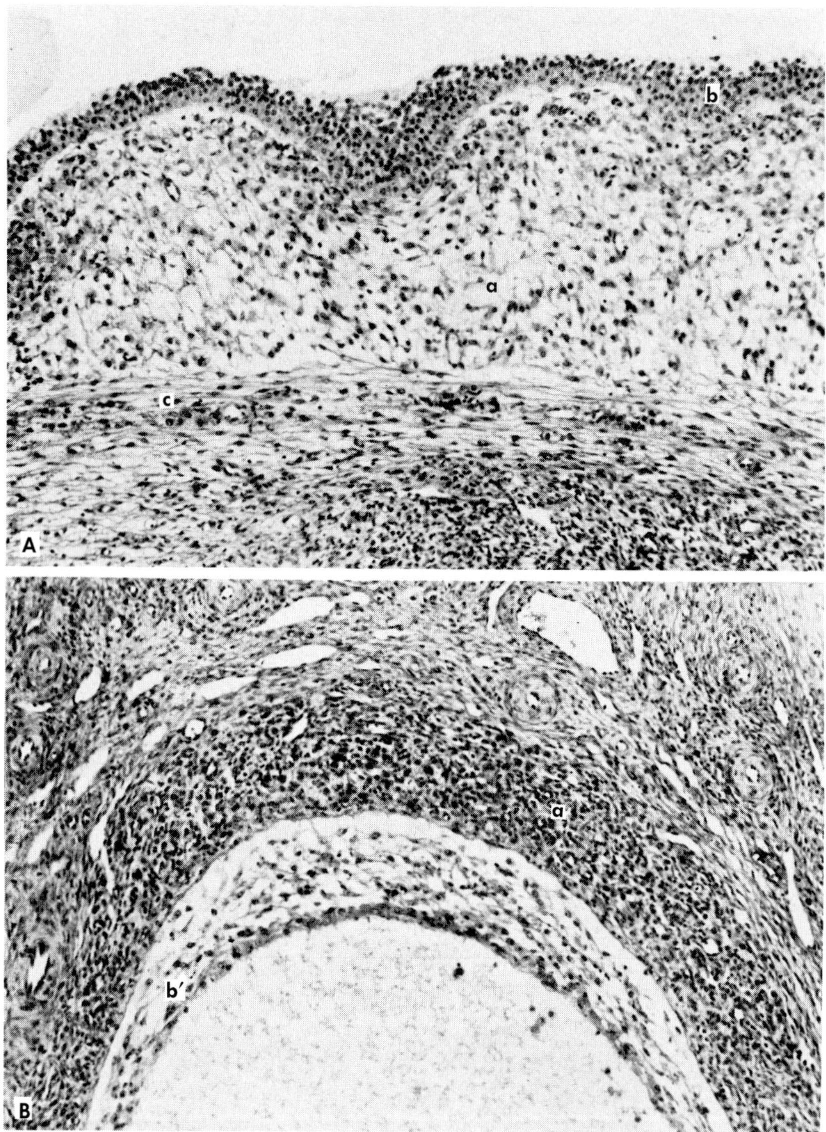

Fig. 13–11. *Atresia of large tertiary ovarian follicles, cow. A, Extensive hyalinization of theca interna (a), and loss or pyknosis of granulosa cells (b). Theca externa (c). ×111. B, Fibrosis of theca interna (a). Granulosa cell remnants (b′). ×139. (From Priedkalns, J.: Effect of melengestrol acetate on the bovine ovary. Z Zellforsch 122:85, 1971.)*

to distinguish. In the cow, the corpus luteum is fully developed and vascularized nine days after ovulation, but continues to grow until the twelfth day, when it attains a diameter of approximately 25 mm (Fig. 13–13).

The *large luteal cells* are polygonal, approximately 40 μm in diameter, with a large spherical vesicular nucleus. They contain numerous metabolic lipid inclusions. During metestrus and diestrus, the cells contain organelles characteristic for steroid-synthesizing cells such as mitochondria with tubular cristae and abundant tubular agranular ER (Fig. 13–14). Evidence suggests that the large luteal cells produce

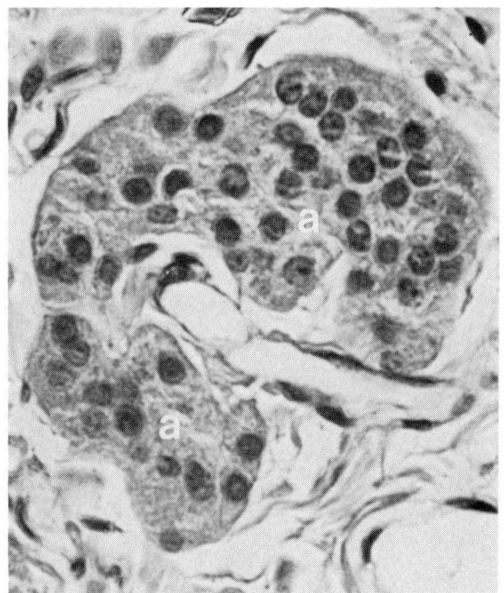

Fig. 13–12. *Ovarian interstitial gland cells (a), mature bitch. ×280. (From Adam, W.S., Calhoun, M.L., Smith, E.M., and Stinson, A.W.: Microscopic Anatomy of the Dog: A Photographic Atlas. Springfield, Ill., C.C Thomas, 1970, Plate 88, Fig. 2, with permission.)*

progesterone during metestrus and diestrus. The *small luteal cells* are more lipid-laden but have fewer steroid cell–type organelles than the large luteal cells (Fig. 13–13).

In cells of the developing and mature corpus luteum, the lipids are mostly phospholipids with traces of triglycerides, cholesterol, and its esters. During regression, cholesterol accumulates in the luteal cells. This suggests decreased cholesterol utilization for steroid hormone synthesis. In active luteal cells, the lipid droplets are small and even in size and distribution, whereas during regression, they are large and unevenly distributed. With the light microscope, they appear as large vacuoles. The first sign of luteal regression occurs in late diestrus and involves condensation of lutein pigment (which then appears reddish), followed by fibrosis. In the cow, these signs are first observed 15 days after ovulation; further regression and shrinkage of the corpus luteum occur rapidly after the eighteenth day and are completed 1 to 2 days after estrus (Fig. 13–15). The loose and vascular connective tissues of the corpus luteum become conspicuous in regression. The connective tissue scar remaining after regression is called the *corpus albicans*.

Functions of the Ovary

In addition to producing oocytes, the ovary has important endocrine functions. It secretes the female sex hormones, estrogens, and progesterone (see pp. 320 and 323). Estrogens are produced primarily by the granulosa cells that convert androgens, secreted by the theca interna cells, to estrogens. Progesterone is produced primarily by the large luteal cells during metestrus, diestrus, and pregnancy and by the placenta. In certain species, the interstitial gland cells secrete large amounts of steroid hormones. Estrogen induces the growth and development of the female reproductive tract and estrous behavior. Progesterone stimulates the development of uterine glands, induces them to secrete, and renders the endometrium receptive to the implantation of the zygote. It also prevents follicular maturation and estrus and promotes behavior appropriate to pregnancy. Estrogens and progesterone promote mammary gland development.

The growth and maturation of ovarian follicles and their estrogen secretion are controlled by pituitary gonadotropins, FSH and LH. Ovarian estrogen secretion, in turn, triggers the release of an ovulatory surge of LH, usually on the day of estrus, which induces the processes leading to ovulation. The formation of the corpus luteum is also initiated by a stimulus of pituitary LH. LH interacts with receptors on cells of the ruptured follicular wall to initiate luteinization and progesterone secretion. In some species, such as the rat and mouse, luteotropic hormone (LTH) is needed to maintain the corpus luteum and its progesterone secretion. Regression of the corpus luteum may follow withdrawal of LH, LTH, or both or may be caused by a uterine luteolytic factor reaching the ovary by local circulation in the ewe, cow, and sow. The

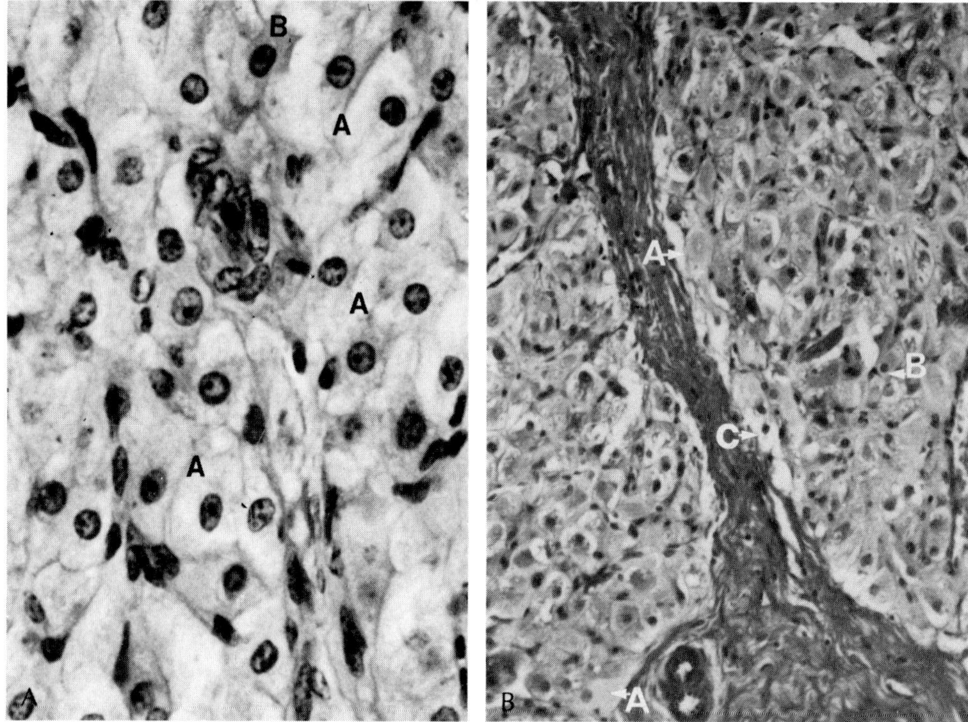

Fig. 13–13. *A, Cow. Active corpus luteum. Large luteal cells (A) with active nuclei and typical foamy cytoplasm. Small luteal cell (B). B, Bitch. Corpus luteum showing large luteal (A), small luteal (B), and regressing luteal cells (C). ×160.*

main luteolytic factor is prostaglandin $F_{2\alpha}$. If pregnancy occurs, the corpus luteum persists as the corpus luteum of pregnancy for different periods of time in various species. In the cow and doe, progesterone production by the corpus luteum continues throughout gestation. The corpus luteum of pregnancy is supported by luteotropic hormones from the pituitary as well as from the placenta. The embryo in the ewe provides, in addition to luteotropic hormones, an antiluteolytic factor that overcomes the luteolytic effect of the uterus. In later stages of pregnancy in most species, the corpus luteum is not important because the placenta secretes the progesterone required for the successful maintenance of pregnancy. Ovarian and placental steroid hormones in turn influence pituitary gonadotropin secretion by a feedback effect on the hypothalamus, regulating mainly the release of the hypothalamic gonadotropin-releasing hormone. Other diencephalic structures, such as the pineal gland, also influence gonadotropic functions.

Vessels and Nerves

The arterial supply of the ovary is derived from the ovarian artery and the ovarian branch of the uterine artery. The arteries enter the ovary at the hilus. In the medulla, they form plexuses and give off branches to the follicular thecae, corpora lutea, and stromal tissue. Around the larger follicles, the branches form a capillary wreath. During the formation of the corpus luteum, capillary loops from the wreath extend inward to form an extensive luteal network. Arteriovenous anastomoses occur in the ovary. During cyclic regression of the corpora lutea and the follicles, cellular hypertrophy and sclerosis occur in the walls of the arteries supplying these structures. The venous return is similar to the arterial supply. Lymph capillaries accom-

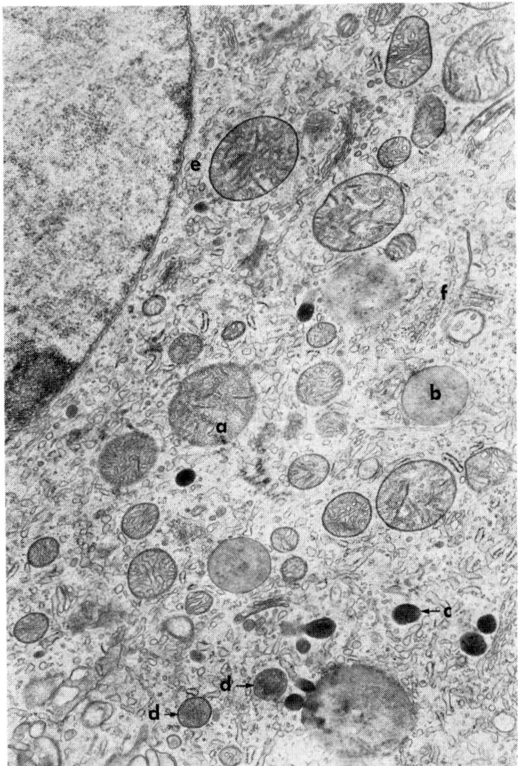

Fig. 13–14. *Electron micrograph of a developing large luteal cell during metestrus, cow. The larger mitochondria (a) contain fine tubular cristae. Lipid bodies (b), dense bodies (c) and "transitional bodies" (d) (with characteristics of both mitochondria and lysosomes) are present. The endoplasmic reticulum (e) is predominantly agranular, and Golgi complexes (f) show vacuolation. ×10,200. (From Priedkalns, J., and Weber, A.F.: Ultrastructural studies of the bovine Graafian follicle and corpus luteum. Z Zellforsch 91*:554, 1968.)

pany blood vessels in follicular thecae and in the corpus luteum, and drain into the lumbar lymph nodes.

The nerves that supply the ovary are generally nonmyelinated. They are vasomotor in nature but include some sensory fibers. The nerves follow blood vessels and terminate on the walls of the vessels and around the follicles, in the corpora lutea, and in the tunica albuginea. They are derived mainly from the sympathetic system through renal and aortic plexuses, but vagal supply to the ovary has also been described. An especially well developed adrenergic innervation of the female repro-

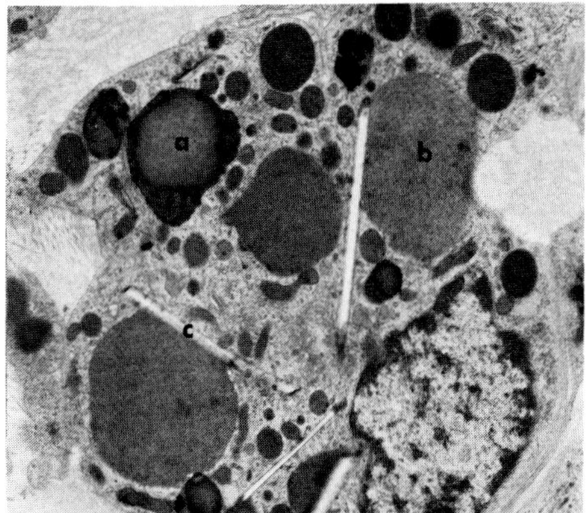

Fig. 13–15. *Electron micrograph of a regressed luteal cell, ovary, cow. Notice the characteristic large remnant lipid bodies (a), granular bodies (b) and crystalloid inclusions (c). ×6,100. (From Priedkalns, J., and Weber, A.F.: Ultrastructural studies of the bovine Graafian follicle and corpus luteum. Z Zellforsch 91:554, 1968.)*

ductive tract has been described in the queen.

UTERINE TUBE (OVIDUCT)

The uterine tubes are bilateral, tortuous structures that extend from the region of the ovary to the uterine horns and convey ova, spermatozoa, and zygotes. Three segments of the uterine tube can be distinguished: (1) the *infundibulum,* a large funnel-shaped portion (Fig. 13–16), (2) the *ampulla,* a thin-walled section extending caudally from the infundibulum (Fig. 13–17), and (3) the *isthmus,* a narrow muscular segment joining the uterus (Fig. 13–18).

Histologic Structure

The epithelium is simple columnar or pseudostratified columnar with motile cilia on a majority of cells. Both ciliated and nonciliated cell types possess microvilli. Morphologic signs of secretory activity are evident in only the nonciliated cells. Ciliated and tall cells occur more commonly in the cranial end of the uterine tube and, in the cow, many of these are seen at estrus. During the luteal phase, the secretory cells

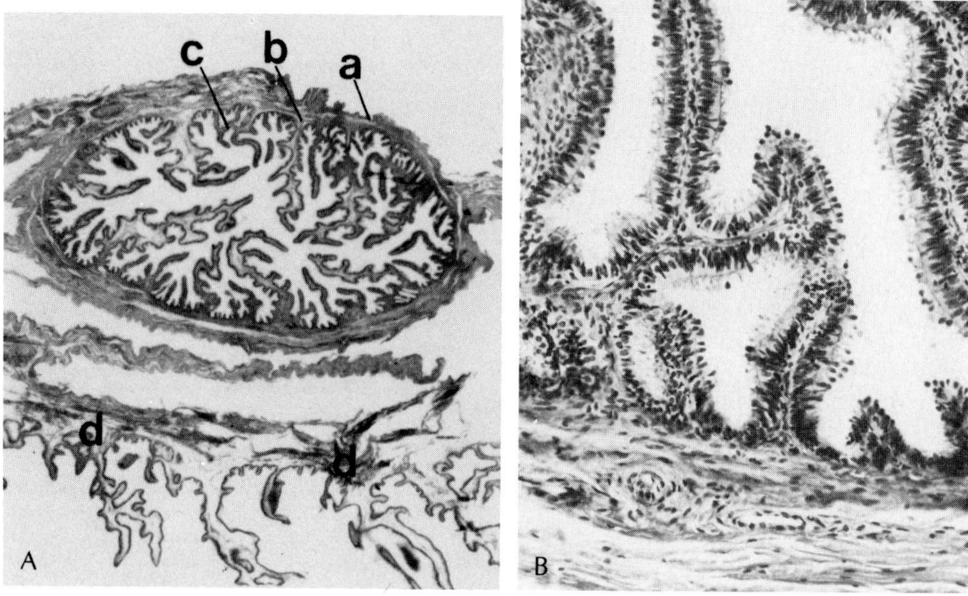

Fig. 13–16. *Sections through the infundibulum of the uterine tube, cow. A, Tunica serosa (a); tunica muscularis (b); extensive mucosal-submucosal folds (c); fimbriae of the free margin of the infundibulum (d). ×14. B, Mucosal-submucosal folds with ciliated columnar epithelium. Notice secretory blebs at cell apices. ×97.*

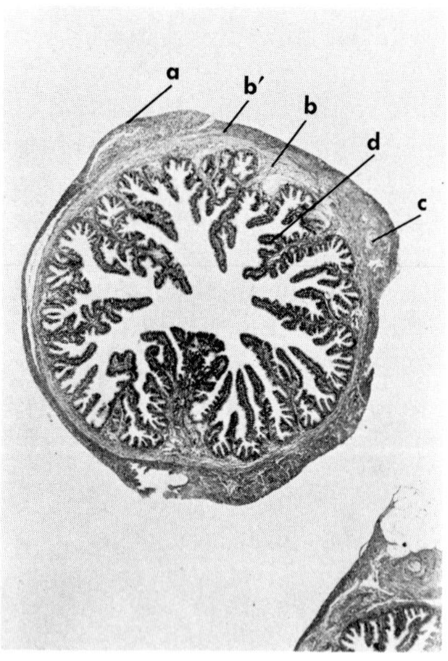

Fig. 13–17. *Section through the ampulla of the uterine tube, cow. Tunica serosa (a); circular muscle layer (b); longitudinal muscle layer (b′); stratum vasculare (c); mucosal-submucosal folds (d). ×20. (Courtesy of A.W. Stinson.)*

become taller than the ciliated cells. Their secretion may provide the ovum with necessary nutrients. Epithelial glands are absent.

The mucosa is continuous with the submucosa in the female reproductive tract because the lamina muscularis is absent. In the uterine tube, the propria-submucosa consists of loose connective tissue with many plasma cells, mast cells, and eosinophils. The tunica mucosa-submucosa of the ampulla is highly folded, especially in the sow and mare. In the cow, about 40 primary longitudinal folds are present in the ampulla, each with secondary and tertiary folds (Fig. 13–17). At the isthmus-uterus junction, where the isthmus is embedded in the uterine wall, only four to eight primary folds and no secondary or tertiary folds are present.

The tunica muscularis consists chiefly of circular smooth muscle bundles, but isolated longitudinal and oblique bundles also occur. The muscle layer gives off radial strands into the mucosa. In the infundibulum and ampulla, the tunica muscularis

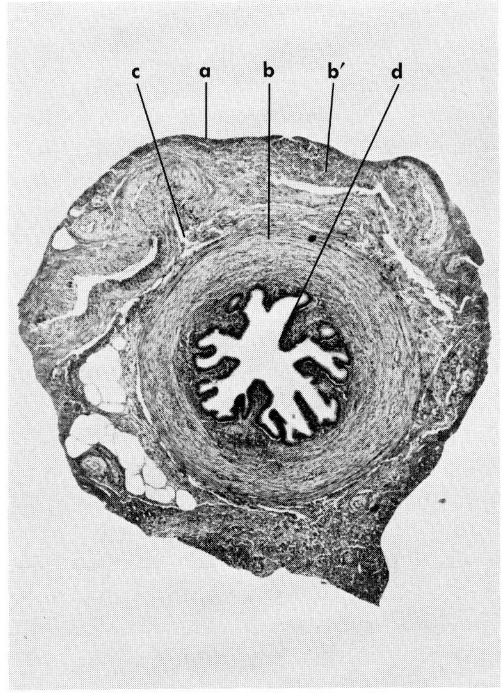

Fig. 13–18. *Section through the isthmus of the uterine tube, cow. Tunica serosa (a); circular muscle layer (b); longitudinal muscle layer (b′); stratum vasculare (c); mucosal-submucosal folds (d). ×36. (Courtesy of A.W. Stinson.)*

is thin and composed of an inner circular layer and a few outer longitudinal bundles of smooth muscle (Fig. 13–17). In the isthmus, the muscle layer is prominent and blends with the uterine circular muscle (Fig. 13–18).

A tunica serosa is present and contains many blood vessels and nerves.

Histophysiology

The infundibulum secures oocytes extruded from the ovary. It is enclosed in the ovarian bursa, or, in species without a definite ovarian bursa (e.g., the mare), it is applied partly around the ovary at estrus. It has fingerlike projections called *fimbriae.* At the time of ovulation in most species, blood vessels in the fimbriae become engorged. The turgid fimbriae move over the surface of the ovary as a result of rhythmic smooth muscle contractions. At the same time, cilia of the infundibular epithelial cells, mostly beating toward the uterus, transport the egg into the ampulla.

The caudal ampulla is the site of fertilization. In the ampulla, ciliary activity is the primary force propelling the egg towards the isthmus, but in some species muscle contractility is also involved. In the isthmus, muscle contractility is the primary force propelling the zygote towards the uterus, with ciliary activity involved in some species. The directionality of isthmus contractions varies according to the phase of the estrous cycle. In the follicular phase, antiperistaltic contractions move the luminal contents towards the ampulla, whereas in the luteal phase segmental contractions gradually propel the zygote towards the uterus. Zygotes require four to five days to traverse the isthmus. This length of time is independent of the isthmus length and the gestation time among species.

The passage of spermatozoa to the ampulla is accounted for by muscular contractions of the uterine and tubal walls. Inert particles and nonmotile spermatozoa can ascend the uterine tube at the same speed as motile spermatozoa, suggesting that the ascent of spermatozoa is not primarily due to their innate motility. In the cow, spermatozoa can reach the ampulla within five minutes after mating. Ascent at this rate is too fast to be accounted for by the motility of spermatozoa and/or the ciliary movement of tubal cells.

Although spermatozoa develop in the male reproductive tract, their ability to fertilize is attained in domestic animals only after capacitation in the uterine tube (see Chapter 12).

Vessels and Nerves

Arterial supply to the uterine tubes is derived from the uterine artery and branches of the ovarian artery. The blood vessels form subepithelial vascular plexuses and proliferate during pregnancy. Lymph vessels have capillary networks in the mucosal and serosal layers and drain into the lumbar lymph nodes.

Both myelinated and nonmyelinated nerve fibers with many subepithelial branches are present. They are derived mainly from the sympathetic system.

UTERUS

The uterus is the site of implantation of the conceptus. It undergoes a definite sequence of changes during the estrous and reproductive cycles. In most species it consists of bilateral horns (cornua) connected to the uterine tubes, and an unpaired body (corpus) and a neck (cervix) which joins the vagina. The cervix will be considered separately. In primates, the entire uterus is a single tube, called the uterus simplex.

Histologic Structure

The uterine wall consists of three layers (Fig. 13–19): (1) the mucosa-submucosa or endometrium, (2) the muscularis or myometrium, and (3) the serosa or perimetrium.

ENDOMETRIUM. The endometrium is composed of two zones differing in structure and function. The superficial layer, called the *functional zone,* degenerates partially or fully during a reproductive, estrous, or menstrual cycle and may be lost in some species. A thin deep layer, the *basal zone,* persists throughout the cycle, and the functional zone, when lost, is restored from this layer (Figs. 13–19 and 13–20).

The Functional Zone. The surface epithelium is simple columnar in the mare, bitch, and queen. It is pseudostratified columnar and/or simple columnar in the sow and ruminants. In isolated areas, the epithelium may be cuboidal. The height and structure of the epithelial cells is related to the secretion of ovarian hormones throughout the cycle. The subepithelial, superficial part of the functional zone consists of a richly vascular, loose connective tissue with many fibroblasts, macrophages, and mast cells. Neutrophils, eosinophils, lymphocytes, and plasma cells enter from the bloodstream; melanophores are present in this area in the sheep. The deep part of the functional zone consists of a loose connective tissue that is less cellular than that of the superficial part. In ruminants, especially during estrus, large irregular tissue spaces containing intercellular fluid are present in the functional zone; this is called *endometrial edema.*

Simple coiled, branched tubular glands, lined by ciliated and nonciliated simple columnar epithelium, are present throughout the functional and basal zones of the endometrium in most species. The glands are absent from the caruncular areas of ruminants (Fig. 13–19B). Rising estrogen levels stimulate the growth and branching of the glands, but coiling and copious secretion of the glands do not generally occur until progesterone stimulation occurs. The branching and coiling of the glands is extensive in the mare, while less branching is seen in carnivores (Fig. 13–20). *Endometrial cups* in the mare occur in early pregnancy after endometrial invasion by fetal cells (see Chapter 14).

Caruncle. In ruminants, circumscribed thickenings of the endometrium known as *caruncles* are present (Fig. 13–19B). They are rich in fibroblasts and have an extensive blood supply. Four rows of approximately 15 caruncles in each are present in each uterine horn in ruminants. They are dome-shaped in the cow and cup-shaped (i.e., a dome with a central depression) in the ewe. Caruncles are the sites of attachment of the maternal placenta to the corresponding sites of the fetal placenta, the cotyledons.

MYOMETRIUM. The myometrium consists of a thick inner layer, which is mostly circular, and an outer longitudinal layer of smooth muscle cells that increase in number and size during pregnancy. Between the two layers, or deep in the inner layer, is a vascular layer consisting of large arteries, veins and lymph vessels (Figs. 13–19 and 13–20). These vessels supply the endometrium. They are especially large in the caruncular regions of ruminants.

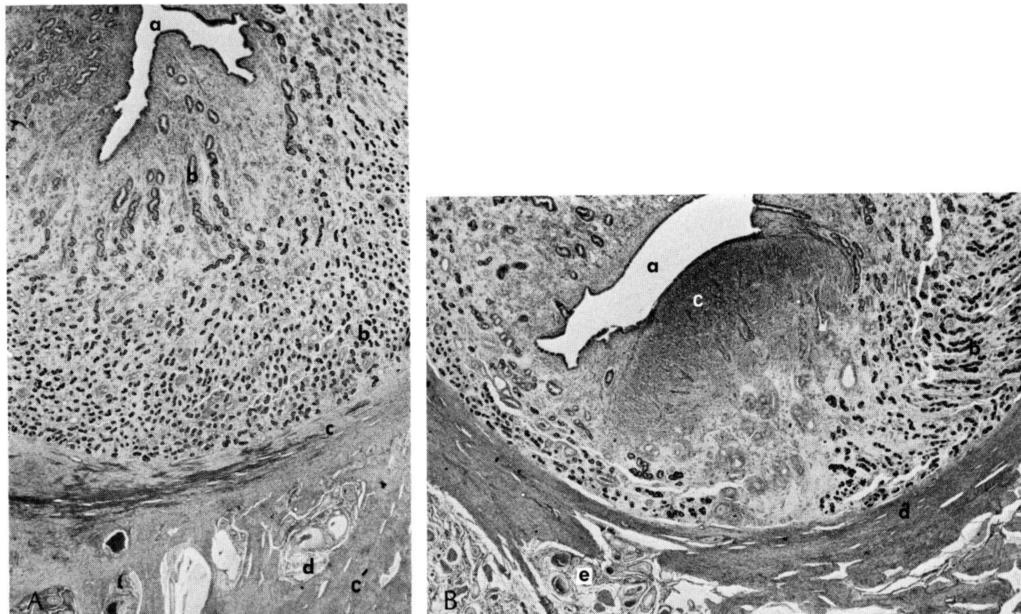

Fig. 13–19. *A, Section through the uterine wall, cow, five days after estrus. Uterine lumen (a); uterine glands (b); circular muscle layer (c); stratum vasculare (d); longitudinal muscle layer (c'). ×10. B, Section through the uterine wall, cow, five days after estrus. Uterine lumen (a); uterine glands (b); caruncle (c); circular muscle layer (d); stratum vasculare (e). ×10. (Courtesy of A.W. Stinson.)*

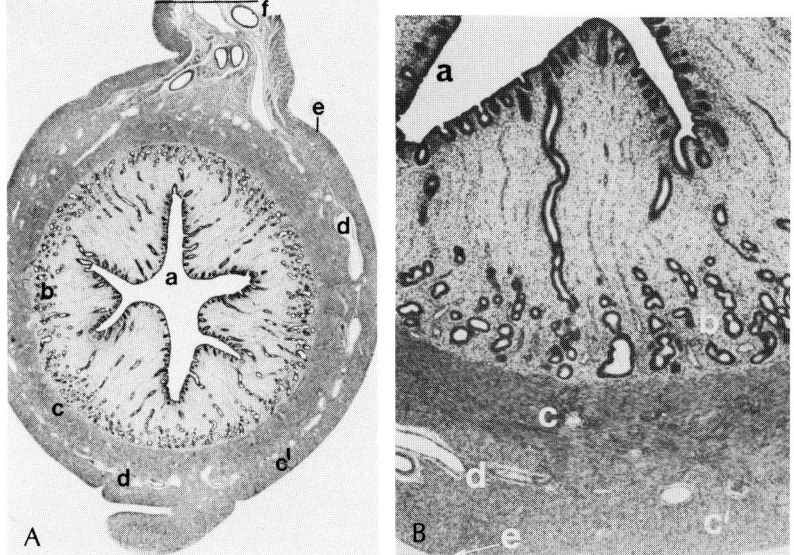

Fig. 13–20. *Sections through the uterine horn, bitch, in estrus. A, Uterine lumen (a); uterine glands (b); circular muscle layer (c), longitudinal muscle layer (c^1); stratum vasculare (d); tunica serosa (e); broad ligament of the uterus (f). ×10. B, Note (a) to (e) as in A. ×38.*

PERIMETRIUM. The perimetrium, or the tunica serosa, consists of loose connective tissue covered by the peritoneal mesothelium. Smooth muscle cells occur in the perimetrium. Numerous lymph and blood vessels and nerve fibers are present in this layer. The perimetrium, the longitudinal layer of the myometrium, and the vascular layer of the myometrium are all continuous with corresponding structures of the broad ligament of the uterus (Fig. 13–20A).

Cyclic Changes in the Endometrium

THE ESTROUS CYCLE. The estrous cycle is regulated by an intrinsic hypothalamo-hypophysial-ovarian rhythm that is modulated by environmental and uterine factors. In domestic animals the estrous cycle is generally divided into the following sequential phases: (1) *proestrus,* the period of follicular maturation and endometrial proliferation following failure of the corpus luteum of the previous cycle. During this phase progesterone level falls, allowing FSH release; rising estrogen levels lead to estrus; (2) *estrus,* the period of sexual receptiveness, during which ovulation occurs in most species. Ovulation is preceded by a surge of LH; at the end of estrus estrogen levels decline; (3) *metestrus,* the period of corpus luteum development and initial progesterone secretion; (4) *diestrus,* the phase of the active corpus luteum when the influence of luteal progesterone on accessory sex structures predominates. Endometrial glandular hyperplasia and secretion are maximal during diestrus; diestrus can be prolonged into pseudopregnancy or gestational and lactational diestrus; (5) *anestrus,* the prolonged period of sexual inactivity. The average duration (in days) of the phases of the estrous cycle in the cow and sow, respectively, is: proestrus—3½, 3; estrus—½ to 1, 2½; metestrus—2½, 3; diestrus—14½, 12.

During proestrus and estrus, large ovarian follicles produce estrogens, whereas during metestrus and diestrus, the corpus luteum produces progesterone. The estrogens and progesterone are to a large extent responsible for the cyclic changes of the endometrium. (During pregnancy, these hormones are produced chiefly by the placenta.)

Some animals, e.g., the bitch and queen, are *monestrous* and have one or two estrous cycles per year, followed by a long anestrous period. Continuously cycling animals, without an anestrous period (e.g., the cow and sow), or seasonally cycling animals (e.g., the mare, ewe, and goat) are *polyestrous.* The endometrium of monestrous animals degenerates and regenerates to a much greater extent than that of polyestrous animals. The immediate factor precipitating uterine degenerative changes is probably local ischemia. Uterine regenerative changes are induced by estradiol and continued by progesterone, which induces glandular secretory activity and causes the endometrium to produce a maternal placenta when stimulated by the presence of the blastocyst.

CYCLIC ENDOMETRIAL CHANGES IN THE COW. In the cow, proestrus lasts about 3½ days, estrus ½ to 1 day, metestrus about 2½ days, and diestrus about 14½ days. Ovulation occurs on the day after estrus, or about 30 hours after the onset of estrus. The day of estrus may be called 'day 0' of the cycle, and the last day of proestrus, 'day 20.' During the last 3 to 4 days of diestrus, the endometrium undergoes regression. The endometrial stroma and epithelium shrink. The glands become shorter, their epithelium lowers and their secretions cease. During proestrus, under the influence of estrogens, the endometrium is again restored. The mucosa becomes thickened, congested, and edematous with a predominance of mucin-filled epithelial cells. However, glandular proliferation is limited to straight lumen growth without significant branching or coiling. During estrus, endometrial edema and hyperemia are maximal. During metestrus, the edema lessens, but a breakdown occurs in some of the congested blood vessels of the mucosa. With the onset of diestrus, under the influence of progesterone, the endometrium transforms from a proliferative to a secretory type, with glandular epithelial growth and glandular branching, coiling, and secretion (Fig. 13–19). During the first 11 days of diestrus, endometrial glandular secretion is greatest. If pregnancy does not occur, the glands again regress along with the corpus luteum during the last 3 to 4 days of diestrus.

Mitotic activity begins in the surface and glandular epithelia and in the interstitial elements during estrus and continues for approximately six days after estrus. Heterophils invade the lamina propria, epithelia, and uterine lumen from late proestrus to about the third or fourth day after estrus. An invasion of agranulocytes, mainly lymphocytes, occurs from the third to the fifth day after estrus. These cells are especially abundant in the basal zone of the endometrium. An eosinophil invasion may occur from estrus to midcycle, but this is not a constant finding. Mast cells, which are usually present in the mucosa, increase in number at the time of maximal edema, especially in the caruncular areas.

Metrorrhagia. Metrorrhagia is the term for microscopic hemorrhages in the functional zone of the endometrium that begin shortly before the time of ovulation in the cow. At ovulation, metrorrhagia becomes widespread and is prominent in the pitted central areas of the caruncles. Metrorrhagia is greatest immediately following maximal endometrial edema. Capillaries rupture in the mucosa and blood accumulates in "blisters" beneath the surface epithelium. The blisters rupture, and blood and shreds of mucosa are liberated into the uterine lumen. Blood in the caruncular areas is mainly phagocytized and resorbed, and generally does not reach the uterine lumen. Tissue fluid as well as blood may be lost at points of rupture in the intercaruncular areas. Metrorrhagia ends abruptly near the end of the second day after estrus.

CYCLIC ENDOMETRIAL CHANGES IN THE BITCH. Proestrus and estrus each last about one to two weeks in the bitch. If pregnancy does not follow estrus, pseudopregnancy and anestrus ensue. Edema, congestion, and hemorrhages occur during proestrus. Ovulation occurs soon after the onset of estrus. On about the sixth day of estrus, corpora lutea become functional, and uterine glands and interstitial elements begin to proliferate. The glandular epithelium becomes tall and the glands coiled (Fig. 13–20). In the nonpregnant state, involution of the endometrial glands and stroma begins about 20 to 30 days after the onset of estrus and lasts throughout anestrus. During anestrus, the endometrium is thin and regressed, and the epithelium is mainly cuboidal. A prolonged and incomplete endometrial regression may occasionally result in pyometra.

RELATION OF METRORRHAGIA TO MENSTRUATION IN PRIMATES. Menstruation in primates is an entirely different phenomenon from the uterine bleeding seen in the bovine and canine species. The uterine hemorrhages in the cow and bitch occur during a *regenerative* phase of the endometrium near estrus, when relatively high levels of estrogens are present.

Menstruation, on the other hand, occurs during a *degenerative* phase of the endometrium, precipitated by the withdrawal of estrogens and, more important, of progesterone after the involution of the corpus luteum. The occurrence of hemorrhages in primates has been related to special coiled arteries in the endometrial functional zone that periodically constrict and dilate as the support of progesterone and estrogens wanes. The arterial constriction causes ischemia and necrosis of tissue, and the dilatation that follows leads to the rupture of the blood vessels, hemorrhage, and loss of tissues of the functional zone. In deeper parts of the functional zone, veins are also involved. However, several species of New World monkeys, known to menstruate, have no coiled endometrial arteries. Neither can experimentally induced menstruation always be ascribed to a preceding period of ischemia.

In certain animal species, the period most analogous to the period of human menstrual regression is the termination of pseudopregnancy. In the bitch, pseudopregnancy invariably follows estrus and spontaneous ovulation if the animal does not become pregnant. In other animals, pseudopregnancy follows estrus and ovulation only if a mating stimulus resulting in a corpus luteum of pseudopregnancy has occurred, i.e., a corpus luteum of prolonged and sometimes greater activity than the corpus luteum of diestrus. Pseudopregnancy is terminated by a cessation of hypophysial luteotropic stimulation. This results in regression of the corpus luteum, decrease of the progesterone and estrogen supply, and consequent regression of the endometrium and the termination of pseudopregnancy. Although no external bleeding occurs in the bitch at this time, microscopic hemorrhages of the endometrium have been observed.

CERVIX

The cervix or neck of the uterus is thick-walled, muscular, and rich in elastic fibers. The mucosa-submucosa forms high primary folds with secondary and tertiary folds. In the cow, 4 large circular folds and 15 to 25 longitudinal folds, each with many secondary and tertiary folds, are present (Fig. 13–21A). The folding may give a false impression of glandular structure. Uterine glands do not extend into the cervix in most species, and the glandular elements present in the cervix are mostly mucigenous.

Histologic Structure

The epithelium is of the simple columnar type with many mucigenous cells (Fig. 13–21B). Goblet cells are present. Increasing quantities of mucus are secreted during estrus and pregnancy, and much of the mucus passes to the vagina. In pregnancy, the mucus thickens to form the cervical seal. A small proportion of the epithelial cells are ciliated in some species. Simple tubular glands are seen in the small ruminants and the sow.

The propria consists of a dense irregular connective tissue, which becomes edematous and assumes a loose areolar structure during estrus. In the mare and bitch, venous plexuses are present in the deep part of the propria-submucosa. Many small bundles of slightly myelinated or nonmyelinated nerve fibers are present in the propria-submucosa and the tunica muscularis.

The tunica muscularis consists of inner circular and outer longitudinal smooth muscle layers. Elastic fibers are prominent in the circular layer. Both muscle and elastic fibers are important in re-establishing cervical structure after parturition. The muscle layers of the cervix are continuous with those of the body of the uterus and the vagina. The cervical circular muscle layer is variously modified in different species. Thickening and infolding of the circular layer occurs in the region of the circular folds or prominences in the small ruminants and the sow. In the mare and cow, the thickened circular layer forms the body of the intravaginal portion of the cervix. The orifice of the intravaginal portion of the cervix in the bitch is surrounded by a loop of the vaginal muscle.

The tunica serosa of the cervix consists of loose connective tissue. A longitudinal duct of the epoophoron (Gärtner's duct) may be present in this layer on one or both sides.

Vessels and Nerves

The uterine artery forms the main arterial supply of the uterus. The arteries are tortuous and thick-walled. They enter the uterus from the broad ligament and form a layer of large, circularly arranged vessels between the circular and longitudinal muscle layers. From this vascular layer, vessels communicate with the endometrium. The veins accompany the arteries and form vascular plexuses. In multiparous animals, the vessels have thickened intimae and an in-

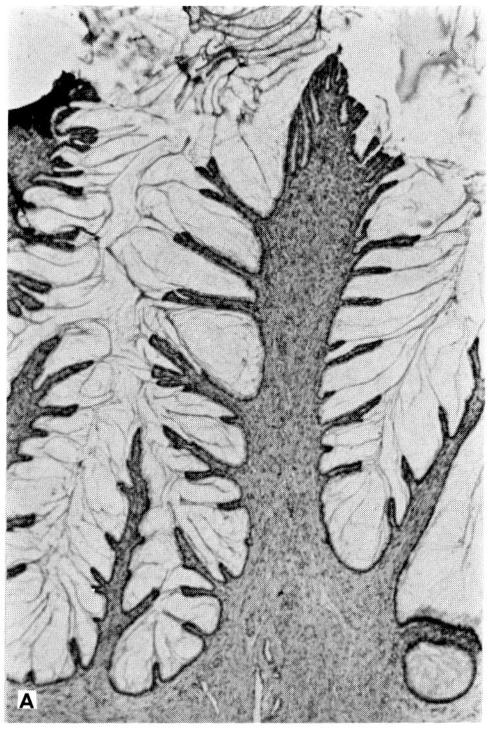

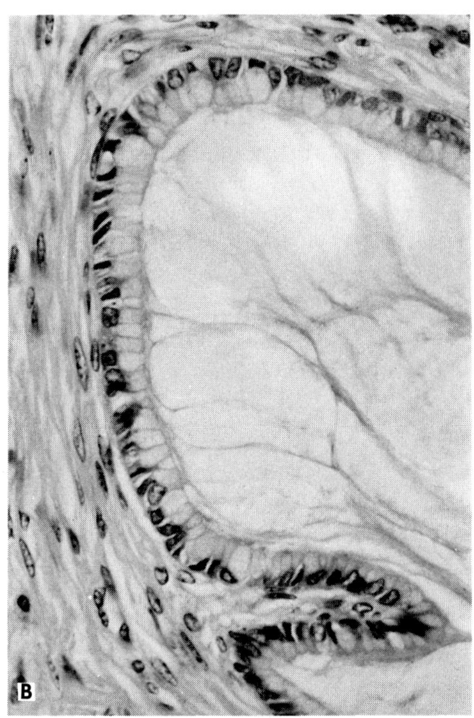

Fig. 13–21. *Cervix uteri, cow. A, Section of a large primary mucosal-submucosal fold with small secondary and tertiary folds projecting into the cervical lumen in which fine strands of coagulated mucus are present.* ×*39. B, Note the mucous secretory activity of the epithelial cells and the coagulated mucus in the cervical lumen.* ×*435.*

creased amount of elastic tissue. Lymph vessels form a subserosal network and drain into mainly the internal iliac and lumbar lymph nodes.

The nerves are derived mainly from the sympathetic system through the uterine and pelvic plexuses. They branch in the muscular and vascular layers and the mucosa. Parasympathetic supply from the sacral segments reaches the uterus through the pelvic plexus. The sympathetic and parasympathetic supplies are not necessarily antagonistic; under central nervous control they may act synergistically to influence certain uterine and possibly placental functions.

VAGINA

The vagina is a muscular tube extending from the cervix to the vestibule. Flat longitudinal mucosal-submucosal folds extend throughout the length of the vagina. In the cow, prominent circular folds are also present in the cranial portion of the vagina. Cyclic variations occur in epithelial height and structure. The increased amounts of vaginal mucus during estrus originate mainly in the cervix. A widespread epithelial cornification is diagnostic of estrus. Cornification is prominent in carnivores and rodents; it does not occur to a great extent in ruminants, probably because of a low estrogen output in most ruminant species.

Histologic Structure

The vaginal wall has three layers: tunica mucosa-submucosa, tunica muscularis, and tunica adventitia or serosa (Fig. 13–22). The vaginal mucosa bears a stratified squamous epithelium that increases in thickness during proestrus and estrus. In the cranial

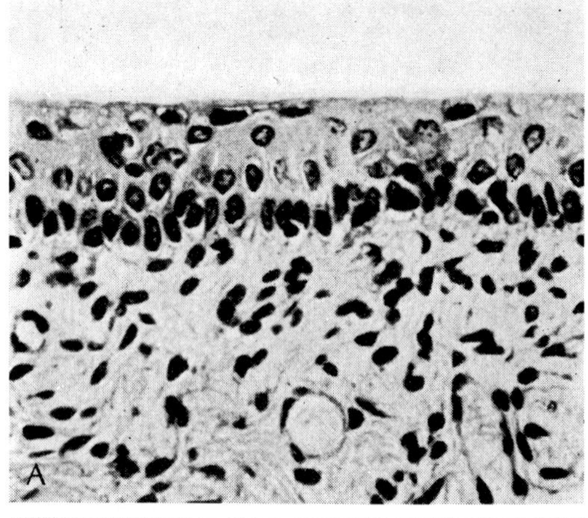

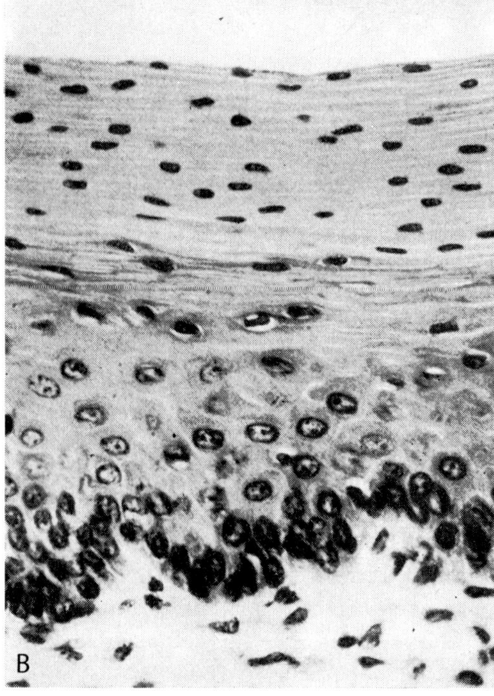

Fig. 13–22. *A, Section of the vagina, bitch, in anestrus. Note the low columnar epithelium. ×530. B, Section of the vagina, bitch, in proestrus. Note the thick cornified epithelium. ×530. (From McDonald, L.E.: Veterinary Endocrinology and Reproduction. 3rd Ed. Philadelphia, Lea & Febiger, 1980.)*

portion of the vagina in the cow, a surface layer of columnar cells and goblet cells is present on the stratified squamous epithelium. Intraepithelial glands occur in the bitch during estrus. In the mare, the epithelial cells are polyhedral with a few layers of flattened cells on the surface. The propria-submucosa consists of loose or dense irregular connective tissue. Lymphatic nodules are present in the propria of the caudal part of the vagina.

The tunica muscularis consists of two or three layers. A thick inner circular smooth muscle layer is separated into bundles by connective tissue and surrounded by a thin outer longitudinal smooth muscle layer. In the sow, the bitch, and to a small extent the queen, there is an additional thin layer of longitudinal muscle inside the circular layer.

The tunica adventitia or, cranially, the tunica serosa, consists of loose connective tissue and contains large blood vessels, nerves, and ganglia. The thin outer longitudinal smooth muscle layer may be considered a part of the tunica serosa and is referred to as muscularis serosae.

Cyclic Changes in the Vaginal Epithelium

THE COW. During early estrus, the superficial layer of columnar and goblet cells in the *cranial part of the vagina* attains maximal height as a result of stored mucus. The underlying polyhedral cells are reduced to less than five layers at estrus.

In the *caudal part of the vagina,* the epithelium increases in height during estrus and reaches maximal height two days after estrus. It remains at maximal height until approximately midcycle. True cornification of the superficial epithelium does not occur; however, between three and ten days after estrus, the surface cells are more squamous than at other times.

Lymphocytes and heterophils invade the vaginal epithelium from estrus until two days after estrus. Attempts to identify the stage of the estrous cycle by the vaginal smear method have not been successful.

THE BITCH. Cyclic cellular changes that occur in the vaginal epithelium of the bitch are clinically useful and important for estimating the times of estrus and breeding. The assessment of cellular changes by the vaginal smear method is widely used (Fig. 13–23). After staining, vaginal smears ap-

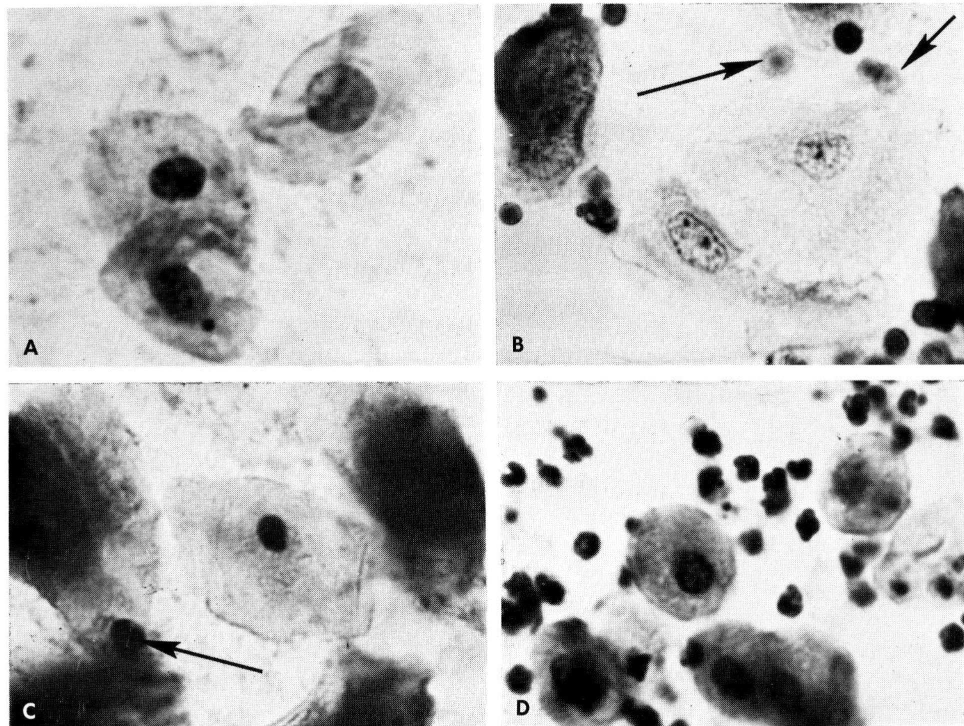

Fig. 13–23. *Cyclic cellular changes in smears from the vaginal epithelium of the bitch. A, Anestrus: typical noncornified epithelial cells. B, Proestrus: noncornified cells in center with cornified cells on both sides; erythrocytes (at arrows). C, Estrus: four cornified epithelial cells and one noncornified cell with pyknotic nucleus; heterophil at arrow. D, Metestrus: noncornified epithelial cells and numerous leukocytes. Shorr's stain. ×950. (Reprinted by permission from* Textbook of Veterinary Clinical Pathology. *William Medway, James E. Prier and John S. Wilkinson, Eds. 1969, Williams & Wilkins, Baltimore.)*

pear as follows: (1) *Anestrus* (about two months' duration): numerous unstained noncornified epithelial cells, a few large stained cells with pyknotic nuclei and a few heterophils and lymphocytes are present. (2) *Proestrus* (about nine days' duration): numerous erythroytes (of uterine origin) and many large flat cornified cells are present. (3) *Estrus* (about nine days' duration): some erythrocytes and numerous cornified cells are present; as estrus progresses, the cornified cells become wrinkled, distorted, and frequently invaded by bacteria. (4) *Metestrus-diestrus* (about three months' duration): epithelial cells are less cornified and appear more like unstained living cells; heterophils are numerous on the third day of metestrus and gradually disappear until the tenth to twentieth day of metestrus.

The epithelial lining of the vagina is thin in anestrus, about 2 to 3 layers of cells. It proliferates during proestrus and may be 12 to 20 cells thick at the beginning of estrus, with cornification of the surface layers. By late estrus, desquamation of the cornified layers begins (Fig. 13–23).

Vessels and Nerves

The arteries and venous plexuses of the vagina are branches of the internal pudendal and uterine vessels. Extensive venous plexuses are present in the tunica serosa or adventitia and in the connective tissue joining the vagina to surrounding structures. Lymph vessels drain mainly into the internal iliac lymph nodes. Numerous nerve bundles and ganglia occur in the tunica serosa or adventitia. The innervation is primarily sympathetic, derived from the pelvic plexus.

VESTIBULE, CLITORIS, AND VULVA

Vestibule

The vestibule is demarcated from the caudal portion of the vagina by a rudimentary fold, the *hymen*. The wall of the vestibule contains the orifices of the urethra, the major and minor vestibular glands, and sometimes the longitudinal ducts of the epoophora (Gärtner's ducts). In the cow, it also contains the suburethral diverticulum. The wall of the vestibule is similar to that of the caudal portion of the vagina, except that more subepithelial lymphatic nodules are present, especially in the region of the clitoris. They appear in the living animal as slight, rounded elevations of the mucosa-submucosa and when inflamed may interfere with reproductive functions.

Major vestibular glands are bilateral compound tubuloacinar mucous glands located in the deep part of the mucosa-submucosa. They occur in ruminants and the queen. The terminal secretory acini contain large mucous cells. The small ducts joining the acini are lined by columnar mucous cells, with isolated areas of goblet cells. The large ducts leading to the vestibule are lined by a thick stratified squamous epithelium. Individual or aggregated lymphatic nodules may surround the large ducts.

Smooth and some striated muscle fiber bundles are present in the interlobular connective tissue. The gland has no capsule but is enclosed in and partly divided by the striated musculature.

The glands provide mucous lubrication of the vestibule. They may be compressed during coitus and secrete mucus, providing mucous lubrication also of the caudal vagina. In the cow, secretory activity increases 1 to 2 days after estrus. They are homologous to the male bulbourethral glands.

Minor vestibular glands are small, branched, tubular mucous glands scattered in the vestibular mucosa of most domestic animals. They are lined by a stratified squamous epithelium containing nests of mucous cells. In the cow, they are concentrated in the median groove cranial to the clitoris. They are homologous to the male urethral glands.

Clitoris

The clitoris corresponds to the dorsal part of the penis and is located in the extreme caudal region of the vestibule, near the ventral commissure of the vulva. It consists of conjoined erectile corpora cavernosa clitoridis, a rudimentary glans clitoridis, and a preputium clitoridis. The corpus cavernosum clitoridis, homologue of the corpus cavernosum penis, is well developed in the mare. The glans clitoridis, homologue of the glans penis, is functionally erectile only in the mare. A nonerectile fibroelastic tissue cover replaces the glans in the queen, sow, and ewe; in the ewe, the cover contains a venous plexus. The preputium clitoridis is a continuation of the vestibular mucosa-submucosa. It has parietal and visceral layers. The visceral layer contains numerous terminal nerve corpuscles, such as the bulbs of Krause, lamellated corpuscles, and genital corpuscles, as well as lymphatic nodules. The space between the parietal and visceral layers of the prepuce is the fossa clitoridis. The fossa is distinct in the bitch and mare but is absent in the cow and sow.

Vulva

The vulva is formed by the labia vulvae. They are covered by skin that is richly supplied with apocrine and sebaceous glands. Fine hairs are distributed over the skin; in the cow they become especially long at the ventral commissure. Striated muscle fibers of the constrictor vulvae are found in the hypodermis. The labia are very well supplied with small blood and lymph vessels, which become congested during estrus, especially in the sow and bitch. This increased blood congestion results in a perceptible increase in the temperature of the labia, thus giving rise to the term "in heat."

Vessels and Nerves

Blood vessels, cavernous tissue, and venous plexuses are abundant in the vestibular wall. An erectile corpus cavernosum, called the *bulbus vestibuli,* is present beneath the vestibular mucosa in the mare and bitch. It resembles the male corpus spongiosum penis. The vestibule and the labia of the vulva are supplied by branches of the internal and external pudendal arteries. Lymphatic nodules are abundant in the region of the clitoris. Lymph vessels from the external genitalia drain into the superficial inguinal nodes. The external genitalia, especially the clitoris, are richly supplied with sensory and autonomic nerve endings.

ACKNOWLEDGMENT

I thank Professor A.F. Weber, Department of Veterinary Anatomy, University of Minnesota, for providing valuable reference material for the writing of this chapter.

REFERENCES

Afzelius, B.A., Camner, P., and Mossberg, B.: On the function of cilia in the female reproductive tract. Fertil Steril *29*:72, 1978.

Austin, C.R., and Short, R.V. (eds.): Reproduction in Mammals, 2nd Ed. Books 1–3. Cambridge, Cambridge University Press, 1982–84. *See* Bk. 1, Ch. 2: 'Oogenesis and ovulation,' pp. 17–45, by T.G. Baker; Bk. 2, Ch. 4: 'The fetus and birth,' pp. 114–141, by G.C. Liggins, and Bk. 3, Ch. 5: 'The ovary,' pp. 91–114, by D.T. Baird.

Beck, I.R., and Boots, L.R.: The comparative anatomy, histology and morphology of the mammalian oviduct. *In* The Oviduct and Its Functions. Edited by A.D. Johnson and C.W. Foley. New York, Academic Press, 1974.

Beller, F.K., and Schumacher, G.F.B. (eds.): The Biology of the Fluids of the Female Genital Tract. Elsevier North Holland, 1979, *See* Chs. 'Morphology of the Fallopian tube,' pp. 299–317, by C.J. Pauerstein and C.A. Eddy; 'Tubal transport,' pp. 319–333, by R.J. Blandau, R. Bourdage and S. Halbert; and 'Tubal secretions,' pp. 335–344, by L. Mastroianni, Jr. and K.J. Go.

Byskov, A.G.S.: Does the rete ovarii act as trigger for the onset of meiosis? Nature *252*:396, 1974.

Eddy, E.M., Clark, J.M., Gong, D., and Fenderson, B.A.: Origin and migration of primordial germ cells in mammals. Gamete Res *4*:332 1981.

Glasser, S.R.: Mechanism of steroid hormone action. *In* Endocrinology of Pregnancy. 3rd Ed. Edited by F. Fuchs and A. Klopper. Philadelphia, Harper and Row, 1983.

Goodman, R.L., and Karsch, F.J.: The hypothalamic pulse generator: a key determinant of reproductive cycles in sheep. *In* Biological Clocks and Seasonal Reproductive Cycles. Colston Papers No. 32. Edited by B.K. Follett and D.E. Follett. Bristol, John Wright, 1981.

Guraya, S.: Biology of Ovarian Follicles in Mammals. Berlin, Springer-Verlag, 1985.

Lincoln, G.A., and Short, R.V.: Seasonal breeding: nature's contraceptive. Recent Prog Horm Res *36*:1, 1980.

Ludwig, H., and Metzger, H.: The Human Female Reproductive Tract, a Scanning Electron Microscopic Atlas. Berlin, Springer-Verlag, 1976.

McCarrey, J.R., and Abbott, K.K.: Mechanisms of genetic sex determination, gonadal sex differentiation, and germ cell development in animals. Adv Genet *20*:217, 1979.

McDonald, L.E.: Veterinary Endocrinology and Reproduction. 3rd Ed. Philadelphia, Lea & Febiger, 1982. *See* Ch. 2: 'The pituitary gland,' Ch. 10: Female reproductive system', Ch. 12: 'Patterns of reproduction', Chs. 13–18: Reproductive patterns of cattle, horses, sheep, swine, dogs, domestic cats, resp.

Moore, R.M., and Seamark, R.F.: Cell Signalling, permeability and microvascularity changes during antral follicle development in mammals. J Dairy Sci *69*:927–943, 1986.

Priedkalns, J.: Pregnancy and the central nervous system. *In* Comparative Placentation. Edited by D.H. Steven. London, Academic Press, 1975.

Priedkalns, J., Weber, A.F., and Zemjānis, R.: Qualitative and quantitative morphological studies of the cells of the membrana granulosa, theca interna, and corpus luteum of the bovine ovary. Z Zellforsch *85*:501, 1968.

Rajakoski, E.: The ovarian follicular system in sexually mature heifers with special reference to seasonal, cyclical and left-right variations. Acta Endocrinol (Kbh.) *34* (Suppl. 52), 1960.

Reiffenstuhl, G.: The Lymphatics of the Female Genital Organs. Philadelphia, J.B. Lippincott, 1964.

Zuckerman, S., and Weir, B.J. (eds.): The Ovary. 2nd Ed. London, Academic Press, 1979.

14

Placentation

NILS BJÖRKMAN
VIBEKE DANTZER

EMBRYOLOGY

The fusion of a female and male gamete results in a *zygote.* After repeated cleavage during the transport through the uterine tube to the uterine cavity, it develops into a fluid-filled vesicle, a *blastocyst,* with a wall of simple epithelium, *trophoblast,* and an eccentrically located *inner cell mass.* The free-living blastocyst is nourished by secretion from endometrial glands (uterine milk). Because the increasing demand from the growing embryo necessitates a more efficient nutritive arrangement, i.e., a vascular transport system, the embryo produces membranes that in a process called *implantation* gradually attach to the endometrial epithelium and thereby establish a close relationship between fetal and maternal circulations for physiologic exchange. As a result, a combined organ, the *placenta,* is formed. In this bimodal structure a *placenta fetalis* and a *placenta uterina* are recognized. The fetus and fetal placenta together are known as the *conceptus.* The manner of formation and attachment of the placenta is termed *placentation.*

The first events in placentation occur in the blastocyst stage. The trophoblast is essential for the transfer of nourishment to the offspring during intrauterine life but has no function after birth of the young and is expelled with the afterbirth (secundinae). The inner cell mass differentiates into three germ layers in two stages, forming, first *ectoderm* and *entoderm* and then between them the *mesoderm.* These layers form the embryo, but they also participate in the formation of the fetal membranes. The ectoderm forms a vesicle enclosing the embryo, the *amnion.* It provides buoyancy and freedom of development to the embryo. The entoderm gives rise to the *yolk sac,* communicating with the midgut, and the *allantois,* a diverticulum from the hindgut (Fig. 14–1).

The further development of the fetal membranes is directed by the mesoderm. The lateral mesoderm splits into a somatic and a splanchnic layer. The resulting intramesodermal cleft gives rise to the body cavity (coelom), which at this stage has an essentially extraembryonic location, *exocoelom.* The somatic mesoderm combines with trophoblast to form the *chorion* or with the ectoderm of the amnion. These membranes constitute the extraembryonic *somatopleure.* The splanchnic mesoderm fuses with the entoderm of the yolk sac and the

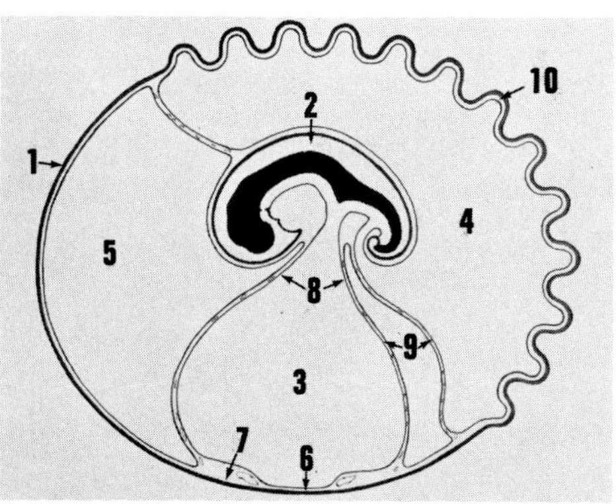

Fig. 14–1. *Diagram of fetal membranes. The arrangement is subject to wide variation in different species. Chorion (1); amniotic cavity (2); yolk sac cavity (3); allantoic cavity (4); exocoelom (5); avascular yolk sac placenta (6); choriovitelline placenta (7); yolk sac entoderm (8); vascular mesenchyme (9); allantochorion (10).*

allantois and together they enter into the extraembryonic *splanchnopleure.*

The somatic mesoderm, and hence the chorion, is avascular, whereas blood islands and vessels first arise in the mesoderm of the yolk sac. Later the allantoic mesoderm also becomes vascularized. To obtain access to the embryonic circulation, the somatic mesoderm of the chorion eventually fuses with the splanchnopleure. The placental vessels, together with the vitelline and allantoic ducts, are contained in the *body stalk,* later to develop into the *umbilical cord.*

CLASSIFICATION

The placenta presents great variations in different species. This has given rise to many different systems of classification; however, three main principles can be used to describe these events: (1) vascular origin, (2) feto-maternal relationship, and (3) morphology.

Vascular Origin

In this context (domestic mammals) there are two fundamental types of placentation, the *omphaloid* or yolk sac–type and the *allantoic type.* The yolk sac and hence the omphaloid placenta develops before the allantois and allantoic placenta. In an early period they are coexistent.

YOLK SAC PLACENTATION. The yolk sac wall, *omphalopleure,* may combine with the chorion, appose to uterine tissue, and form a *choriovitelline* placenta (Fig. 14–2). The yolk sac develops early but undergoes rapid or gradual involution. In some species (e.g., the rabbit) the yolk sac placenta participates in passive immunization by absorbing immunoglobulins.

CHORIOALLANTOIC PLACENTATION. A more widespread vascularization is effected by the allantoic vessels. When the allantois fuses with the chorion an *allantochorion* is formed, resulting in a *chorioallantoic* placenta. This is the most efficient organ for mediating physiologic exchange between parent and offspring.

Feto-Maternal Relationship

The degree to which the fetal membranes are anchored to the endometrium determines the amount of uterine tissue lost at parturition. On this basis, two different types of allantoic placentation, *nondeciduate* and *deciduate,* are recognized. In the former type, the fetal components interlock with relatively intact uterine tissue, from which they can be separated without much defect (ungulates). In the deciduate placenta, part of the endometrial stroma, the *decidua,* is shed with the fetal membranes after parturition. Decidual cells are enlarged and rounded or polyhedral cells derived from fibroblasts in the endometrium. They exhibit differences of size, contents (lipid and glycogen), and structure in different animal species. Decidual cells are found in the carnivore placenta.

Morphologic Classification

The structural variations of the placenta are immense. There are intermediate forms, and the placenta also changes its internal structure during intrauterine life.

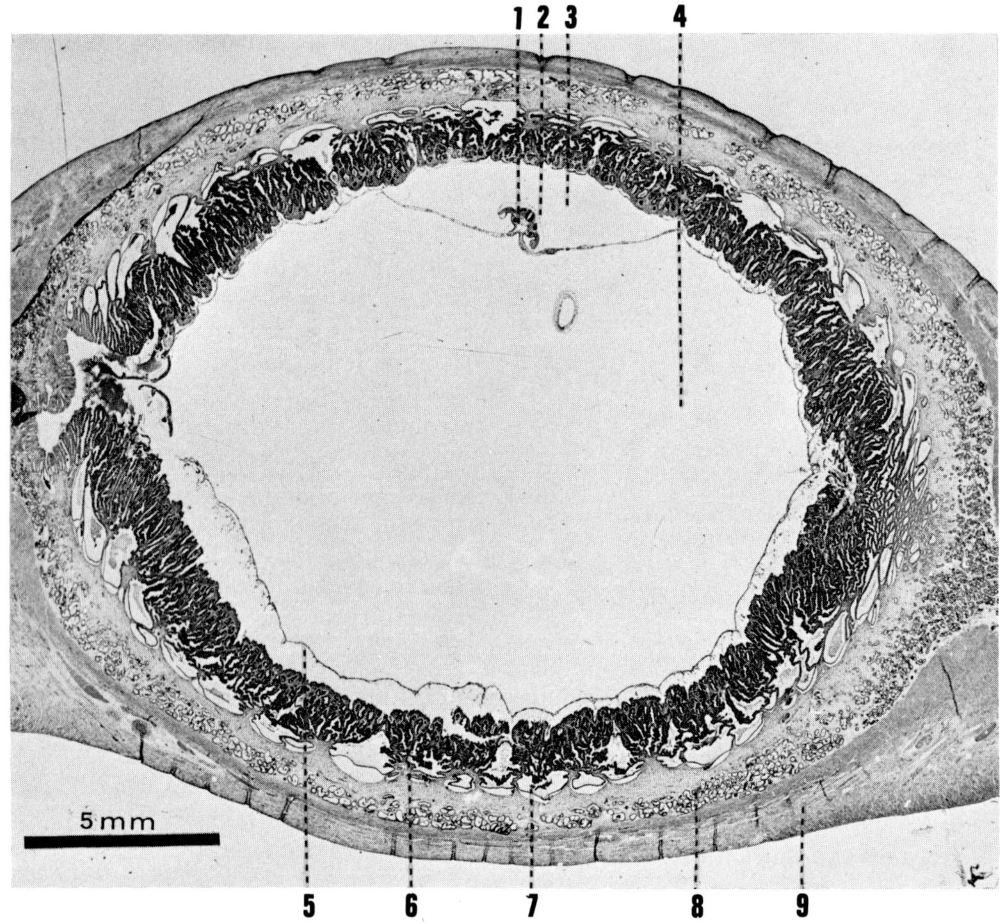

Fig. 14–2. *Cross section of a uterine horn, bitch, three weeks pregnant. Embryo (1); amnion (2); exocoelom (3); yolk sac cavity (4); yolk sac wall (omphalopleure) (5); hypertrophied epithelial surface of the endometrium containing chorionic villi (choriovitelline placenta) (6); spongy zone (7); glandular zone (8); muscular coat (9). ×5. (Courtesy of A. Hansen.)*

Although a morphologic classification cannot always be exact, three criteria do provide a basis for such a classification—shape, internal structure, and number of layers of the interhemal membrane.

The principle of providing a vast feto-maternal area of interchange determines the structure on gross and microscopic levels. The part of the chorion with an accordingly increased area is called *chorion frondosum,* and the smooth part, when present, *chorion laeve.*

SHAPE. Three types of the chorion frondosum and its uterine counterpart are recognized macroscopically in domestic mammals:

(1) Diffuse placenta *(placenta diffusa)*—most of the chorionic sac forms a chorion frondosum attached to the endometrial epithelium (sow, mare).

(2) Cotyledonary placenta *(placenta multiplex)*—tufts of chorionic protrusions, *cotyledons,* attach to preformed endometrial prominences, *caruncles.* The chorionic and uterine structures combine to form *placentomes.* In the intercaruncular area a chorion laeve is apposed to the endometrial epithelium (ruminants).

(3) Zonary placenta *(placenta zonaria)*—the chorium frondosum forms a band around the equator of the chorionic sac. Outside the girdle the chorion laeve ap-

poses to the endometrial epithelium (carnivores).

(4) Discoid placenta *(placenta discoidalis)* (not present in domestic mammals)—the chorion frondosum forms a disc shaped area of fusion (e.g., man, apes, rodents).

INTERNAL STRUCTURE. Enhancement of the capacity for feto-maternal exchange by enlargement of the surface area is effected in three ways, producing folded, villous, and labyrinthine types of placentation.

(1) In folded placentation the enlargement takes place by macroscopic folds, *plicae,* of different orders, and by microscopic folds or ridges, *rugae,* also of different orders (sow).

(2) The fetal component in villous placentation forms arborizing *chorionic villi* with vascular mesenchymal cores, which fit into corresponding caruncular *crypts* (mare, ruminants) (see Fig. 14–10).

(3) In labyrinthine placentation the allantochorion forms an intercommunicating maze, containing anastomosing fetal blood channels (carnivores, rodents).

NUMBER OF LAYERS OF THE INTERHEMAL MEMBRANE. Because the fetal component of the chorioallantoic placenta is made up of chorionic tissue vascularized by allantoic vessels, it consists of three tissue layers: endothelium, mesenchyme, and trophoblast. The maternal counterpart consists basically of three corresponding layers in reverse order: uterine surface epithelium, connective tissue, and endothelium. When they intervene between the fetal and maternal blood streams, these layers form the placental or interhemal membrane, which is a combined, highly selective barrier and transport avenue in the fetal-maternal exchange (Fig. 14–3).

Although constant in the fetal placental membrane, the number of tissue layers of the maternal component varies with the species. Therefore, placentae are classified on the basis of the number of uterine tissue layers:

(1) Epitheliochorial *(placenta epitheliochorialis)*—all three layers persist.

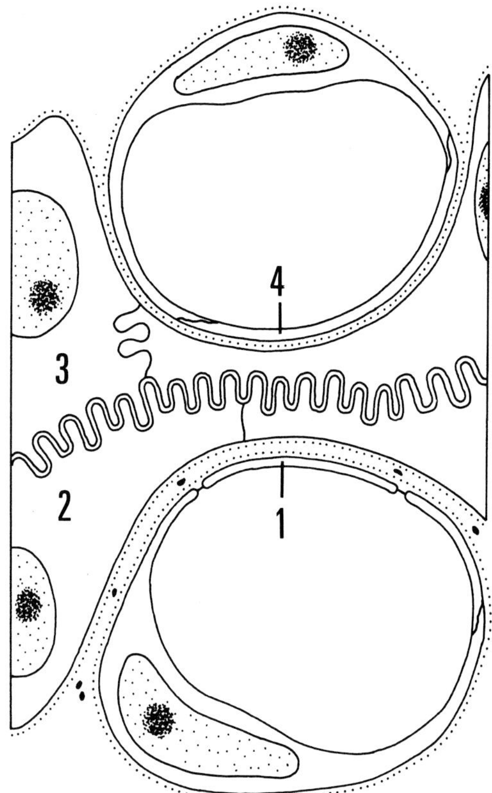

Fig. 14–3. *Schematic drawing of the epitheliochorial interhemal membrane in an advanced stage. Uterine capillary endothelium (1); uterine surface epithelium (2); trophoblast (3); fetal capillary endothelium (4). Dotted lines represent basal laminae between which collagen fibers may be seen. (Courtesy of P. Hyttel.)*

(2) Syndesmochorial *(placenta syndesmochorialis)*—the uterine epithelium is reduced, leaving connective tissue and maternal endothelium intact.

(3) Endotheliochorial *(placenta endotheliochorialis)*—the uterine epithelium and the connective tissue are absent, and endothelium alone separates the maternal blood from trophoblast.

(4) Hemochorial *(placenta hemochorialis)*—all three layers are absent, rendering the trophoblast freely exposed to maternal blood.

Macroscopically, the epitheliochorial placenta generally conforms to the diffuse (e.g., sow, mare) or cotyledonary (ruminants) types. The syndesmochorial relationship may occur locally in ruminant placentae. The endotheliochorial placenta is found primarily in carnivores; it is a zonary placenta in the bitch and queen as well as in furred carnivores (e.g., mink). The hemochorial type generally coincides with the discoid shape (e.g., man, rodents).

HISTOLOGIC DESCRIPTION

The main physiologic principle of the chorioallantoic placenta is the exchange between maternal and fetal blood. The substance that nourishes the offspring is termed *embryotrophe.* It comes from both maternal blood, the *hemotrophe,* and uterine glandular secretions and cell fragments, the *histiotrophe.* The circulations remain morphologically separated by a varying number of tissue layers. The placenta contains various tissue elements, but circulating blood and trophoblast are functionally the most important. Fetal blood circulates in a closed system in the placenta. The fetal capillaries generally have relatively wide lumina and partly attenuated endothelial walls, which may be surrounded by basal laminae.

In the uterine placenta, the blood either is contained in maternal vessels or bathes the trophoblast directly. When the endothelium is absent (hemochorial placenta), the blood flows through trophoblastic tubules or intervillous spaces. In fact, trophoblast and fetal endothelium are always present in the placental membrane.

The parenchymal part of the fetal placenta consists of the trophoblast, which carries out many different functions. This is reflected in a complex structure of the individual cells or in a diversity of cell types developed by differentiation. Trophoblast consisting of discrete cells is termed *cytotrophoblast.* If the cells fuse, they form a *syncytiotrophoblast.* When both types of trophoblasts are present, as in carnivores, the cellular form is primitive and the syncytial form is more advanced with respect to the development of organelles. Another form of differentiation of the trophoblast is the formation of trophoblastic giant cells, e.g., in ruminants.

The increase in surface area mentioned previously is supplemented by microvilli or an irregular cell surface where the trophoblast is in contact with maternal tissue or blood. In the epitheliochorial placenta, trophoblastic microvilli interdigitate with corresponding microvilli from uterine surface epithelium (see Figs. 14–13 and 14–18). In the endotheliochorial placenta, the trophoblast lacks microvilli, but the cell surface is very irregular.

The placenta continuously changes in size, shape, and internal structure throughout gestation. After implantation, it grows with a rapid although gradually decreasing rate and may be subject to minor involution before term. Rearrangements on the cellular level are reflected in cell destruction and mitotic activity. Another expression of the changing of placental structure is the progressive attenuation of the physical barrier between the maternal and fetal circulations.

VASCULAR SUPPLY

The supply of oxygenated blood to the placenta is derived from the uterine artery and anastomoses from the ovarian and vaginal arteries. The arteries are enlarged during pregnancy, and their placental capillaries have a diffuse or localized distribution or lose their endothelium and form blood spaces. The uterine placenta is drained by satellite veins.

The fetal placenta is vascularized for the uptake of oxygen and nutrients and for delivery of waste products. To facilitate exchange, the placental circulation frequently performs countercurrent flow between allantoic and uterine vessels. The yolk sac placenta receives blood from the *omphalomesenteric* or *vitelline* arteries, which arise from the abdominal aorta. The oxygenated blood is returned to the heart by the omphalomesenteric veins.

The allantoic placenta receives blood from the paired *umbilical* arteries, from the caudal part of the aorta, and returns oxygenated blood through the umbilical veins. The left umbilical vein carries blood to the heart via the liver; the right vein undergoes involution within the fetus.

FUNCTIONAL-STRUCTURAL RELATIONSHIP

Structural differences in the various placental types do not necessarily reflect their function. The rate of simple diffusion is inversely related to membrane thickness, but the permeability of living cells is related to their thickness to a limited extent only. Furthermore, capillaries from both fetal and uterine sides of the placenta may bypass the connective tissue and indent the epithelial coverings (see Fig. 14–13). Thus, the fetal and maternal blood can be in close spatial relation, despite a varying number of layers in the interhemal membrane.

The villi and microvilli constitute areas of increased fetal-maternal contact, providing an extensive surface for interchange. Furthermore, adhesiveness between the cells, mainly reinforced by divalent cations, plays a role in anchoring the conceptus. The contact between trophoblast and maternal epithelium, as in the epitheliochorial placenta, provides a vast area for the adhesive forces.

The most important structure in cellular transport is the plasma membrane. It is impermeable to some elements but serves as a diffusion membrane for others or even facilitates transport. However, membranes of living cells contain molecules or aggregates of polypeptides or proteins, called carriers with enzymatic capability to participate in active transport. The substantial increase in the dimensions of the plasma membrane of cells with microvilli provides accommodation for membrane-bound enzymes. Transcytosis is another form for transport and is a common feature of the placental membrane.

From the preceding discussion, it is evident that the number of plasma membranes to be traversed is important for the function of the placental membrane as a selective barrier and transport avenue. As parts of the placental barrier, the plasma membranes are present only in epithelium and endothelium, whereas the maternal connective tissue, when present, and the fetal placental mesenchyme do not offer any such obstacles. In order to traverse a cell (or syncytium), a substance has to pass the plasma membrane twice. The number of plasma membranes in the placental barrier gives an indication of permeability. Other structural features related to function may be the thickness of the cells and their internal physiologic properties. The attenuation of the trophoblast, as gestation proceeds, renders the placental membrane more permeable toward term.

The most immediate demand from the conceptus is for oxygen. The transfer mechanism of the respiratory gases implies essentially simple diffusion under gradient pressure. Therefore, the thickness of the diffusion barrier is of major importance to the efficiency in this respect.

In general, the placental membrane is freely permeable to water and electrolytes. Among important inorganic elements, e.g., calcium, phosphorus, iodine, and iron, a directional preference from mother to fetus generally exists. This is especially characteristic of iron; there is no retrograde transfer of iron from fetus to mother. However, in different species the iron transfer takes place by different mechanisms. In carnivores and in the ewe, iron is absorbed from blood hemoglobin in maternal hemorrhages, whereas in the sow the source is glandular secretion.

The hemoglobin of the growing offspring contains different types of polypeptide chains during different phases of development. The earliest (nucleated) erythrocytes from the yolk sac mesoderm contain embryonic hemoglobin. Later, in intrauterine life, hepatic and splenic eryth-

Table 14–1.
Implantation and Gestation in Domestic Animals

	Beginning of Implantation Day	Gestation Time Days
Bitch	17–18	58–63
Queen	12½–14	63–65
Mare	35–40	329–345
Sow	13–14	112–115
Cow	16–18	279–285
Ewe	15–20	144–152

rocytes carry fetal hemoglobin, and near the time of birth a gradual change in bone marrow cells with adult hemoglobin takes place. Embryonic and fetal hemoglobin have a higher affinity for oxygen than the adult form and thus are able to extract oxygen diffusing across the placental barrier more efficiently than adult hemoglobin. This is an adaptation for intrauterine life with low oxygen pressure.

SPECIES DIFFERENCES

The beginning of implantation and length of gestation vary considerably in different species (Table 14–1).

Bitch and Queen

The yolk sac forms a choriovitelline placenta, with trophoblastic villi invading eroded uterine mucosa. This transient placenta is originally extensive (Fig. 14–2) but eventually disappears. The yolk sac, however, persists until term.

The allantoic placenta is deciduate, zonary, labyrinthine, and endotheliochorial. Implantation in the queen begins at day 13 with the formation of junctions between trophoblast and maternal epithelium. At day 14 the trophoblast of the girdle area has intruded into the endometrium forming an endotheliochorial placenta with syncytio- and cyto-trophoblast. At the periphery an extravasate zone develops into the marginal hematoma in the bitch. This zone is diffuse in the queen. The chorion frondosum and uterine capillaries form lamellae, which are localized in a girdle around the equator of the chorionic sac. Outside the girdle, a chorion laeve is apposed to the uterine surface epithelium in early stages. Located beneath the labyrinth is a spongy *junctional zone,* containing terminal parts of placental lamellae, maternal vessels, cell debris, and glandular secretions. It is connected with the *glandular zone* formed by the dilated upper parts of the uterine glands (Fig. 14–4).

Hemorrhage of uterine blood within and outside the placental girdle gives rise to hematomas. After breakdown of the blood, they become brown or green (in the bitch) because of degradation of hemoglobin. In the bitch, distinct *marginal hematomas* with large blood compartments are formed (Fig. 14–4), whereas in the queen, smaller hemorrhages occur in irregular positions in the placental girdle and between the chorion laeve and the endometrium. The columnar trophoblast lining the compartments is involved in absorption of iron from destroyed maternal erythrocytes. In the bitch, the trophoblast presents evidence of phagocytosis.

The fetal part of the placental labyrinth is composed of lamellae of trophoblast and mesenchyme, which contain small thin-walled capillaries. Enclosed by trophoblast, relatively wide and thick-walled capillaries form the maternal constituent of the labyrinth (Fig. 14–5). The capillaries are surrounded by a thick amorphous layer, which is especially irregular in the queen. The maternal endothelial cells are prominent. In addition to the maternal vessels, giant decidual cells occur in the queen (Fig. 14–6) and, less frequently, in the bitch. In the bitch, the lamellae are branched and have a tubular appearance (Fig. 14–6), whereas in the queen, the lamellae are more regularly stacked.

The trophoblast originally consists of discrete cells. A syncytium is formed by the coalescing of some cells. Thus the trophoblast includes cytotrophoblast and syncy-

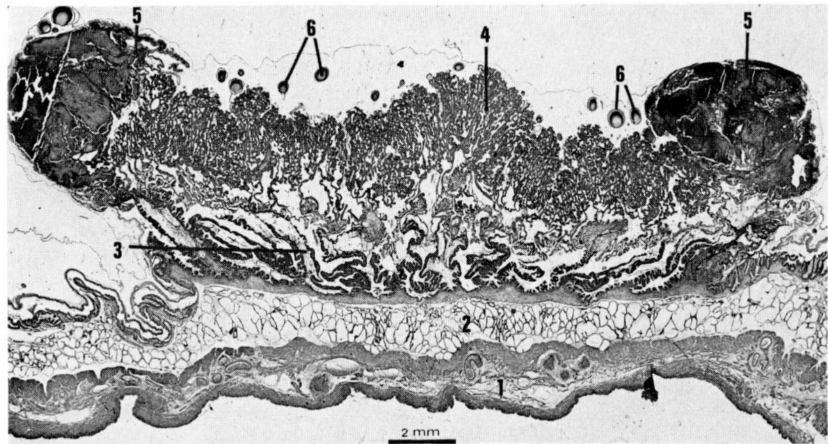

Fig. 14–4. *Cross section of placental girdle, bitch, near term. Myometrium (1); glandular zone (2); spongy zone (3); placental labyrinth (4); marginal hematomas (5); fetal vessels in mesenchyme (6). ×2.7. (Courtesy of A. Hansen.)*

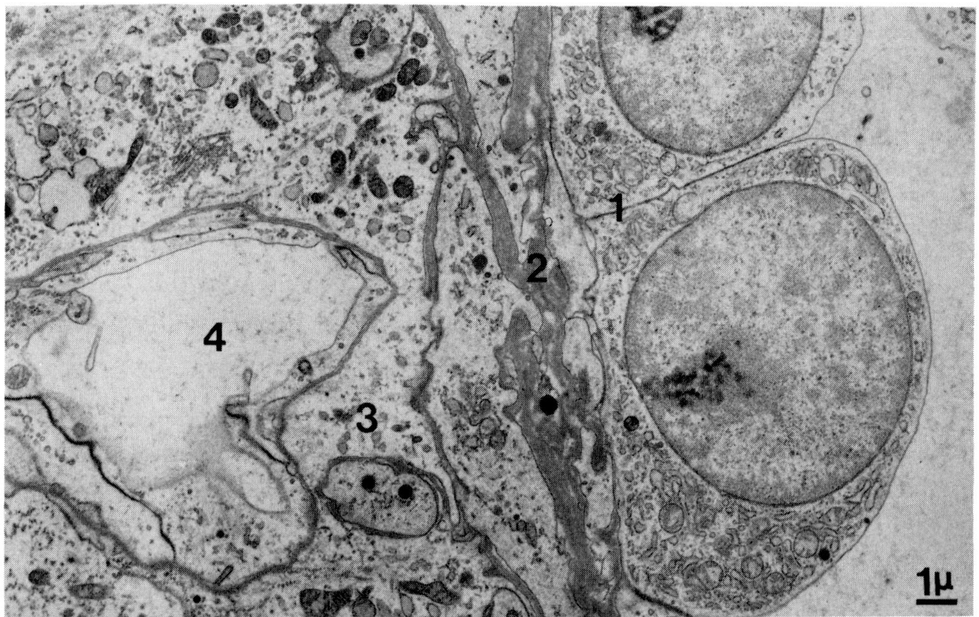

Fig. 14–5. *Electron micrograph of placental labyrinth, bitch, late pregnancy. Maternal endothelium (1); basal lamina (2); syncytial trophoblast (3); fetal capillary (4). ×5740.*

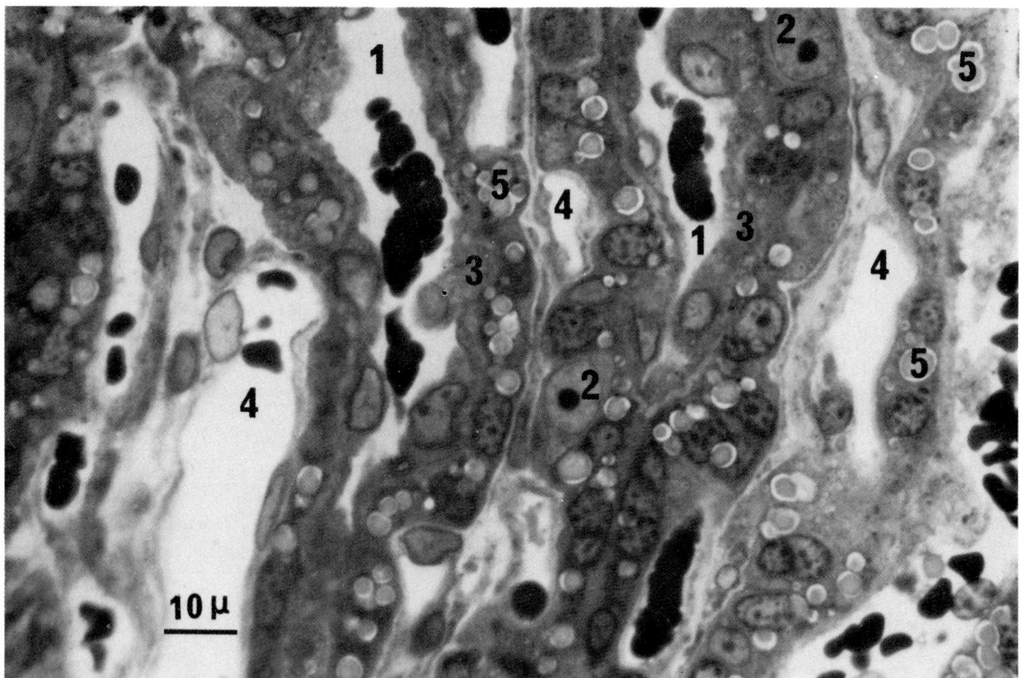

Fig. 14–6. *Placental labyrinth, queen, late pregnancy. Maternal capillaries (1); decidual cell (2); syncytial trophoblast (3); fetal capillaries (4); lipid droplets (5). Epon. Toluidine blue. ×1000.*

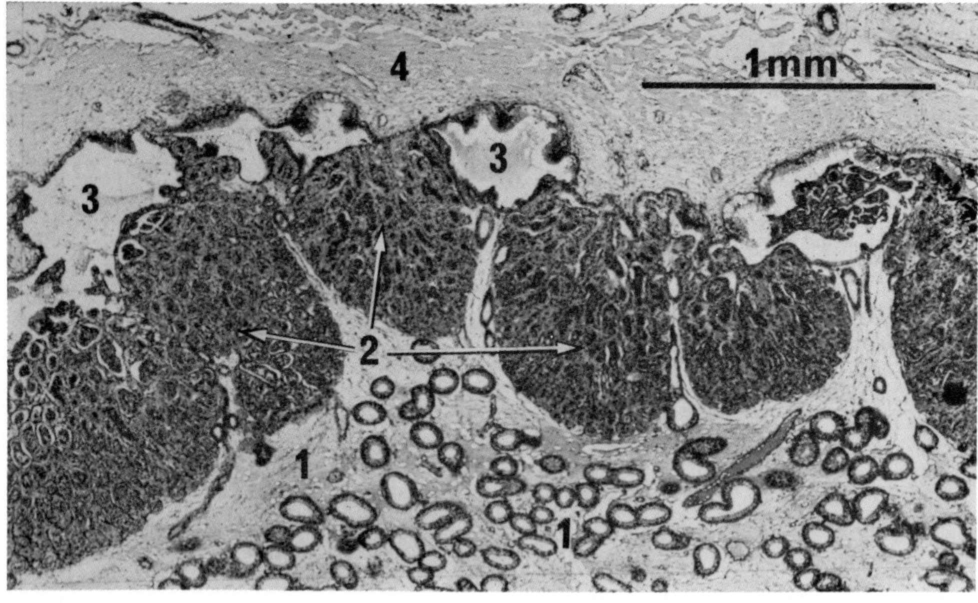

Fig. 14–7. *Cross section of placenta, mare, late pregnancy. Endometrium with glands (1), microplacentomes (2); areolae (3); chorionic mesenchyme (4). ×40. (From Björkman, N.: An Atlas of Placental Fine Structure. London, Baillère, Tindall & Cassell, 1970.)*

tiotrophoblast. The syncytium constitutes the major part of the lamellae and forms a continuous interhemal barrier. The cytotrophoblast is discontinuous, and the cells occur mainly along the mesenchymal parts of the lamellae. The discrete cells contain free ribosomes and a poorly developed ER. The syncytium possesses a conspicuous ER, numerous mitochondria, and dense bodies, apparently lysosomes. In the queen the syncytium contains numerous lipid droplets.

At parturition, the placenta separates from the endometrium through the spongy zone above a layer of condensed connective tissue (Fig. 14–4).

Mare

A big yolk sac is present three weeks after insemination and becomes an important fetal-maternal interchange medium, temporarily composed of an avascular yolk sac wall and, in a marginal zone, a choriovitelline placenta. About the end of the sixth week, the change from the vitelline to the allantoic circulation is effected, and the yolk sac, although persisting until term, undergoes gradual involution.

The allantoic placenta of the mare is nondeciduate, diffuse, villous, and epitheliochorial. Although the embryo hatches from the zona pellucida at day 8 to 9, it remains completely encapsulated in a second noncellular translucent membrane until at least day 17. Until 40 to 45 days the conceptus remains spherical and lies unattached in the uterine lumen, held in place merely by a pronounced increase in uterine tone. Then villi of the allantochorion begin to enter corresponding crypts in the endometrium, and by day 90 to 100 the typical microcotyledonary placenta has developed over the entire surface of the endometrium. Except in minor smooth areas, the membrane is attached by small tufts of branched chorionic villi that fit into corresponding endometrial crypts arranged in a honeycomblike manner. The tufts and corresponding crypts form placental units, *microplacentomes* (Fig. 14–7).

The villi consist of vascular mesenchyme covered with trophoblast. The villi fit into crypts lined with simple uterine epithelium of varying height. The crypts are separated by *septa* consisting of vascular uterine connective tissue. Indentations of capillaries into the trophoblast and maternal epithelium are seen in later pregnancy (Fig. 14–8).

Normal cryptal cells are light. The trophoblast cells are slightly darker and have a more compact ER. In both the trophoblast and uterine epithelial cells, the Golgi complex is inconspicuous and the mitochondria are small and sparse. The apical surface of the trophoblast and the uterine epithelium bear microvilli that interdigitate and form a dark border as seen with the light microscope (Fig. 14–8). The lateral and basal surfaces of these cells are comparatively even. Sites of local degeneration of trophoblast and cryptal epithelium are indicated by dark cytoplasm. They are seen in later stages of gestation. Between the microplacentomes, there are openings of uterine glands, and small areolae are formed in which a simple columnar trophoblast lines the areolar lumen (Fig. 14–7).

At the junction of the developing allantochorion and the regressing yolk sac, the chorion forms an annulate *chorionic girdle* consisting of projections of rapidly proliferating trophoblast cells. Between days 36 and 38 the girdle cells invade the endometrium by amoeboid movements. They destroy the uterine epithelium almost completely and implant themselves in the endometrial stroma, where they form *endometrial cups.* The cups measure from a few millimeters to approximately 5 cm in diameter. The uterine surface epithelium regenerates quickly. The cup cells become densely packed and intermingled with uterine glands (Fig. 14–9). They grow to large polyhedral cells with two nuclei and an rER as the dominating cytoplasmic organelle. The cup cells elaborate horse cho-

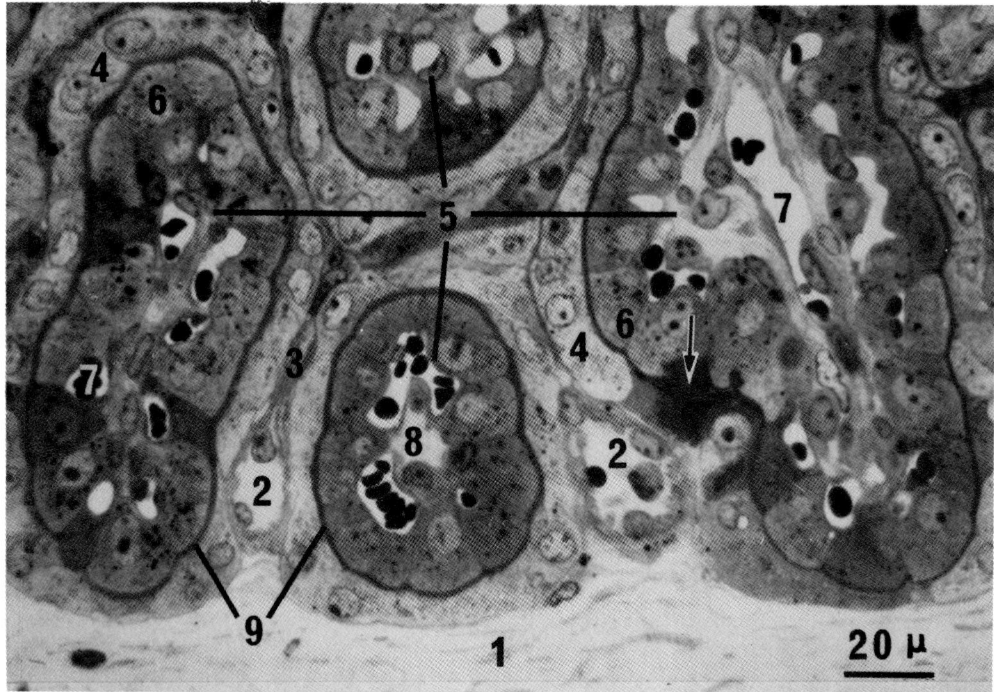

Fig. 14–8. *Detail of microplacentome, mare, late pregnancy. Uterine connective tissue (1); uterine capillaries (2); maternal septum (3); cryptal epithelium (4); chorionic villi (5); trophoblast (6); fetal capillaries (7); mesenchyme (8); border of microvilli (9). The dark parts of trophoblast and cryptal epithelium (arrows) are apparently degenerated. Epon. Toluidine blue. ×630.*

rionic gonadotropin (equine CG) (formerly called PMSG), which can be used in pregnancy diagnosis.

The endometrial cups eventually become surrounded by leukocytes, which invade and destroy the cup cells as they begin to degenerate after about 80 days of gestation. From the 120th to the 150th day their remnants are rejected. After detachment the cups are encapsulated by chorionic folds and form allantochorionic pouches. There are also flattened oval bodies of disputed origin, *hippomanes,* which are floating freely in the allantoic fluid.

Sow

In early stages, the yolk sac is unusually large and well vascularized with its maximal development about day 20. A choriovitelline placenta of insignificant extent is formed but disappears as the yolk sac rapidly decreases in size.

The allantoic placenta is nondeciduate, diffuse, folded, and epitheliochorial. The fusiform chorionic sac adheres over its whole area except at the avascular extremes and over the uterine gland openings.

The blastocyst undergoes extremely rapid elongation from day 10 to 12. It changes from a sphere of about 2 mm in diameter to a membranous thread about 100 cm long. At day 12 to 14 the blastocysts are evenly distributed in both uterine horns along the mesometrial side. Placentation begins close to the embryo, where the endometrium at day 13 to 14 forms epithelial proliferations covered with corresponding caplike formations of the chorion, thus giving an anchoring effect until interdigitating microvilli between uterine

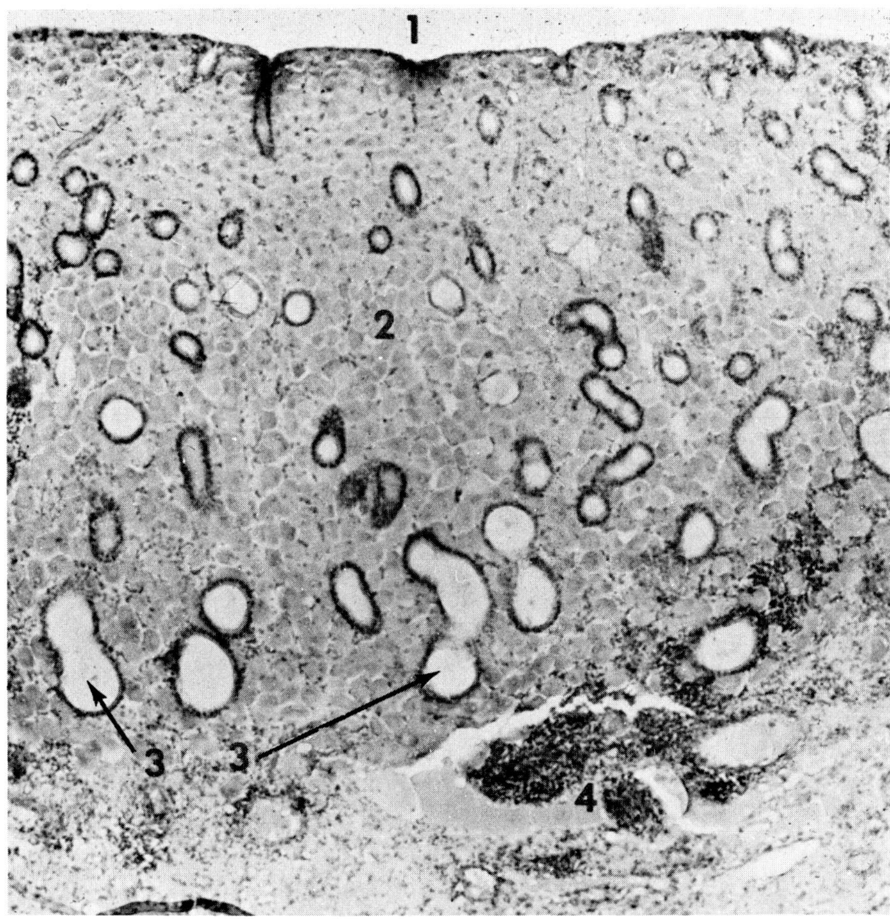

Fig. 14–9. *Endometrial cup, mare, 50 days pregnant. Uterine lumen (1); large epithelioid cup cells (2); uterine glands (3); lymphocytes (4).* ×*45. (From Allen, W.R., Hamilton, D.W., and Moor, R.M.: The origin of equine endometrial cups. Anat Rec 177:503, 1973.)*

epithellium and trophoblast begin to develop at day 15.

The chorionic-endometrial contact area is increased about three times by primary and secondary macroscopic circular folds, *plicae,* which are permanent on the maternal side and mainly nonpermanent on the fetal side (Fig. 14–10). When the whole chorionic sac is spread out it measures about three times the length of the corresponding permanently folded endometrium. The microscopic folds, which increase the exchange area about four times, form irregular *rugae* separated by *fossae* in the early stage of placentation after day 20 and are permanent on both the maternal and the fetal side. These rugae develop into more regular circular primary rugae that have the same direction as the macroscopic folds (Figs. 14–10, 14–11, and 14–12). In the late third of gestation the fossae on the maternal side become subdivided by low secondary rugae perpendicular to the primary rugae, thereby subdividing the fetal rugae into bulbous protrusions in late gestational stages. The epithelial cells are further differentiated as the trophoblast lining the chorionic fossae forms arcades of high columnar epithelium, which is apposed to the low columnar

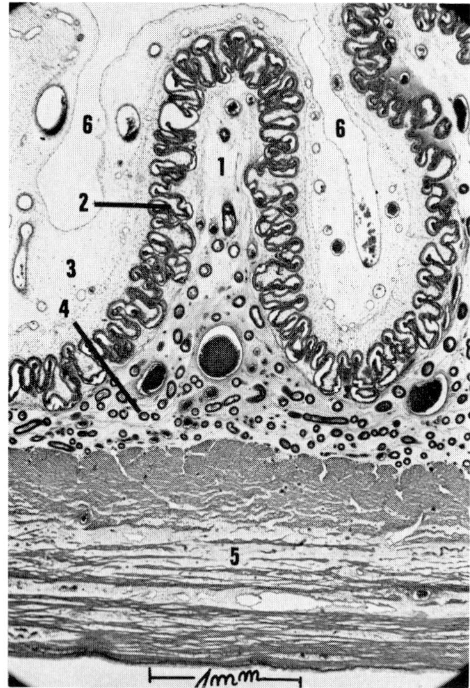

Fig. 14–10. *Longitudinal section of uterine horn with placenta, sow, late midpregnancy. Primary fold (1); rugae (2); allantochorion (3); endometrium with glands (4); myometrium (5); allantoic cavity (6). ×16. (Courtesy of A. Hansen.)*

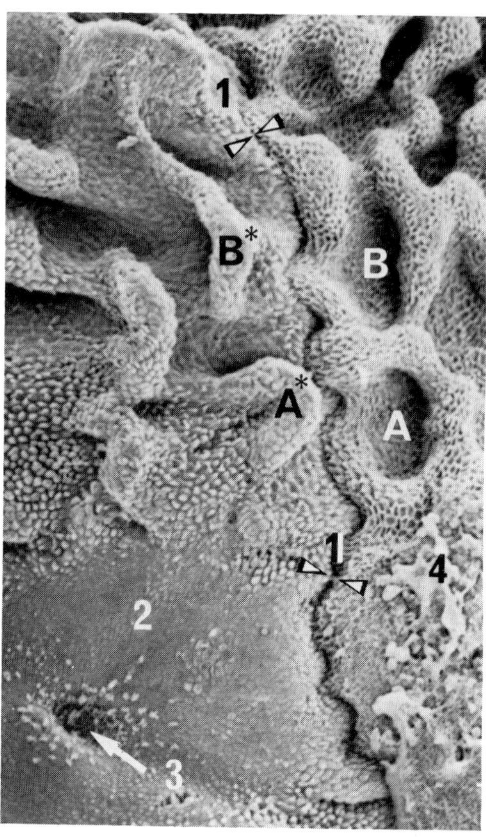

Fig. 14–11. *Placenta, sow, day 35. Partly separated. The line of separation is indicated by the waving dark line (1) with the maternal side to the left and the fetal side to the right. Maternal rugae (A* and B*) and the complementary fetal fossae (A and B). Maternal areola (2) with uterine gland opening (3) and the corresponding fetal areola (4) covered by uterine milk. Scanning electron micrograph ×45. (From Dantzer, V.: Scanning electron microscopy of exposed surfaces of the porcine placenta. Acta Anat 118:96, 1984, with permission.)*

epithelium of the summit of the endometrial rugae. The remaining chorionic and uterine epithelia are cuboidal or flattened (Fig. 14–13).

As gestation proceeds, allantoic and uterine capillaries indent those parts of the respective rugae where the trophoblast and endometrial epithelium are low. Thus the connective tissue interposed between the capillaries and epithelia on both sides is bypassed and the originally six-layered interhemal membrane is reduced to four layers. In advanced stages the thickness can be less than 2 μm.

The trophoblastic and uterine epithelial cells are provided with interdigitating microvilli increasing the area of exchange additionally by a factor of about 10. Furthermore, the plasma membranes of the uterine epithelium have complex basal infoldings, and between trophoblastic cells the lateral plasma membranes form mutual infoldings.

The uterine epithelial cells contain spherical nuclei with small nucleoli. The ER is mainly of the rough type. The Golgi complex is extensive with many stacks in each cell. Small mitochondria are scattered in the cytoplasm. An extensive lysosomal complex consisting of membrane whorls and dense bodies is characteristic for the maternal epithelial cells from 40 to 80 days (Fig. 14–14).

The trophoblastic cells have rounded

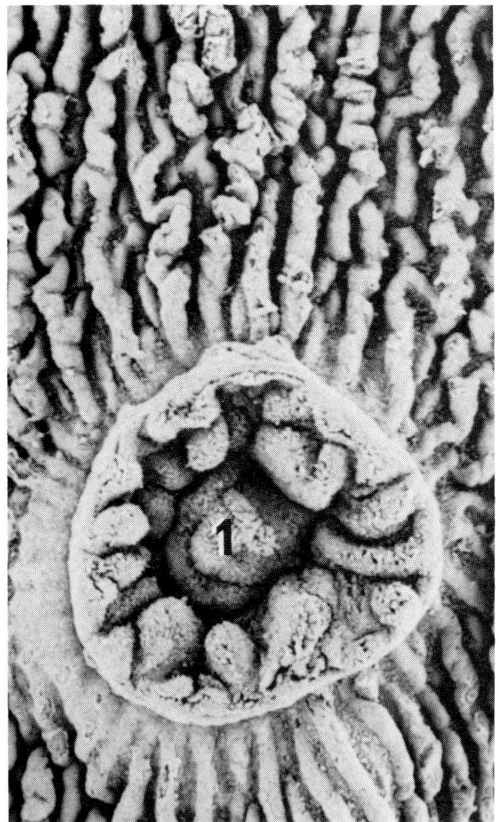

Fig. 14–12. *Surface of the porcine allantochorion from midgestation with a fetal areola (1). The chorionic rugae radiating from its periphery fuse with parallel chorionic rugae after a short distance. Scanning electron micrograph ×130. (From Dantzer, V.: Scanning electron microscopy of exposed surfaces of the porcine placenta. Acta Anat 118:96, 1984, with permission.)*

nuclei with distinct nucleoli. The composition of the ER varies. The ER occurs mainly in the basal part of the cells intermingled with electron-dense PAS-positive bodies. Soon after 80 days, aggregations of smooth ER are seen basally and laterally in the cells, and their occurrence is correlated with high estrogen synthesis. The supranuclear Golgi complexes are small. The mitochondria are larger than on the maternal side and located apically in the cells, where coated pits and vesicles, tubular and vacuolar endosomes give evidence of high endocytic activity.

The macroscopically visible areolae contain uterine milk and are subdivided into maternal areolae and fetal areolae (Fig. 14–11). The maternal areolae form smooth surfaced shallow cups around the openings of uterine glands. The fetal areola forms a rosette-like structure composed of villi (Fig. 14–12). The main transfer of iron from mother to fetus takes place via the areola-gland complex. The uterine glands secrete an iron containing glycoprotein, *uteroferrin,* subsequently taken up by the areolar trophoblast supplied with an extensive capillary net. The interareolar histiotrophe, visible microscopically, is located in the intermicrovillous space between uterine and fetal epithelia.

Cow

The yolk sac at first has a rather large vascular area and forms a functional choriovitelline placenta. The yolk sac is rapidly outgrown by the allantois, and after three weeks it begins to degenerate.

The allantoic placenta is nondeciduate, cotyledonary, villous, and epitheliochorial. The elongated blastocyst begins placentation close to the embryo at day 18 to 19 and gradually proceeds peripherally. In the intercotyledonary areas the trophoblast develops papillae that extend into the uterine gland openings, possibly functioning as an anchor. They occur until day 21. At day 22 the blastocyst extends equally into both uterine horns, and by day 27 intimate contact between trophoblast and maternal epithelium by interdigitating microvilli is established. In later stages of gestation and under pathologic conditions, sites of syndesmochorial fetal-maternal relationship may also occur. The fetal-maternal connection is initiated when simple villi develop from areas of the chorionic sac in contact with caruncles. The chorionic villi are retained in developing caruncular crypts to establish the initial interlocking. The originally simple villi ramify within the caruncles and the placentomes grow ap-

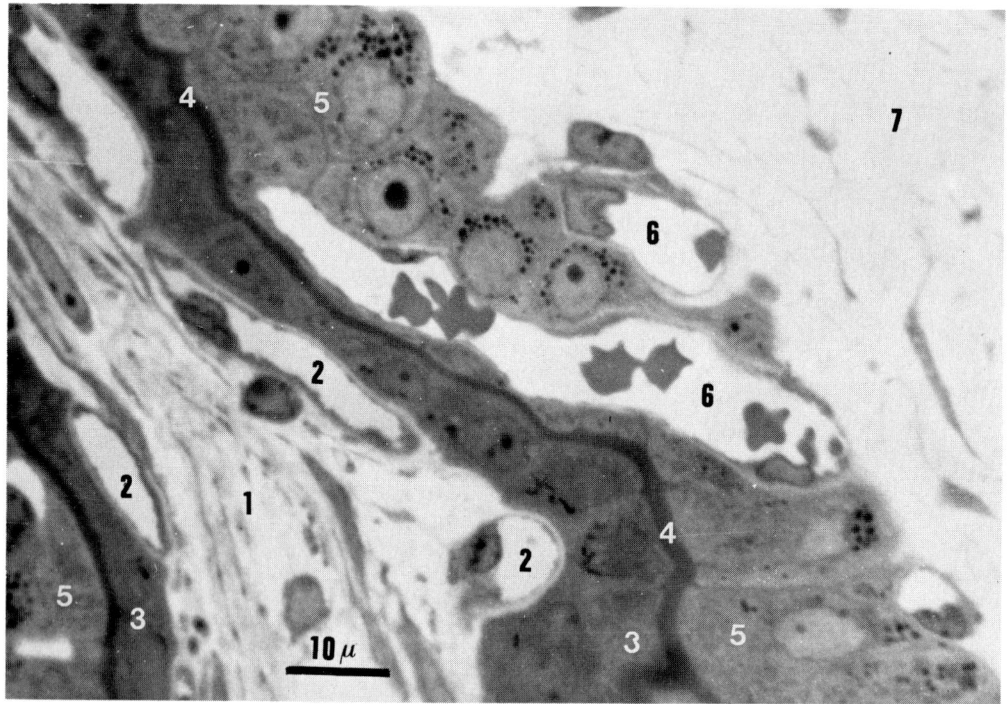

Fig. 14–13. *Placental fold, sow, late pregnancy. Uterine connective tissue (1); uterine capillaries (2); uterine epithelium (3); border of microvilli (4); trophoblast with dense colloid droplets (5); fetal capillaries (6); mesenchyme (7). Epon. Toluidine blue. ×1300. (From Björkman, N.: Fine structure of the fetal-maternal area of exchange in the epitheliochorial and endotheliochorial types of placentation. Acta Anat (Basel), 86, Suppl 1:1, 1973.)*

proximately 5000-fold but undergo a slight involution towards term.

The bovine placentome is a slightly elongated convex structure provided with a stalk containing maternal vessels (Fig. 14–15). A chorionic villus consists of a main stem that ramifies progressively into villi of higher orders. The villi generally fit into corresponding crypts, where main septa give off septa of secondary and higher orders to form the maternal constituent.

The cryptal epithelium is cuboidal or flattened (Fig. 14–16). The cells have spherical nuclei with distinct nucleoli. The ER varies considerably in appearance from the irregularly distributed scarce cisternae (see Fig. 14–18) to regularly stacked lamellae. Infranuclear whorls are also present. Most of the membranes are rough surfaced, but the whorls consist, to a minor extent, of smooth membranes. Free ribosomes, an inconspicuous Golgi complex, and a few small mitochondria are also present. Adjacent cell surfaces generally do not interdigitate. The basal lamina may project between adjacent cells (Fig. 14–17). The borders of interdigitating microvilli are more irregular than those in the mare and sow. Spaces between the uterine and trophoblastic microvilli contain a dense granular material. Most cells contain lipid inclusions in the infranuclear region.

Among the uterine cuboidal cells are a few cryptal giant cells. They contain two or three closely apposed nuclei and little cytoplasm (Fig. 14–16). The apical surfaces of these cells have microvilli.

The chorionic villi consist of vascular mesenchyme covered with a simple layer of trophoblast. The villi are branched and fit tightly into the crypts of the caruncles.

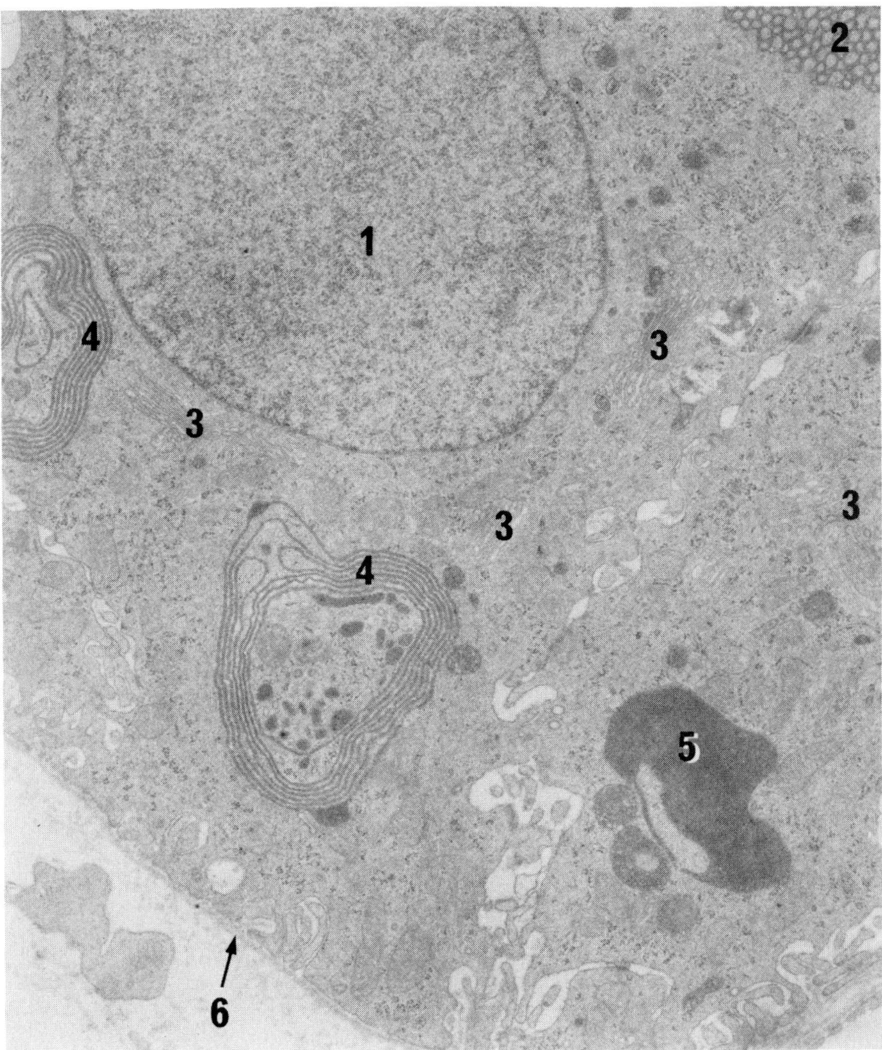

Fig. 14–14. *Electron micrograph of maternal epithelium, porcine placenta, late pregnancy. Nucleus (1); microvilli (2); Golgi complex (3); membrane whorls (4); dense body (5); basal lamina (6). ×15,000.*

The trophoblast is composed of mononuclear columnar or irregularly shaped cells and giant cells with two or more nuclei. The mononuclear cells have rounded or irregularly shaped nuclei with large nucleoli. They have a sparse rER and conglomerations of smooth tubules. Free ribosomes are scattered throughout most of the cytoplasm. Relatively numerous, moderately large mitochondria occur mainly in the apical portion of the cells (Fig. 14–18). The plasma membranes of adjacent cells interdigitate but are straight along the basal lamina. In some cells numerous transcytotic vesicles are seen in the vicinity of the apical microvilli.

The trophoblastic giant cells are considered to have differentiated from columnar trophoblast or from common stem cells through karyokinesis without accompanying cytokinesis. Accordingly, there are two pairs of centrioles in the cytoplasm. The giant cells lack desmosomes and appear to be mobile within the chorionic epithelium.

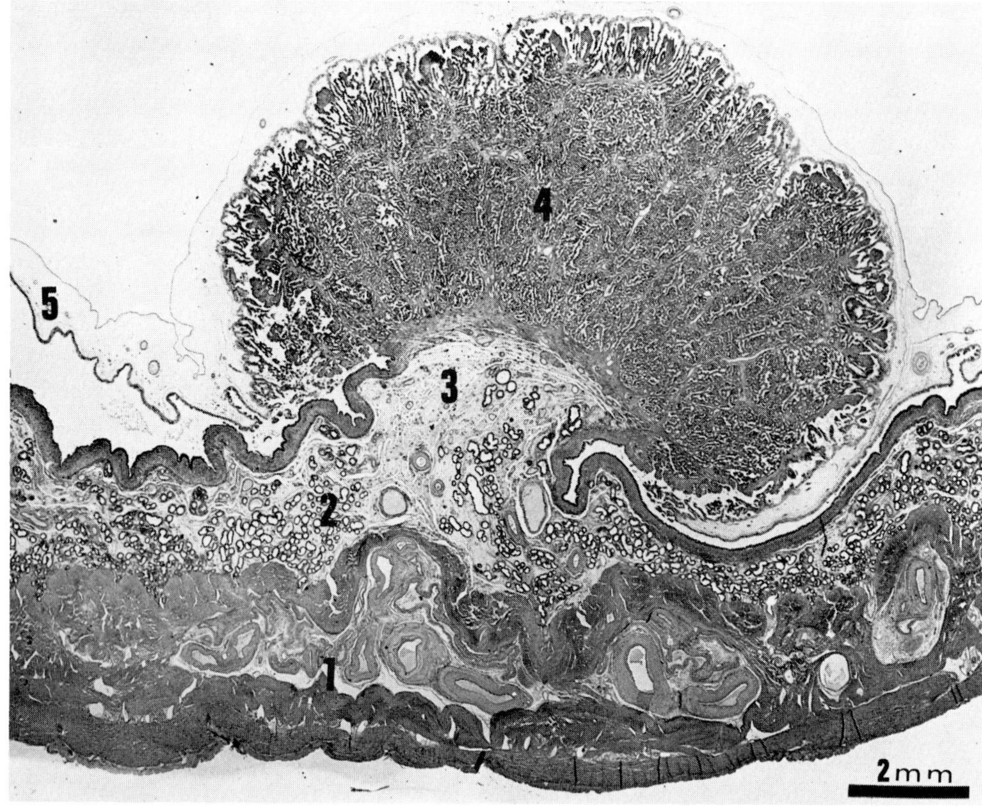

Fig. 14–15. *Cross section of placentome, cow, mid-pregnancy. Myometrium (1); endometrium with glands (2); stalk of placentome (3); placentome (4); chorion laeve (5). ×8. (Courtesy of A. Hansen.)*

They have also been reported to migrate into the cryptal epithelium, where they fuse with uterine epithelial cells to form trinucleate hybrid cells. Trophoblastic giant cells have spherical, widely separated nuclei with conspicuous nucleoli, and the cytoplasm is voluminous. Furthermore, the cell surface lacks microvilli. In contrast to the mononuclear cells, giant cells show no morphologic evidence of absorption.

At the fine-structural level, the cytoplasm displays a great diversity of organelles and inclusions. The ER is rough-surfaced and sparse, and free ribosomes are numerous. The Golgi complex is well developed; the mitochondria are numerous and moderate in size. There is a varying number of dense bodies, multivesicular bodies, and light secretory granules. The cells produce chorionic gonadotropin, progesterone, and prostanoids.

Regressive changes occur frequently in the placentome. They occur mainly in cryptal epithelium (Fig. 14–16), but trophoblastic cells of both varieties are also involved. Degenerating giant cells have a tendency to multiply their nuclei further. After parturition, the chorionic villi are pulled out of the crypts. Normally, the separation occurs at the line of interdigitating microvilli, and the trophoblast and cryptal epithelium remain intact. However, a common complication of parturition in cattle is retained afterbirth *(retentio secundinarum)*, in which the villi are trapped in the crypts and the adhesiveness between the fetal and maternal tissues remains high.

In the intercotyledonary area, a chorion

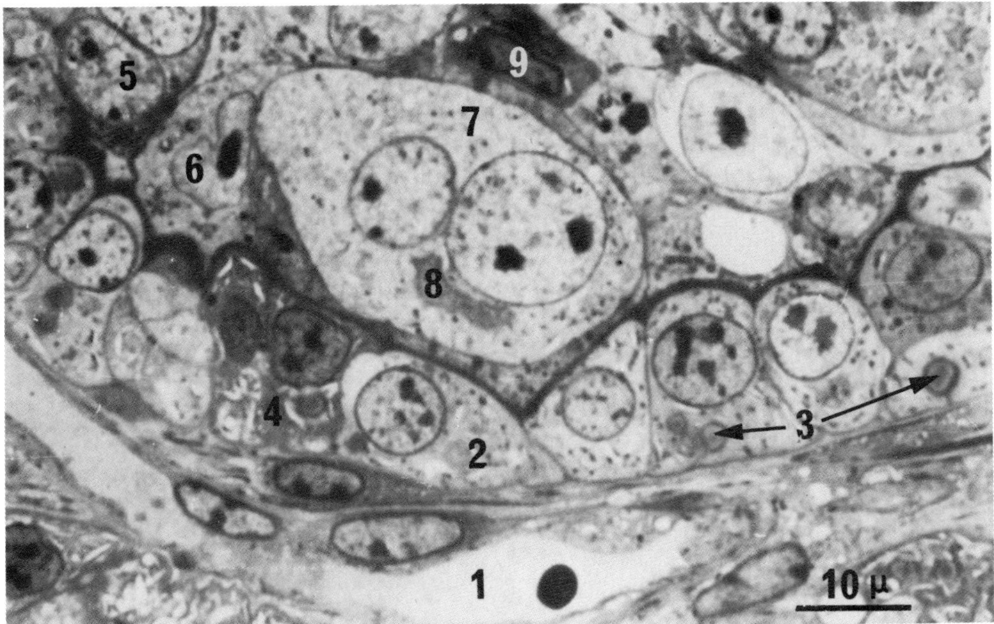

Fig. 14–16. *Detail of placentome, cow, mid-pregnancy. Maternal capillary (1); viable cryptal epithelial cells (2); lipid droplets (3); degenerated cryptal epithelial cells (4); cryptal binuclear giant cell (5); mononuclear trophoblastic cells (6); binuclear trophoblastic giant cell (7); Golgi complex (8); fetal capillary (9). The dark dots in the cryptal and trophoblastic cells are mitochondria. Epon. Toluidine blue. ×1600. (From Björkman, N.: Light and electron microscopic studies on cellular alterations in the normal bovine placentome. Anat Rec 163:17, 1969.)*

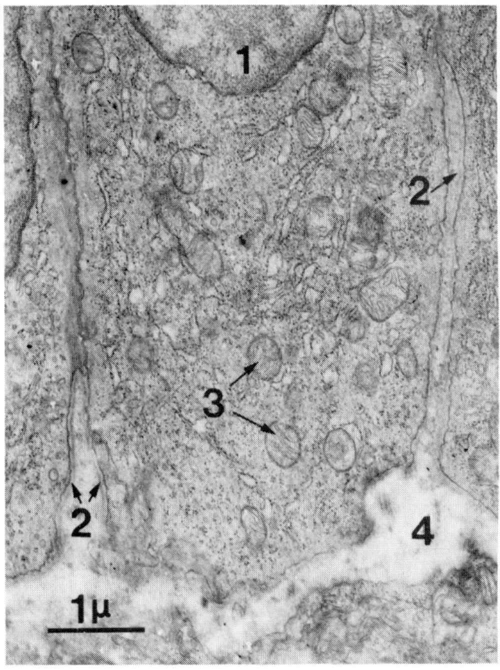

Fig. 14–17. *Electron micrograph of infranuclear portions of cryptal epithelial calls, cow, early pregnancy. Nuclei (1); basal lamina (2); mitochondria (3); uterine connective tissue (4). ×13,400.*

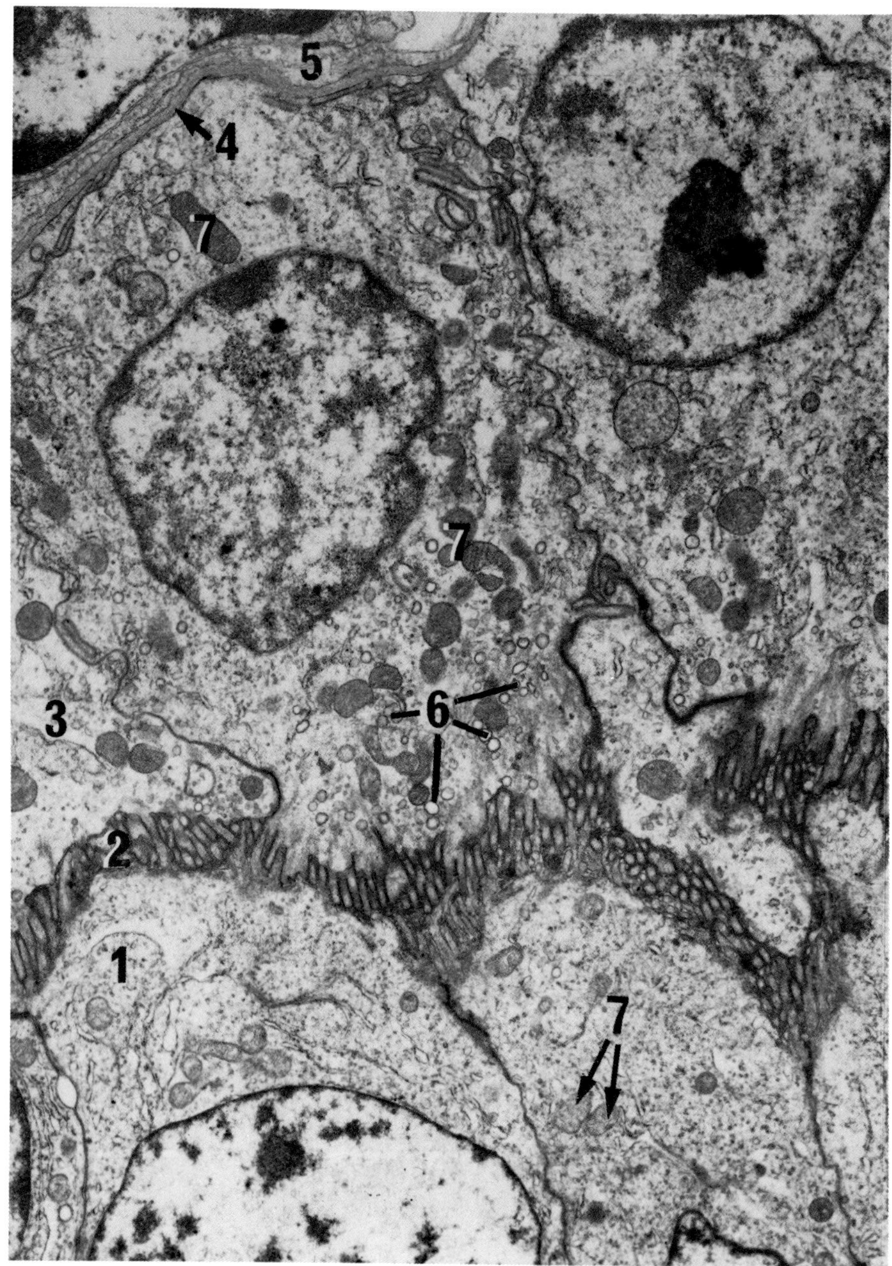

Fig. 14–18. *Electron micrograph of part of placentome, cow, late pregnancy. Cryptal epithelium (1); interdigitating microvilli (2); columnar trophoblast (3); basal lamina (4); fetal endothelium (5); transcytotic vesicles (6); mitochondria (7). ×8000.*

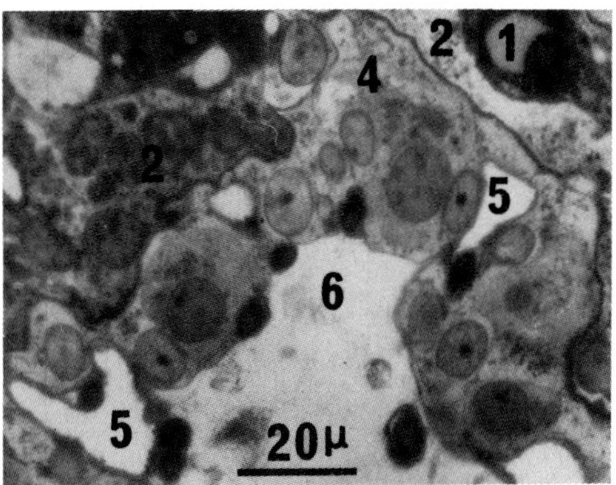

Fig. 14–19. *Section of placentome, ewe, mid-pregnancy. Maternal capillary (1); maternal syncytium (2); border of microvilli (3); trophoblast (4), fetal capillaries (5); mesenchyme (6). Epon. Toluidine blue.* ×*655.*

laeve adheres to the endometrium, except over the glandular openings where areolae are formed. The simple columnar trophoblast and the simple uterine epithelium are both provided with interlocking brush borders (microvilli).

Amniotic plaques are yellow irregular elevations of ectodermal epithelium on the inner surface of the amnion. They measure from a fraction of a millimeter to a few millimeters and are loaded with glycogen.

Ewe

The placenta of the ewe is similar to that of the cow but differs in some respects. Implantation, occurring as in the cow, begins at day 14 to 15, with development of interdigitating microvilli at day 16 to 18 between trophoblast and maternal epithelium of the developing placentomes. Trophoblastic papillae are seen from day 13 to 20. Grossly, the placentome has a concave surface. Microscopically, the villi are more irregular (Fig. 14–19). The cryptal lining consists of multinucleated cell masses of disputed origin. The arrangement of microvilli is similar to that in the cow, which makes it plausible that the syncytium is derived from maternal epithelium. However, selective staining provides circumstantial evidence that binucleate giant cells migrate across the microvillous junction to fuse with and become part of the syncytium.

Hematomata are present at the bases of the chorionic villi. Erythrocytes are phagocytized by trophoblastic cells and broken down by lysosomes, whereupon the hemoglobin is digested. Amniotic plaques are also present in the ewe.

Goat

The placentome of the goat is flatter than that of the ewe, but has a similar internal structure.

REFERENCES

Allen, W.R.: Immunological aspects of the endometrial cup reaction and the effect of xenogeneic pregnancy in horses and donkeys. J Reprod Fertil (Suppl.) *31*:57, 1982.

Amoroso, E.C.: Placentation. *In* Marshall's Physiology of Reproduction. 3rd Ed., Vol. II. Edited by A.S. Parkes. London, Longmans, Green and Co., 1952, pp. 127–311.

Anderson, J.W.: Ultrastructure of the placenta and fetal membranes of the dog. 1. The placental labyrinth. Anat Rec *165*:15, 1969.

Björkman, N.: An Atlas of Placental Fine Structure. London, Baillère, Tindall & Cassell, 1970.

Björkman, N.: Fine structure of the fetal-maternal area of exchange in the epitheliochorial and endotheliochorial types of placentation. Acta Anat (Basel), *86* (Suppl. 1):1, 1973.

Carlson, R.M.: Patten's foundations of embryology. 4th Ed. New York, McGraw-Hill Book Company, 1981.

Dantzer, V.: An extensive lysosomal system in the maternal epithelium of the porcine placenta. Placenta *5*:117, 1984.

Dantzer, V., Björkman, N., and Hasselager, E.: An electron microscopic study of histiotrophe in the interareolar part of the porcine placenta. Placenta *2*:19, 1981.

Dantzer, V., and Nielsen, M.H.: Intracellular pathways of native iron in the maternal part of the porcine placenta. Eur J Cell Biol *34*:103, 1984.

Dantzer, V., and Svenstrup, B.: Relationship between ultrastructure and oestrogen levels in the porcine placenta. Anim Reprod Sci 1986 (in press).

Friess, A.E., Sinowatz, F., Skolek-Winnisch, R., and Träuter, W.: The placenta of the pig. Anat Embryol *158*:179, 1980.

Friess, A.E., Sinowatz, F., Skolek-Winnisch, R., and Träutner, W.: The placenta of the pig. II: The ultrastructure of the areolae. Anat Embryol *163*:43, 1981.

Grosser, O.: Vergleichende Anatomie und Entwicklungs geschichte der Eihäute und der Placenta. Vienna, Braumüller, 1909, pp. 1–314.

Guillomot, M., Fléchon, J.-E., and Wintenberger-Torres, S.: Conceptus attachment in the ewe: An ultrastructural study. Placenta *2*:169, 1981.

Guillomot, M., and Guay, P.: Ultrastructural features of the cell surfaces of uterine and trophoblastic epithelia during embryo attachment in the cow. Anat Rec *204*:315, 1982.

King, G.J., Atkinson, B.A., and Robertson, H.A.: Implantation and early placentation in domestic ungulates. J Reprod Fertil (Suppl.) *31*:17, 1982.

Leiser, R.: Kontaktaufnahme zwischen Trophoblast und Uterusepithel während der frühen Implantation beim Rind. Anat Histol Embryol *4*:63, 1975.

Leiser, R.: Funktionelle Morphologie der Implantation und der frühen Plazentation bei der Hauskatze. Licht- und elektronenmikroskopische Untersuchung mit histocytochemischer Ergänzung. Thesis, Kanton Bern, 1980.

Myagkaya, G., and Schellens, J.P.M.: Final stages of erythrophagocytosis in the sheep placenta. Cell Tissue Res *214*:501, 1981.

Ramsey, E.M.: The placenta. Human and Animal. New York, Praeger Publishers, 1982.

Reimers, T.J., Ullmann, M.B., and Hansel, W.: Progesterone and prostanoid production by bovine binucleate trophoblastic cells. Biol Reprod *33*:1227, 1985.

Steven, D.H.: Comparative Placentation. New York. Academic Press, 1975.

Wooding, F.B.P.: Role of binucleate cells in fetomaternal cell fusion at implantation in the sheep. Am J Anat *170*:233, 1984.

Wooding, F.B.P., Staples, L.D., and Peacock, M.A.: Structure of trophoblast papillae on the sheep conceptus at implantation. J Anat *134*:507, 1982.

15

Endocrine System

H.-DIETER DELLMANN

The endocrine organs are ductless glands whose parenchymal cells secrete their products, the hormones, directly into the intercellular or perivascular connective tissue spaces whereby they reach the circulatory system. The circulating hormones regulate the functions of cells in general or of specific tissues or organs, referred to as target organs. The endocrine glands, together with the nervous system, participate in the maintenance of a steady physiologic state, called homeostasis. Their functions are intimately linked, coordinated, and sometimes even integrated as, for example, in the hypothalamo-hypophysial systems.

The parenchymal cells predominate in most endocrine organs; they are usually large epithelioid cells in contact with a blood or lymph capillary. The blood supply of the endocrine organs is among the densest in the organism and reflects both the high metabolic activity and the route of secretion.

The major endocrine functions are carried out by cell groups or single cells that are part of a nonendocrine organ. For example, scattered among the intestinal epithelial lining cells are peptide synthesizing cells, so-called APUD cells, characterized by amine precursor uptake and decarboxylation, with local rather than distant endocrine functions.

The following endocrine glands will be discussed in this chapter: hypothalamo-hypophysial systems, pineal gland, thyroid gland, parathyroid glands, adrenal glands, and pancreatic islets. The endocrine glands of the testis and ovary are dealt with in Chapters 12 and 13, respectively.

HYPOTHALAMO-HYPOPHYSIAL SYSTEMS

The hypophysis has two major portions, the adenohypophysis and the neurohypophysis. During ontogenetic development, the adenohypophysis originates as a dorsal evagination of the roof of the embryonic pharynx and establishes contact with the neurohypophysis, a ventral outgrowth of the diencephalic (hypothalamic) floor. The result is an intimate structural and functional relationship between hypothalamus and hypophysis, best described as two units: the hypothalamo-adenohypophysial system and the hypothalamo-neurohypophysial system. These two systems consist of the following parts (Figs. 15–1 and 15–2):

1. Hypothalamo-adenohypophysial system
   a. Hypothalamic portion: hypophysiotropic (parvicellular)

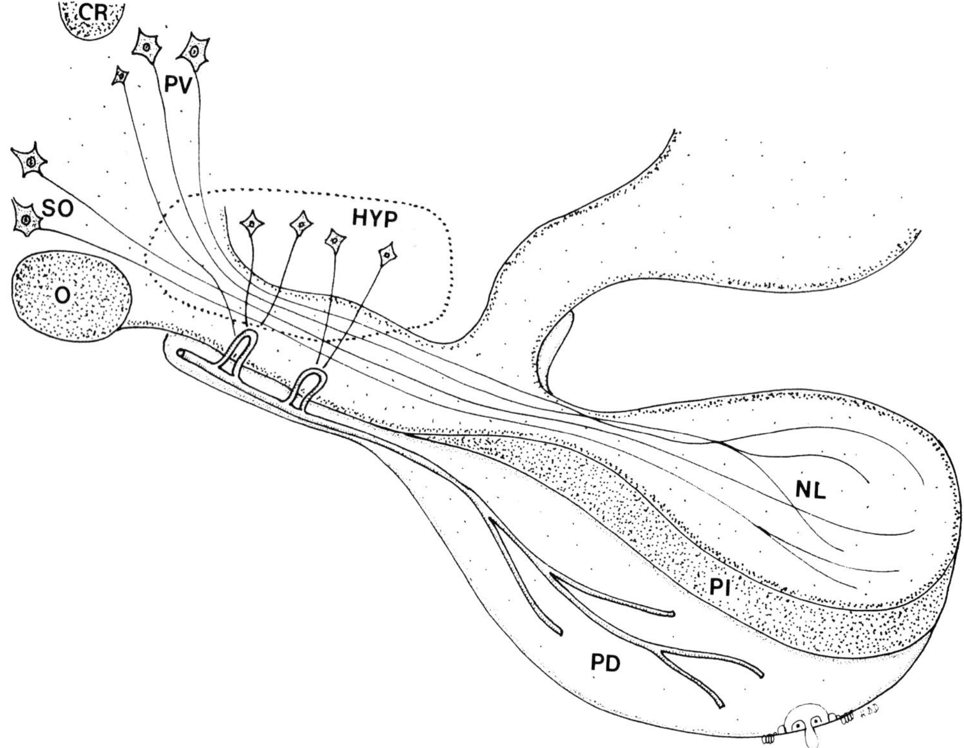

Fig. 15–1. *Schematic drawing of the hypothalamo-adenohypophysial and the hypothalamo-neurohypophysial systems. Optic chiasm (O); rostral commissure (CR); dotted line delineating the hypophysiotropic area (HYP); axons from the parvicellular nuclei of this region terminate in contact with the primary capillary loops of the hypophysial portal system in the external zone of the median eminence. Various releasing hormones reach the pars distalis through the portal system. Neural lobe (NL); pars distalis of the adenohypophysis (PD); pars intermedia of the adenohypophysis (PI); paraventricular nucleus (PV); supraoptic nucleus (SO); the axons of these two nuclei terminate in the neural lobe and store and release oxytocin and antidiuretin.*

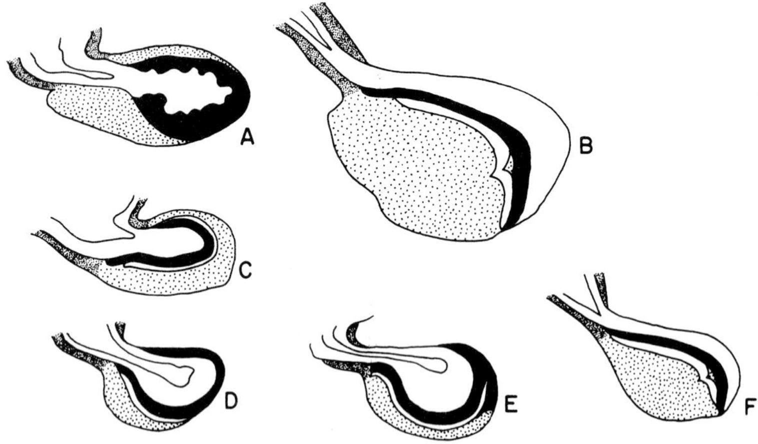

Fig. 15–2. *Schematic drawing of a midline sagittal section through the hypophysis of A, horse; B, large ruminant; C, dog; D, pig; E, cat; F, small ruminant (sheep). White, neurohypophysis with hypophysial cavity; small dots, pars tuberalis of the adenohypophysis; large dots, pars distalis of the adenohypophysis; black, pars intermedia of the adenohypophysis. (From Dellmann, H.-D.: Veterinary Histology: An Outline Text-Atlas. Philadelphia, Lea & Febiger, 1971.)*

hypothalamic nuclei
b. Neurohypophysial portion:
axon terminals of the hypophysiotropic neurons in median eminence
c. Adenohypophysial portion:
pars distalis
pars intermedia
pars tuberalis
2. Hypothalamo-neurohypophysial system
a. Hypothalamic portion:
supraoptic and paraventricular nuclei
b. Neurohypophysial portion:
median eminence
infundibular stem
pars nervosa or neural lobe

The neural lobe, pars intermedia, and pars distalis are surrounded by a common capsule of dense irregular connective tissue of variable thickness that blends dorsally with the diaphragma sellae.

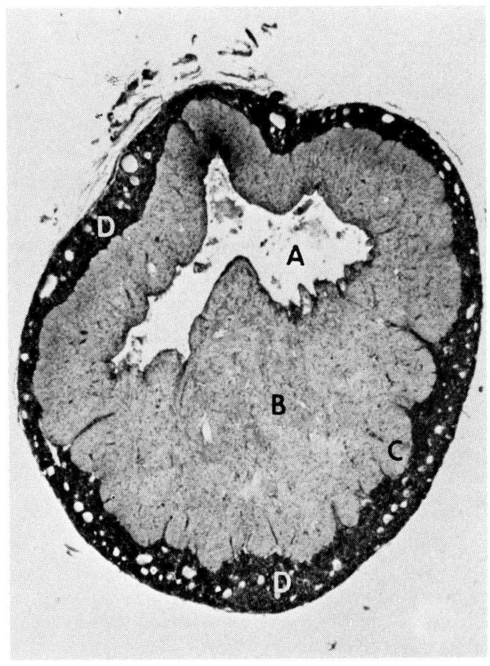

Fig. 15–3. *Horizontal section through the median eminence, large ruminant. Hypophysial cavity (A); internal zone (B); external zone (C); pars tuberalis of the adenohypophysis with numerous portal vessels (D). Masson's trichrome. ×19.*

Hypothalamo-Adenohypophysial System

HYPOTHALAMIC PORTION

The hypophysiotropic area is that portion of the basal hypothalamus within which most of the neurosecretory cells are located and whose axons project to the external zone of the median eminence (Fig. 15–1). Individual neuronal cell bodies and axons containing specific hypophysiotropic-releasing or -inhibiting hormones have been identified with immunohistochemical methods throughout this area.

NEUROHYPOPHYSIAL PORTION

The axons of the hormone-synthesizing nerve cells of the hypophysiotropic area terminate in the external zone of the median eminence (Figs. 15–1 and 15–3), where they establish neurovascular contacts with the primary capillaries of the hypophysial portal system (Fig. 15–4) to regulate hormone release by releasing or inhibiting hormones from the pars distalis. In addition, aminergic axons of hypothalamic and extrahypothalamic origin influence hormone release. Ependymal (tanycyte) or glial cell processes terminate at the same level (Fig. 15–5).

ADENOHYPOPHYSIAL PORTION

Pars Distalis

The pars distalis consists of clusters and cords of cells in close apposition to a dense network of sinusoidal capillaries.

The classic tinctorial distinction and classification of the various cell types into acidophils, basophils, and chromophobes is useful for routine examinations of the pars distalis (Fig. 15–6). However, unequivocal identification of specific cell types in a given species is not a routine matter and, because of species-specific staining affinities, is sub-

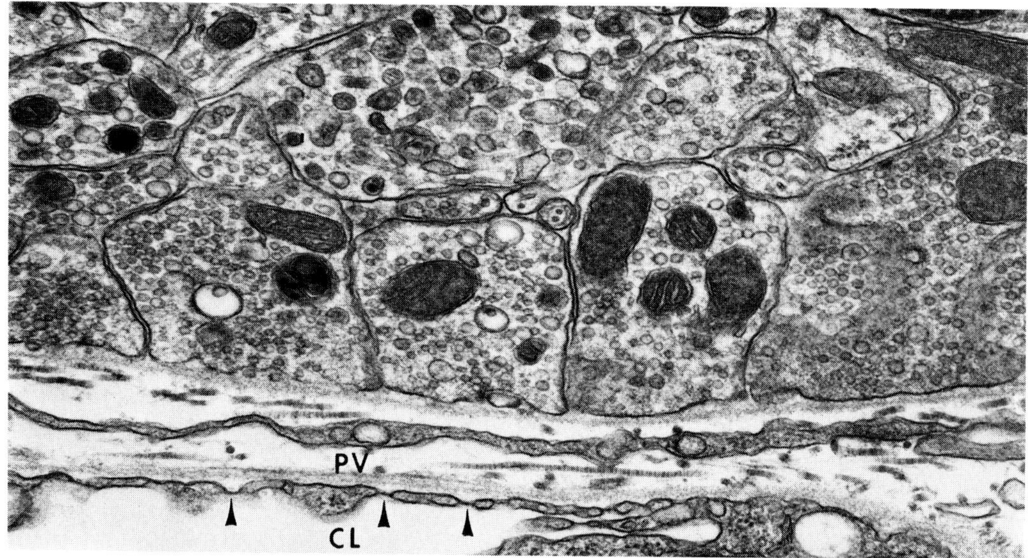

Fig. 15–4. *Axon terminals contacting the perivascular connective tissue space of the external zone of the median eminence, rat. Notice the presence of clear and granular vesicles of varying sizes and densities, possibly indicative of various functions, fenestrations in the capillary endothelium (arrows), and reticular fibers in the perivascular connective tissue space (PV). Capillary lumen (CL).*

ject to wide variations. By use of immunohistochemical methods it has been possible to classify adenohypophysial cells according to the hormone (or hormones) they contain. The following hormones are synthesized by the pars distalis: growth hormone or somatotropin (STH); prolactin; thyrotropin (TSH); gonadotropins: follicle-stimulating hormone (FSH) and luteinizing hormone (LH); procorticolipotropin that is cleaved into adrenocorticotropin (ACTH), β and γ lipotropin (LPH), endorphins, melanocyte-stimulating hor-

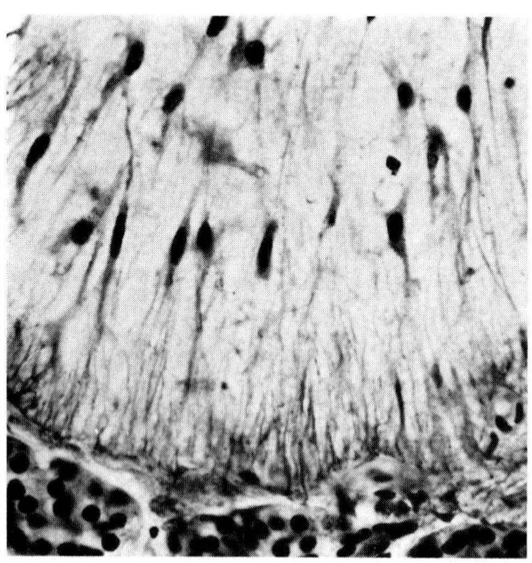

Fig. 15–5. *External zone of the median eminence, large ruminant. Glial cell and ependymal cell processes terminate at the contact zone between median eminence and pars tuberalis of the adenohypophysis. Silver impregnation. ×435.*

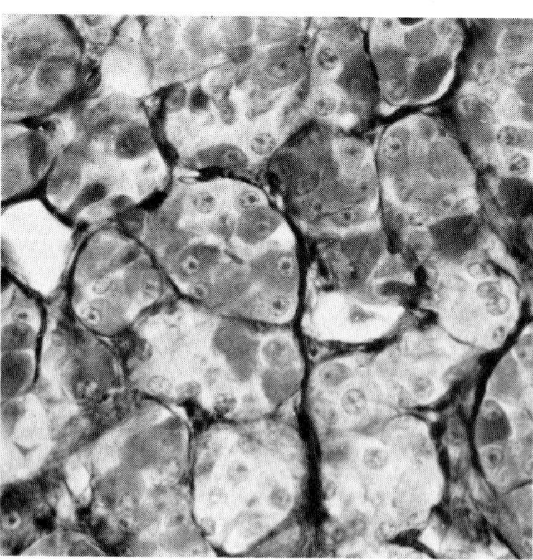

Fig. 15–6. *Pars distalis of the adenohypophysis, large ruminant, with groups of basophilic (dark-staining) and acidophilic (light-staining) cells. Azan. ×435.*

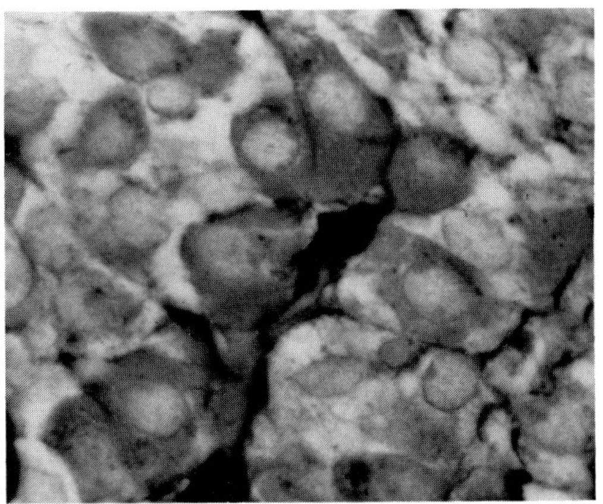

Fig. 15–7. *Pars distalis of the adenohypophysis, rat, somatotropes. Herlant's tetrachrome method.* ×*428. (Courtesy of N. Chang.)*

mone (MSH), and corticotropin-like intermediate lobe peptide (CLIP).

ACIDOPHILS. The granules of acidophils are eosinophilic and may be visible individually with the light microscope (dog or cat). With immunohistochemical methods and the electron microscope, two types of acidophils are distinguished. The *somatotropes* predominate in the lateral portions of the pars distalis; their abundant granules (see Figs. 15–9 and 15–10) have a distinct affinity for orange G (Fig. 15–7). They measure 300 to 400 nm in diameter and stain immunohistochemically for growth hormone (STH).

Lactotropes or *prolactin cells* stain with erythrosin and carmoisin L, especially when the cells are hypertrophied and contain many granules, as in pregnancy and lactation, or when nonpregnant animals are treated with estrogen. An extensive Golgi complex, long ER cisternae and lysosomes, as well as large granules (up to 800 nm in diameter), and a positive immunohistochemical reaction for prolactin also characterize these cells.

BASOPHILS. All basophilic cells give a strong PAS reaction owing to the presence of glycoprotein hormones. Furthermore, all basophilic granules have some degree of affinity for alcian blue. The use of electron microscopy and immunohistochemistry has identified the basophil cell types thyrotropes, gonadotropes, and corticotropes.

The *thyrotropes* are irregularly shaped or angular cells that predominate in the midventral region of the pars distalis and stain with aldehyde-fuchsin and are also PAS-positive. Their granules are the smallest among all adenohypophysial cells (maximum diameter 150 nm). They are immunoreactive for TSH.

Gonadotropes are relatively small cells that are not always readily identified with routine histologic methods. Their granules stain with alcian blue, aldehyde thionin, and, weakly, with PAS, and measure about 200 nm in diameter. The rER of these cells is extensive and its cisternae sometimes dilated. The gonadotropes are immunoreactive for FSH and/or LH.

Following castration, the gonadotropes enlarge considerably (Figs. 15–8 and 15–9). The absence of an inhibitory feedback causes an initial increase in the number of granules, with a concurrent increase in the FSH and LH content. Eventually, "signet ring" cells are formed (Fig. 15–8–1) with a peripheral rim of cytoplasm surrounding one or several large vacuoles.

The *corticotropes* are dispersed throughout the pars distalis and are usually difficult to identify with the light microscope. The cells may be spherical, ovoid, or stellate, depending on the species. Their granules average 150 to 200 nm in diameter and frequently are located peripherally (Fig. 15–10). They stain immunohistochemically for ACTH and β-lipotropin (β-LPH).

CHROMOPHOBIC CELLS. The chromophobes comprise three cell types. The *follicular cells* line follicles of unknown significance; *stellate cells* with numerous fine processes are interspersed between the other cells of the pars distalis. These two types do not contain any granules. A third cell type of varying shape and size contains a few specific granules and is considered to

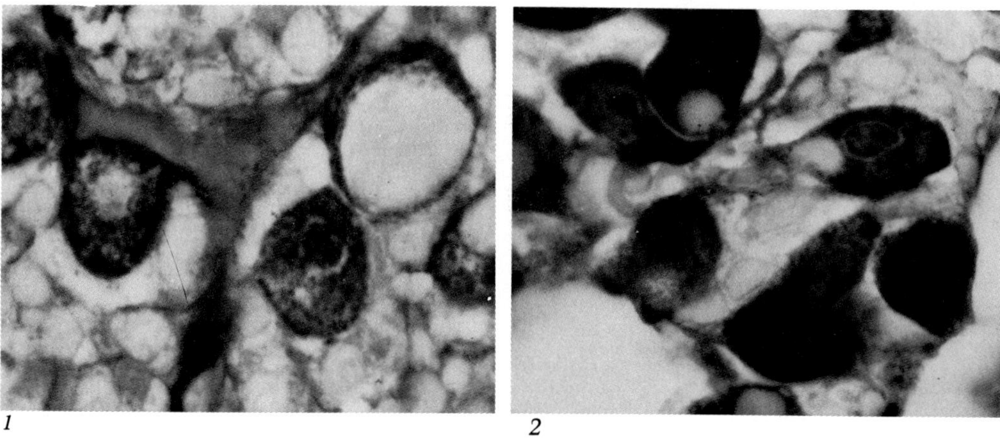

Fig. 15–8. *1. These enlarged cells stain purple with Herlant's tetrachrome and are possibly FSH cells; notice a signet ring cell in the upper right hand corner. 2. Enlarged cells that stain red are considered to be LH cells. Herlant's tetrachrome method. ×1240. (Courtesy of N. Chang.)*

be a *resting degranulated form* of all the other granulated cells.

PARS INTERMEDIA

The pars intermedia is closely associated with the neurohypophysis and is almost completely separated from the pars distalis by the hypophysial cleft (Figs. 15–2 and 15–11). Pars intermedia cells may penetrate into the neural lobe, and neurosecretory and aminergic axons are observed in the pars intermedia. Blood vessels and interstitial connective tissue are generally sparse.

The number of cell types is subject to species variation. However, the most abundant cell type of the pars intermedia is a large, pale-staining cell that may surround colloid-filled follicles (Fig. 15–12). Other cell types include typical pars distalis cells (especially ACTH cells), follicular cells, interstitial cells, and low cuboidal epithelial cells that line the hypophysial cleft.

The main cell type of the pars intermedia produces melanocyte-stimulating hormone (MSH) and β-LPH.

PARS TUBERALIS

The pars tuberalis surrounds the median eminence like a sleeve (Fig. 15–3) and consists of clusters of epithelial cells often forming small follicles. It is traversed longitudinally by the wide hypophysial portal vessels that receive tributaries mainly from the primary capillary plexus in the median eminence.

In addition to a few gonadotropes and thyrotropes, the pars tuberalis contains secretory cells that are not found in any other portion of the adenohypophysis. Their functional significance is unknown.

BLOOD AND NERVE SUPPLY

The main blood supply is provided by the portal vessels, which irrigate the neuro- and adenohypophysial portions; the hypothalamic portion receives an independent blood supply. The *hypophysial portal system* consists of a primary capillary plexus in and around the median eminence, a secondary capillary plexus in the pars distalis, and connecting portal vessels in the pars tuberalis (Figs. 15–1 and 15–3). The primary capillary plexus comprises two types of primary capillary loops and a superficial plexus. The short capillary loops are located in the external zone of the median eminence. The long capillary loops penetrate the inner zone deeply and often oc-

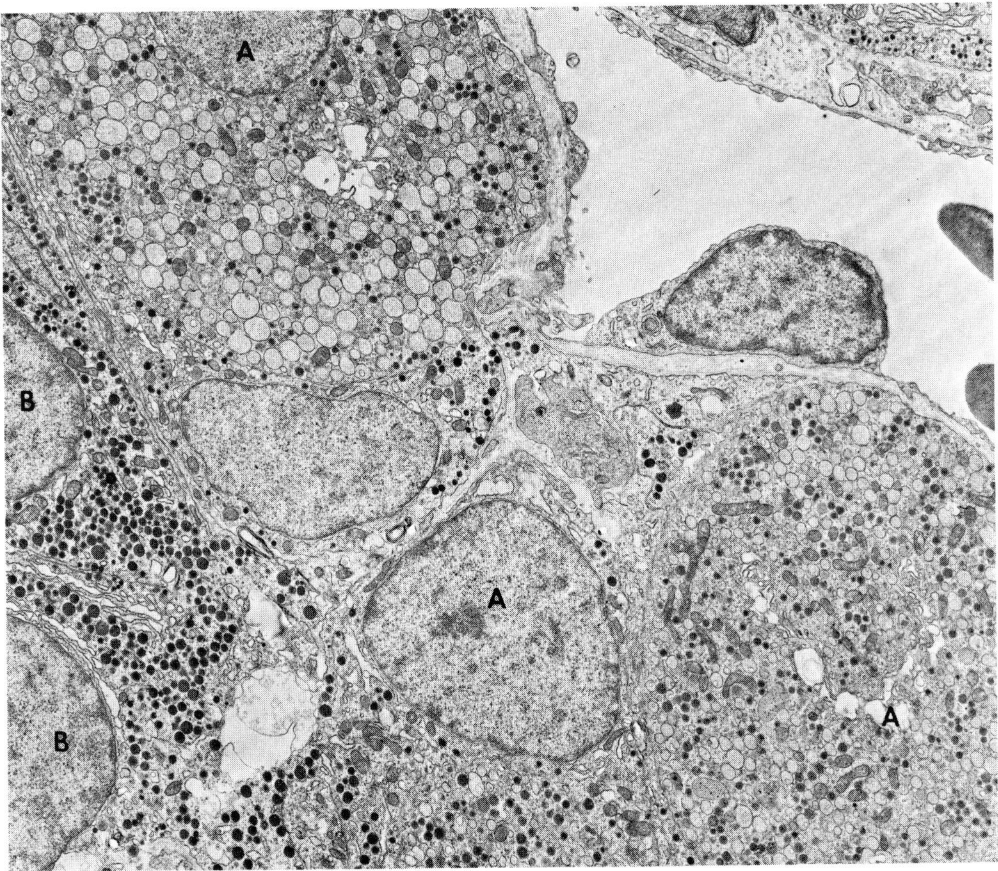

Fig. 15–9. *Electron micrograph of pars distalis of the adenohypophysis, female rat, ovariectomized 40 days. Gonadotropes (two of them are enlarged and have a prominent Golgi complex with dilated cisternae) (A); somatotropes (B).* ×3977. *(Courtesy of N. Chang.)*

cupy a subependymal position. The superficial plexus lies between the median eminence and the pars tuberalis. The capillary loops and the superficial plexus connect with fenestrated portal vessels and capillaries, which course longitudinally through the pars tuberalis and continue into the secondary capillary plexus. This plexus receives additional blood through accessory vessels.

The blood supply of the pars intermedia is restricted to a plexus of vessels within the connective tissue that separates the neurohypophysis from the pars intermedia (plexus intermedius). A few capillaries may be found in the sparse connective tissue (dog, cat). However, the most rostral part (rostral zone) of the pars intermedia, at the level of its junction with the partes distalis and tuberalis, has a rich blood supply.

A few nerve fibers regularly course from the neurohypophysis into the adenohypophysis, but only those that terminate in the pars intermedia are considered to be of functional significance. The inhibitory role of these hypothalamic nerve fibers is spectacularly demonstrated by the accumulation of secretory granules in and the size increase of the pars intermedia cells following transection of these nerve fibers.

Autonomic nerve fibers reach the adenohypophysis within the perivascular connective tissue sheaths.

HISTOPHYSIOLOGY

Releasing hormones (RH), releasing factors (RF), and inhibitory factors (IF) are

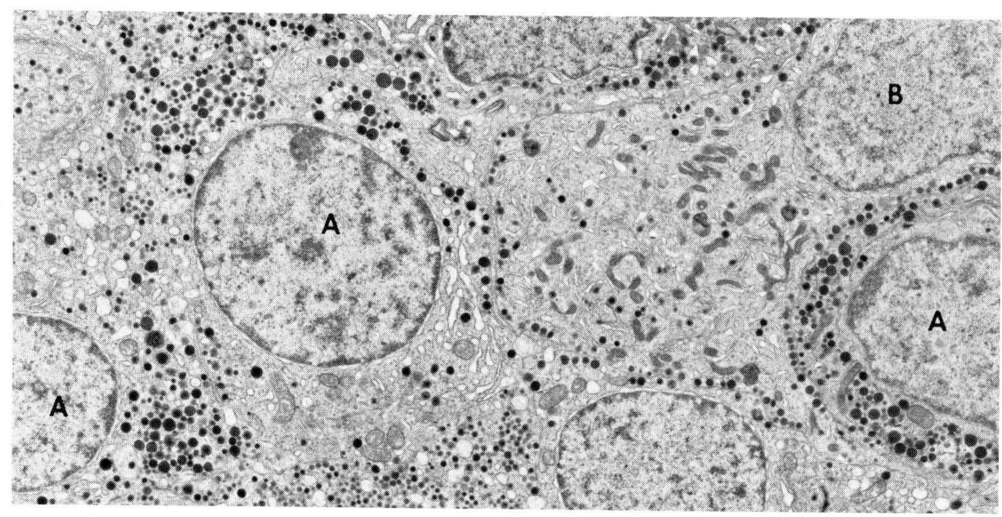

Fig. 15–10. *Electron micrograph of pars distalis of the adenohypophysis, rat. STH cells (A); ACTH cells (B).* ×*4375. (Courtesy of N. Chang.)*

synthesized by neuronal perikarya in the hypophysiotropic region of the hypothalamus. These substances are transported intra-axonally into the median eminence, where they are released into the hypophysial system. They are responsible for the regulation of adenophypophysial functions and include the following: CRH (for corticotropin), TRH (for thyrotropin), PRF (for prolactin) and PIF (for prolactin), GnRH (for luteinizing hormone and for follicle-stimulating hormone), MIF (for melanocyte-stimulating hormone), and

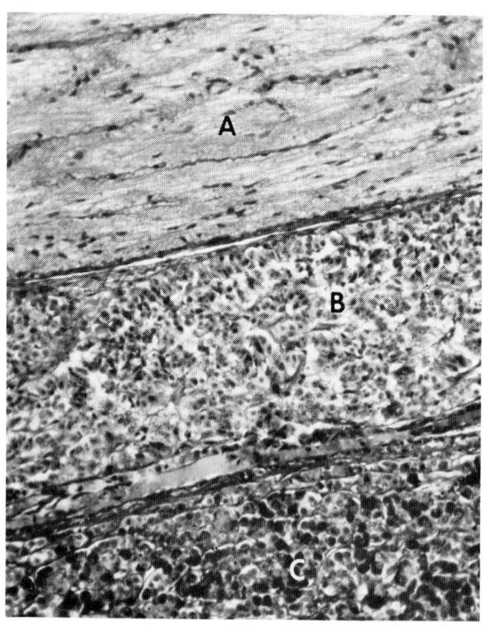

Fig. 15–11. *Hypophysis, large ruminant. Neural lobe (A); pars intermedia (B); pars distalis (C). Azan.* ×*135.*

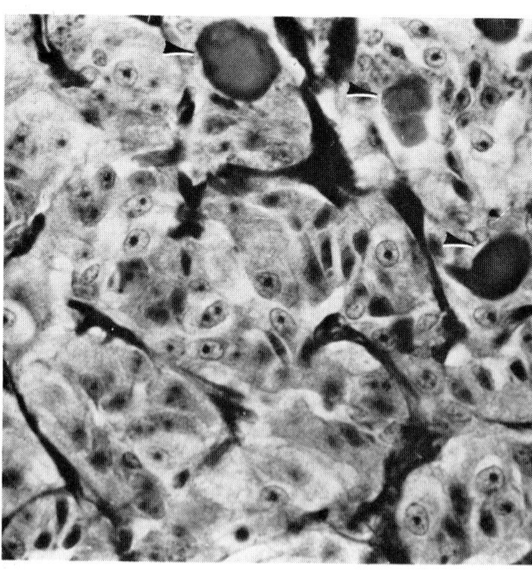

Fig. 15–12. *Pars intermedia of the adenohypophysis, large ruminant. Notice the presence of colloid-filled follicles (arrows) and a relatively large amount of connective tissue, characteristic for large ruminants. Azan.* ×*435.*

GHRF (for growth hormone) and somatostatin (for growth hormone).

Prolactin induces secretion in the mammary gland (lactogenic activity), stimulates growth and secretory activity of the pigeon crop sacs (crop-stimulating activity), activates the corpus luteum in some mammalian species (rat), and, finally, has prelactational mammogenic activity. Prolactin cells are prominent when prolactin secretion is high. Prolactin secretion is predominantly under inhibitory hypothalamic control.

Somatotropic hormone promotes growth after birth. A decrease in the number of somatotropes results in dwarfism, and hypersecretion leads to gigantism in young and acromegaly in adult animals.

Thyrotropin acts almost exclusively on the thyroid gland, inducing the synthesis and release of thyroxine.

In female animals, FSH stimulates the growth of primary and older follicles. LH is required for the follicle to reach full size and to secrete estrogen. LH, in conjunction with FSH, causes ovulation and is necessary for the subsequent development of a corpus luteum and the secretion of progesterone.

In male animals, FSH stimulates the growth of the seminiferous tubules and promotes the first phases of spermatogenesis. The late phases of spermatogenesis (spermiogenesis), as well as the full development of the testis, and synthesis and release of androgens depend on the presence of LH.

Adrenocorticotropin (ACTH) affects primarily the adrenal cortex by stimulating growth of the zonae fasciculata and reticularis and by regulating their secretory activity, i.e., the secretion of glucocorticoids. In the pars distalis corticotropes, the prohormone procorticolipotropin is cleaved into ACTH and LPH (β and γ). In the pars intermedia, ACTH is further cleaved to α MSH and CLIP, and LPH to β MSH and β endorphin. MSH causes dispersion of melanophores in amphibians and promotes melanization of growing hair in some mammals, and there is evidence for its participation in learning and memory control and fetal growth. There is no known function for LPH, while β endorphin action is similar to that of morphine.

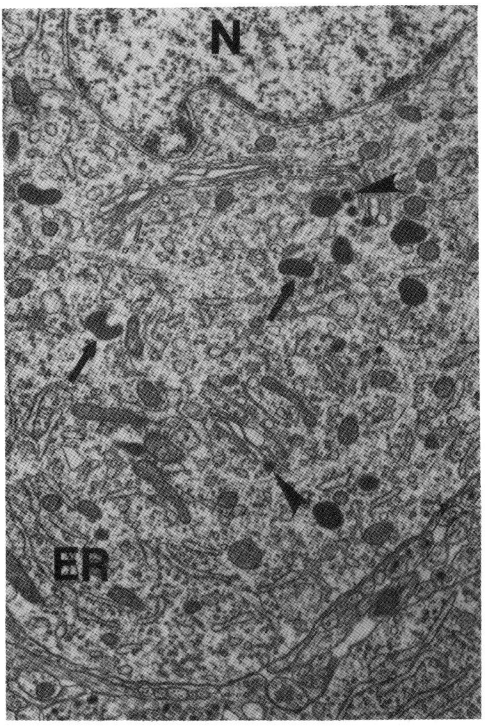

Fig. 15–13. *Portion of a neurosecretory cell from the supraoptic nucleus, mouse. Notice the presence of neurosecretory granulated vesicles (arrowheads) in the vicinity of the Golgi complex, lysosomes (arrows) and rough ER (ER); (N) nucleus. ×11,000.*

Hypothalamo-Neurohypophysial System

HYPOTHALAMIC PORTION

The magnocellular hypothalamic supraoptic and paraventricular nuclei are characterized by large cells that have a positive immunohistochemical reaction for either antidiuretic hormone (ADH) or oxytocin. At the electron microscopic level these hormones are localized within neurosecretory granulated vesicles (Fig. 15–13). These are transported within the

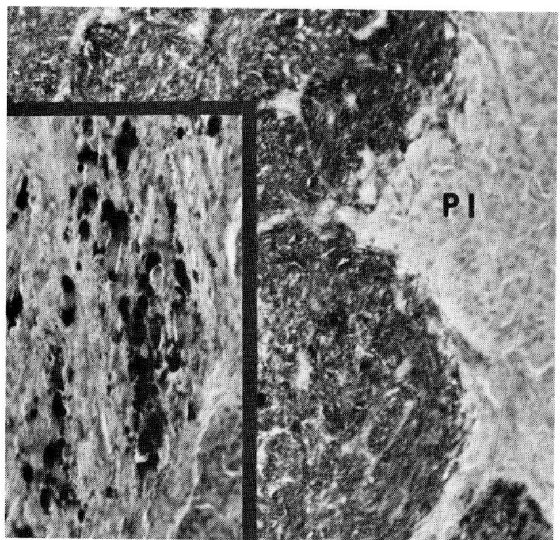

Fig. 15–14. *Portion of the neural lobe of a large ruminant adjacent to the pars intermedia (PI) of the adenohypophysis. Notice the abundant neurosecretory material (black). The inset shows a portion of the neural lobe where Herring bodies are particularly numerous. Aldehyde-fuchsin. ×135.*

axons of the supraoptico- and paraventriculo-neurohypophysial tracts, coursing through the hypothalamus and median eminence into the neural lobe.

NEUROHYPOPHYSIAL PORTION

Most axons of the hypothalamo-neurohypophysial tract merely traverse the *median eminence* in the internal zone. Others, originating from the parvocellular PVN, terminate in the external zone (Fig. 15–1).

In the *neural lobe,* axon terminals abut the perivascular spaces; they store and release neurosecretory vesicles (see Fig. 15–15). With certain dyes, such as aldehydefuchsin, large numbers of these neurosecretory vesicles are visualized at the light microscopic level as intensely blue staining *neurosecretory material* (Fig. 15–14). Some axons penetrate the pars intermedia and end in contact with its cells.

Large axon dilatations containing neurosecretory vesicles and other organelles in varying quantities are referred to as Herring bodies (Fig. 15–14). They are considered places of storage and disposal of hormones.

The neuroglial cells of the neural lobe, the pituicytes, form an extensive, three-dimensional framework among axons and capillaries. Their functional significance is unknown.

BLOOD AND NERVE SUPPLY

In the hypothalamic neurosecretory nuclei, a dense network of capillaries is present. The neural lobe is supplied by a plexus of sinusoidal capillaries into which the neurohormones are released.

Perivascular sympathetic nerve fibers encircle the blood vessels of the neurohypophysis; their function is assumed to be vasomotor.

HISTOPHYSIOLOGY

Neurophysin-oxytocin and neurophysin-ADH complexes represent the major component of the neurosecretory granules. Their biosynthesis takes place in separate neurons from a larger precursor molecule that is enzymatically cleaved during its transport from perikarya to the axon terminals in the neural lobe. Release of the hormones takes place by exocytosis of the neurosecretory vesicular content. Subsequent endocytosis of the vesicular membrane leads to the formation of vacuoles and microvesicles in the axon terminals (Fig. 15–15). With immunocytochemical methods a variety of biogenic amines, acetylcholine, GABA, enkephalin, dynorphin, α-neoendorphin, and other peptides have been found in neural lobe axon terminals either coexisting with oxytocin and vasopressin or in independent neural systems. There is evidence that these substances modulate the release of vasopressin or oxytocin.

ADH, also referred to as vasopressin, is released in response to an increased plasma osmolality or hypovolemia and acts specifically on the lining epithelium of the distal convoluted tubules and collecting ducts, rendering them permeable to water. Ab-

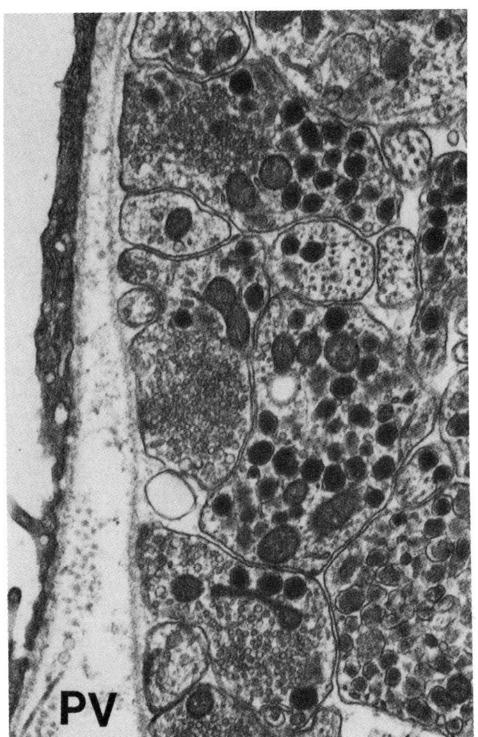

Fig. 15–15. *Electron micrograph of neural lobe, rabbit. Neurosecretory axons terminate at the perivascular connective tissue space (PV). In addition to large membrane-bounded neurosecretory granules, the axons contain small clear vesicles and mitochondria. ×22,000.*

sence or failure of ADH release leads to diabetes insipidus.

Oxytocin stimulates contractions of the myoepithelial cells of the mammary gland, and subsequent milk ejection. Stimulation of the teat results in afferent impulses being sent to the hypothalamus, which in turn causes oxytocin release from the neurohypophysis.

During parturition, stimuli from the genital area cause the hypothalamo-neurohypophysial system to release oxytocin, which stimulates the contractions of the uterus necessary for delivery.

PINEAL GLAND

The mammalian pineal gland is a solid or follicular parenchymatous organ surrounded by a thin layer of loose connective

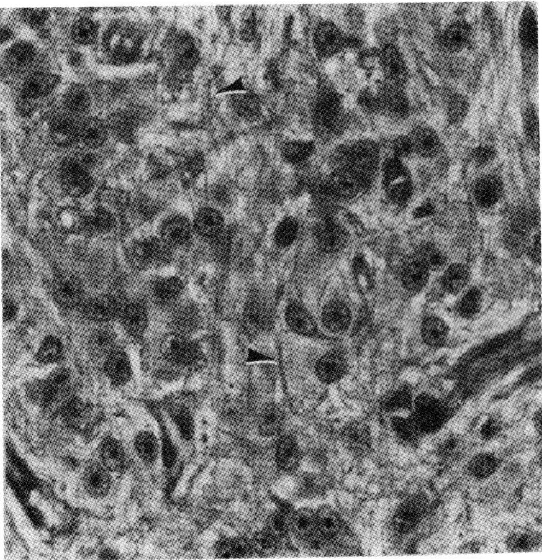

Fig. 15–16. *Pineal gland, large ruminant. The pinealocytes are intermingled with numerous astrocyte processes (arrows). Azan. ×435. (From Dellmann, H.-D.: Veterinary Histology: An Outline Text-Atlas. Philadelphia, Lea & Febiger, 1971.)*

tissue. Connective tissue trabeculae of varying thickness contain occasional melanocytes, striated muscle cells, blood vessels, and nerve fibers. Frequently, calcium deposits (brain sand; corpora arenacea) occur within the parenchyma, which consists of pinealocytes and glial cells.

The dominating cells of the mammalian pineal gland are pinealocytes, which often occur in clusters (Fig. 15–16). They possess numerous long and winding processes that terminate at follicular lumina, or among other pinealocytes and in the perivascular or interstitial connective tissue. Morphologic evidence suggests that these cells have a secretory activity.

In addition, the pineal gland contains astrocytes, whose processes (Fig. 15–16) surround pinealocytes and contact the perivascular basal lamina. The pineal gland is permeated by a capillary network whose perivascular spaces are bordered by pinealocyte and astrocyte processes.

The mammalian pineal gland is innervated exclusively by sympathetic nerve fibers (from the cranial cervical ganglion) that establish synaptic contacts with the pinealocytes.

The circadian rhythmic secretory activity of the pineal gland is driven by the hypothalamic suprachiasmatic nucleus, which receives information from the retina and relays it via the midbrain tegmentum and cervical spinal cord to the cranial cervical ganglion and its postganglionic fibers to the pineal gland.

Function

The pineal gland secretes methoxyindoles, the most prominent of which is melatonin, and peptidic and polypeptidic compounds. The reported actions of these substances are diverse among the investigated species. Among the most important actions are direct or indirect involvement in daily and seasonal photoperiodically induced rhythms, in sexual behavior and reproduction, in thermoregulation, and in color changes.

THYROID GLAND

The thyroid gland is surrounded by a thin *capsule* of dense irregular connective tissue. Thin trabeculae extend from the capsule into the parenchyma. In large ruminants and swine, the capsule and trabeculae are thick. The collagen fibers of the trabeculae continue into the sparse, loose interstitial connective tissue.

The thyroid gland consists of numerous *follicles* (Fig. 15–17) (20 to 500 μm in diameter), usually filled with colloid and lined by follicular cells. In various physiologic conditions, the simple epithelial cells assume different shapes. When resting, they are low cuboidal or even squamous cells, and the colloid appears dense and uniformly stained; when stimulated, the cells become cuboidal or columnar, and the colloid is nonuniformly stained and often contains vacuoles (see Fig. 15–19).

The follicular colloid stains red with azocarmine and blue with aniline blue when

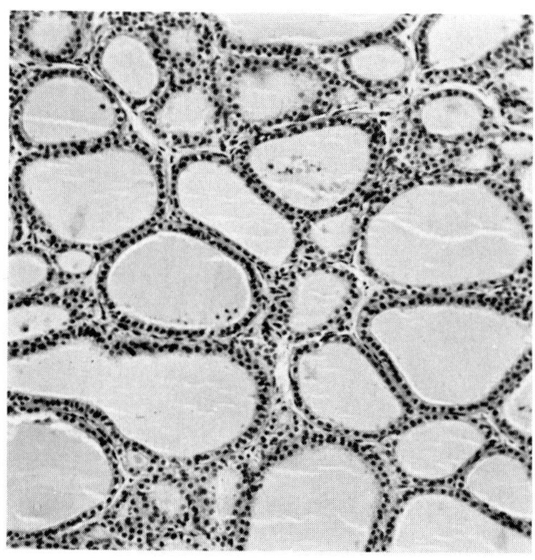

Fig. 15–17. *Thyroid gland, pig. H & E. ×135.*

the colloid is diluted; it is PAS-positive because of its content of glycoprotein (thyroglobulin). The follicles are surrounded by a basement membrane, sparse connective tissue, and a dense network of capillaries and lymph capillaries, which very likely participate in hormone transport.

The shape of the nucleus of *follicular cells* varies with that of the cell; it is located in the cell base. Mitochondria, rER, ribosomes, and polysomes are distributed throughout the cytoplasm. The Golgi complex lies between the nucleus and the microvillous apical cell surface. The apical cytoplasm also contains two types of vesicles: *apical vesicles,* which originate from the Golgi complex and contain thyroglobulin, which is secreted by exocytosis into the follicular lumen; and large membrane-bounded *colloid droplets.* These arise through sequestration by pseudopods that form at the luminal surface and, through merging with lysosomes, form phagolysosomes, in which thyroglobulin is broken down (see below).

Parafollicular or *C cells* derive from the neural crest and reach the thyroid during development via the ultimobranchial body. They usually occur as single cells within the basement membrane of the follicles (Fig.

15–18) but may also form groups in the same location or outside the follicles (Fig. 15–19), especially in the dog. These cells are the source of calcitonin (thyrocalcitonin) and are characterized by light-staining cytoplasm, little endoplasmic reticulum, abundant Golgi complex, many mitochondria, and especially numerous, small membrane-bound vesicles (Fig. 15–18).

Histophysiology

The first step in thyroid hormone biosynthesis is thyroglobulin formation in the usual rER-Golgi complex sequence and its secretion, via apical vesicles, into the follicular lumen. By way of the same synthetic steps and very likely the same route, thyroperoxidase is synthesized, packaged, and released into the follicular lumen, where it is responsible for the iodination of thyroglobulin, i.e., the attachment of iodine to the tyrosyl radicals of thyroglobulin. During the second phase of secretion, this stored thyroglobulin is taken up by follicular cells (see above) and broken down by proteolytic digestion within phagolysosomes to yield the active hormones (thyroxine and triiodothyronine [T3]) that diffuse out of the cell base into the perivascular space.

Hormone synthesis and uptake are regulated by TSH and occur simultaneously in active follicles, so that hormone release is a continuous process.

The cellular actions of thyroid hormones, their physiologic and metabolic functions, as well as their morphologic effects, are too varied and numerous to even be enumerated in this context. The student is referred to specialized texts.

The C cells produce thyrocalcitonin, which lowers the blood calcium level by suppressing bone resorption. Therefore, the effect of thyrocalcitonin is opposite to that of parathormone.

PARATHYROID GLANDS

The parathyroid gland is surrounded by a *capsule* of dense irregular connective tis-

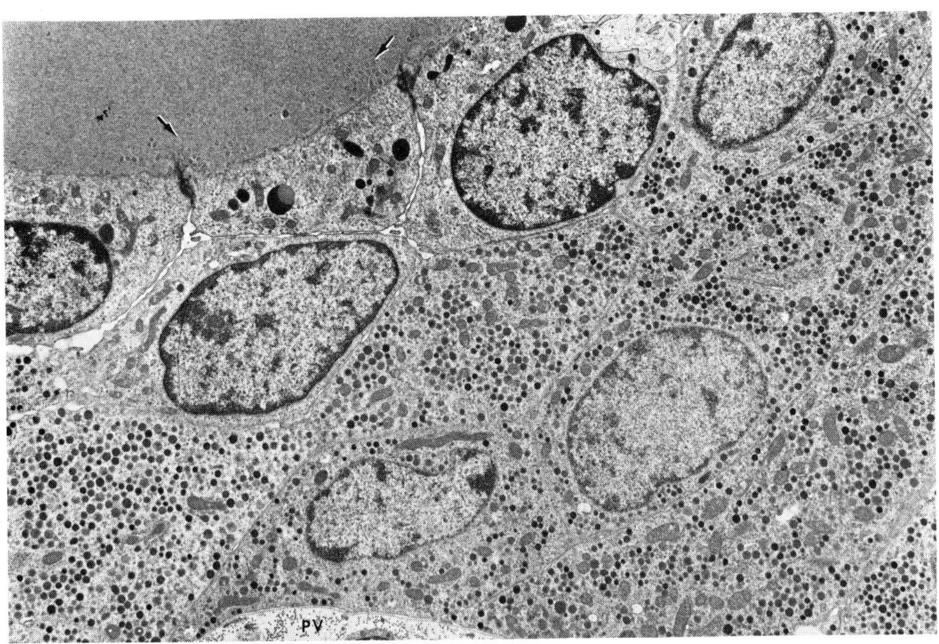

Fig. 15–18. *Electron micrograph of thyroid gland, dog. Microvilli of the follicular lining cells (arrows) project into the colloid. The C cells are packed with secretory granules and do not reach the follicular lumen. Perivascular connective tissue space (PV). ×5640. (Courtesy of K.R. Moore and S.L. Teitelbaum.)*

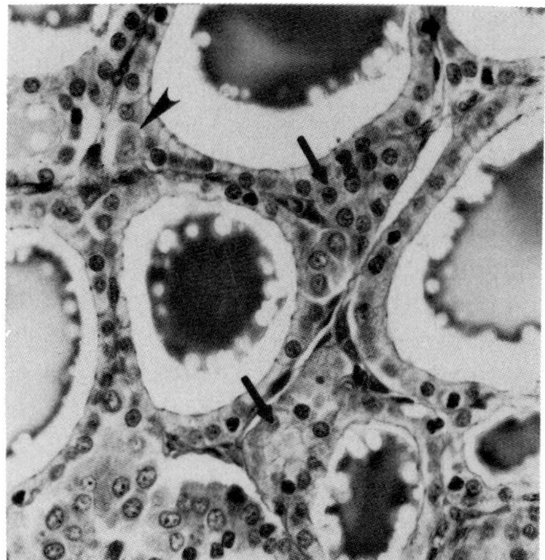

Fig. 15–19. *Thyroid gland, dog. Single C cells (arrowhead) or groups of them (arrows) are readily identified by their location outside the follicular epithelium. Trichrome. ×200.*

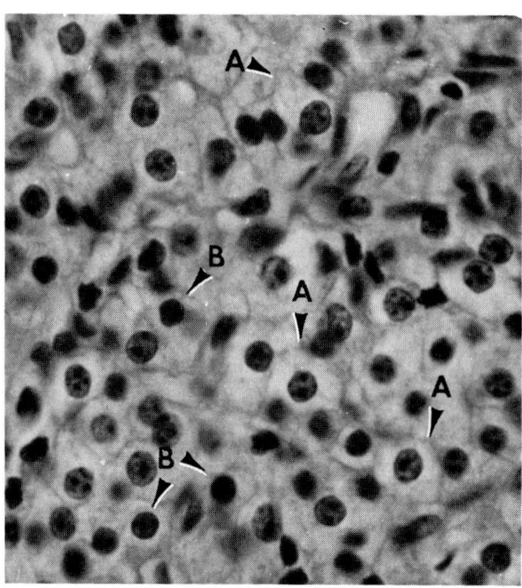

Fig. 15–20. *Parathyroid gland, horse. Inactive (A) and active (B) principal cells are readily distinguishable. H & E. ×750. (From Dellmann, H.-D.: Veterinary Histology: An Outline Text-Atlas. Philadelphia, Lea & Febiger, 1971.)*

sue, which is thick in large ruminants and swine and thin in the dog and cat. Trabeculae and interstitial connective tissue are abundant in large ruminants and swine and sparse in the other domestic mammals. They contain a dense capillary network.

The parenchyma is generally arranged in clusters, strands, or cords and contains mainly a single basic cell type, the principal cell. Principal cells are in various stages of secretory activity and designated as inactive (light) and active (dark) principal cells. The inactive (light) principal cells usually are the most frequent cell type (Fig. 15–20). They are considered to be in a resting stage or at the end of a secretory cycle. They are relatively large, acidophil cells. The Golgi complex is inconspicuous, the rER is concentrated in small areas, and there are occasional secretory granules; lipid droplets and lipofuscin inclusions (cattle) or glycogen (cat) may be present. The nucleus is large and light-staining.

The active (dark) principal cells (Fig. 15–20) contain a nucleus with condensed chromatin, surrounded by dark cytoplasm containing an extensive Golgi complex, abundant rER, and numerous mitochondria and secretory granules. The entire appearance is that of a stimulated cell. In addition, a second cell type, the oxyphil cell, is present rather regularly in the horse and large ruminants but is rare in other domestic mammals. These large cells (up to 27 μm in the horse) occur either singly or in clusters. They possess a small and at times pyknotic nucleus and a light-staining cytoplasm, which is literally filled with mitochondria, whereas Golgi complex, granular ER, and secretory granules are scarce. These cells are obviously in an inactive stage of secretion. Their functional significance is unknown.

A transitional cell type with structural characteristics intermediate between those of principal and oxyphil cells, i.e., with many mitochondria, relatively abundant rER, Golgi complex, and secretory granules, is likewise present.

In all domestic mammals except the goat and sheep, the dark and light principal cells are distributed randomly with one or the other form prevailing, depending on the functional phase of the glands. Colloidal cysts with ciliated lining cells are frequent.

In the sheep and goat, the periphery of

the gland is occupied by light principal cells, whereas the dark principal cells are in the center.

In the dog and sometimes in the horse, the parenchymal cells form a simple pericapillary epithelial layer with occasional rosette-like formations.

Function

The parathyroid glands produce parathormone, which maintains the normal blood calcium level. In severe parathyroid hormone deficiencies (after parathyroidectomy, for example), the decreased blood calcium level causes fibrillary twitching in various muscles (increase in neuromuscular irritability), followed by clonic movements of the limbs and, finally, by rigid spasms (tetany) and death.

The principal role of the parathyroid hormone is to maintain normal levels of calcium and phosphorus in the blood. It does this by inducing an increased absorption of calcium from the intestine, a resorption of calcium from bones (activation of osteoclasts), and a decreased loss of calcium in the urine. Parathyroid hormone acts directly on the proximal tubules of the kidney to inhibit the reabsorption of phosphate and to promote the reabsorption of calcium.

ADRENAL GLANDS

The adrenal gland is composed of two distinct portions, an outer cortex of mesodermal origin, and an inner medulla, derived from neuroectoderm. They are surrounded by a common thin capsule of dense irregular connective tissue, occasionally with some smooth muscle fibers (Fig. 15–21). Thin trabeculae originate from the capsule and penetrate the cortex but rarely enter the medulla. Frequently, clusters of cortical cells, resembling undifferentiated cortical cells that may differentiate into the cells of the zona glomerulosa, are seen in the capsule (Fig. 15–22).

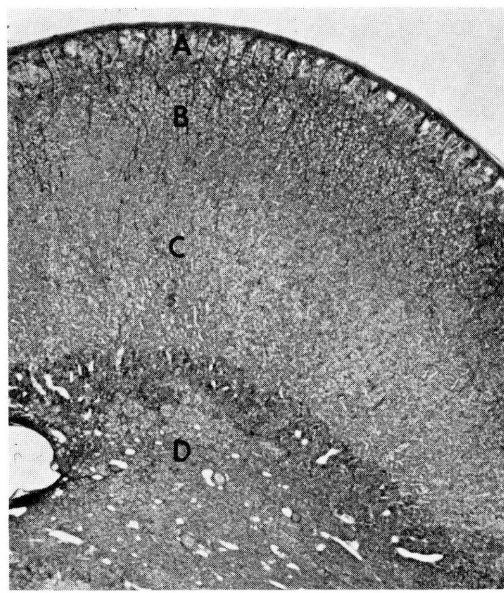

Fig. 15–21. *Adrenal gland, horse. The organization of the cortex into zona glomerulosa (A), zona fasciculata (B) and zona reticularis (C) is readily distinguishable. Notice the high vascularity of the medulla (D). H & E. ×15. (From Dellmann, H.-D.: Veterinary Histology: An Outline Text-Atlas. Philadelphia, Lea & Febiger, 1971.)*

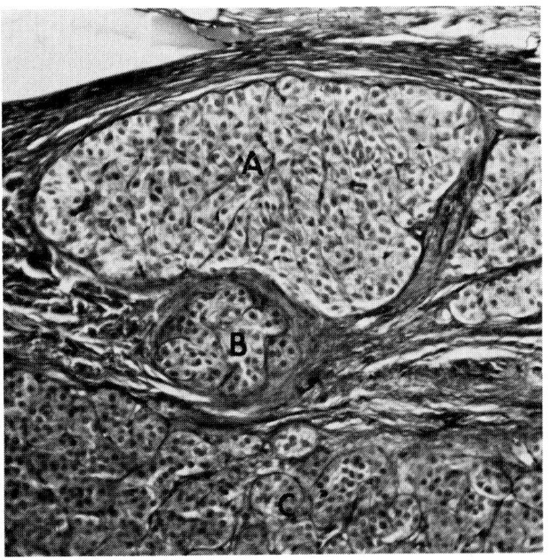

Fig. 15–22. *Adrenal gland, large ruminant. Clusters of "undifferentiated" cells (A) are located superficially in the capsule. The slightly deeper cells (B) closely resemble the cells of the zona glomerulosa (C). H & E. ×133. (From Dellmann, H.-D.: Veterinary Histology: An Outline Text-Atlas. Philadelphia, Lea & Febiger, 1971.)*

Cortex

The adrenal cortex is subdivided into three distinct zones (Fig. 15–21): (1) the outermost zona glomerulosa, followed by (2) the zona fasciculata and (3) the zona reticularis, which lies adjacent to the medulla.

The *zona glomerulosa* in ruminants (Fig. 15–23–1) is formed of irregular clusters and cords of cells. In the horse, donkey (Fig. 15–23–2), carnivores, and pig, this zone is called the zona arcuata because the cells are arranged in arcs, with their convexity directed toward the periphery.

In the horse and donkey, the cells are tall columnar cells (Fig. 15–23–2); they are much smaller in the other domestic mammals (Fig. 15–23–1). They have spherical or ovoid nuclei surrounded by a homogeneous cytoplasm. Their ultrastructural characteristics are those of steroid-secreting cells, i.e., abundant smooth ER, tubular-type mitochondria, little rER, a multilocular Golgi complex usually in the vicinity of the nucleus, and a few lipid droplets. Acidophilic granules of unknown significance are present in the bovine zona glomerulosa.

A *zona intermedia* occurs in the horse, dog, and cat, and to a lesser degree in the cow, sheep, and goat. It is a transitional zone of small undifferentiated cells between the zona glomerulosa and the zona fasciculata.

The *zona fasciculata* consists of radially arranged cords of cuboidal or columnar cells usually one cell-layer thick (Fig. 15–24). The foamy appearance of the cells (spongiocytes) is due to the presence of numerous vacuoles from the dissolution of lipid droplets during routine tissue processing. Furthermore, the cytoplasm contains a large Golgi complex, mitochondria with tubular cristae, lysosomes, and lipofuscin. The granular ER and smooth ER are more abundant than in the cells of the zona glomerulosa.

The *zona reticularis* is an irregular network of anastomosing cell cords (Fig. 15–25). The cells are polyhedral and have roughly the same morphologic features (Fig. 15–26) as the cells of the zona fasciculata. However, they contain fewer lipid droplets and more lipofuscin, and their nuclei are generally heterochromatic and often pyknotic.

Medulla

The endocrine cells of the adrenal medulla are modified postganglionic sympa-

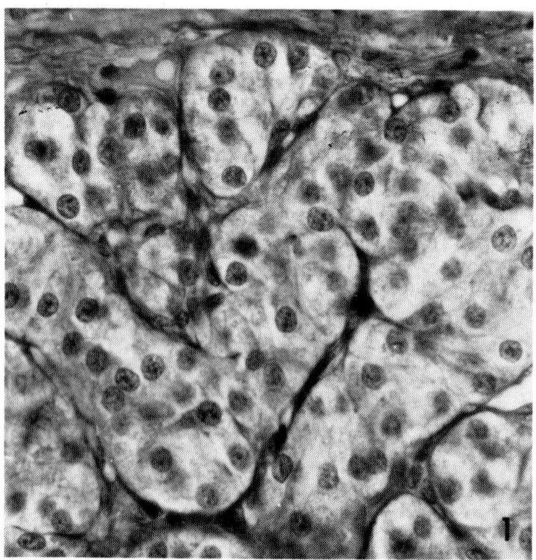

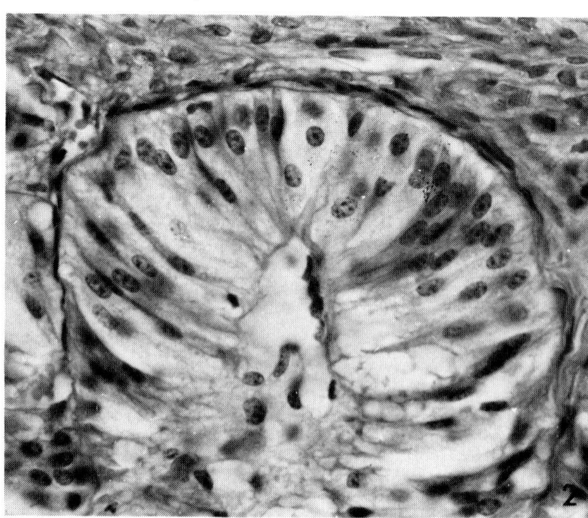

Fig. 15–23. *Adrenal gland, zona glomerulosa. 1, Large ruminant; 2, donkey. H & E. ×435. (From Dellmann, H.-D.: Veterinary Histology: An Outline Text-Atlas. Philadelphia, Lea & Febiger, 1971.)*

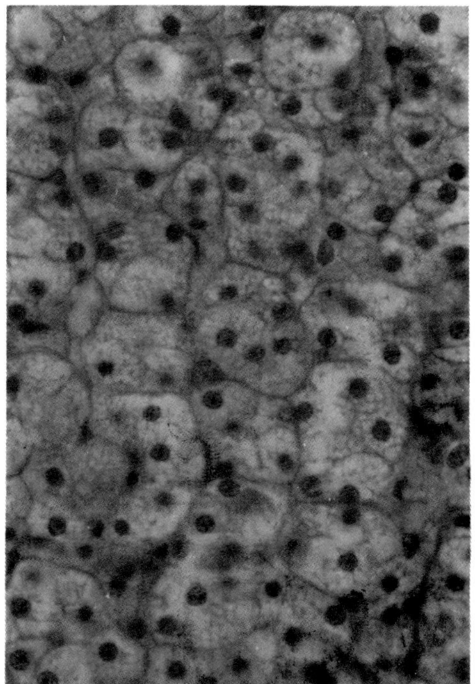

Fig. 15–24. *Adrenal gland, zona fasciculata, large ruminant. The dissolved lipid gives the cells a vacuolated appearance. H & E. ×435.*

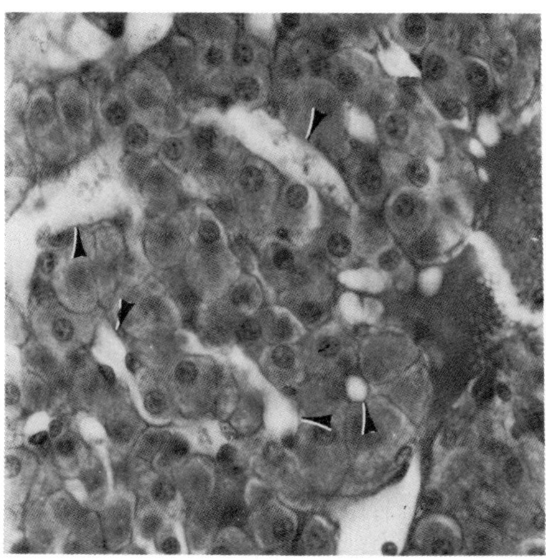

Fig. 15–25. *Adrenal gland, zona reticularis, large ruminant. Irregular cords of polyhedral cells are separated by wide sinusoidal capillaries (arrows). H & E. ×435. (From Dellmann, H.-D.: Veterinary Histology: An Outline Text-Atlas. Philadelphia, Lea & Febiger, 1971.)*

thetic nerve cells with an abundant preganglionic sympathetic innervation that regulates the secretory activity of these cells. When treated with fixatives containing chromium salts, the large cells stain dark brown. This chromaffin reaction is due to oxidation and polymerization of the catecholamines, epinephrine and norepinephrine, synthesized within these cells. Therefore, these cells are often referred to as chromaffin cells; this affinity is shared with cells of similar function and origin in other organs (paraganglia, enterochromaffin cells).

The *norepinephrine* cells contain a large spherical nucleus and argentaffin granules. Ultrastructurally, membrane-bounded, highly electron-dense granules are present together with numerous mitochondria, an abundant rER, and a Golgi complex.

The *epinephrine* cells are similar to the norepinephrine cells; however, their granules are less electron-dense and are distinguished from the norepinephrine granules by a small empty space located between the granule and the bounding membrane.

The chromaffin cells in the adrenal medulla are arranged in irregular cords and clusters, separated by a dense network of sinusoidal capillaries. Single sympathetic ganglion cells or clusters of cells may occur among the chromaffin cells (Fig. 15–27).

In the horse, cow, sheep, and pig, the medulla is subdivided into two distinct zones: an outer zone made up of large, intensely stained epinephrine cells, and an inner zone of clusters of small, polyhedral cells with low staining affinities that secrete norepinephrine (Fig. 15–27).

Blood, Lymph, and Nerve Supply

Numerous arteries penetrate the adrenal gland to give origin to a dense arteriolar network that extends into the sinusoidal capillaries of the cortex. This network in turn connects with the large sinusoidal capillaries of the medulla, which is also supplied by direct arterioles that course

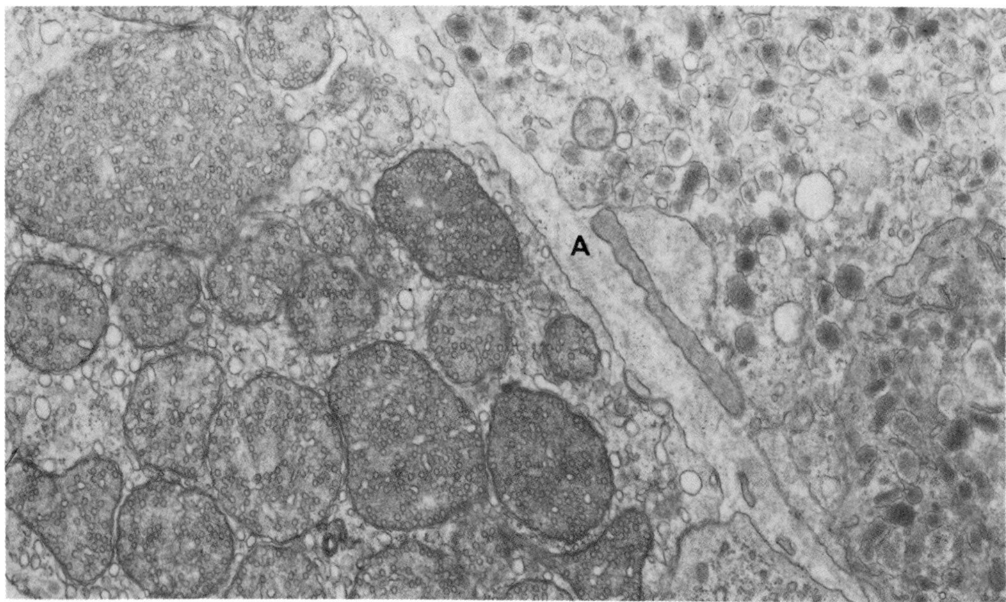

Fig. 15–26. *Electron micrograph of adrenal gland, rat. The cell in the zona reticularis contains numerous mitochondria with tubular cristae and cisternae of smooth ER and is separated by a basement membrane (A) from cells of the medulla with membrane-bounded dense granules, the sites of storage of catecholamines.* ×*16,322. (From Dellmann, H.-D.: Veterinary Histology: An Outline Text-Atlas. Philadelphia, Lea & Febiger, 1971.)*

through the cortex without branching. These vessels become constricted by epinephrine secretion, causing an increased blood supply to the cortex and thus increased secretion of cortical hormones. On the other hand, glucocorticoids that reach the medulla are believed to influence epinephrine synthesis, since they stimulate the methylation of norepinephrine to epinephrine.

Lymph vessels are found only in the capsule, trabeculae, and perivascular connective tissue.

The main nerve supply consists of exclusively preganglionic sympathetic nerve fibers that end in the medulla, forming a close network around the medullary cells. A small number of nerve fibers is present in the adrenal cortex, but nothing is known about their possible function.

Function

CORTEX. The zona glomerulosa produces mineralocorticoids, deoxycorticosterone, and aldosterone, which maintain the electrolyte level in extracellular body fluids by controlling the retention and the excretion of sodium and potassium by the kidney tubules. After adrenalectomy, release of sodium and retention of potassium in the distal tubules increase. Aldosterone secretion is regulated primarily by the renin-angiotensin system (see p. 278) and is largely independent of the adenohypophysis. Hypophysectomy alters neither the function nor the structure of the zona glomerulosa.

Both the zona fasciculata and the zona reticularis are involved in the production of the glucocorticoids (cortisol and corticosterone), which participate in protein, fat, and carbohydrate metabolism. The physiologic effects of corticosteroids include facilitation of protein catabolism and gluconeogenesis, release of fatty acids from adipose tissue, destruction of lymphocytes and concomitant release of gamma globulin, decrease of circulating eosinophils, and inhibition of cellular and fibrous proliferation (anti-inflammatory effect).

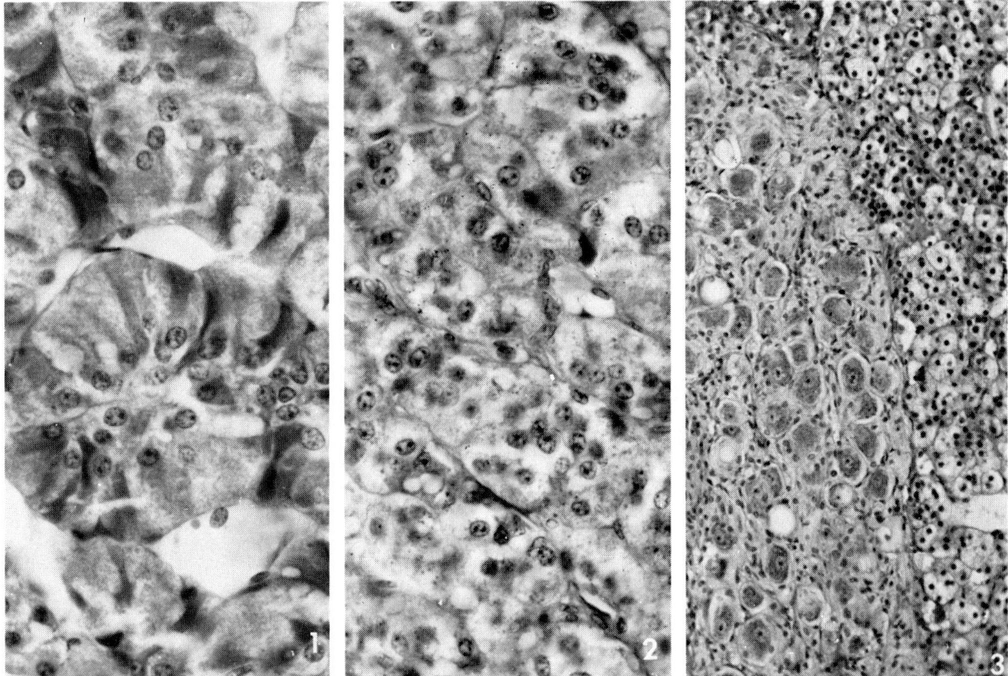

Fig. 15–27. *Adrenal gland, medulla, large ruminant (1). Tall cells are characteristic for the outer zone. H & E. ×435. (2) Small polyhedral cells; and (3) groups of nerve cells make up the inner zone. H & E. (2) ×435; (3) ×135.*

Extracts of normal adrenal cortex contain estrogens, androgens, and progesterone.

Glucocorticoid secretion is controlled by hypothalamic corticotropin-releasing hormone (CRH) and ACTH, whose release is influenced by a wide variety of internal and external factors, such as stressors, and by a negative feedback control by glucocorticoids. Hypophysectomy causes atrophy of the zonae fasciculata and reticularis and a decline in secretory activity.

MEDULLA. Secretion of the adrenal medullary hormones is under the direct control of acetylcholine released from preganglionic sympathetic nerve terminals. Norepinephrine and epinephrine have a wide variety of functions, too numerous to be enumerated here, with a primary role in homeostasis.

PANCREATIC ISLETS

The endocrine cells of the pancreas are clustered in pancreatic islets. These are variously shaped structures, generally spherical or oval, intermingled with the exocrine pancreatic tissue. The islet cells are arranged in irregular anastomosing cords composed of five different cell types: A(α), B(β), C, D(δ), and F cells.

The A cells contain granules insoluble in alcohol that stain brilliant red with Masson's trichrome method and Gomori's aldehyde-fuchsin. They are also argyrophilic. At the electron microscopic level, these granules are membrane-bounded and have a dark, electron-dense center surrounded by a lighter peripheral zone. The granules, little granular ER, a small Golgi complex, and a few long slender mitochondria are concentrated at the vascular pole of the cell. The nucleus is generally deeply indented or lobulated. The A cells represent approximately 5 to 30% of the islet population; in the pig, their number decreases from about 50% in the newborn animal to between 8 and 20% in the adult. The pancreatic islets of the dog's uncinate

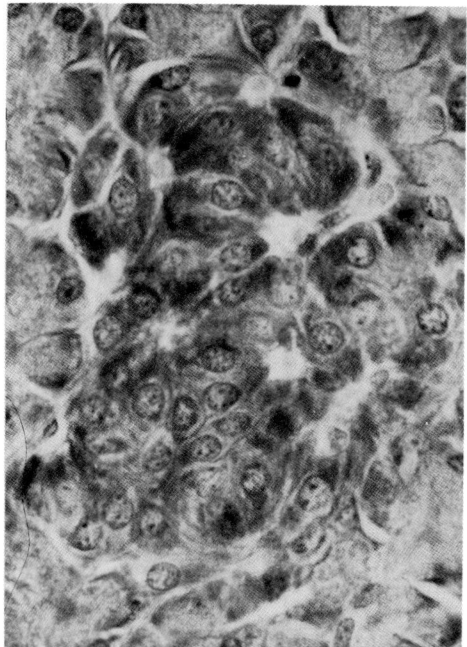

Fig. 15–28. *Pancreatic islet, dog. The majority of the cells are B cells and contain granules stained deep purple. Aldehyde-fuchsin. ×350.*

process are devoid of A cells. These cells are often located in the core of the islets in the horse; in cattle they tend to be arranged at the periphery.

B cells have indistinct boundaries, are polyangular, and are nonargyrophilic. They are by far the most numerous cells in the pancreatic islets and contain granules soluble in alcohol that stain dark orange with Mallory's trichrome and deep purple with Gomori's aldehyde-fuchsin stain (Fig. 15–28). In some species the B-cell granules are only slightly different in size and electron density from the A-cell granules. In the dog (and some other species) they contain crystalloid structures of variable shapes (crystalline insulin) embedded in a pale matrix. The ER of B cells is less abundant than that of A cells, the Golgi complex is more extensive, and the mitochondria are larger. Generally, the nucleus is spherical and smaller than that of A cells. B cells make up approximately 60 to 80% of the total islet cell population (up to 98% in sheep). They predominate in the periphery of the pancreatic islets of the horse and in the center of the islets in cattle.

C cells are nongranulated or sparsely granulated cells that are immature precursor cells to the other types of islet cells. They do not give any positive light-microscopic staining reaction and can be identified unequivocally only with the EM.

D cells are of relatively rare occurrence (approximately 5% in the dog) and are located mainly in the periphery of the islets. They synthesize somatostatin which apparently has an inhibitory action on the secretion of insulin and glucagon.

In addition, there occurs a heterogeneous population of small-granulated cells, considered precursors to a variety of cells that produce various gastroentero-pancreatic hormones (e.g., pancreatic polypeptide, vasoactive intestinal polypeptide and cholecystokinin-pancreozymin [CCK]). These cells, referred to as F cells in the dog, produce pancreatic polypeptide that stimulates gastric secretion and inhibits intestinal motility and bile secretion.

At this point, the letter designation of the pancreatic islet cells, with the exception of A and B cells, is far from being generally accepted; it is preferable to name these cells according to the hormones that they produce.

Blood, Lymph, and Nerve Supply

The pancreatic islets are supplied by a dense capillary network. Lymph vessels are found only around the pancreatic islets. Sympathetic nerve fibers from the celiac plexus reach the pancreatic islets with the blood vessels. Parasympathetic fibers of vagal origin penetrate the islets independently of the blood supply and occasionally terminate in contact with the islet cells. Axons in juxtaposition to islet cells are referred to as neuroinsular complexes. The functional significance of the innervation of the pancreatic islets has not been elucidated. In the dog and cat, lamellar corpuscles are observed regularly.

Function

Pancreatectomy results in diabetes mellitus, a severe disturbance of carbohydrate metabolism, characterized by an increased blood glucose level (hyperglycemia) and excess sugar in the urine (glycosuria). Insulin, the hormone produced by the B cells, reduces the blood sugar level (and subsequently the urine sugar level) by facilitating the storage of glycogen in the liver and muscle and converting it into fat for storage as adipose tissue.

In the absence of insulin, the blood sugar level rises, with a concurrent depletion of the glycogen stores in the liver and other tissues. This condition can be produced experimentally by the administration of alloxan, which almost selectively destroys the B cells. An excess of insulin may result in a rapid decrease of the blood sugar level and subsequent convulsions and death, unless the effect is counteracted by the administration of sugar.

The A cells of the pancreatic islets produce glucagon, which counteracts the effect of insulin by breaking down liver glycogen and increasing the blood glucose level. A selective destruction of the A cells is obtained by the administration of cobalt chloride.

REFERENCES

Allen, M.B., and Mahesh, V.B. (eds): The Pituitary. A Current Review. New York, Academic Press, 1977.

Bhatnagar, A.S. (ed): The Anterior Pituitary Gland. New York, Raven Press, 1983.

Gale, T.F.: An electron microscopic study of the pars distalis of the dog adenohypophysis. Z Anat Entwicklungsgesch *137*:188, 1972.

Ganong, W.F., and Martini, L. (eds): Frontiers in Neuroendocrinology 1973. New York, Oxford University Press, 1973.

Ganong, W.F., and Martini, L. (eds.): Frontiers in Neuroendocrinology. Vol. V. New York, Raven Press, 1978.

Ganong, W.F., and Martini, L. (eds.): Frontiers in Neuroendocrinology. Vol. VII. New York, Raven Press, 1982.

Ganong, W.F., and Martini, L. (eds.): Frontiers in Neuroendocrinology. Vol. 9. New York, Raven Press, 1986.

Harris, G.W., and Donovan, B.T. (eds.): The Pituitary Gland. Vol. I, Anterior Pituitary; Vol. II, Anterior Pituitary; Vol. III, Pars Intermedia and Neurohypophysis. Berkeley, University of California Press, 1966.

Holmes, R.L., and Ball, J.N.: The Pituitary Gland. A Comparative Account. New York, Cambridge University Press, 1974.

James, V.H.T. (ed.): The Adrenal Gland. New York, Raven Press, 1979.

Jeffcoate, S.L., and Hutchinson, J.S.M. (eds.): The Endocrine Hypothalamus. New York, Academic Press, 1978.

Knigge, K.M., Scott, D.E., Weindl, A. (eds.): Brain Endocrine Interaction. Median Eminence; Structure and Function. Basel, S. Karger, 1971.

Martini, L., and Ganong, W.F. (eds.): Frontiers in Neuroendocrinology 1971. New York, Oxford University Press, 1971.

Martini, L., and Ganong, W.F. (eds.): Frontiers in Neuroendocrinology. Vol. IV. New York, Raven Press, 1976.

Martini, L., and Ganong, W.F. (eds.): Frontiers in Neuroendocrinology. Vol. VI. New York, Raven Press, 1980.

Martini, L., and Ganong, W.F. (eds.): Frontiers in Neuroendocrinology. Vol. VIII. New York, Raven Press, 1984.

Motta, P.M. (ed.): Ultrastructure of Endocrine Cells and Tissues. Boston, Nijhoff, 1984.

Müller, E.E., and MacLeod, R.M. (eds.): Neuroendocrine Perspectives. Amsterdam, Elsevier, 1982.

Nunez, E.A., and Gershon, M.D.: Cytophysiology of thyroid parafollicular cells. Int Rev Cytol *52*:1, 1978.

Nussdorfer, G.G., Mazzocchi, G., and Meneghelli, V.: Cytophysiology of the adrenal zona fasciculata. Int Rev Cytol *55*:291, 1978.

Reichlin, S., Baldessarini, R.J., and Martin, J.B. (eds.): The Hypothalamus. New York, Raven Press, 1978.

Relkin, R. (ed.): The Pineal Gland. New York, Elsevier, 1983.

Van Blerkom, J., and Motta, P.M. (eds.): Ultrastructure of Reproduction. Boston, Nighoff, 1984.

Werner, S.C., and Ingbar, S.H. (eds.): The Thyroid: A Fundamental and Clinical Text. Hagerstown, Harper and Row, 1978.

16

Integument

M. LOIS CALHOUN
AL W. STINSON

The skin, or integument, is composed of the epidermis, dermis (corium), hair follicles, sweat and sebaceous glands, the digital organs (hoof, claw), and a wide variety of specialized glandular structures (Fig. 16–1). It is one of the largest organs in the body.

Functionally, it protects against mechanical injuries, noxious agents, and irradiation; secretes sweat and sebum; acts as a sensory organ; aids in temperature regulation; elaborates vitamin D, so vital for phosphorus and calcium metabolism; and reflects the condition of the body. Although absorption is not a primary function of stratified squamous epithelium, it is well established that many substances can cross the epidermal barrier. Because disease conditions are reflected in the skin, histologic examination is an integral part of diagnostic procedures.

Generally, the skin is thickest over the dorsal surface of the body and on the lateral surfaces of the limbs. It is thinnest on the ventral side of the body and medial surfaces of the limbs. There are area, sex, breed, and species differences. Of the skin measurements available for the domestic animal species (horse, ox, sheep, goat, pig, dog, and cat), the thinnest areas range from 0.4 mm (cat) to 2.4 mm (Holstein cow), and the thickest from 1.9 mm (cat) to 10.7 mm (stallion).

A subcutaneous or hypodermal layer of loose and adipose connective tissue binds the dermis to the underlying fascia and skeletal muscles. Occasionally, some of the muscle fibers invade the dermis.

DEVELOPMENT

Both ectoderm and mesoderm give rise to the integumentary system. The epithelial covering and its derivatives, the hair follicles, sweat and sebaceous glands, and nervous tissues, originate from ectoderm (Fig. 16–2). The connective tissue and vascular elements are contributed by mesoderm.

LAYERS OF THE SKIN

Epidermis

The epidermis, the outermost layer of the skin, is a keratinized stratified squamous epithelium (Fig. 16–3). At least four layers can be identified, the *stratum basale, stratum spinosum, stratum granulosum,* and *stratum corneum.* In such areas as the

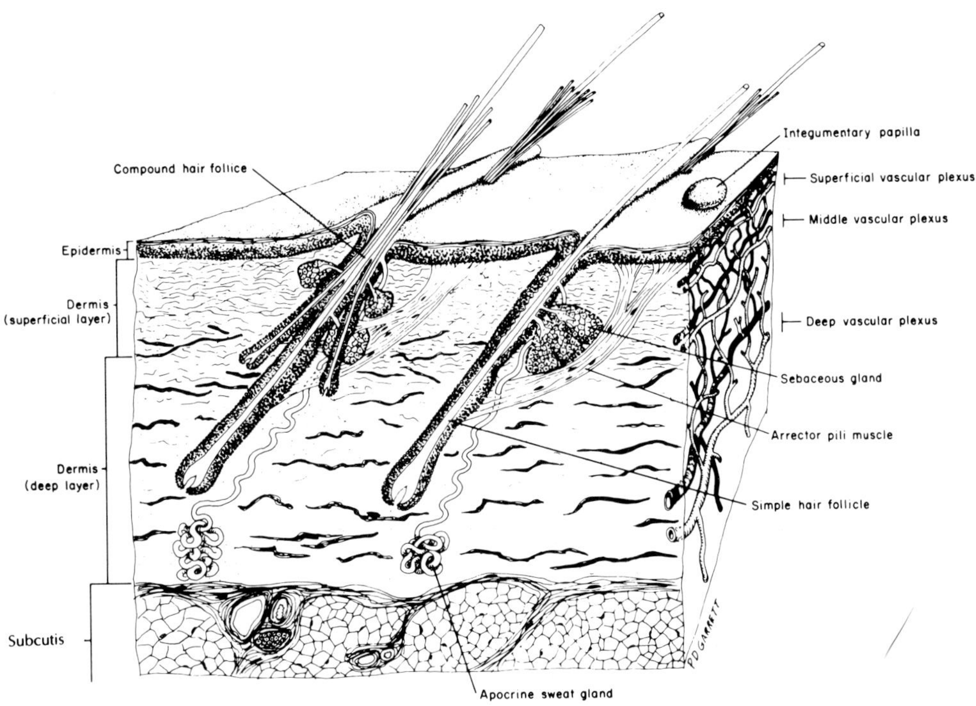

Fig. 16–1. *Schematic drawing of skin. For the sake of simplification, the vascular supply is shown on only one face.*

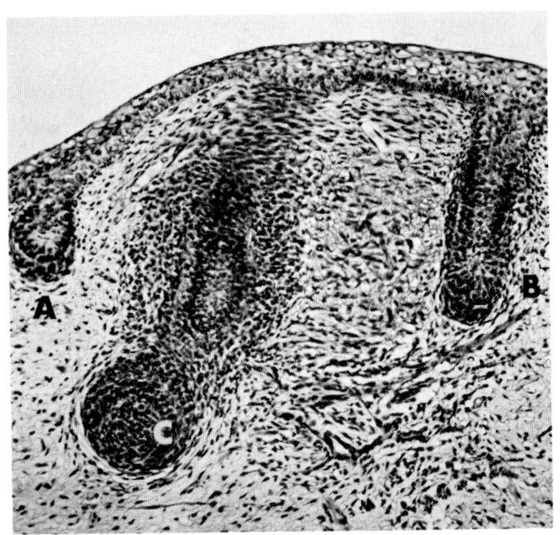

Fig. 16–2. *Developing hair follicles, pig. Epithelial bud (A); later stage of hair growth (B); hair papilla (C). H & E. ×75. (From Fowler, E.H., and Calhoun, M.L.: The microscopic anatomy of developing fetal pig skin. Am J Vet Res 25:156, 1964.)*

planum nasale and foot pads, a lighter stained *stratum lucidum* is interposed between the stratum granulosum and the stratum corneum. The surface cells from the stratum corneum become loose and detach, forming a layer that is called the *stratum disjunctum* (Fig. 16–3).

The epidermal surface is smooth in some areas, but in others it has ridges or folds that reflect the contour of the underlying superficial dermal layer (Fig. 16–3–1).

The thickness of the epidermis varies with its location. In regions where there is a heavy protective coat of hair, the epidermis is thin (Fig. 16–3–1), but in nonhairy skin, such as that of the mucocutaneous junctions, the epidermis is thicker (Fig. 16–3–2). On the foot pads, where there is considerable abrasive action, the stratum corneum is considerably thickened (Fig. 16–3–3). For more details, see Chapter 2.

There are four distinct cell types that occur in the epidermis. The most numerous type is the *keratinocyte,* which is respon-

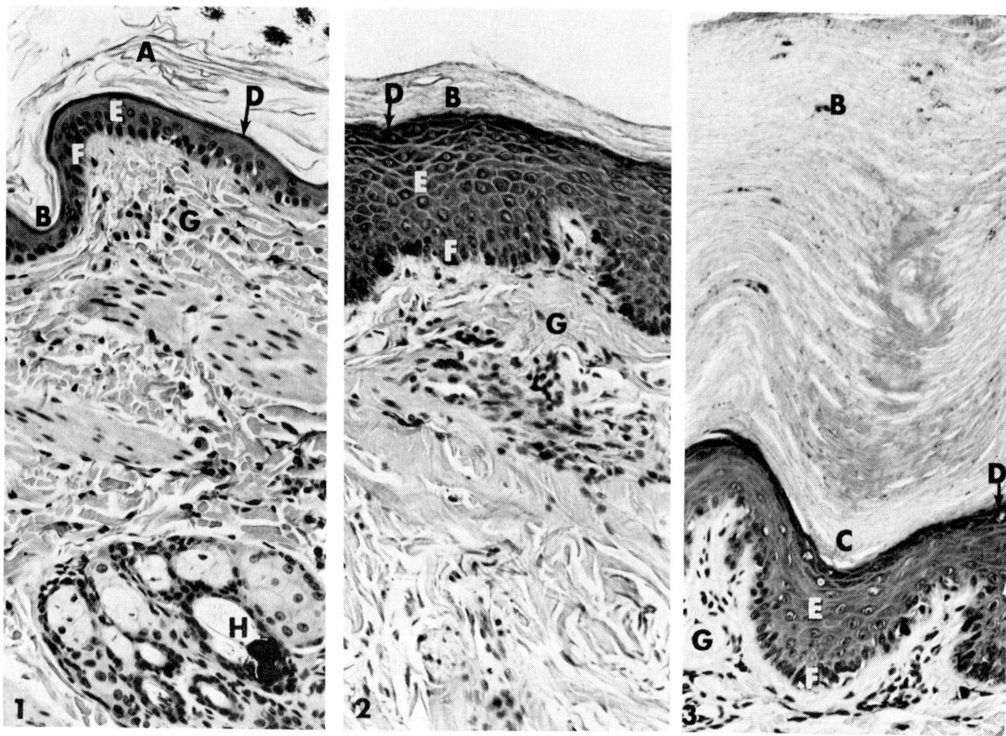

Fig. 16–3. *Epidermis, cat. 1, Hairy skin with thin epidermis, lumbar region. 2, Nonhairy skin with thicker epidermis, nose. 3, Footpad with thick stratum corneum. Stratum disjunctum (A); stratum corneum (B); stratum lucidum (C); stratum granulosum (D); stratum spinosum (E); stratum basale (F); superficial layer of the dermis (G); hair follicle (H). H & E. ×200.*

sible for the production of keratin, an insoluble protein that fills the cells of the stratum corneum. Three stages of activity of this cell type are recognized: (1) a proliferative phase in which the cells located just above the basal lamina undergo mitotic division; (2) a maturation phase during which the cells migrate toward the surface and accumulate *keratin filaments* (tonofilaments) and irregular, nonmembrane-bound *keratinohyaline granules,* which increase in number as the cells reach the upper surface of the epithelium; and (3) an inactive phase during which the nuclei disappear and the keratin filaments and keratohyaline granules are compacted into the flattened, squamous cells. *Melanocytes* are cells of neural crest origin that migrate into the epidermis during the embryonic period. They are located among the cells of the stratum basale and send dendritic processes among the keratinocytes of the stratum spinosum (Fig. 16–4). The melanin granules produced by the melanocytes give rise to skin and hair color. The black or dark brown pigment is generally called eumelanin, and the light brown, orange and yellow varieties, phaeomelanin. The melanin granules are transferred from the melanocyte to the keratinocyte by cytocrine secretion. During this process the keratinocytes phagocytize the terminal portion of the melanocyte processes containing the melanin granules. Eventually the granules migrate within the keratinocyte to form caplike aggregates just above the nucleus (Fig. 16–5). As the keratinocytes migrate to the surface, the number of granules decreases, possibly as a result of lysosomal degradation. The lack of melanin in the epidermis of some animals may be due to an absence of melanocytes, as in albinos, or

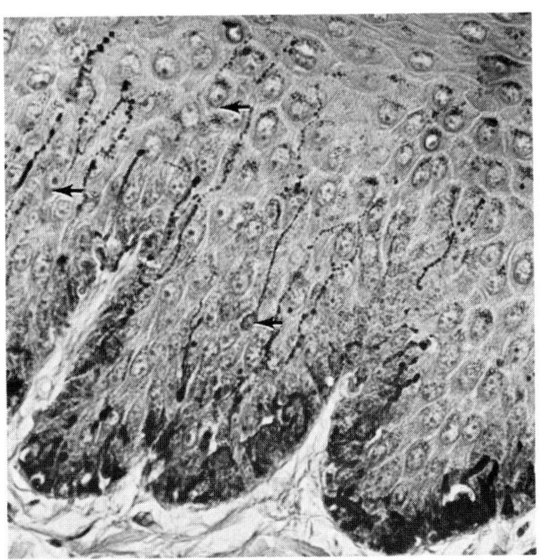

Fig. 16–4. *Melanocytes with dendritic processes (arrows), lip, horse. H.& E. ×330. (From Talukdar, A.H., Calhoun, M.L., and Stinson, A.W.: Microscopic anatomy of the skin of the horse. Am J Vet Res 33:2365, 1972.)*

to the inability of the melanocytes to produce melanin, as in the white spots of some animals. *Langerhans cells* (agranular dendritic cells) are bone marrow–derived immune cells of the epidermis. They represent the most peripheral outpost of the immune system and function as a link between the extracutaneous environment

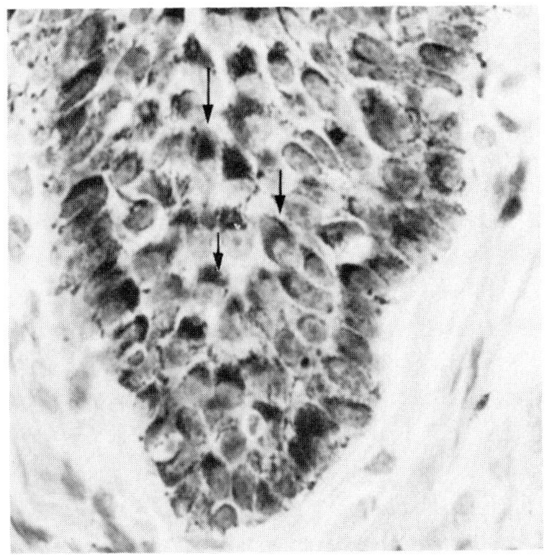

Fig. 16–5. *Aggregates of melanin granules shielding the epidermal cells (arrows), planum nasale, dog. H & E. ×630.*

and the organism. In light microscopy, they appear as "clear" cells in the stratum basale and stratum spinosum. At the fine-structural level, the cytoplasm is relatively electron-lucent and contains no tonofilaments, desmosomes, or melanin granules; however, the presence of racket-shaped granules (Birbeck granules) is the distinguishing characteristic of this cell type. *Tactile epithelioid cells* (Merkel cells) occur in the epidermis of the *tactile elevations* or *dome corpuscles* of many species (most widely studied in the cat). These areas consist of a thickened epidermis with a row of tactile epithelioid cells enclosing the terminal ends of nerve fibers that penetrate the basement membrane (see Fig. 6–24).

The junction between the epidermis and dermis is generally smooth in skin protected by a dense coat of hair (Fig. 16–3–1). In areas subjected to mechanical stress, such as the foot pads and lips, the epidermal projections interdigitate with dermal papillae and ridges (Fig. 16–4).

Dermis

The dermis (corium) is a feltwork of collagen, elastic, and reticular connective tissue fibers. Hair follicles, sweat and sebaceous glands, blood and lymph vessels, and nerves are embedded at various levels throughout the dermis.

The dermis is generally divided into a superficial (papillary) layer that blends into a deep (reticular) layer without a clear line of demarcation (Fig. 16–6). The *superficial layer* is in contact with the epidermis and conforms to the contour of the stratum basale. It is composed of a network of fine collagen, reticular, and elastic fibers, fibrocytes, macrophages, plasma cells, and mast cells. Occasionally, chromatophores and fat cells may be present. The superficial layer is wider in horse (Fig. 16–6) and cattle skin than in that of carnivores (Fig. 16–7) and encompasses the hair follicles and adjacent sweat glands. The *deep layer* of the dermis is much more coarse and dense than the

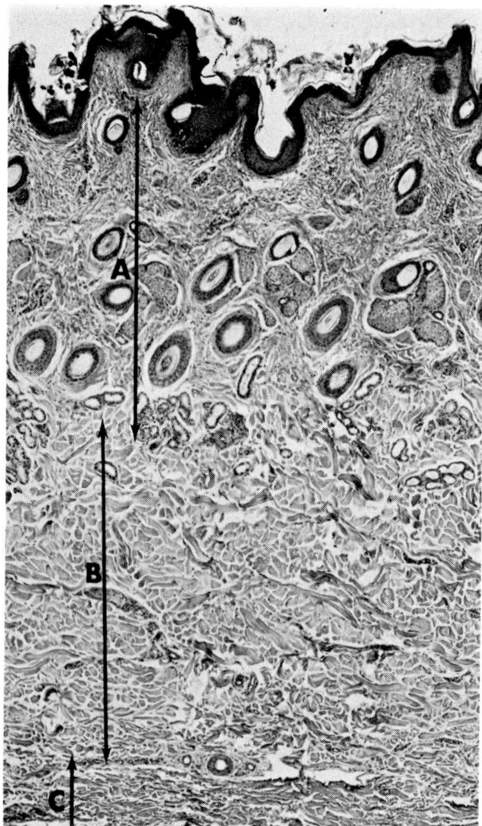

Fig. 16–6. *Layers of the dermis characteristic of the horse, lateral neck. Superficial layer (A); deep layer (B); deeper dense parallel collagen layer (C). H & E. ×40. (From Talukdar, A.H., Calhoun, M.L., and Stinson, A.W.: Microscopic anatomy of the skin of the horse. Am J Vet Res 33:2365, 1972.)*

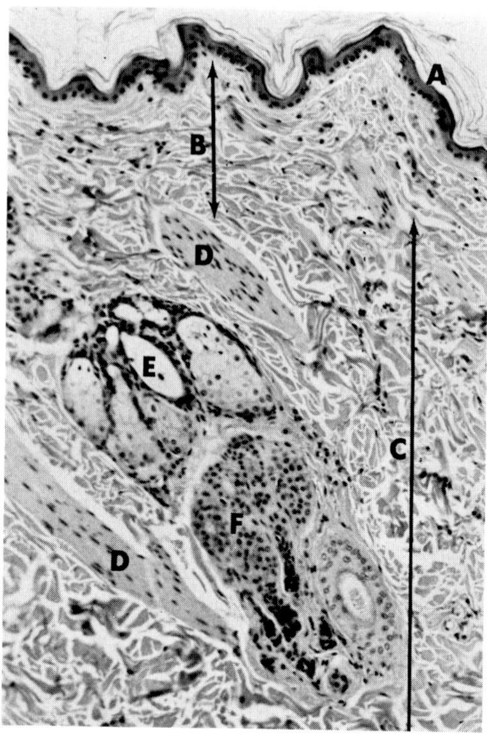

Fig. 16–7. *Skin of lumbar region, cat. Epidermis (A); superficial layer of dermis (B); deep layer of dermis (C); arrector muscle (D); hair follicle surrounded by sebaceous glands (E); cluster of sweat glands (F). H & E. ×120.*

superficial layer and contains large bundles of collagen fibers aligned parallel to the surface. In some regions of horse skin, a third layer is present beneath the deep layer. In the lateral neck region, this additional layer may consist of very dense, parallel collagen fiber bundles, while in the gluteal and sacral regions, collagen bundles are oriented perpendicularly. There are fewer connective tissue cells in the deep layer than in the superficial layer.

Smooth muscle fibers may be present in the dermis in such specialized areas as the scrotum, teat, and penis. Skeletal muscle fibers of the cutaneous muscle (panniculus carnosus) penetrate the dermis and allow voluntary movement of the skin. There may also be skeletal muscle fibers associated with the large sinus hairs of the facial region.

Subcutis

The subcutis (tela subcutanea) is a layer of connective tissue that anchors the dermis to the underlying muscle or bone. It consists of a loose arrangement of collagen and elastic fibers that allows the skin flexibility and free movement over the underlying structures. Adipose tissue is also present in this layer and may take the form of small clusters of cells or large masses that make up a cushion or pad of fat, called the *panniculus adiposus* (Fig. 16–8). Pork bacon and fatback are derived from the panniculus adiposus, and large fat deposits in the hypodermis are characteristic of the foot

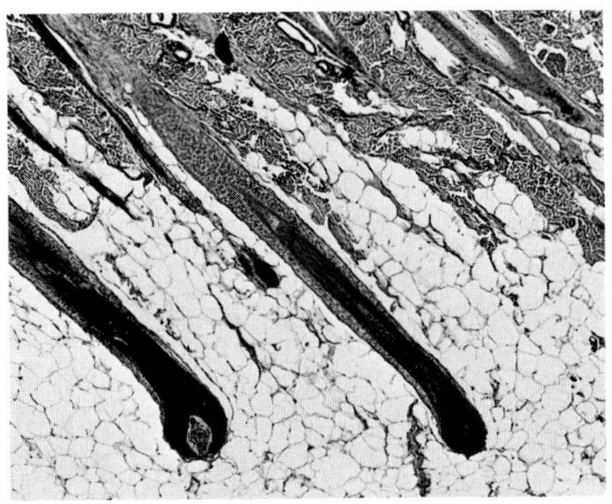

Fig. 16–8. *Subcutis with two large primary hair follicles extending into the subcutaneous fat (panniculus adiposus), dog. H & E. ×30.*

pads and digital cushions, where they serve as shock absorbers.

SKIN APPENDAGES

Hair

In domestic animals, hair covers the entire body with the exception of the foot pads, hoofs, glans penis, mucocutaneous junctions, and the teats of some species. Hair is a flexible, keratinized structure produced by a hair follicle.

The distal or free part of the hair above the surface of the skin is the hair *shaft.* The part within the follicle is the hair *root,* which has a terminal, hollow knob, the hair *bulb,* attached to a dermal papilla. The hair shaft is composed of three layers: an outermost *cuticle,* a *cortex* of densely packed keratinized cells and a *medulla* of loose cuboidal or flattened cells (Fig. 16–9). The cuticle is formed by a single layer of flat keratinized cells whose free edges, which overlap like shingles on a roof, are directed toward the distal end of the shaft. The cortex consists of a layer of dense, compact, keratinized cells with their long axes parallel to the hair shaft. Nuclear remnants and pigment granules are present within the cells. Desmosomes hold the cells firmly together. Near the bulb the cells are shorter, more oval, and contain spherical nuclei. The medulla forms the center of the hair and is loosely filled with cuboidal or flattened cells (Fig. 16–9). In the root, the medulla is solid; in the shaft, air-filled spaces occur among the cells. The pattern of the surface of the cuticular cells, together with the cellular arrangement of the medulla, is characteristic for each species (Fig. 16–10) and is used for medicolegal purposes.

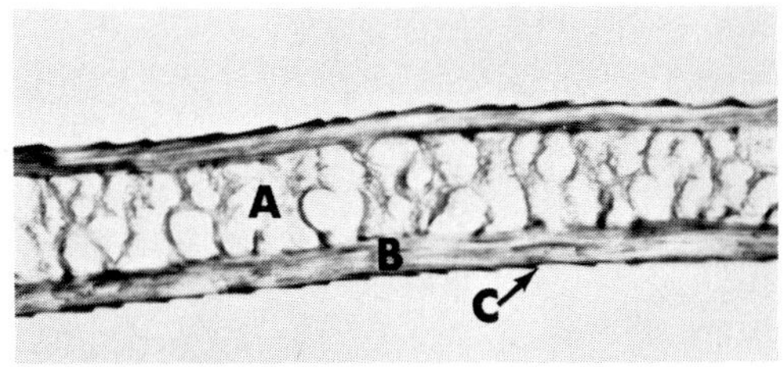

Fig. 16–9. *Hair, sheep. Medulla (A); cortex (B); cuticle (C). H & E. ×300. (From Kozlowski, G.P.: The Microscopic Anatomy of the Integument of Sheep. M.S. thesis, Michigan State University, East Lansing, Mich., 1966.)*

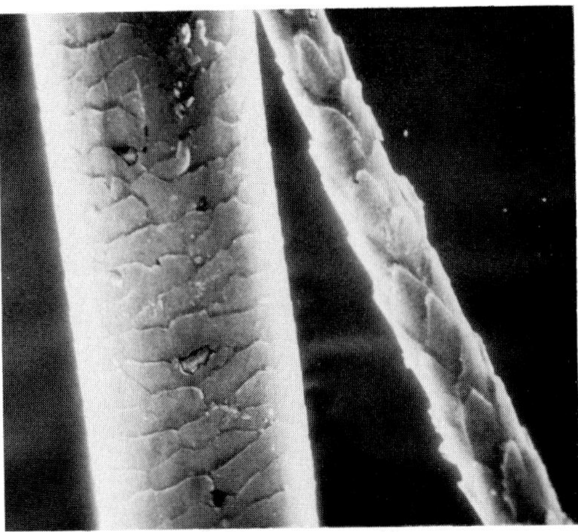

Fig. 16–10. *Scanning electron micrograph of primary and secondary hairs, cat. ×500.*

The hair or fleece of sheep is referred to as fibers. There are three types of fibers: (1) wool fibers, tightly crimped fibers of small diameter lacking a medulla; (2) kemp fibers, coarse and with a characteristic medulla; and (3) coarse fibers of intermediate size relative to wool and kemp fibers. The various breeds of sheep produce wools with different characteristics, and these various

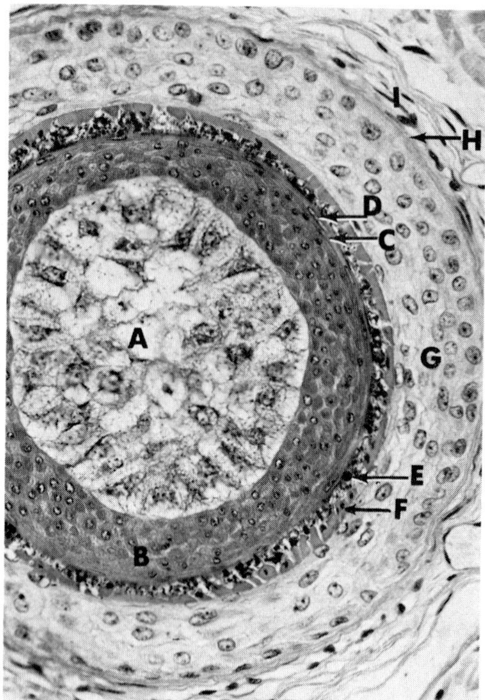

Fig. 16–11. *Hair follicle, goat. Medulla (A); cortex (B); cuticle of hair (C); cuticle of the internal root sheath (D); granular epithelial layer of the internal root sheath (E); pale epithelial layer of the internal root sheath (F); external root sheath (G) glassy membrane (H); connective tissue sheath (I). H & E. ×170. (From Sar, M., and Calhoun, M.L.: The microscopic anatomy of the integument of the common American goat. Am J Vet Res 27:444, 1966.)*

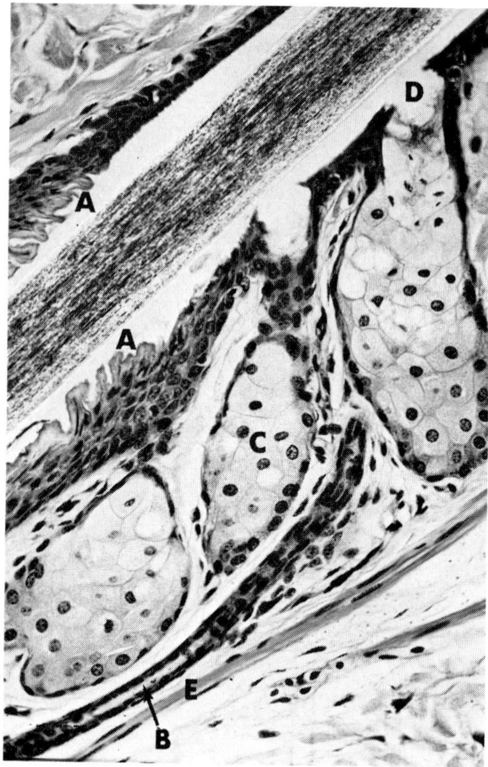

Fig. 16–12. *Follicular folds just below the openings of the sebaceous glands, forehead, cow. Follicular folds (A); sweat duct (B); sebaceous gland (C); opening of sebaceous gland into the hair follicle (D); arrector muscle (E). H & E. ×165.*

kinds of fleece are utilized for different purposes.

Hair Follicles

The hair follicle is formed by growth of the ectoderm into the underlying mesoderm of the embryo (Fig. 16–2). The epithelial downgrowth becomes canalized and the surrounding cells differentiate into several layers or sheaths that surround the hair root. The follicle is embedded in the dermis, usually at an angle, and the bulb may extend as deep as the subcutis (Fig. 16–8). The innermost layer, next to the hair root, is the internal epithelial root sheath (Fig. 16–11). It is composed of the inner cuticle, middle granular epithelial, and outer pale epithelial layers. The cuticle of the internal root sheath is formed by overlapping keratinized cells similar to those of the cuticle of the hair, except that the free edges are oriented in the opposite direction or toward the hair bulb. This arrangement results in a solid implantation of the hair root in the hair follicle. The granular epithelial layer is composed of one to three layers of keratinized cells rich in trichohyaline granules. The pale epithelial layer is the outermost layer of the internal root sheath and is composed of a single layer of keratinized cells. Just below the opening of the sebaceous glands, the internal root sheath of the large follicles becomes corrugated, forming several circular or follicular folds (Fig. 16–12). The sheath then becomes thinner and the cells fuse, disintegrate, and become part of the

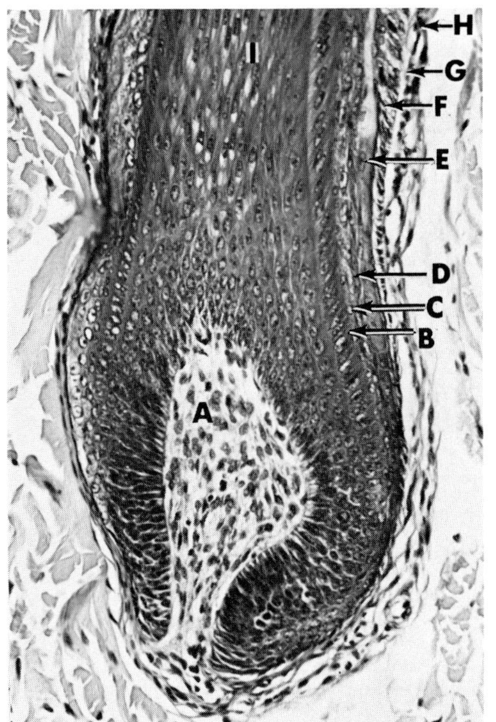

Fig. 16–13. *Hair bulb, lateral carpal region, boar. Papilla (A); hair cuticle (B); inner sheath cuticle (C); granular epithelial layer (D); pale epithelial layer (E); external root sheath (F); glassy membrane (G); connective tissue of the hair follicle (H); cortex (I). H & E. ×200.*

sebum. The outer epithelial root sheath is composed of several layers of cells similar to those of the stratum spinosum in the epidermis, with which it is continuous in the upper portion of the follicle. The entire epithelial sheath is enclosed by a dermal sheath composed of inner and outer layers of collagen fibers.

The cells covering the dermal papillae and composing most of the hair bulb are the *hair matrix cells.* They are comparable to germinative cells of regular epidermis and give rise to the cells that keratinize to form the hair (Fig. 16–13). There are several important differences in the potency of these cells, however. They differ from the keratinocytes of surface epidermis with respect to the type of keratin produced. Surface keratinocytes produce during the course of their development a "soft" form of keratin that passes through a keratohyaline phase. The cells containing "soft" keratin have a high lipid content and a low sulfur content, and they desquamate when they reach the surface. Conversely, the matrix cells of the hair follicle produce a "hard" keratin that is characteristic of hair, horn, and feather. The keratinocytes do not go through a keratohyaline phase, do not desquamate, and have a low lipid content and a high sulfur content. In the surface epidermis, the process of keratinization is continuous because of the uninterrupted production of new keratinocytes, but in the hair follicle, the matrix cells undergo periods of quiescence in which no mitotic activity occurs. When the matrix cell proliferation is reinstituted, a new hair is formed. This cyclic activity of the hair bulb allows for the seasonal change in the hair coat of domestic animals.

The period during which the cells of the hair bulb are mitotically active is called *anagen.* Following this growth phase, the hair follicles go through a regressive stage, referred to as *catagen.* During this period, cellular proliferation slowly decreases and finally ceases altogether, until all that remains of the bulb is a flimsy, disorganized column of cells, or club hair. The hair follicle then enters a resting or quiescent phase known as *telogen.* The club hair remains anchored by keratogenous rootlets, and the dermal papilla is reduced to a ball of cells located below the capsule of the germ cells of the bulb.

Following the resting phase, mitotic activity and keratinization start again and a new hair is formed. As the new hair grows, the root of the old hair gradually moves toward the surface, where it is eventually shed (Fig. 16–14). This intermittent mitotic activity and keratinization of the hair matrix cells constitutes the hair cycle and may be controlled by several factors, among which are length of daily periods of light, ambient temperature, and hormones, particularly estrogen, testosterone, adrenal steroids, and the thyroid hormone.

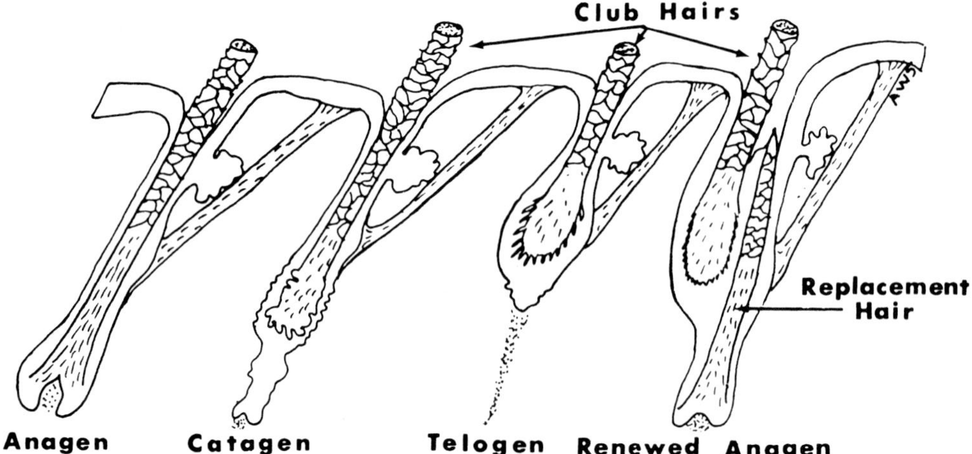

Fig. 16–14. *The three main stages of hair follicle growth and replacement.*

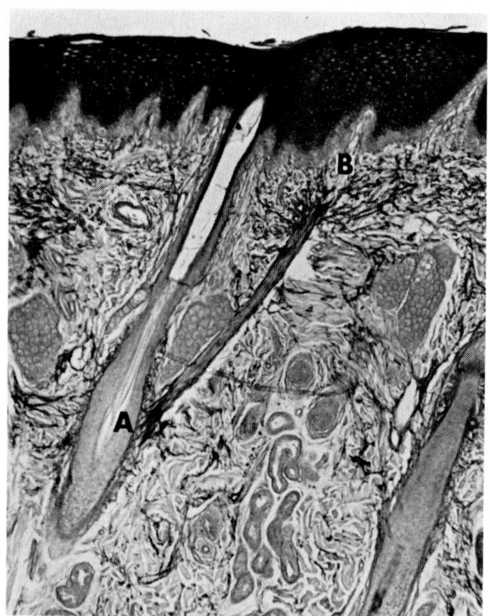

Fig. 16–15. *Hair follicle complex, mare. The elastic connective tissue fibers of the arrector muscle are attached to the hair follicle (A) and to the superficial dermis (B). Aldehyde fuchsin. ×48. (From Talukdar, A.H., Calhoun, M.L., and Stinson, A.W.: Microscopic anatomy of the skin of the horse. Am J Vet Res 33:2365, 1972.)*

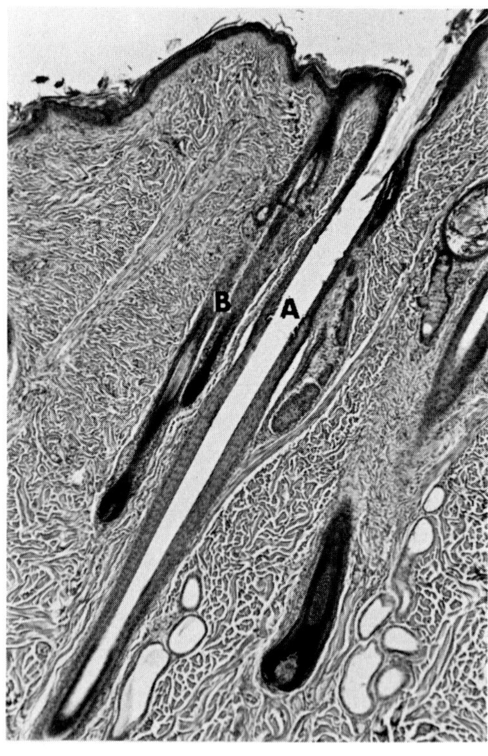

Fig. 16–16. *Hair follicles, primary (A) and secondary (B), flank, goat. H & E. ×40.*

Hair pigment is derived from the epidermal melanocytes located over the dermal papillae. Gray hair results from the inability of melanocytes in the hair bulb to produce tyrosinase.

The epidermal portion of the follicle is separated from the dermis by a thickened basal lamina associated with reticular fibers. Because of its shiny appearance, this is called the glassy membrane (Fig. 16–11). The connective tissue sheath is a feltwork of circular and longitudinal collagen and elastic fibers richly supplied with blood vessels and nerves, especially in the dermal papillae.

Bundles of smooth muscle cells form the arrector muscle (arrector pili), which inserts in the connective tissue sheath of the hair follicle and extends toward the epidermis, where it attaches to the superficial layer of the dermis (Fig. 16–15). These muscles are anchored by elastic fibers at their insertions and attachments and are innervated by autonomic nerve fibers. The arrector muscles are especially well developed along the back of the dog, where they cause the hair to "bristle" when they contract. The contraction of the arrector muscles during cold weather elevates the hairs, allowing minute air pockets to form in the coat. This dead-air space provides significant insulation that helps to maintain internal body temperature.

Hair follicles are classified into several types. A primary hair follicle is one of large diameter, is rooted deep in the dermis, and is usually associated with sebaceous and sweat glands and an arrector muscle (Fig. 16–16). The hair that emerges from such a follicle is called a *primary hair.* A secondary follicle is smaller in diameter than a primary follicle, and the root is near the surface. It may have a sebaceous gland but lacks a sweat gland and an arrector muscle. Hairs from these follicles are *secondary,* or underhairs. Those follicles with only one hair emerging to the surface are called *single* or *simple follicles.*

Compound follicles are composed of clusters of several hair follicles located in the dermis. At the level of the sebaceous gland opening, the follicles fuse and the various hairs emerge through one external follicular orifice (Fig. 16–1). Compound hair follicles usually have one primary hair follicle and several secondary hair follicles.

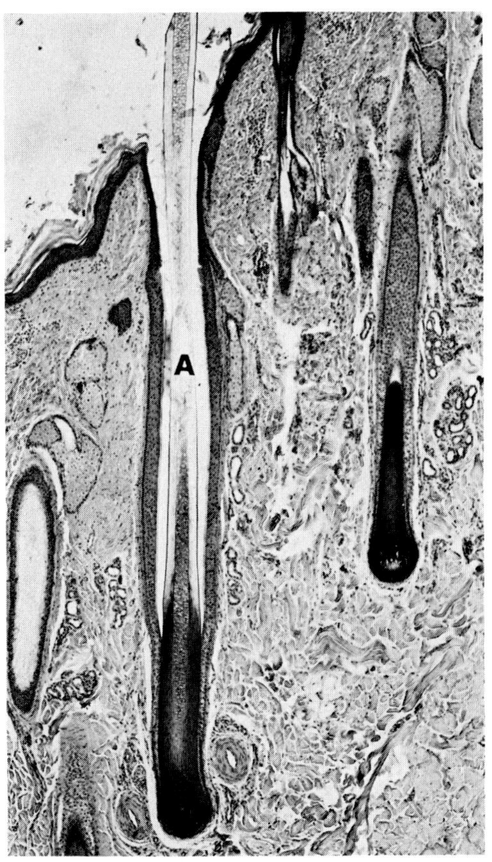

Fig. 16–17. *Dorsal neck region illustrating single hair follicle distribution, horse. Large mane hair (A) with smaller hairs adjacent. H & E. ×30. (From Talukdar, A.H., Calhoun, M.L., and Stinson, A.W.: Microscopic anatomy of the skin of the horse. Am J Vet Res 33:2365, 1972.)*

Many differences exist in the arrangement of the hair follicles among the domestic animals. Horses and cattle have single hair follicles distributed evenly (Fig. 16–17). Pigs have single follicles grouped in clusters of two to four follicles, with three being most common (Fig. 16–18). This cluster is usually surrounded by dense connective tissue. The compound follicle

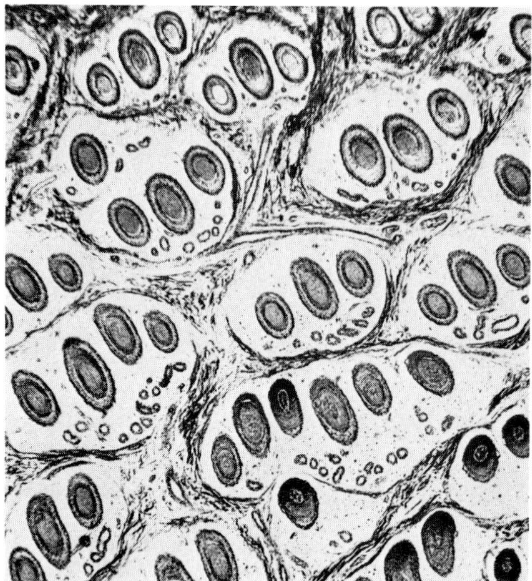

Fig. 16–18. *Hair follicle groups, pig. Notice the numbers of follicles per cluster and the position of the sweat glands. H & E. ×30. (From Smith, J.L., and Calhoun, M.L.: The microscopic anatomy of the integument of newborn swine. Am J Vet Res 25:165, 1964.)*

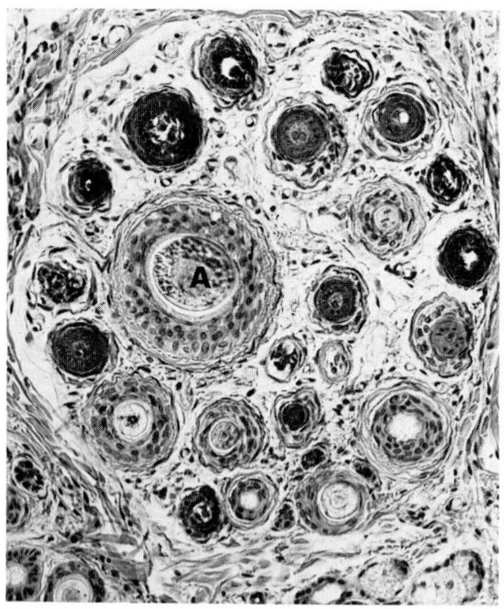

Fig. 16–19. *Compound hair follicle, dog. Primary hair follicle (A). Except for a few blood vessels, the structures are all secondary follicles. H & E. ×175. (From Adam, W.S., Calhoun, M.L., Smith, E.M., and Stinson, A.W.: Microscopic Anatomy of the Dog: A Photographic Atlas. Springfield, Ill., Charles C Thomas, 1970.)*

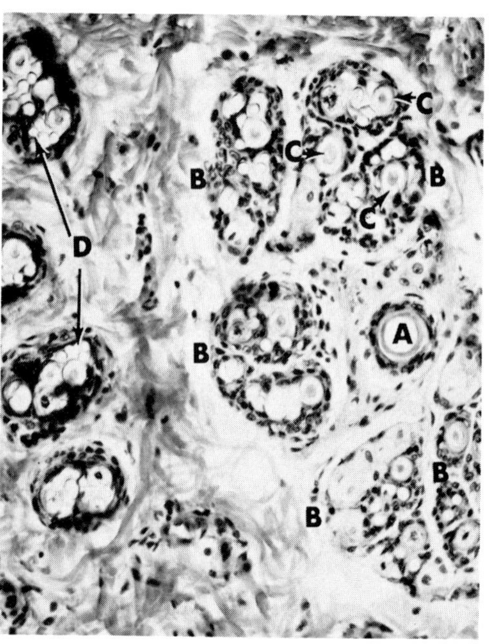

Fig. 16–20. *Hair follicle cluster, cat. Primary hair follicle (A) surrounded by five compound follicle clusters (B), each composed of three small primary hair follicles (C), surrounded by 6 to 12 fine secondary hair follicles seen best in adjacent clusters (D). H & E. ×170. (From Strickland, J.H., and Calhoun, M.L.: The integumentary system of the cat. Am J Vet Res 24:1018, 1963.)*

of dogs consists of a single long primary hair and a group of smaller secondary underhairs (Fig. 16–19). As many as 15 hairs may emerge from a single opening in the skin. The compound follicles occur in clusters of three, with the center one slightly larger. The arrangement of the follicles in the cat consists of a single large primary (guard) hair follicle surrounded by clusters of two to five compound follicles (Fig. 16–20). In each compound follicle there are 3 coarse primary hairs and 6 to 12 fine or secondary hairs. The skin of sheep has hair-growing regions such as the face, the distal part of the limbs, and the pinna of the ear, and has wool-growing regions that cover most of the body. The hair-growing regions contain mostly single follicles, whereas the densely covered wool-growing regions have large numbers of compound follicles. The typical follicle cluster contains

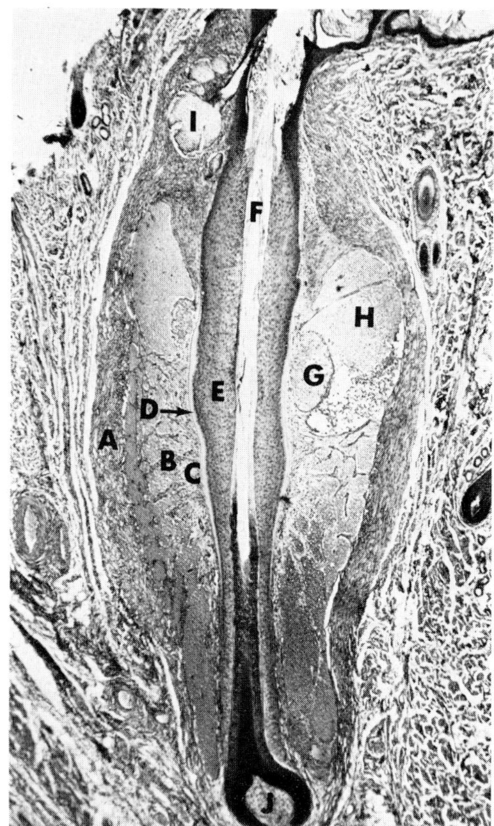

Fig. 16–21. *Sinus hair follicle, dog. Outer layer of the dermal sheath (A); cavernous blood sinus with trabeculae (B); inner layer of the dermal sheath (C); glassy membrane (D); external root sheath (E); hair (F); sinus pad, an enlargement of the inner dermal sheath (G); annular sinus filled with blood (nontrabecular) (H); sebaceous glands opening into the pilosebaceous canal (I); hair papilla (J). H & E. ×35. (From Adam, W.S., Calhoun, M.L., Smith, E.M., and Stinson, A.W.: Microscopic Anatomy of the Dog: A Photographic Atlas. Springfield, Ill., Charles C Thomas, 1970.)*

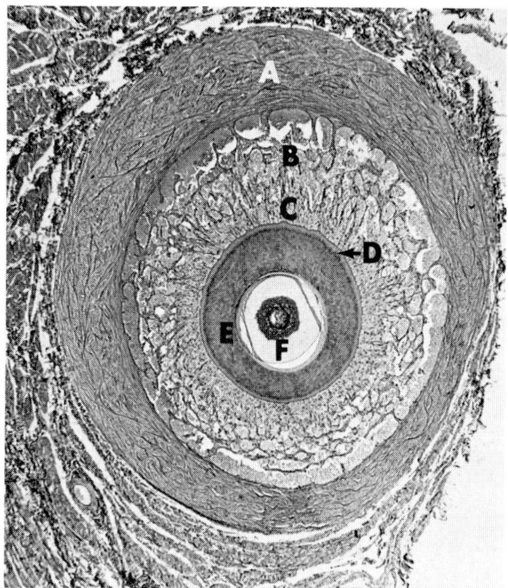

Fig. 16–22. *Sinus hair follicle, cross section at level B in Figure 16–21, dog. Outer layer of the dermal sheath (A); cavernous blood sinus with trabeculae (B); inner layer of the dermal sheath (C); glassy membrane (D); external root sheath (E); hair (F). H & E. ×30. (From Adam, W.S., Calhoun, M.L., Smith, E.M., and Stinson, A.W.: Microscopic Anatomy of the Dog: A Photographic Atlas. Springfield, Ill., Charles C Thomas, 1970.)*

three primary follicles and a number of secondary follicles. In the goat, the primary follicles occur in groups of three, with three to six secondary follicles associated with each group.

Sinus Hair Follicles

Sinus or *tactile hair follicles* of the head are highly specialized for tactile sense. They are very large single follicles characterized by a blood-filled annular sinus between the inner and outer layers of the dermal sheath (Fig. 16–21). In the horse and ruminants, the annular sinus is traversed by fibroelastic trabeculae throughout its length (Fig. 16–22). However, in the pig and carnivores, the upper portion of the sinus hair follicles is somewhat different. The inner layer of the dermal sheath thickens, forming a sinus pad, and this is surrounded by an annular sinus free of trabeculae (Fig. 16–21). Skeletal muscles are attached to the outer sheath of the follicle, allowing some voluntary control (Fig. 16–23). Numerous nerve bundles penetrate the outer sheath and ramify in the trabeculae and inner dermal sheath.

Skin Glands

SWEAT GLANDS. Based on their morphologic and functional characteristics, sweat (sudoriferous) glands are classified into two types: apocrine and merocrine (eccrine).

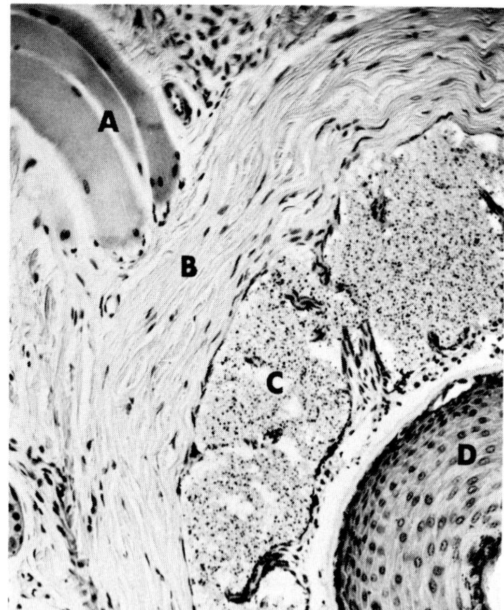

Fig. 16–23. *Sinus hair follicle, goat, with skeletal muscle attached (A); outer dermal sheath (B); blood sinus (C); external sheath (D). H & E. ×105. (From Sar, M., and Calhoun, M.L.: The microscopic anatomy of the integument of the common American goat. Am J Vet Res 27:444, 1966.)*

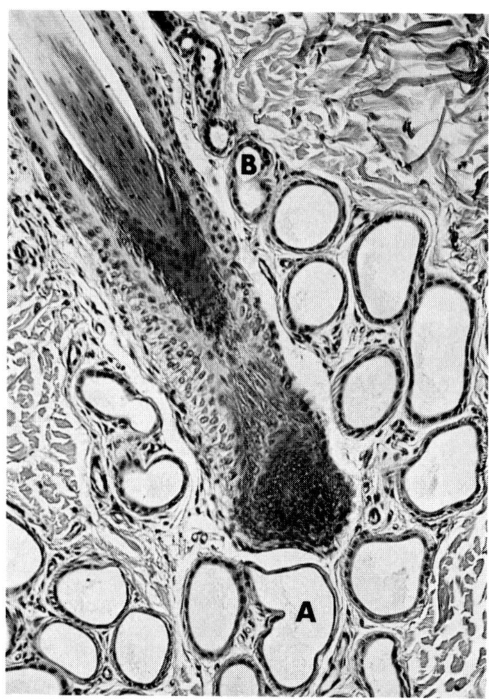

Fig. 16–24. *Saccular apocrine sweat glands, goat. Coiled secretory portion (A) lined with flattened cuboidal epithelium. Excretory duct (B). H & E. ×105. (From Sar, M.: The Microscopic Anatomy of the Integument of the Common American Goat. M.S. thesis, Michigan State University, East Lansing, Mich., 1963.)*

The apocrine type is the most extensively developed in the domestic mammals. They are simple saccular or tubular glands with a coiled secretory portion and a straight duct (Figs. 16–24 and 16–25). The secretory portion has a large lumen lined with flattened cuboidal to low columnar epithelial cells, depending on the stage of their secretory activity. The cytoplasm may contain glycogen, lipid, or pigment granules. The free surface of cells in apocrine sweat glands has cytoplasmic protrusions, indicative of their secretory activity (Fig. 16–26). Myoepithelial cells are located between the secretory cells and the basement membrane (Fig. 16–27). The duct portion pursues a straight course toward the upper part of the dermis. It has a narrow lumen and two layers of flattened cuboidal cells (Fig. 16–28). Most frequently, the duct penetrates the epidermis of the hair follicle just before it opens onto the surface of the skin. The apocrine glands in the domestic animals are located throughout most of the skin. This contrasts with their distribution in man, where they are mainly in the axillary, pubic, and perianal regions. In the horse, these glands are quite active and produce visible sweat during exercise and at high temperature. In other species, the secretion is scant and rarely perceptible. In the dog and cat, the glands may be tortuous or serpentine, and in ruminants the lumen is dilated, giving the appearance of large saccules (Fig. 16–24). The apocrine glands are least active in the goat and cat.

There are several areas where the apocrine glands are specialized in structure and function. These special apocrine sweat glands will be discussed later in this chapter.

The merocrine (eccrine, atrichial) glands are found mainly in special skin areas such as the footpads of the dog and cat, the frog

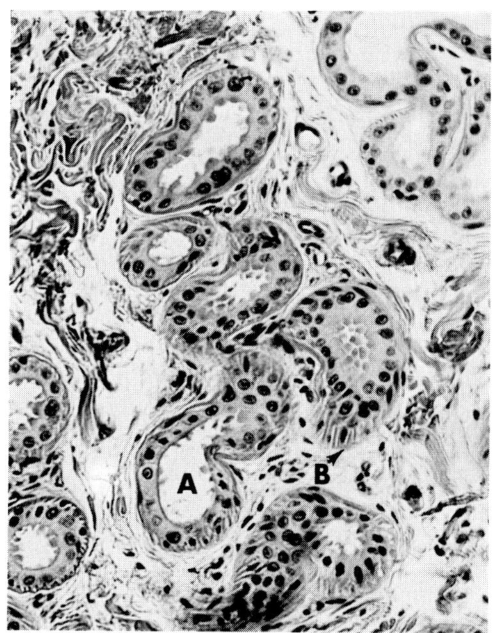

Fig. 16–25. *Tubular apocrine sweat gland, goat. Coiled glands (A); myoepithelial cells (B) H & E. ×160. (From Sar, M.: The Microscopic Anatomy of the Integument of the Common American Goat. M.S. thesis, Michigan State University, East Lansing, Mich., 1963.)*

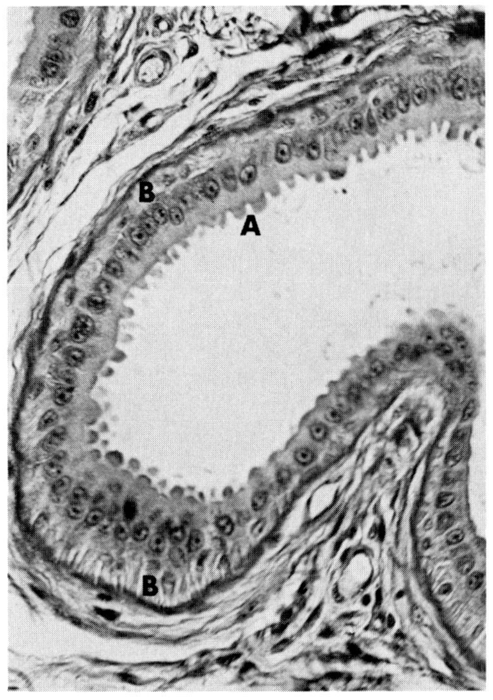

Fig. 16–26. *Apocrine sweat gland, goat. Apical secretory caps projecting into the lumen (A); myoepithelial cells (B). H & E. ×240.*

of ungulates, the planum nasale of the pig, the planum nasolabiale of the ox, and the carpal glands of swine. They are coiled simple tubular glands that open directly onto the skin surface rather than into hair follicles. Studies involving low level sweat gland activity of cat footpads indicate that friction increases with epidermal hydration. The presence of sweat on the external nasal surfaces may be associated with the improved tactile sense that results from a moist epidermis. The secretory portion is composed of cuboidal epithelium with two distinct cell types (Fig. 16–29). The dark or mucoid cells have more ribosomes than the clear cells, and numerous droplets occur in the apical part of the cell. The clear cells lack cytoplasmic basophilia and are thought to be involved in fluid transport. Intercellular canaliculi occur between adjacent clear cells and course from the lumen to the base of the epithelium. Myoepithelial cells surround the secretory units. The duct is relatively straight and opens directly onto the surface of the epidermis. It is composed of two layers of cuboidal epithelial cells resting on a basement membrane.

SEBACEOUS GLANDS. Sebaceous glands

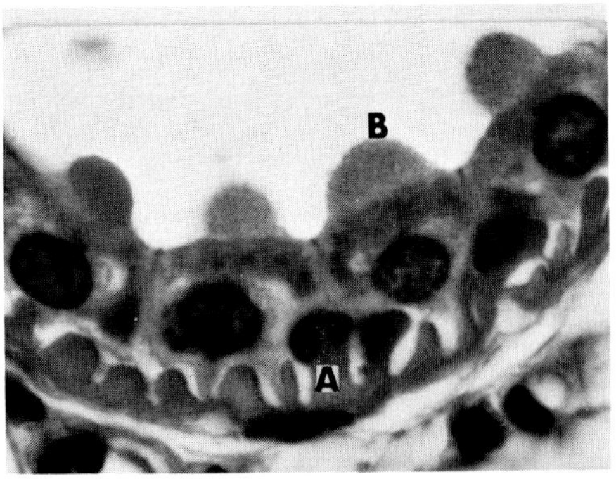

Fig. 16–27. *Apocrine sweat gland, pig, illustrating myoepithelial cells (A) and apical secretory caps (B). H & E. ×1200.*

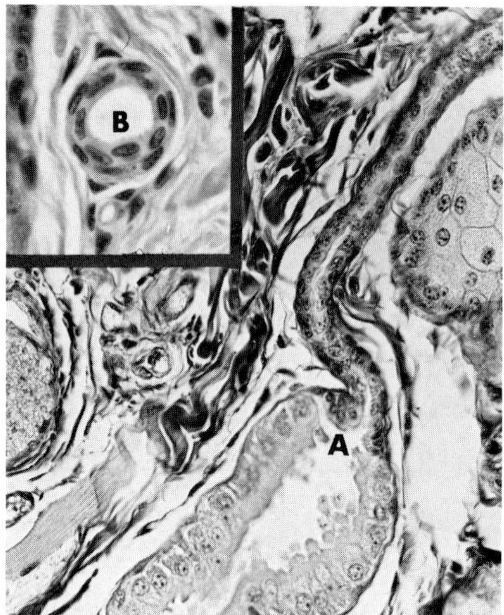

Fig. 16–28. *Junction of an apocrine gland with the collecting duct (A). H & E. ×200. Inset, cross section of a collecting duct showing two layers of flattened cuboidal epithelium (B). ×480. (From Sar, M., and Calhoun, M.L.: The microscopic anatomy of the integument of the common American goat. Am J Vet Res 27:444, 1966.)*

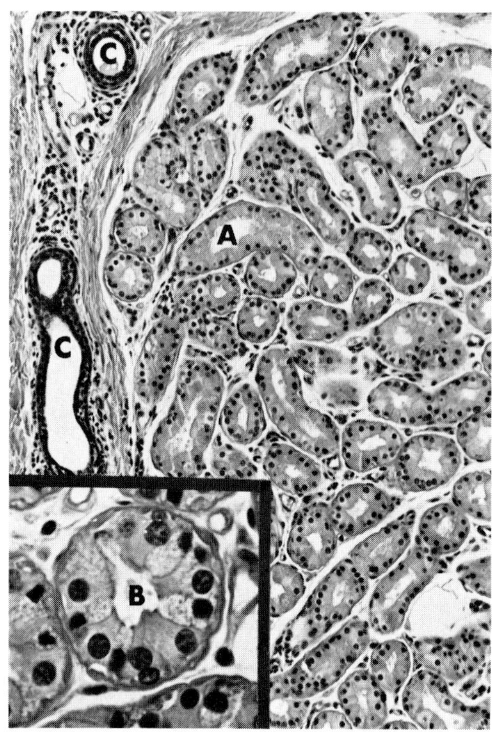

Fig. 16–29. *Merocrine sweat gland, carpal gland (A), and ducts (C), pig. Inset, higher magnification of a single acinus (B) showing light and dark cells. H & E. ×480.*

may be simple, branched, or compound alveolar glands that release their secretory product, sebum, by the holocrine mode. They originate from the external epithelial root sheath of the hair follicle and invade the dermis. They are most frequently associated with hair follicles, into which their ducts empty to form the pilosebaceous canal of the hair follicle (Fig. 16–30). In certain hairless areas such as the anus, the teat of the horse, and the internal layer of the prepuce of some species, sebaceous glands empty directly onto the skin surface through a duct lined with stratified squamous epithelium (Fig. 16–31). The secretory unit consists of a solid mass of epidermal cells, enclosed by a connective tissue sheath that blends with the surrounding dermis (Fig. 16–30). At the periphery of the glandular mass, a single layer of low cuboidal cells rests on a basal lamina. Most of the mitotic activity takes place in this layer, and as the cells move inward they enlarge, become polygonal, and accumulate numerous lipid droplets. The cells near the duct contain pyknotic nuclei. The sebum is derived from the disintegration of the cells and passes into the lumen of the hair follicle through a short duct lined with stratified squamous epithelium.

Many areas of the body of certain species have especially well developed accumulations of sebaceous glands, some associated with modified sweat glands. These sites include the infraorbital, inguinal, and interdigital regions of sheep, the base of the horn of goats, anal sacs of cats, and the prepuce and circumanal regions, and will be discussed later in this chapter.

BLOOD VESSELS, LYMPH VESSELS, AND NERVES

Terminal branches of the cutaneous arteries give rise to three plexuses: (1) the

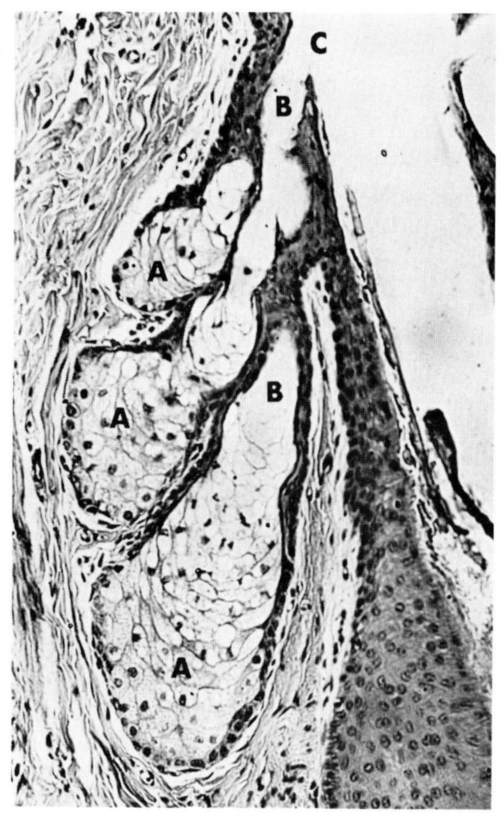

Fig. 16–30. *Sebaceous glands, swine. Sebaceous glands (A) and ducts (B), one of which opens into the pilosebaceous canal (C). H & E. ×120. (From Marcarian, H.Q., and Calhoun, M.L.: The microscopic anatomy of the integument of the adult swine. Am J Vet Res 27:765, 1966.)*

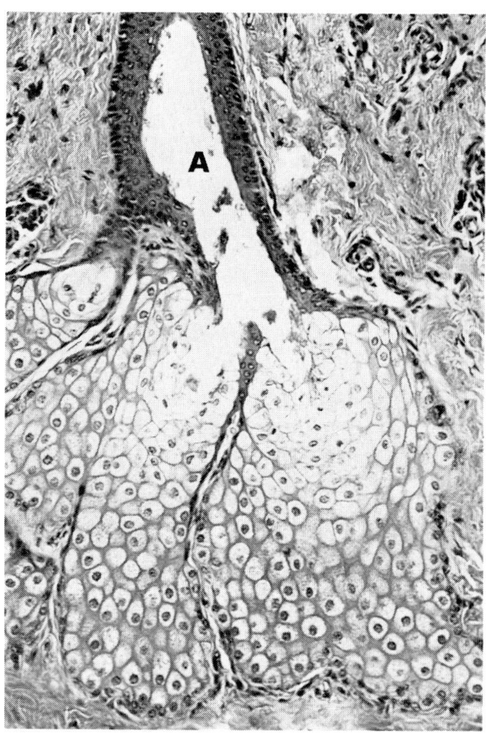

Fig. 16–31. *Multilobulated sebaceous glands (horse teat) opening into a duct lined with stratified squamous epithelium (A). H & E. ×150. (From Talukdar, A.H., Calhoun, M.L. and Stinson, A.W.: Microscopic anatomy of the skin of the horse. Am J Vet Res 33:2365, 1972.)*

deep or subcutaneous plexus, which in turn gives off branches to the (2) middle or cutaneous plexus, which provides branches to make up the (3) superficial and subpapillary plexus (Fig. 16–1). The reverse applies for venous return to the cutaneous veins. By this arrangement, all components of the skin are assured an adequate blood supply. The superficial plexus also furnishes the capillary loops that extend into the dermal papillae when present. Lymph capillaries arise in the superficial dermis and form a network that drains into a subcutaneous plexus.

The nerve supply to the skin varies in different parts of the body. Small subcutaneous nerve trunks give rise to a nerve plexus that pervades the dermis, supplies the glands, muscles, and hair, and sends small branches to the epidermis. The nerve fiber terminates in several kinds of endings: free endings in the epidermis, and lamellated and nonlamellated endings, particularly in the lips. The large lamellated corpuscles are rarely present in the skin of domestic animals but have been observed in the frog of the hoof of the horse, the digital cushion of the dog and cat, and the anal sac wall of the cat.

SPECIAL SKIN STRUCTURES

External Ear

The external ear is composed of the auricula and the external ear canal (auditory meatus). The auricula consists of a flat perforated plate of elastic cartilage and the

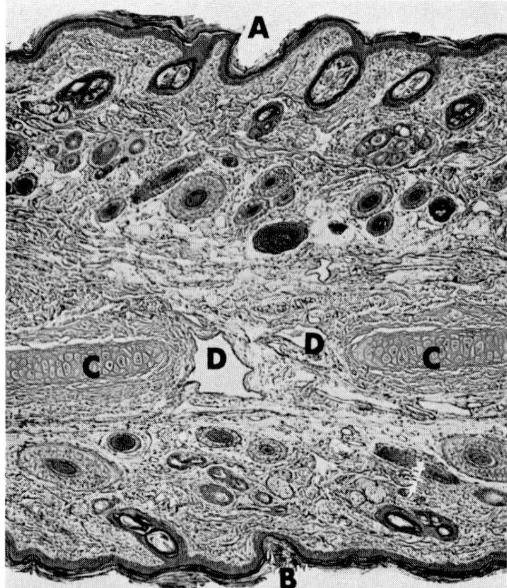

Fig. 16–32. *Auricula of the ear, dog. Outer surface (A); inner surface (B); auricular elastic cartilage (C); blood vessels (D) traversing one of the many foramina in the cartilage plate. H & E. ×38. (From Adam, W.S., Calhoun, M.L., Smith, E.M., and Stinson, A.W.: Microscopic Anatomy of the Dog: A Photographic Atlas. Springfield, Ill., Charles C Thomas, 1970.)*

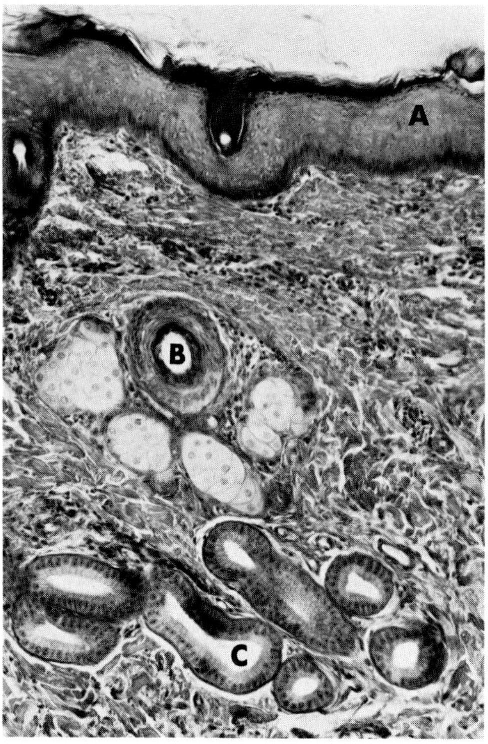

Fig. 16–33. *External auditory canal, cow. Stratified squamous epithelium (A); hair follicle with associated sebaceous glands (B); ceruminous glands (C). H & E. ×120.*

attached auricular muscles. It is covered on both sides by thin skin containing sweat and sebaceous glands and hair follicles. The convex surface of the ear has more hair follicles per unit area than the thinner concave surface (Fig. 16–32). Blood vessels traverse the perforations in the cartilage. It has been conjectured that severe trauma causes the cartilage to impinge on the blood vessels and might account for the hematomas frequently observed on the lateral surface of the cartilage in dog ears.

The lumen of the *external auditory canal* is irregular in contour, the result of a number of permanent skin folds with fatty central cores. The skin that lines the canal contains small hair follicles, sebaceous glands, and ceruminous glands. Ceruminous glands are simple coiled tubular glands that resemble apocrine sweat glands (Fig. 16–33). The ceruminous glands open either into the hair follicle or onto the surface. They increase in number in the lower third of the meatus. The combination of sebum with the ceruminous gland secretion and the desquamating stratified squamous epithelium forms the cerumen or ear wax. The external auditory canal is supported by elastic cartilage in the outer portion and by bone near the tympanic membrane.

Eyelids

Upper and lower eyelids protect the eyeball and aid in maintaining a moist surface. The outermost covering of both lids is typical skin containing sweat and sebaceous glands and hair follicles (Fig. 16–34). Special hairs, the eyelashes, are numerous in the upper lid of all species except the cat. In the lower eyelid, the eyelashes are fewer in number in ruminants and the horse, and are generally absent in the cat, dog, and

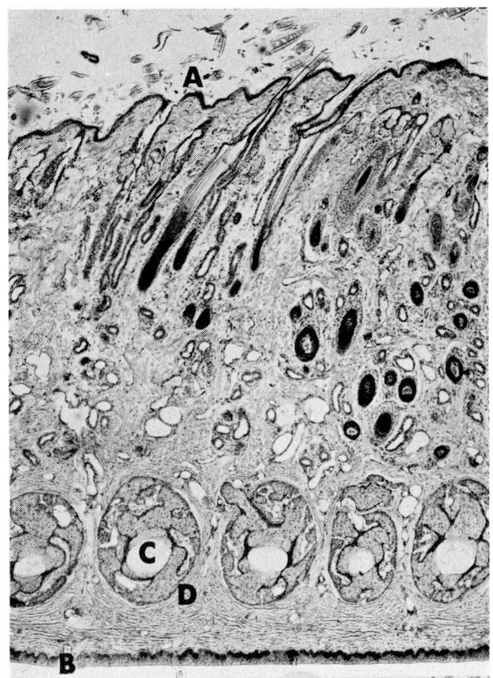

Fig. 16–34. *Upper eyelid, cat. External or skin surface (A); internal or conjunctival surface (B); tarsal glands (C); tarsal plate (D). H & E. ×26. (From Strickland, J.H., and Calhoun, M.L.: The integumentary system of the cat. Am J Vet Res 24:1018, 1963.)*

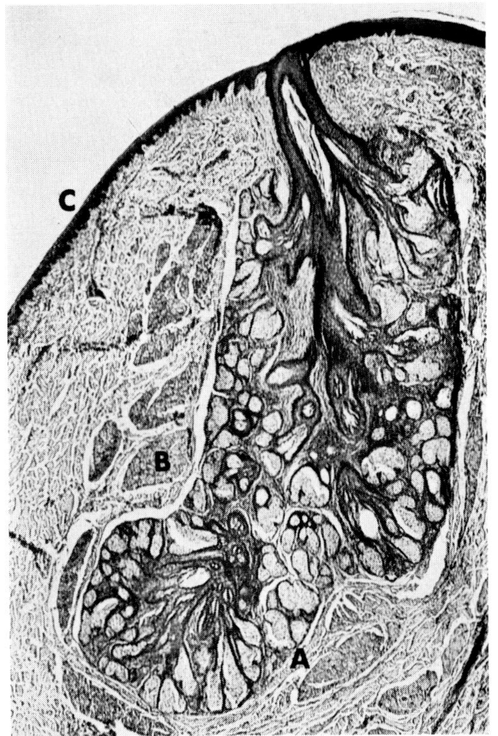

Fig. 16–35. *Tarsal gland in the lower eyelid, cow. Multilobulated sebaceous tarsal gland in longitudinal section surrounded by the tarsal plate (A), and skeletal muscle (B). Conjunctival surface (C). H & E. ×15. (From Goldsberry, S.: Histologic and Histochemical Studies of the Protective Apparatus of the Eyes in Hereford and Aberdeen Angus Cattle. Ph.D. thesis, Michigan State University, East Lansing, Mich., 1965.)*

pig. Tactile hairs may be present on or near the eyelids. The inner surface of the eyelids, the palpebral conjunctiva, is a mucous membrane. Its epithelial covering varies with the area and species, from stratified squamous epithelium near the edge of the eyelid to various combinations of columnar, cuboidal, polyhedral, and squamous cells. As a result, it is variously described as stratified squamous, stratified cuboidal, stratified columnar, and transitional or pseudostratified. Goblet cells are often present.

The most characteristic feature of the eyelids is the tarsal glands, which are better developed in the upper lid (Fig. 16–34). They are multilobular sebaceous glands with a central duct, which opens onto the palpebral surface at the margin of the eyelid (Fig. 16–35). These glands are most highly developed in the cat and poorly developed in swine. The tarsal glands are surrounded by the *tarsal plate,* a compact layer of collagen and elastic fibers. Skeletal muscle fibers from the orbicular muscle (orbicularis oculi) penetrate the eyelid, and scattered bundles of smooth muscle fibers are also present.

Apocrine sweat glands, referred to as ciliary glands, open cranially to the tarsal gland and near the eyelashes or into the follicle of the eyelashes (Fig. 16–36). Unlike ordinary sweat glands, the terminal portions of ciliary glands are only slightly coiled, and the gland lumina are more dilated. They have the typical cylindric secretory and myoepithelial cells surrounded by a basement membrane. Their structure and location are similar in all domestic animals but their function is obscure.

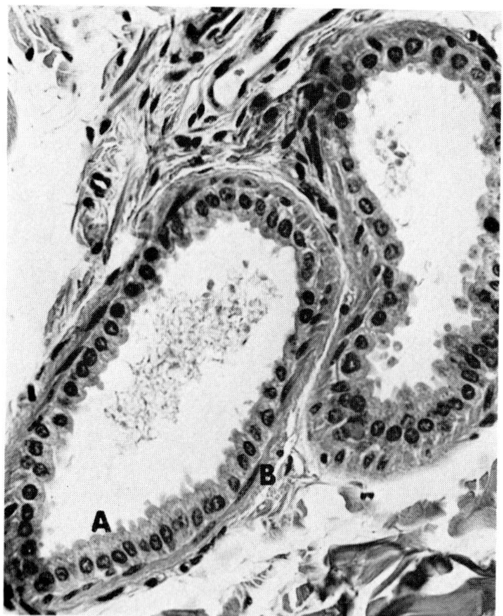

Fig. 16–36. *Ciliary glands, cow. Secretory cells (A); myoepithelial cells (B). H & E. ×600. (From Sinha, R.D.: The Microscopic Anatomy of the Integument of Holstein Cattle. M.S. thesis, Michigan State University, East Lansing, Mich., 1964.)*

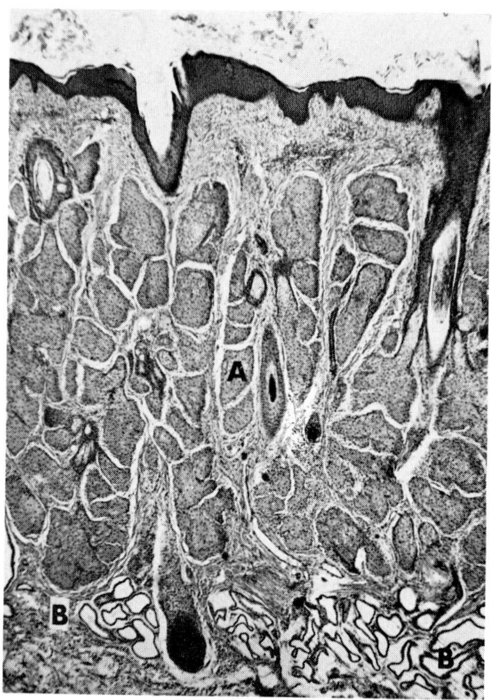

Fig. 16–37. *Wall of infraorbital sinus, sheep. Large sebaceous glands (A); peripheral apocrine sweat glands (B). H & E. ×30. (From Sinha, R.D.: A Gross, Histologic and Histochemical Study of the Eye Adnexa of Sheep and Goats. Ph.D. thesis, Michigan State University, East Lansing, Mich., 1965.)*

Infraorbital Sinus

The infraorbital sinus of sheep, located medially and cranially to the eye, is lined with thin skin that contains few hairs but large sebaceous glands that form a continuous layer around the sinus (Fig. 16–37). A few apocrine sweat glands are located peripherally.

Nose

The skin around the external openings of the nasal cavity is slightly modified in each species of domestic animals. The planum nasale of the dog and cat is composed of a thick, keratinized epidermis with distinct elevations and grooves, which provide the basis for identification by nose printing, similar to fingerprinting (Fig. 16–38). There are no sweat or sebaceous glands associated with this area. The skin around the nostril of the horse is usually thin and contains fine hairs and numerous sebaceous glands. The planum rostrale of the pig has fine hairs sparsely distributed over the surface and numerous, well-developed merocrine sweat glands. The planum nasale of small ruminants (Fig. 16–39) and the planum nasolabiale of large ruminants (Fig. 16–40) contain no hair follicles but have large merocrine glands with intercellular secretory canaliculi.

Mental Organ

The mental organ of pigs is a large, spherical mass of apocrine glands located midway between the jaws behind the angle of the chin.

Submental Organ

The submental organ of the cat, located in the intermandibular space, is composed

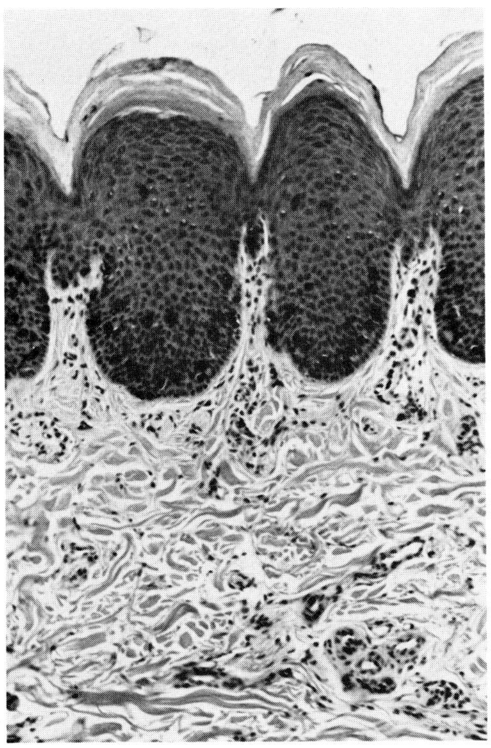

Fig. 16–38. *Planum nasale, cat. Notice the thickened keratinized epithelium with grooves and ridges. H & E. ×120.*

of sebaceous gland lobules, each containing a central collecting space. The lobules are surrounded by skeletal muscle. The fatty excretion collects in a sebum-filled depression.

Carpal Glands

The carpal glands of pigs are large accumulations of merocrine sweat glands on the medial surface of the carpus (Fig. 16–41). They open to the skin surface through three to five diverticula, lined with stratified squamous epithelium, that are visible to the naked eye. The glandular tissue located in the subcutis consists of numerous lobules of densely packed secretory units typical of merocrine sweat glands. Both secretory cell types, the dark and clear cells, and myoepithelial cells are present. Each lobule is drained by a duct lined with a two-layered cuboidal epithelium, which pursues a serpentine course through the dermis. The duct passes through the epidermis in a tortuous course and opens onto the inner surface of the diverticulum.

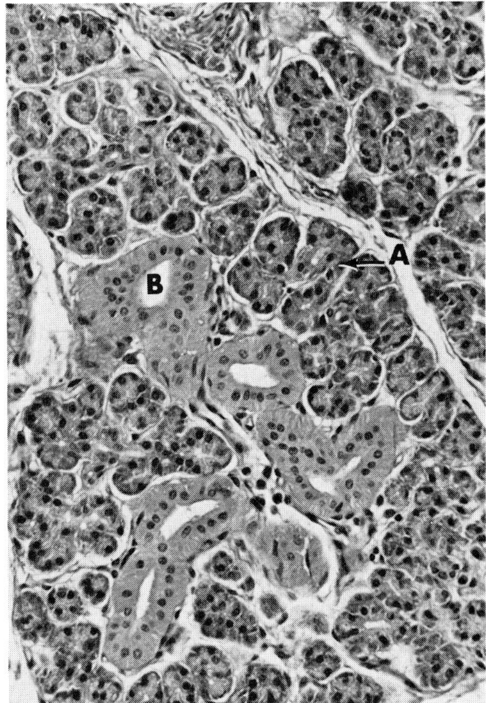

Fig. 16–39. *Merocrine nasolabial glands, goat. Serous glands (A); collecting ducts (B). H & E. ×185.*

Interdigital Sinus

The interdigital sinus of sheep is located between the digits just above the hoofs (Fig. 16–42). The opening of the sinus is at the dorsal tip of the interdigital space. The sinus is lined with a stratified squamous epithelium, and the dermis contains a scattering of hair follicles and sebaceous glands. The deep part of the wall is filled with large apocrine glands, with blebs of cytoplasm projecting from the surface of the epithelial cells. These are collectively referred to as the *interdigital glands.*

Inguinal Sinus

The inguinal sinus of sheep is a cutaneous diverticulum in the inguinal region

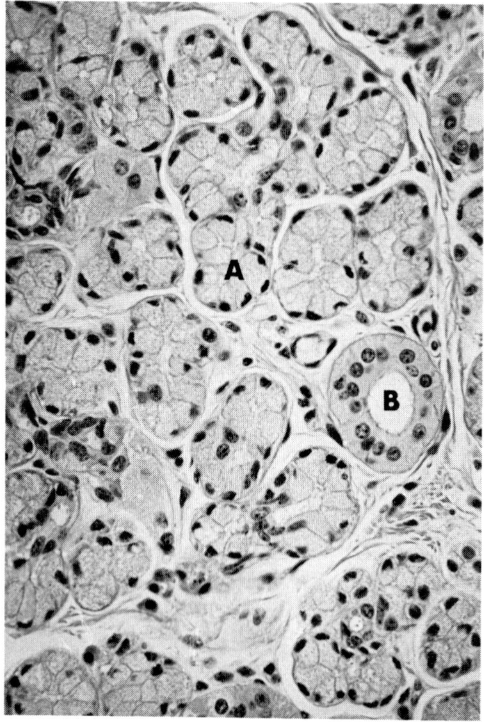

Fig. 16–40. *Merocrine nasolabial glands, cow. Mucous glands (A); collecting duct (B). H & E. ×300.*

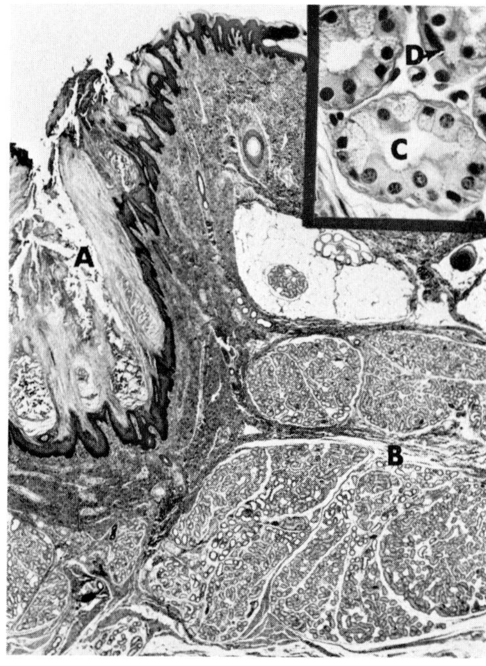

Fig. 16–41. *Carpal glands, pig. Diverticulum lined with keratinized stratified squamous epithelium (A) into which the merocrine glands (B) open. H & E. ×12. Inset, a secretory unit with dark and clear cells (C). Myoepithelial cell (D). H & E. ×300.*

of both sexes. The skin of the diverticulum contains scattered small hair follicles and well-developed sebaceous glands. Exceedingly large coiled apocrine glands are also characteristic. An elastic lamina from the abdominal tunic is attached to the skin in the deepest portion of the sinus.

Scrotum

Generally, scrotal skin is thinner than that on other parts of the body. Sebaceous and apocrine sweat glands are present but differ in size and number in various species. The boar has only a few small apocrine glands in the scrotal skin, whereas the stallion has large sebaceous and well-developed apocrine sweat glands. Mast cells are prominent in the scrotum of sheep and cattle. The amount of pigment varies with species and breed. Short fine hair is characteristic of all species. The tunica dartos is a unique layer of smooth muscle and fibroelastic connective tissue associated with the dermis of the scrotum (Fig. 16–43). These muscle fibers are responsive to the environmental temperature and facilitate the regulation of internal testicular temperature by changing the position of the testes in relation to the body wall. When the environmental temperature is high, the muscle is relaxed and the weight of the testes stretches the fibroelastic elements of the scrotum. At this time, the testes are farther from the body and the skin surface is smooth, thin, and pliable. During colder temperatures, the muscle contracts, bringing the testes closer to the body, and the scrotum has a corrugated appearance and is thicker and less pliable. Mechanical or tactile stimulation of the scrotum also results in contraction of the dartos muscle.

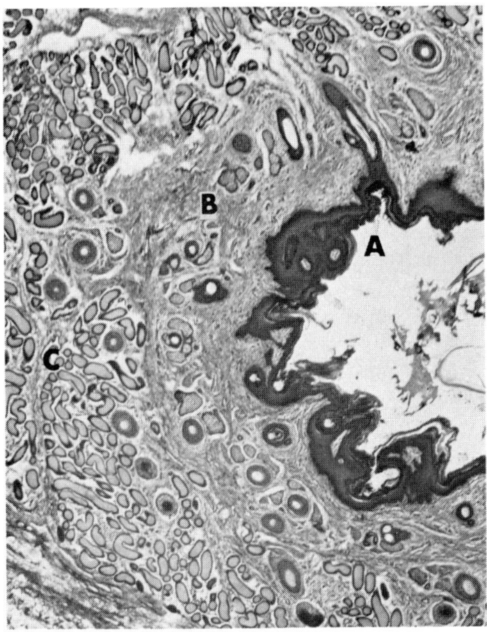

Fig. 16–42. *Wall of interdigital sinus, sheep. Lumen lined with stratified squamous epithelium (A); region of hair follicles and sebaceous glands (B); peripherally located tubular sweat glands (C), which open into the hair follicles. H & E. ×15. (From Kozlowski, G.P., and Calhoun, M.L.: Microscopic anatomy of the integument of the sheep. Am J Vet Res 30:1267, 1969.)*

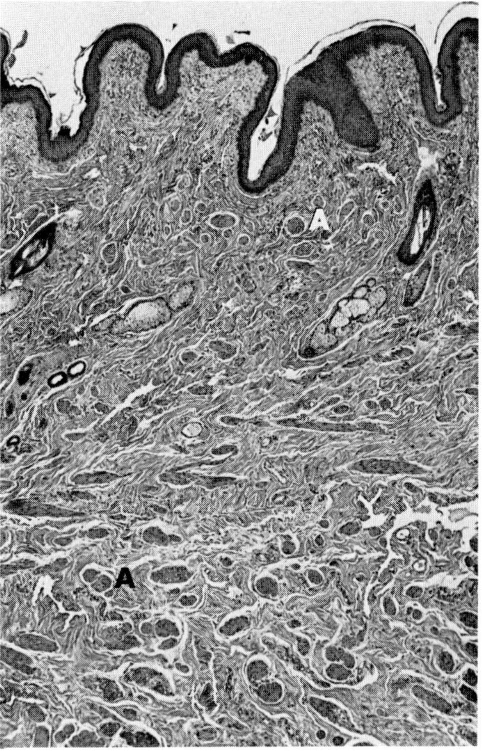

Fig. 16–43. *Scrotum, dog. Few hairs and sweat glands are present in this section; smooth muscle bundles are prominent (A). H & E. ×30.*

Anal Sacs

The anal sacs (sinus paranales) are cutaneous diverticula located between the inner smooth and outer striated sphincter muscles of the anus. The duct opens into the anus at the level of the anocutaneous junction. The ducts and sacs are lined by stratified squamous epithelium. The wall of the anal sac contains both sebaceous and apocrine sweat glands in the cat, but in the dog only large apocrine glands are present (Figs. 16–44 and 16–45). The anal sac duct of the dog is prone to occlusion, resulting in its engorgement with secretory material and detritus. Infection frequently follows this occlusion, necessitating either the expression of the sac's content or the surgical removal of the sac. Because this is rarely if ever a problem in the cat, it may be that the sebaceous glands within the wall of the sac add sufficient amounts of lipid to the secretory material, consequently decreasing the possibility of occlusion of the duct.

Circumanal Glands

The circumanal glands are lobulated, modified sebaceous glands located in the dermis and subcutaneous muscles of the zona cutanea of the anus (Fig. 16–46). They extend from the mucocutaneous junction peripherally for about one to three centimeters in all directions. Similar glands have been described in the skin of the prepuce, tail, loin, and groin. These glands are present shortly after birth, increase in size throughout adult life, and tend to atrophy during or at senility. They are clinically important because they rank third in frequency as the site of all canine tumors.

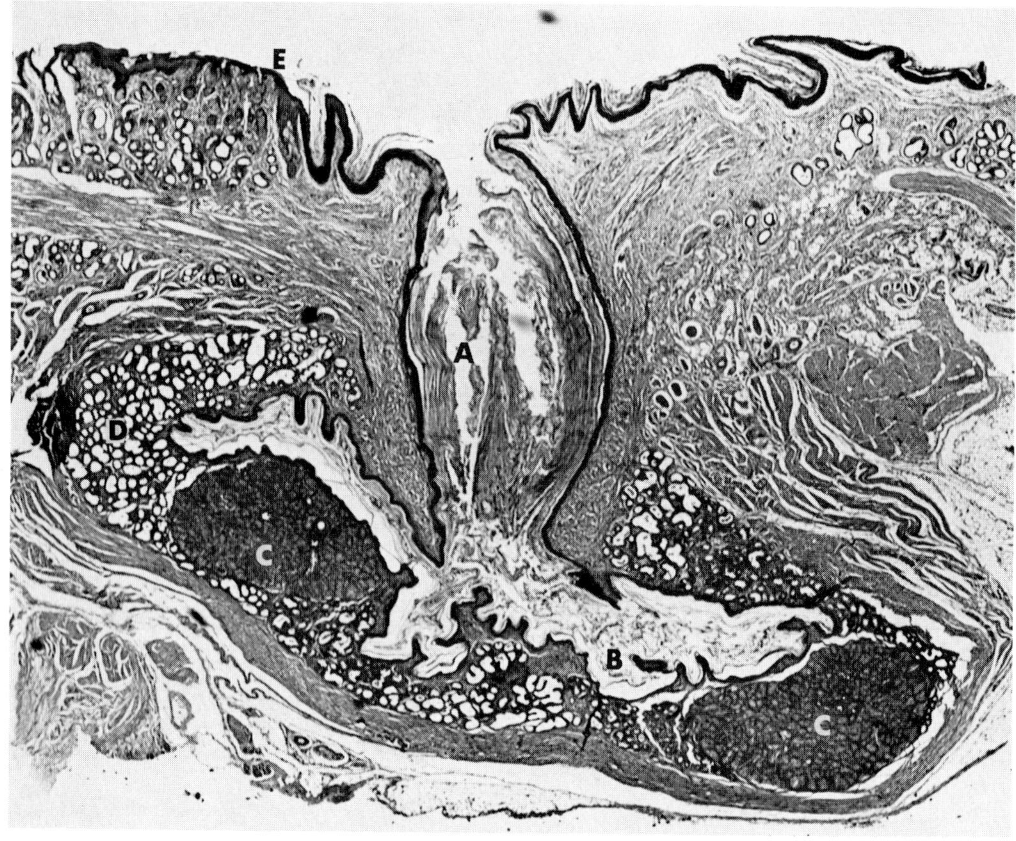

Fig. 16–44. *Anal sac and associated glands, cat. Duct (A) and lumen (B) of the anal sac filled with keratinized epithelial fragments and secretory material. Sebaceus gland masses (C); apocrine anal sac glands (D); linea anocutanea (E). H & E. ×17. (From Greer, M.B., and Calhoun, M.L.: The anal sacs of the domestic cat—Felis domesticus. Am J Vet Res 27:773, 1966.)*

This lobulated gland is composed of solid, compact masses of cells resembling closely packed liver cells. The term "hepatoid" has been used to describe the glandular parenchyma. Three cell types are present: 1) the basal or peripheral cells, which are cuboidal with little eosinophilic cytoplasm and a deeply staining basophilic nucleus, and 2) light and 3) dark polyhedral cells, which have granular eosinophilic cytoplasm and make up the main mass of each lobule. Since there is no duct system to drain the lobule, it may be considered a type of endocrine gland. Numerous capillaries are located in the connective tissue surrounding the lobules. A precise function for this gland has not been determined; however, recent investigations indicate that it is probably involved in steroid hormone metabolism.

Between the circumanal glands and the skin surface are regular lipid-producing sebaceous glands whose ducts empty either into the hair follicle or directly onto the skin surface.

Supracaudal Gland

The supracaudal gland, located in an oval circumscribed area on the dorsum of the tail (3 to 9 cm from base of the tail) in the dog and cat, is an accumulation of well-developed sebaceous glands that empty into single hair follicles (Fig. 16–47). The secretion is a waxy substance that may cause a matting of the hair of the region,

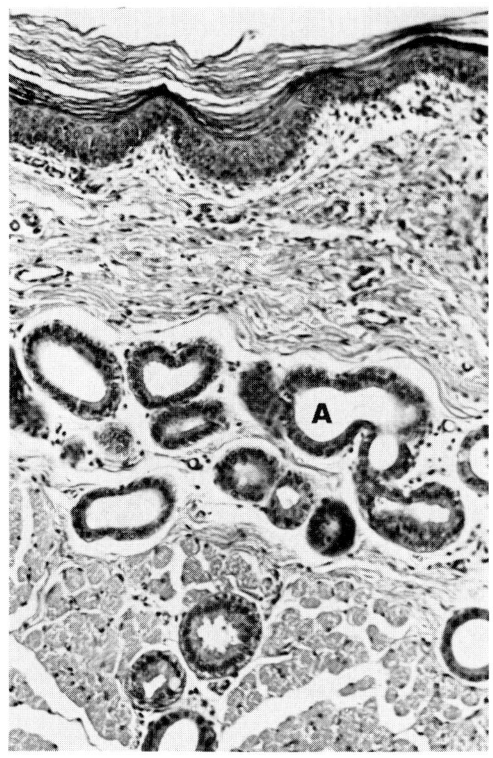

Fig. 16–45. *Wall of anal sac, dog. Only apocrine tubular glands (A) are present. H & E. ×120.*

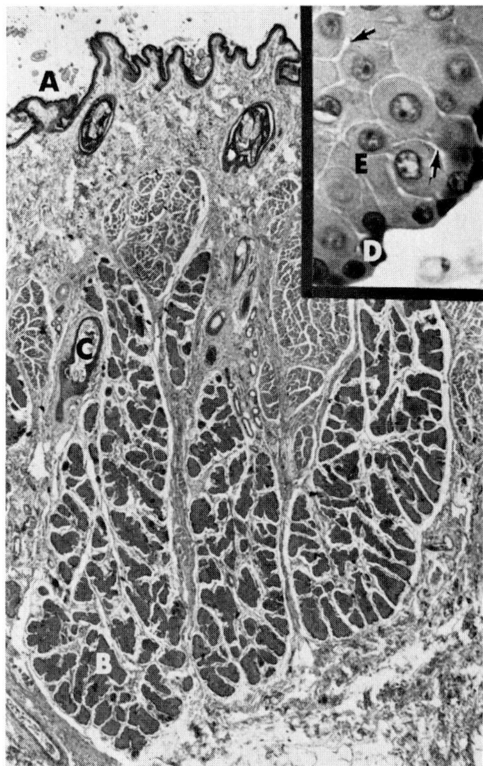

Fig. 16–46. *Circumanal glands, dog. Zona cutanea (A); nonsebaceous circumanal gland (B); ducts (C). H & E. ×20. Inset, proliferative polyhedral cells (D); nonsebaceous gland cells (E); intercellular canaliculi (arrows). H & E. ×480.*

especially if the glands are overactive. This can present a problem in show cats, because the appearance of the hair coat of the tail is affected.

Mammary Gland

Mammary glands are specialized skin organs derived embryologically by the invagination of ectodermal buds into the underlying mesoderm. Their development begins in the embryo and continues at a very slow rate during the prepuberal period. In the female, their growth rate is increased following puberty as a result of cyclic hormonal stimulation. With the onset of pregnancy, growth is greatly accelerated and reaches its greatest development during the lactation period shortly after parturition. Rudimentary mammary glands are present in the male and consist only of a few primary and secondary ducts embedded in fat.

The mammary gland is a compound tubuloalveolar gland (Fig. 16–48). Groups of tubuloalveolar secretory units form lobules separated by connective tissue septa.

The secretory unit is lined by a layer of simple cuboidal epithelium that varies markedly in height during various stages of secretory activity (Fig. 16–49). Shortly after milking, the alveolus begins a new secretory phase. At this time the lumen is partially collapsed and irregular in outline. The basal portion of the columnar epithelial cells contains a well-developed rER. The spherical nuclei are located near the center of the cell. Fat droplets in close association with mitochondria and membrane-bounded vesicles filled with micelles

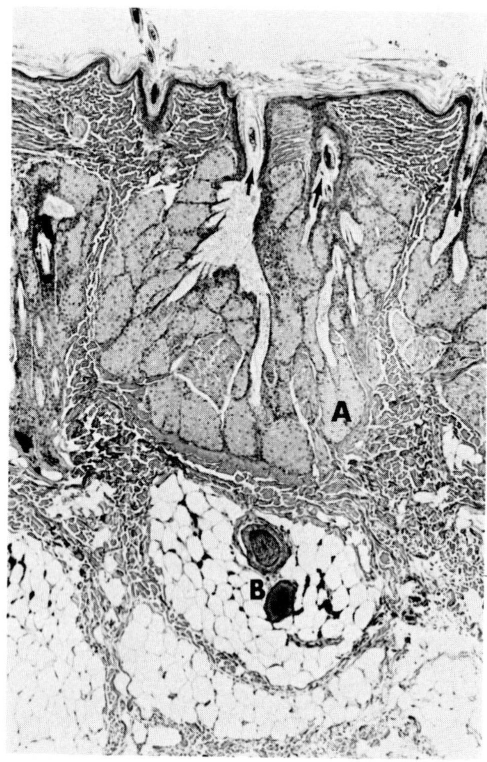

Fig. 16–47. *Supracaudal gland region, tail, cat. Sebaceous gland (A); ducts opening into hair follicles (arrows); roots of hair follicles extending into the hypodermis (B). H & E. ×48.*

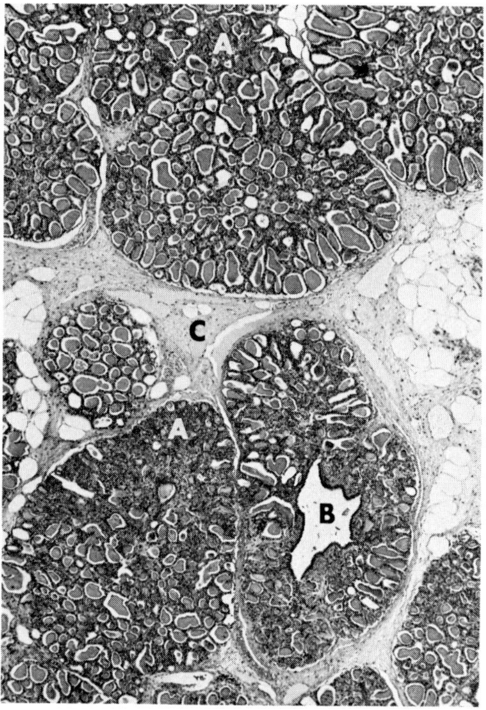

Fig. 16–48. *Mammary gland at parturition, sow. Gland lobules with alveoli filled with colostrum (A); intralobular collecting duct (B); interstitial loose connective tissue and fat (C). H & E. ×30.*

of milk protein occur throughout the upper part of the cell. As the secretory cycle continues, the lipid droplets move toward the surface and finally project from the cell as apical secretory caps. They are released from the cell surrounded by varying amounts of cytoplasm, along with cell-derived plasmalemma. The vesicles filled with protein micelles move toward the surface where the membrane fuses with the cell membrane, and they are released into the lumen. This process is typical of the merocrine mode of secretion. Therefore, milk is produced by both apocrine and merocrine secretion. Continuous milk production enlarges the lumen. At the end of the secretory cycle, the epithelial cells are the low cuboidal type. All the lobules within the gland are not in the same secretory phase at the same time. Some lobules may complete their secretory cycle and be filled with milk before others begin. Therefore, a single histologic section may contain lobules in various stages of activity. Usually all of the secretory units within a lobule are in approximately the same secretory phase.

Stellate and spindle-shaped myoepithelial cells are between the epithelial cells and the basement membrane of the alveolus. The release of oxytocin by the neurohypophysis results in the contraction of the myoepithelial cells, forcing the milk from the secretory units into the duct system. This phenomenon is called "milk letdown" by the dairyman.

The interstitial tissue of the mammary gland provides important structural support for the secretory units and contains the blood and lymph vessels and nerves. Surrounding each secretory unit is loose connective tissue with an extensive plexus of blood and lymph capillaries. Plasma cells

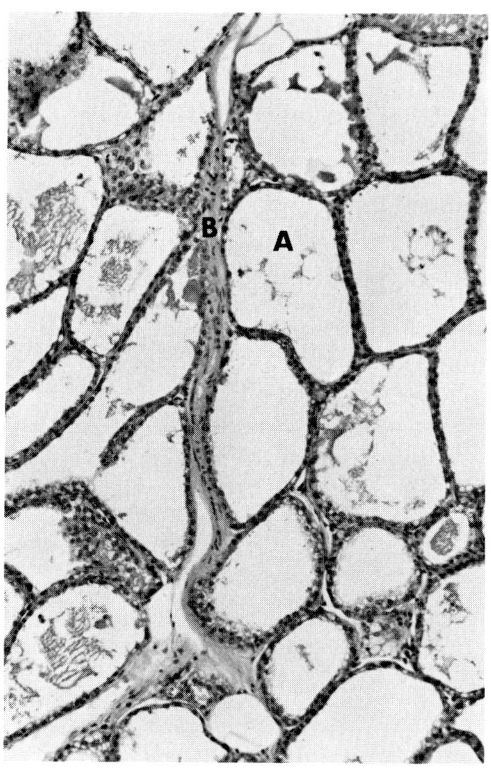

Fig. 16–49. *Lactating mammary gland, just before milking, cow. Alveolus (A); interlobular septum (B). H & E. ×120.*

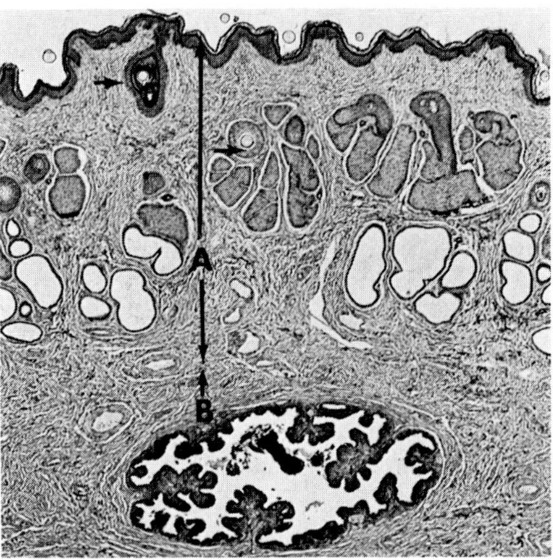

Fig. 16–50. *Teat, goat. Skin of teat with hair follicles (arrow) (A); wall of teat sinus lined with two-layered cuboidal epithelium (B). H & E. ×18. (From Sar, M., and Calhoun, M.L.: The microscopic anatomy of the integument of the common American goat. Am J Vet Res 27:444, 1966.)*

and lymphocytes are common constituents, particularly at parturition when the colostrum is being secreted. The connective tissue surrounding each lobule is thick, forming a dense septum containing the interlobular ducts and larger blood and lymph vessels. In the cow, these interlobular septa are continuous with the thick, heavy internal suspensory ligament and the thinner lateral (external) suspensory ligament, and support the large mammary gland characteristic of this species.

The duct system begins within the lobule as an intralobular duct. The epithelium is simple cuboidal without secretory activity. Spindle-shaped myoepithelial cells may be associated with these intralobular ducts. As the duct enters the interlobular connective tissue septa, it becomes the interlobular duct and consists of two layers of cuboidal cells. Longitudinal smooth muscle fibers become associated with these ducts as they merge with other interlobular ducts to form the large lactiferous ducts. The two-layered cuboidal epithelium continues in these larger ducts, and smooth muscle becomes more prominent. Sacculations result from variations in the diameter of the lumen. The constrictions between these sacculations may have an annular fold containing smooth muscle. In ruminants, several lactiferous ducts empty into a lactiferous sinus at the base of the teat. This sinus is continuous with the teat sinus that opens into the papillary duct leading to the external surface of the teat. The lactiferous ducts of the other species open separately onto the teat surface; in the cat there are 4 to 7, in the dog 7 to 16, and in the pig and horse 2 to 3 ducts opening onto the teat surface.

The teat or nipple contains the terminal part of the duct system and is lined with a mucous membrane that lies next to the dermis of the skin (Fig. 16–50). Numerous blood vessels are in this area, forming a stratum vasculare. The teat of ruminants has a large lumen, the teat sinus, lined by a two-layered cuboidal epithelium. An annular fold of the mucosa extends into the opening between the lactiferous and teat sinuses. The size of this opening is somewhat variable from one animal to another. Occasionally, trabeculae of connective tissue may extend across the opening, resulting in a slowing of the milk flow from the lactiferous sinus to the teat sinus. These trabeculae are called "spiders," and frequently veterinarians find it necessary to cut them surgically.

The lamina propria beneath the epithelium of the teat sinus may contain small clusters of rudimentary glands. Smooth muscle bundles oriented parallel to the long axis are prominent in some species and form the boundary between the teat mucosa and the dermis. The numerous large blood vessels in the dermis become engorged with blood during the milking or suckling process; thus, the skin is stretched, resulting in a smooth surface. Following milking, when the blood has drained from the teat vessels and the longitudinal smooth muscle has contracted, the teat surface returns to its typical corrugated appearance. The papillary duct is a small duct lined with a stratified squamous epithelium and opens onto the skin surface at the apex of the teat. Circularly oriented bundles of smooth muscle in the mucosa form a sphincter to hold the milk until it is forced out by milking or suckling.

The skin of the teat may be composed of only an epidermis and dermis without any hair follicles or sweat and sebaceous glands, such as in the cow and sow, or it may contain fine hairs and well-developed sweat and sebaceous glands, such as in other domestic animals.

After the lactation period, the secretory activity of the gland ceases and the process of involution begins. This is initiated to remove the accumulated milk when the internal pressure increases as the result of the cessation of suckling or milking. The alveoli are distended, and no further secretion occurs until they are emptied. If the

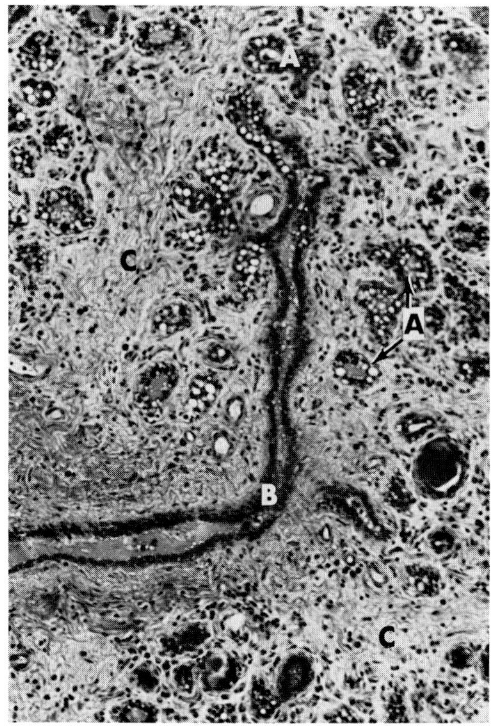

Fig. 16–51. *Nonlactating mammary gland, cow. Involuted alveolus (A); collecting duct (B). Notice the increased amount of interstitial loose connective tissue (C). H & E. ×120.*

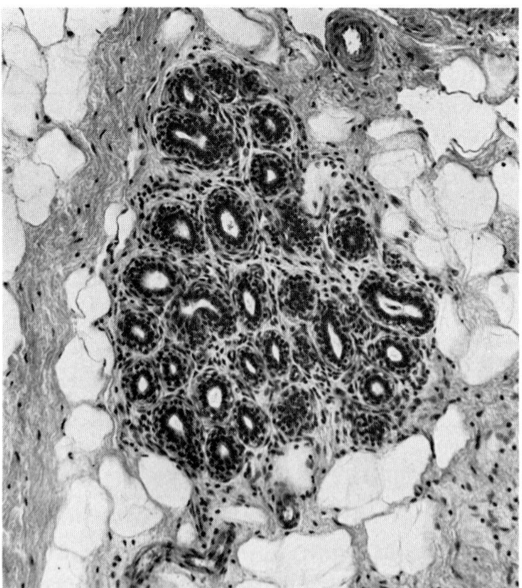

Fig. 16–52. *Developing duct system in the prepuberal mammary gland, heifer. The cluster of ducts is surrounded by fat and stroma. H & E. ×120.*

secretory product is not removed for several days, the epithelial cells begin to degenerate, and the residual milk in the lumen is gradually absorbed. Characteristically, the involuted mammary gland has more interstitial tissue than glandular elements, and isolated clusters of branched tubules with a few small alveoli are all that remain of the parenchyma (Fig. 16–51). They are lined by a low cuboidal epithelium with prominent underlying myoepithelial cells. The connective tissue septa are thicker, and fat cells may occur singly or in clusters. Lymphocytes and plasma cells are present in significant numbers. Small, dark-staining bodies of casein (corpora amylacea) may be found in the alveoli, ducts, or interstitial tissue.

The development and structure of the mammary gland parenchyma are markedly dependent on multiple hormonal influences. During fetal development and the prepuberal period, the growth of the primary and secondary duct system is proportional to the growth of the body as a whole (Fig. 16–52). Following puberty, growth of the duct system depends on estrogen, but progesterone is required for alveolar development. The hypophysis has a direct effect on mammary gland growth through the influence of prolactin and somatotropin. The continued secretion of prolactin is necessary for the maintenance of lactation.

DIGITAL ORGANS AND HORN

The digital organ consists of a keratinized portion, the underlying connective tissue or dermis, the subcutis, the bones and associated structures, and the digital pads. The keratinized portion is made up of a hard keratin or horn such as in the hoofs of the horse, ruminants, and pigs and the claws of carnivores. The dermis or corium contains blood vessels and nerves. The bones or phalanges and their ligaments and tendons form the supportive structure

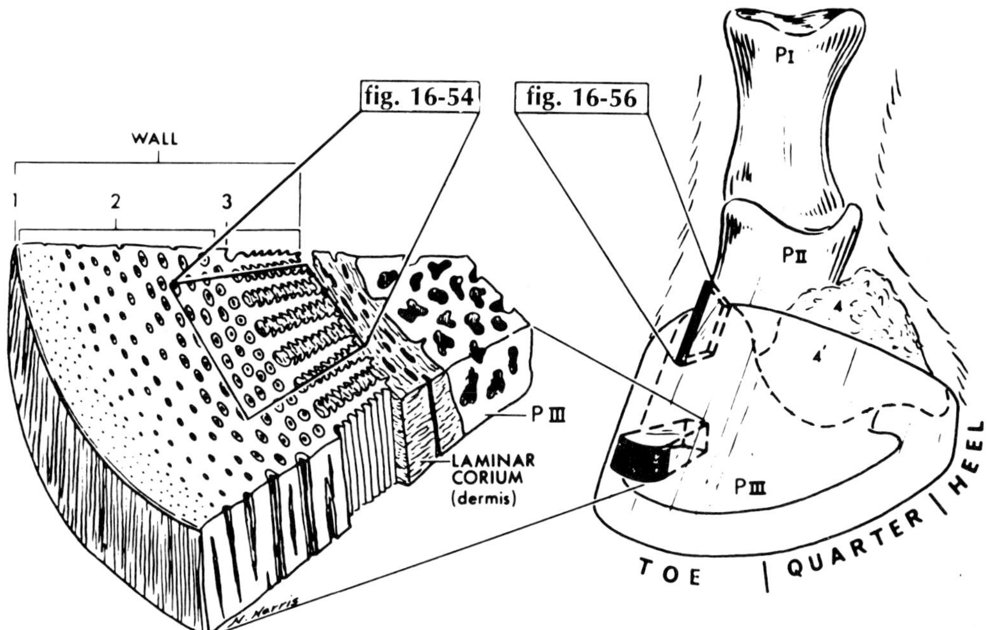

Fig. 16–53. *Frontolateral view, equine foot. The wall of the hoof is composed of three layers: stratum externum (1), stratum medium (2), stratum internum (3); proximal (PI), medial (PII), distal (PIII) phalanges; lateral cartilages of the hoof (4) and (4'). (From Stump, J.E.: Anatomy of the normal equine foot, including microscopic features of the laminar region. J Am Vet Med Assoc 151:1588, 1967.)*

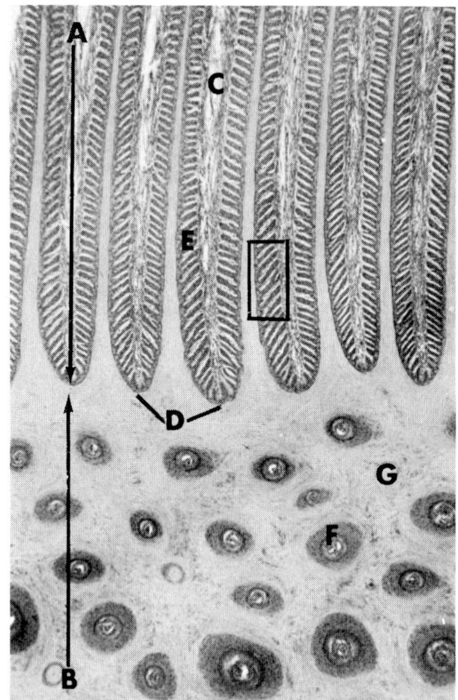

Fig. 16–54. *Wall of hoof, horse, from area marked in Figure 16–53, horse. Stratum internum (A); stratum medium (B); laminar corium (C); primary lamina (D); secondary laminar (E); tubular horn (F); intertubular horn (G). H & E. ×38. (From Dellmann, H.-D.: Veterinary Histology: An Outline Text-Atlas. Philadelphia, Lea & Febiger, 1971.)*

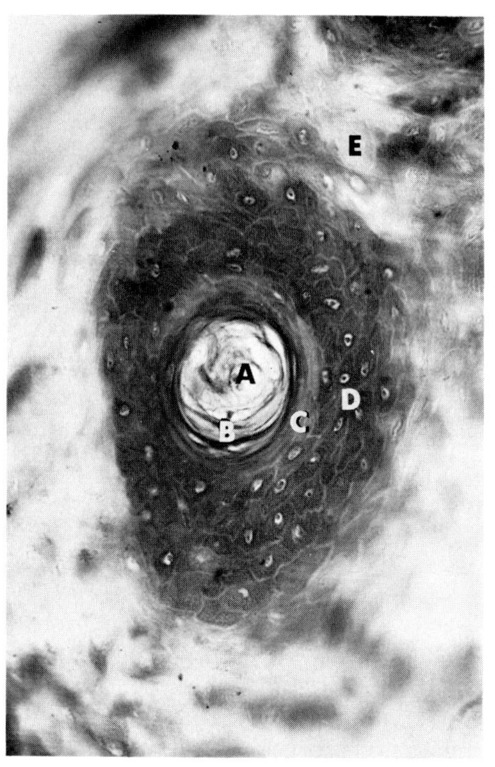

Fig. 16–55. *Cellular arrangement of tubular horn, hoof, horse. Medulla (A); inner zone of cortex (B); middle zone of cortex (C); outer zone of cortex (D); intertubular horn (E). Trichrome. ×300.*

of the digital organ. The digital organ in carnivores includes the digital pads, thick cushionlike structures that rest on the ground.

Equine Hoof

The soliped hoof is the keratinized portion of the digital organ and is composed of three main parts. The wall (paries) is that portion visible when the foot is placed on the ground. The sole (solea) forms the greatest part of the ventral surface of the foot; the frog (cuneus ungulae) is a wedge-shaped mass medial and caudal to the sole.

The wall of the hoof is formed of three layers (Fig. 16–53). From the outside inward they are the *stratum externum* (tectorium), the *stratum medium,* and the *stratum internum* (lamellatum). Each of these is structurally distinct and will be discussed separately.

The *stratum externum* is a thin layer of soft, flaky horn, which originates from the germinal layers of the epidermis of the periople (epidermis limbi), a roll of modified skin just above the coronary border of the hoof (see Fig. 16–56). Toward the back of the foot, the periople widens into a broad keratinized layer or bulb (heel). The corium beneath the periople is papillated and continuous with the dermis of skin above and the coronary corium below.

The *stratum medium* consists of tubular and intertubular horn and is the main supportive structure of the wall (Fig. 16–54). The horny tubules are oriented parallel to the outer surface of the hoof, and their keratinized cells have a highly ordered ar-

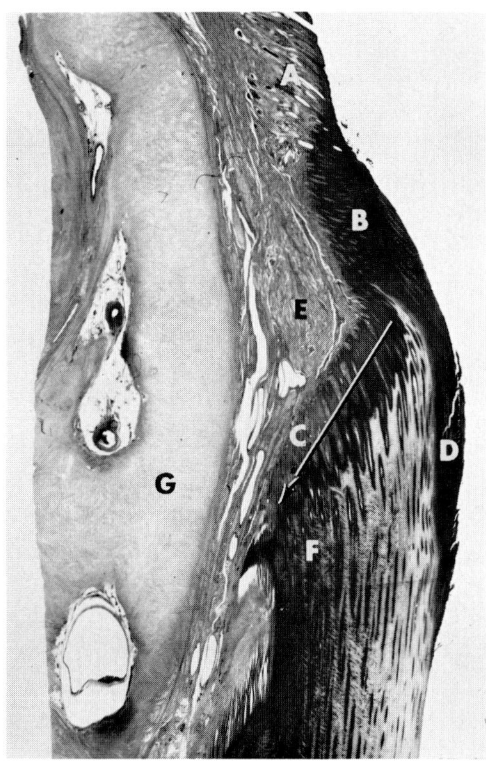

Fig. 16–56. *Vertical section of hoof, horse. See area marked in Figure 16–53. Skin (A); periople (B); epidermis lining the coronary groove (C); stratum externum (D); coronary corium (E); stratum medium (F); hyaline cartilage (G). Trichrome.* ×*3.*

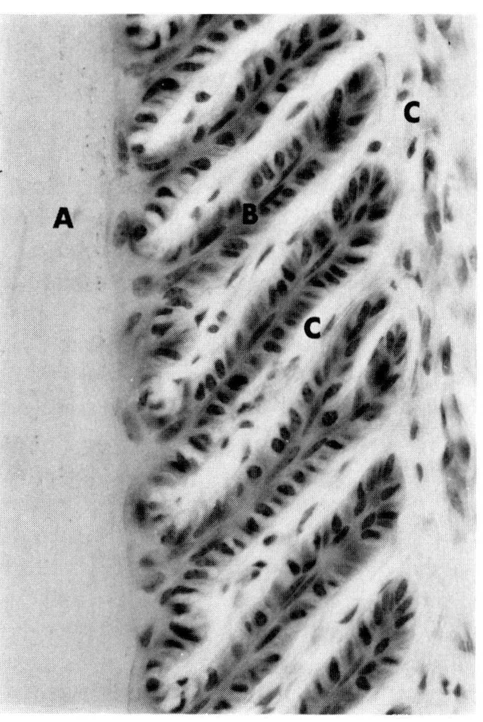

Fig. 16–57. *Secondary laminae, hoof, horse. See area marked in Figure 16–54. Primary lamina of the wall (A); secondary lamina (B); laminar corium (C). H & E.* ×*435. (From Dellmann, H.-D.: Veterinary Histology: An Outline Text-Atlas. Philadelphia, Lea & Febiger, 1971.)*

rangement. The cross-sectional profiles of the tubules may be circular, oval, or wedge-shaped, and have a central region of loose elements similar to the medulla of the hair shaft (Fig. 16–55). The cortex of the tubule has three zones. The inner zone contains keratinized cells oriented around the medulla in fairly tight coils; those of the middle zone form loose spirals, and the outer zone is another layer of tight coils. This coiled, springlike arrangement of the cells of tubular horn helps to dampen the compression of the hoof when it strikes a hard surface. The intertubular horn fills the spaces between the tubular horn.

The tubular and intertubular horn of the stratum medium is produced by the stratum germinativum of the epidermis lining the coronary groove (Fig. 16–56[C]). This epidermis covers the coronary corium, a bed of vascularized connective tissue with long, well-developed papillae that extend for a short distance into the medulla of the tubular horn of the stratum medium. The germinal cells covering the tips of the papillae give rise to loose cellular components of the medulla of the tubule, whereas those over the sides and base of the papillae proliferate to form the horny cells of the cortex. The germinal cells covering the interpapillary part of the coronary corium give rise to the intertubular horn. The deeper connective tissue of the coronary corium is composed of dense bundles of collagenous connective tissue and numerous large blood vessels.

The *stratum internum* (lamellatum) consists of approximately 600 primary, vertically oriented, keratinized laminae extending inward from the stratum medium with which they are continuous (Fig. 16–54). One hundred to two hundred secondary laminae project at right angles from each primary lamina (Fig. 16–57). These laminae interdigitate with similar laminae of the corium and anchor the keratinized hoof to the underlying sensitive connective tissue. The primary epidermal laminae are part of the stratum corneum (hard keratin) produced by the stratum germinativum located between the proximal ends of the dermal laminae at the deep edge of the coronary groove. The cells keratinize as they move downward at about the same rate as those of the stratum medium. The secondary epidermal laminae are composed of stratum germinativum that is only partially keratinized. The stratum basale of each secondary lamina rests on the connective tissue of each secondary dermal lamina, forming the interdigitation between the two laminae. The central core of each secondary epidermal lamina is composed of stratum spinosum, 1 to 3 cell-layers thick, that attaches to the sides of the primary epidermal lamina (Fig. 16–57). The germinal cells of the secondary laminae multiply throughout the length of the laminae and give rise to the keratinized cells that move downward at the same pace as those of the primary laminae, but at an oblique angle. The interdigitation between the nonpigmented wall laminae with the pigmented tubular and intertubular horn of the sole is referred to as the white zone.

The laminar corium fills the space between the horny laminae of the stratum internum and the bone of the distal phalanx. It is composed of bundles of coarse collagen connective tissue and a massive network of large arteries and veins without valves. This vascular bed helps to dampen the compressive forces from the hard inflexible hoof to the bone of the phalanx.

The sole is composed of tubular and intertubular horn. Its superficial layers are not firmly attached and can be peeled off in the form of small flakes. The corium of the sole bears long papillae whose epidermal covering gives rise to the tubular horn of the sole. It blends with the periosteum of the ventral surface of the distal phalanx.

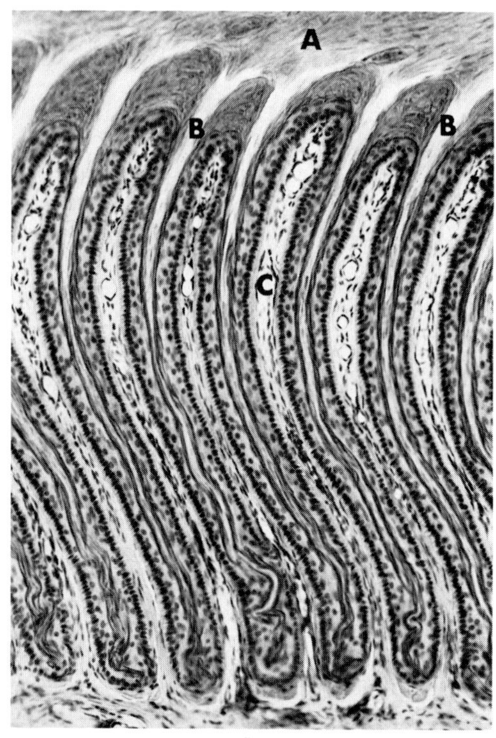

Fig. 16–58. *Stratum internum, hoof, sheep. Stratum medium (A); primary laminae (B); laminar corium with numerous capillaries (C). H & E. ×120.*

The frog is composed of incompletely keratinized tubular and intertubular horn and is therefore somewhat softer than the wall and sole. The corium of the frog is molded to the deep surface and contains small short papillae. The connective tissue blends with the digital cushion, which is a wedge-shaped mass of collagen and elastic connective tissue fibers among masses of fat. Branched coiled merocrine glands occur chiefly in the part that overlies the central ridge of the frog. Their ducts pursue a slightly tortuous course through the corium and pass in a spiraling manner through the epidermis of the frog.

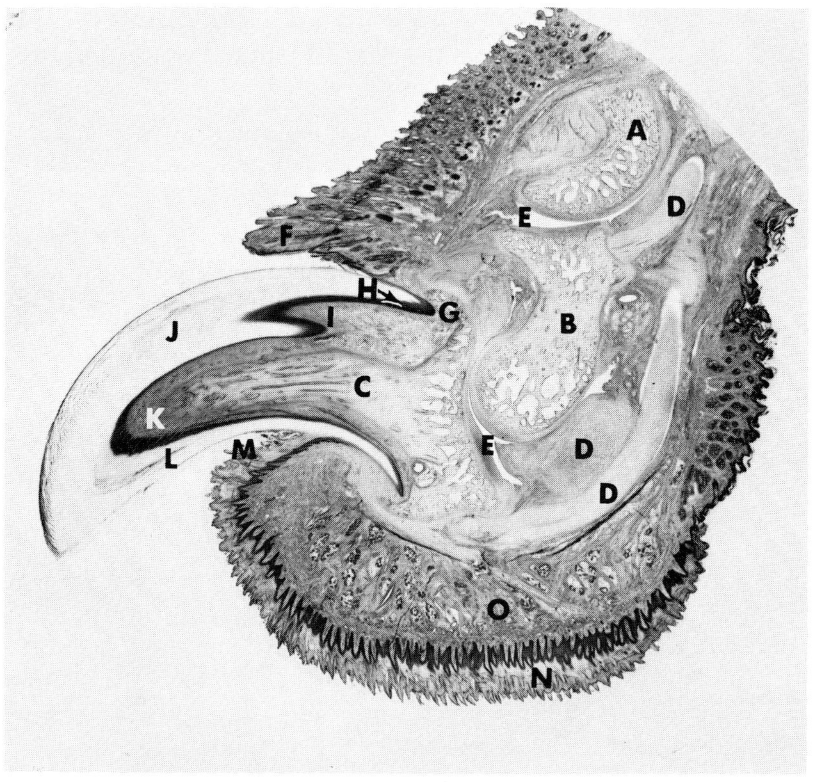

Fig. 16–59. *Claw, dog. Proximal phalanx (A); middle phalanx (B); distal phalanx (C); tendons (D); joint cavities with accompanying joint capsules and articular cartilages (E); fold of skin overlying claw (F); ungual crest (G); nonkeratinized epidermal layers of the claw (H); dorsal ridge (I); stratum corneum of the claw epidermis (J); dermis (K); sole (L); limiting furrow between the sole and digital pad (M); epidermis of the digital pad (N); dermis of the digital pads with clusters of coiled merocrine sweat glands and fat (O). H & E. ×4. (From Adam, W.S., Calhoun, M.L., Smith, E.M., and Stinson, A.W.: Microscopic Anatomy of the Dog: A Photographic Atlas. Springfield, Ill., Charles C Thomas, 1970.)*

Ruminant and Swine Hoofs

The digital organs of ruminants and pigs are similar to those of the horse, with a few exceptions. The stratum internum and corresponding laminar corium do not possess the secondary laminae characteristic of the horse (Fig. 16–58). The sole consists of a narrow rim next to the wall and is histologically similar to that of the horse. There is no frog, but a prominent bulb of soft thin horn is continuous with the skin and makes up a large part of the ventral surface of the hoof.

Claw

The claws of dogs and cats are shields of hard keratin, curved in both directions, which cover the distal phalanges. They consist of a wall and sole (Fig. 16–59).

The *wall* or *claw plate* covers the coronary corium and the wall corium. It is thickest in the area of the dorsal ridge and gradually thins out along the side. Its thin ventral margins extend beyond the junction of the wall with the sole. The stratum spinosum in the dorsal ridge region is thicker than along the sides. The inner surface of the epidermis at the margin of the dorsal ridge has a few rudimentary laminae, but these do not have the strong attachment function of those of the horse and ruminants.

The epidermis of the *sole* is thick and produces a softer, more flaky form of keratin than that of the wall. A stratum granulosum and a stratum lucidum are present.

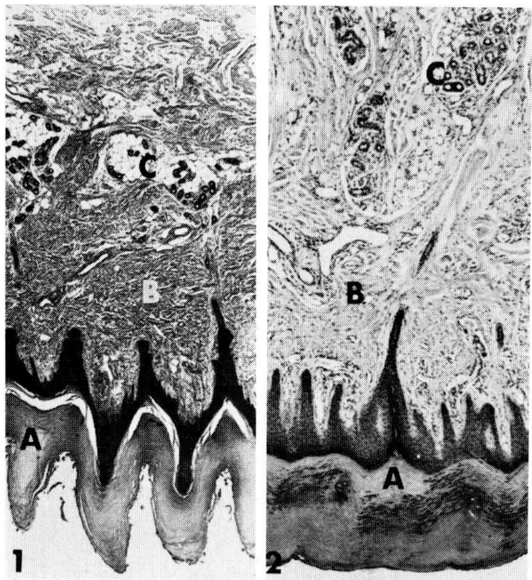

Fig. 16–60. *1, Foot pad, dog. 2, Foot pad, cat. The horny epidermis (A) is rough in the dog and smooth in the cat. The dermis (B) is papillated and contains coiled merocrine sweat glands and fat (C). H & E. ×20. (1, From Adam, W.S., Calhoun, M.L., Smith, E.M., and Stinson, A.W.: Microscopic Anatomy of the Dog: A Photographic Atlas. Springfield, Ill., Charles C Thomas, 1970. 2, From Strickland, J.H., and Calhoun, M.L.: The integumentary system of the cat. Am J Vet Res 24:1018, 1963.)*

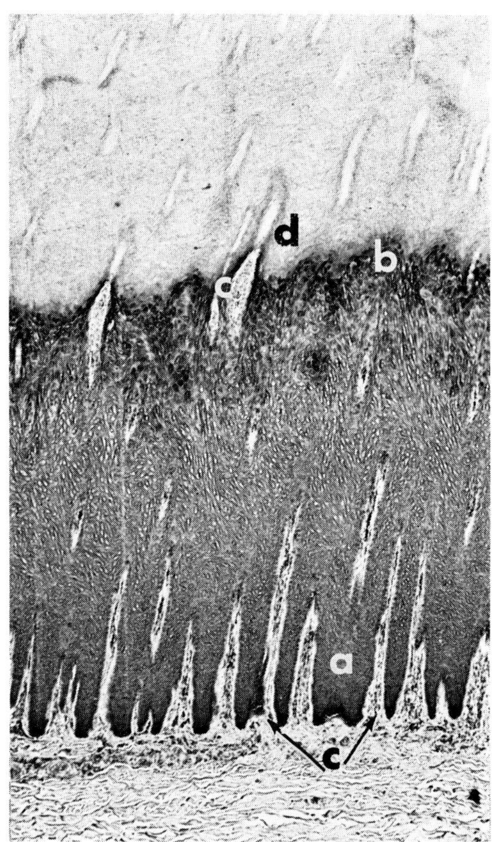

Fig. 16–61. *Chestnut, horse. Epidermal papillae (a); stratum granulosum (b); dermal papillae (c) extending into horny tubules (d). H & E. ×33. (From Talukdar, A.H., Calhoun, M.L.: and Stinson, A.W.: Microscopic anatomy of the skin of the horse. Am J Vet Res 33:2365, 1972.)*

The corium of the claw is composed of dense collagen and elastic connective tissue with numerous blood vessels. It is thickened over the dorsal surface of the distal phalanx, forming the dorsal ridge.

The claw fold is a fold of skin, similar to the periople of the hoof, that covers the claw plate for a short distance on its dorsal and lateral margins. As the plate grows, it carries with it a thin layer of flaky keratin comparable to the stratum externum of the hoof. This is produced by the epidermis of the inner surface of the claw fold.

Digital Pads

The hairless *digital pads* of the dog and cat are similar in structure with the exception of the surface, which is smooth in the cat but roughened by horny conical papillae in the dog (Fig. 16–60). The epidermis is the thickest of any in the entire skin of both species, and contains all the layers, including a stratum lucidum. The dermis has prominent dermal papillae that interdigitate with the epidermal pegs. The dermis of both species contains the usual dermal structures. Coiled merocine glands are present in both the dermis and the *digital cushion,* the subcutis. Subcutaneous masses of adipose tissue are separated, and they are enclosed by collagen and elastic fibers. The footpads of the cat are used frequently in physiologic and pharmacologic studies of drug action and sweating.

Chestnut and Ergot

Horny protuberances, the supracarpal and tarsal chestnuts on the medial surface of the limbs and the ergot at the flexion of the fetlocks, are considered to be vestiges of the first, second and fourth digits. They have similar histologic features, both having a thick keratinized epidermal layer composed of horn tubules (Fig. 16–61). The underlying dermis has long highly vascular papillae. Sebaceous glands are well developed around the ergot but sweat glands are absent. Arrector muscles are absent around both structures.

Horn

Horns of ruminant species are composed of a hard, keratinized epidermis, a dermis, and a subcutis, all of which form the covering over the cornual process of the frontal bone.

The epidermis has a thick stratum corneum of hard keratin in the form of tubular and intertubular horn. A thin, outermost layer of soft keratin, the epikeras, forms at the root of the horn and extends only a short distance. It becomes flaky and desquamates as horny scales, similar to the stratum externum of the hoofs. The basal layer of the epidermis interdigitates with connective tissue papillae and gives rise to the tubular and intertubular horn. The dermis and hypodermis are beds of well-vascularized connective tissue that fill the space between the epidermis and the periosteum of the bone.

REFERENCES

Budsberg, S.C., and Spurgeon, T.L.: Microscopic anatomy and enzyme histochemistry of the canine anal canal. Zbl Vet Med C Anat Histol Embryol *12*:295, 1983.

Fowler, E.H., and Calhoun, M.L.: The microscopic anatomy of developing fetal pig skin. Am J Vet Res *25*:156, 1964.

Goldsberry, S., and Calhoun, M.L.: The comparative histology of the skin of Hereford and Aberdeen-Angus cattle. Am J Vet Res *20*:61, 1959.

Greer, M.B., and Calhoun, M.L.: The anal sacs of the domestic cat—*Felis domesticus*. Am J Vet Res *27*:773, 1966.

Jenkinson, D.M.: The skin of domestic animals. *In* Comparative Physiology and Pathology of the Skin. Edited by R.J. Rook and G.S. Walton. Philadelphia, F.A. Davis Co., 1965.

Kozlowski, G.P., and Calhoun, M.L.: Microscopic anatomy of the integument of the sheep. Am J Vet Res *30*:1267, 1969.

Marcarian, H.Q., and Calhoun, M.L.: The microscopic anatomy of the integument of the adult swine. Am J Vet Res *27*:765, 1966.

Meyer, W., Neurand, K., and Radke, B.: Collagen fibre arrangement in the skin of the pig. J Anat *134*:139, 1982.

Montagna, W.: The Structure and Function of Skin. New York, Academic Press, Inc., 1962.

Montgomery, I., Jenkinson, D. McE., and Elder, H.Y.: The effects of thermal stimulation on the ultrastructure of the fundus and duct of the equine sweat gland. J Anat *135*:13, 1982.

Sar, M., and Calhoun, M.L.: The microscopic anatomy of the integument of the common American goat. Am J Vet Res *27*:444, 1966.

Silver, I.A.: The anatomy of the mammary gland of the dog and cat. J Small Anim Prac 7:689, 1966.

Smith, J.L., and Calhoun, M.L.: The microscopic anatomy of the integumentum of newborn swine. Am J Vet Res. *25*:165, 1964.

Strickland, J.H., and Calhoun, M.L.: The integumentary system of the cat. Am J Vet Res *24*:1018, 1963.

Stump, J.E.: Anatomy of the normal equine foot, including microscopic features of the laminar region. J Am Vet Med Assoc *151*:1588, 1967.

Talukdar, A.H., Calhoun, M.L., and Stinson, A.W.: Sensory end organs in the upper lip of the horse. Am J Vet Res *31*:1751, 1970.

Talukdar, A.H., Calhoun, M.L., and Stinson, A.W.: Sweat glands of the horse: a histologic study. Am J Vet Res *31*:2179, 1970.

Talukdar, A.H., Calhoun, M.L., and Stinson, A.W.: Specialized vascular structures in the skin of the horse. Am J Vet Res *33*:335, 1972.

Talukdar, A.H., Calhoun, M.L., and Stinson, A.W.: The microscopic anatomy of the skin of the horse. Am J Vet Res *33*:2365, 1972.

Warner, R.L., and McFarland, L.Z.: Integument. *In* The Beagle as an Experimental Dog. Edited by A.C. Anderson. Ames, Iowa, The Iowa State University Press, 1970, p. 126.

Webb, A.J., and Calhoun, M.L.: The microscopic anatomy of the skin of mongrel dogs. Am J Vet Res *15*:274, 1954.

Wolff, K., and Stingl, G.: The Langerhans cell. J Invest Dermatol *80*:17 (Suppl.) 1983.

17

Eye

H.-DIETER DELLMANN
LINDA L. COLLIER

The eye is located in the bony orbit along with extraocular muscles, ligaments, adipose tissue, blood vessels, nerves, and glands. The lacrimal apparatus, the eyelids, and the third eyelid provide protection to the eye. The globe consists of three tunics that enclose compartments containing refractive media.

The three tunics of the eye are (Fig. 17–1): (1) *the outer,* or *fibrous, tunic* (tunica fibrosa bulbi), which is in turn subdivided into (a) the sclera, the white tough posterior portion of the globe, and (b) the cornea, the transparent portion of the fibrous tunic, which bulges slightly in the center of the rostral pole of the eye; (2) *the middle,* or *vascular, tunic* (tunica vasculosa bulbi), referred to as the uveal tract, composed of (a) the choroid, (b) the ciliary body, and (c) the iris; and (3) *the inner,* or *neuroepithelial, tunic of the eye* (tunica interna bulbi) with (a) an optic portion, the retina, containing the sensory receptors and (b) a blind portion that is epithelial in nature and covers the ciliary body and the posterior surface of the iris.

The globe encloses several compartments that contain refractive media. The anterior compartment is filled with aqueous humor and is located between the cornea and the vitreous body. It is further subdivided into (1) the anterior chamber (camera anterior bulbi) located between the cornea and the iris and (2) the posterior chamber (camera posterior bulbi) located between the iris and the vitreous body. The posterior compartment (camera vitrea bulbi) of the eye, located between the lens and the retina, is filled with the vitreous body.

TUNICA FIBROSA

Sclera

The sclera is a white, tough layer of dense irregular connective tissue that protects the eye and maintains its form (shape). Thickness of the sclera varies in different parts of the eye and among species. Bundles of collagen fibers containing a few elastic fibers and elongated fibroblasts, as well as melanocytes in some areas, are arranged parallel to the surface of the globe. These bundles are intricately interwoven and arranged predominantly in an equatorial direction near the junction between sclera and cornea, the so-called limbus, and around the optic nerve. In the other portions of the eye, meridional bundles pre-

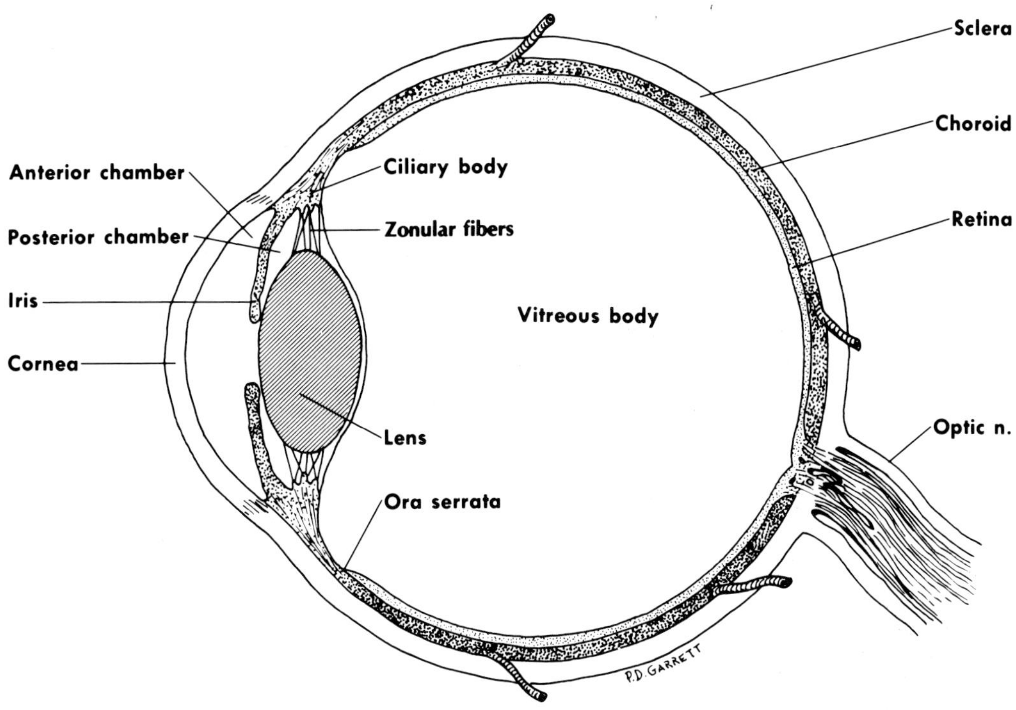

Fig. 17–1. *Schematic drawing of a longitudinal section through the eye.*

dominate. In the layer of the sclera adjacent to the choroid, elastic fibers predominate and fibroblasts and melanocytes are more numerous; this layer is referred to as the *lamina fusca sclerae.*

A firm attachment to the sclera is provided for the tendons of the extrinsic eye muscles through the interweaving of tendon and scleral fibers. The optic nerve leaves the eye through numerous perforations in a disklike area referred to as the *area cribrosa sclerae.*

Cornea

The transparent cornea is a convex-concave lens, thicker at the center than at the periphery, and with a smaller radius of curvature centrally than peripherally. Because it also has a smaller radius of curvature than the sclera, it is more curved than the sclera. The normal cornea is completely devoid of blood vessels.

The cornea is composed of five layers: (1) the anterior epithelium, (2) subepithelial basement membrane, (3) substantia propria, or stroma, (4) posterior limiting membrane (Descemet's membrane), and (5) posterior epithelium (corneal endothelium).

ANTERIOR EPITHELIUM. The corneal epithelium is stratified nonkeratinized squamous, between 4 and 12 layers in thickness (Fig. 17–2). The epithelial cells are tightly packed, interdigitate profusely, and adhere through numerous desmosomes. They contain abundant microfilaments, little rER, and a small Golgi complex. The basal cell layers are rich in glycogen. The numerous microvilli on the surface of the superficial cells probably function to retain the tear film on the corneal surface. Numerous free nerve endings are present among the epithelial cells. The regenerative capability of the corneal epithelium is pronounced and, together with cell movements, assures a rapid return to normal of injured epithelium. An intact epithelium is

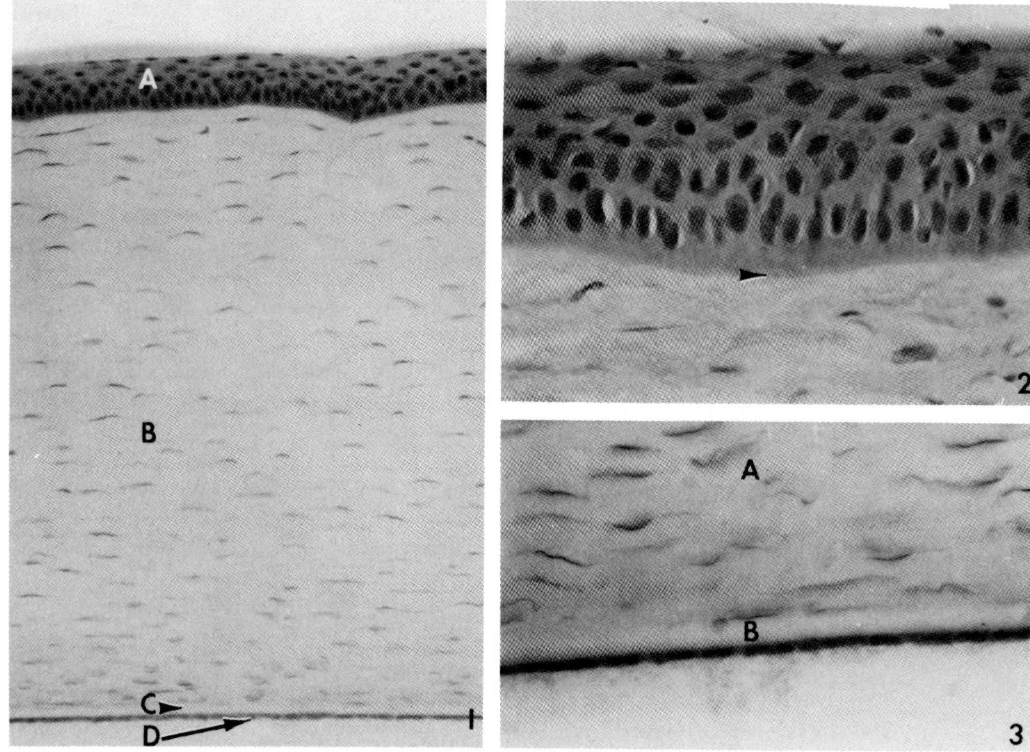

Fig. 17–2. *Cornea, dog. 1, Anterior epithelium (A); substantia propria (B); posterior limiting membrane (C); corneal endothelium (D). H & E. ×176. 2, The corneal stratified squamous epithelium is separated from the substantia propria by a subepithelial basement membrane (arrow). H & E. ×435. 3, Collagen fibers and fibrocytes are in the substantia propria (A), followed by the caudal limiting membrane (B) and the corneal endothelium. H & E. ×435.*

necessary for maintenance of corneal transparency.

SUBEPITHELIAL BASEMENT MEMBRANE. The subepithelial basement membrane consists of a basal lamina and an underlying layer of reticular fibers. Frequently, this layer can be distinguished with the light microscope (Fig. 17–2). It should not be confused with the anterior limiting lamina (Bowman's membrane), a modified outermost layer of the substantia propria, which is present only in primates.

SUBSTANTIA PROPRIA. The corneal propria, or stroma, consists of a varying number (about 100 in the cat) of collagen fiber layers or lamellae (Fig. 17–2). Within one layer the fibers are always parallel with the corneal surface; in successive layers the fibers cross each other at right angles. Adjacent lamellae are held together firmly by fibers that deviate from their parallel course. Occasional elastic fibers are observed at the periphery of the cornea.

The predominating cell type of the corneal substantia propria is the fibroblast, located mainly between the collagen layers rather than within them. These cells are elongated and branched, with little cytoplasm (Fig. 17–2). Toward the limbus, other cells such as histiocytes are present.

Cells and fibers are embedded in the amorphous ground substance that stains metachromatically owing to the presence of sulfated glycosaminoglycans (chondroitin sulfate, keratan sulfate). The ground substance plays an essential role in the transparency of the cornea by maintaining an optimal degree of hydration; excessive water content causes opacification of the cornea.

POSTERIOR LIMITING LAMINA. With the light microscope (H & E–stained preparations), the posterior limiting lamina appears as a highly refractile, thick amorphous layer that gives a positive PAS reaction and stains with dyes specific for elastic fibers (Fig. 17–2). However, at the fine-structural level, the lamina consists only of collagen fibrils that lack the characteristic periodicity and are arranged in a regular, hexagonal array. In the vicinity of the corneal endothelium, the lamina consists only of basal lamina material.

CORNEAL ENDOTHELIUM. A single layer of flat hexagonal cells covers the caudal surface of the cornea (Fig. 17–2). The cells interdigitate heavily and contain numerous mitochondria and pinocytotic vesicles. The endothelium functions in the maintenance of the transparency of the cornea; indeed, defects in the endothelium cause edema and opacification of the cornea, which disappear rapidly after regeneration of the endothelium. Endothelial regeneration occurs through increased mitosis in the vicinity of the wound. The regenerative ability appears to vary with species and the age of the animal.

Corneoscleral Junction (Limbus)

At the junction between sclera and cornea, there is a slight rostral lapping of the sclera over the cornea. The corneal epithelium gradually changes into conjunctival epithelium, which rests on a propria of loose connective tissue. The characteristically layered collagen fibers of the substantia propria assume a more irregular arrangement, become associated with elastic fibers, and are continuous with the equatorial bundles of the sclera. The posterior limiting lamina splits and is continuous with the connective tissue trabeculae of the corneoscleral trabeculae. The corneal endothelial cells become flatter and larger and surround these trabeculae.

The only blood vessels supplying the cornea are located at the level of the limbus. The corneal nerves originate from a marginal dense nerve fiber plexus at the same level, or from the ciliary plexus of the vascular tunic.

TUNICA VASCULOSA

The tunica vasculosa, or uveal tract, comprises three portions: the choroid, the ciliary body, and the mesodermal components of the iris.

Choroid

The choroid is a thick, highly vascularized layer that is continuous with the ciliary body stroma anteriorly and extends posteriorly around the globe. The ora serrata (junction between retina and ciliary epithelium) overlies the junction between choroid and ciliary body. The outer side of the choroid is connected with the sclera; the inner side is adjacent and intimately attached to the pigmented epithelium of the retina. The choroid is subdivided into five layers as follows.

SUPRACHOROID LAYER. The suprachoroid layer, the most peripheral layer (see Fig. 17–11) of the choroid, is loosely structured, consisting of bundles of collagen and some elastic fibers. Toward the sclera these bundles assume an oblique course, are separated by numerous spaces, the perichoroidal spaces, and are continuous with the connective tissue of the sclera. The cell population of this layer consists of fibroblasts, numerous flat melanocytes, and occasional macrophages.

VESSEL LAYER. Numerous large arteries and veins, separated by a stroma, similar to that of the suprachoroid, make up this layer (see Fig. 17–11).

TAPETUM LUCIDUM. The tapetum lucidum is a light-reflecting layer, supposedly increasing light perception under conditions of poor illumination. The tapetum is not present throughout the choroid but is located mainly in the dorsal half of the fundus of the eye. In herbivores the tapetum is fibrous, consisting of intermingling collagen fibers and a few fibroblasts. In carnivores the tapetum consists of a varying number of layers of flat polygonal cells that appear bricklike in cross section (Figs. 17–3 and 17–8). The thickness of the tapetum varies, being multilayered at its center (up to 15 cell-layers thick in the dog and 35 in the cat) and thinning to a single cell at its periphery. The tapetal cells are packed with bundles of parallel small rods, all of which are oriented with their long axes parallel to the retinal surface. In the cat, the rods may be modified melanosomes, and the tapetal cells at the outer periphery (next to the sclera) contain both rods and normally shaped melanosomes. Zinc is associated with the rods in both dogs and cats and may contribute to the reflection of light. Diffraction of light as a result of the spatial orientation of the rods (or of the collagen fibrils in herbivores) is probably responsible for producing the light reflection of the tapetum. In swine, the tapetum is absent.

CHORIOCAPILLARY LAYER. The choriocapillary layer (lamina choroidocapillaris) is a dense network of capillaries immediately adjacent to the pigmented epithelial layer of the retina (see Figs. 17–8, 17–9, 17–10, and 17–11). The wide capillaries often deeply indent these cells and are thus intimately related to them. Furthermore, the endothelium is fenestrated, endothelial nuclei and pericytes are located only toward the choroidal side of the capillaries, and the capillary and pigmented epithelial basement membranes are fused (see Figs. 17–9 and 17–10). These features indicate transport from the capillaries to the pigmented epithelium.

BASAL COMPLEX. The basal complex (complexus basalis) is also referred to as Bruch's membrane. It separates the choroid from the retina. There is species variation among domestic animals with respect to the degree of development and thickness of the basal complex. When fully developed, the basal complex consists of five layers: (1) the basement membrane of the retinal pigment epithelium, (2) the inner collagenous zone, (3) the elastic layer, (4) the outer collagenous zone, and (5) the basement membrane of the choriocapillary layer. In the area over the cellular tapetum, the basement membranes of the retinal pigment epithelium and choriocapillaris often fuse, obliterating the other three layers.

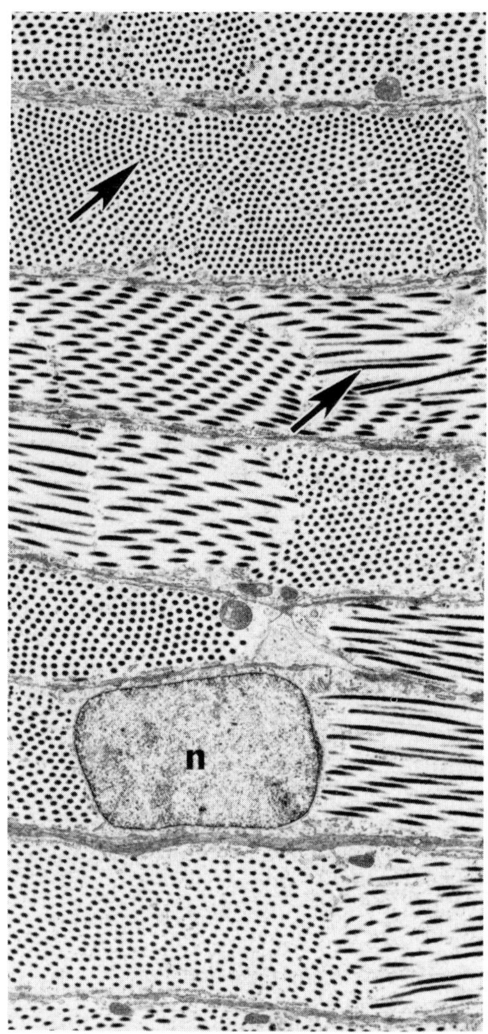

Fig. 17–3. *Tapetum lucidum, cat. Electron micrograph illustrating the bricklike arrangement of cells and bundles of parallel rods (arrows) oriented in various directions with their long axes perpendicular to the angle of incident light and a tapetal cell nucleus (n). ×3780. (Courtesy of E.J. King.)*

Ciliary Body

The ciliary body is the direct rostral continuation of the choroid (Fig. 17–1). It begins caudally at the ora serrata, a sharply outlined dentate border that marks the transition between the optic part (pars optica retinae) and the blind or ciliary part (pars ciliaris retinae) of the retina. Rostrally, it is continuous with the iris and participates in the formation of the trabecular meshwork of the iris angle (see below).

In a longitudinal section through the globe, the ciliary body is a triangle with the narrow base oriented toward the anterior chamber and the iris, and with the narrow angle gradually merging into the choroid (Fig. 17–1). The caudal outer portion contains the ciliary muscle. The rostral outer and inner portions form a connective tissue plate, the basal plate. Rostrally, the inner surface is differentiated into the ciliary processes, which protrude into the posterior chamber. This region is the ciliary crown (corona ciliaris), also called pars plicata. The innermost portion, within the ciliary processes, is a highly vascularized connective tissue. Caudally, the ciliary body is flat and smooth and is referred to as the pars plana or orbiculus ciliaris.

Because of the close topographic and functional relationship between the ciliary body and the pars ciliaris retinae, these two structures will be discussed together. The outermost layer of the ciliary body is merely a continuation of the suprachoroid layer of the choroid. Adjacent to it are the muscle bundles of the *ciliary muscle* (see Fig. 17–7). Usually three predominant fiber directions are distinguishable. The outermost fibers are the meridional fibers that originate from the substantia propria of the cornea, the adjacent connective tissue of the trabecular meshwork of the iris angle and the sclera. They are attached by elastic tendons to the basal complex of the choroid. These muscle fibers predominate in the temporal portion of the globe in the pig. They make up practically the entire muscle in carnivores. In other domestic mammals, the main portion of the ciliary muscle consists of meridional fibers in the posterior portion of the ciliary body that are rostrally and peripherally continuous with circular fibers located partially within the sclera. Radiate fibers have the same origin as meridional fibers; they are located inside these fibers and radiate into the circular fibers.

Circular fibers are less numerous than meridional fibers. However, they predominate in the nasal portion of the ciliary body, where in the pig they are the only existing fibers.

The *vessel layer* of the ciliary body is a continuation of the same layer of the choroid. Veins are predominant and are interspersed with some capillaries. Some arteries are located in the periphery. This layer extends as a dense network of capillaries into the ciliary processes. The meshes of this network are filled with loose connective tissue (Fig. 17–7). The basal plate is a moderately dense, irregular connective tissue.

The basal complex of the choroid continues into the ciliary body. However, it gradually disappears toward the rostral third of the ciliary body.

The ciliary body is covered by two layers of cuboidal epithelial cells of neuroepithelial origin. The *pigmented epithelial layer* is continuous with the pigmented epithelium of the retina. It consists of heavily pigmented, simple cuboidal epithelium (Fig. 17–4) on a basement membrane next to the stroma. These cells have deep basal invaginations of the plasma membrane. The apical surface of the pigmented and the adjacent nonpigmented epithelial layers are connected through fingerlike processes and junctional complexes.

The inner *nonpigmented epithelial layer* consists of cuboidal or columnar cells (Fig. 17–4) with a basal lamina, continuous with the inner limiting membrane of the retina, that separates it from the posterior chamber. The basal portions of the cells thus face

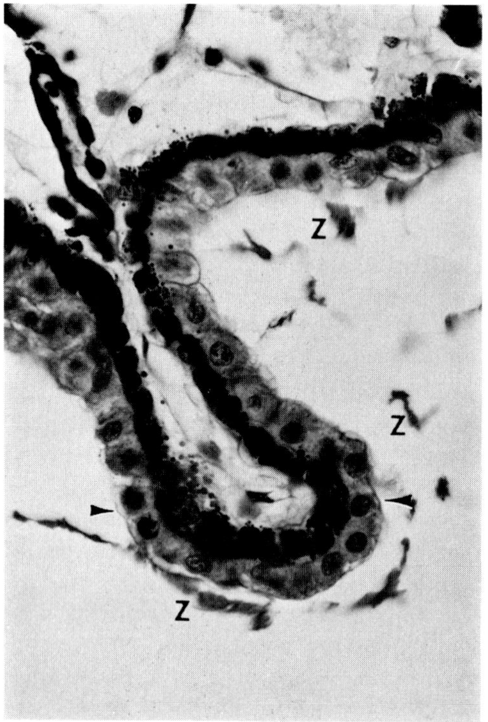

Fig. 17–4. *Ciliary process, dog. Notice the pigmented and nonpigmented epithelial layers, the ciliary inner limiting membrane (arrows) and remnants of zonular fibers (Z). Masson's trichrome. ×435.*

the posterior chamber. They possess numerous deep plasmalemmal invaginations and associated mitochondria, and well-developed rER and Golgi complexes are present in the cell apices. Gap junctions occur not only between adjacent epithelial cells within one layer, but also between the cell apices of the two layers. These structural characteristics are those of actively transporting epithelia and suggest a role in the transport of aqueous humor. This is a thin, clear fluid similar to blood plasma, though its composition is somewhat different. It has a considerably lower protein content. Elaborated by the capillaries of the ciliary processes and their connective tissue cells, the aqueous humor is transported via the epithelial layers into the posterior chamber. This transport is selective in that certain molecules are excluded from transepithelial passage.

The nonpigmented epithelial cells also give rise to the zonular fibers (Fig. 17–5). The zonular fibers insert into the basal lamina of these cells, which is continuous with the inner limiting membrane of the retina.

Iris

The iris is located rostrally to the lens and separates the anterior and posterior chambers, which communicate through the central opening, the *pupil.* The iris consists of a *stroma* of pigmented, highly vascularized loose connective tissue, the sphincter and dilator muscles, and the posterior (pigmented) epithelium. Toward the anterior chamber, fibroblasts and melanocytes form a discontinuous lining; thus, open communication exists between the anterior chamber and channel-like spaces in the anterior limiting layer, and crypts that often permeate deep into the stroma, especially at the pupillary margin. The *anterior limiting layer* (or anterior border layer) is avascular and differs from the stroma of the iris in that it is particularly rich in proteoglycans and pigment cells (Fig. 17–6). The latter, along with stromal melanocytes, determine the color of the iris. In a blue iris, they are essentially absent, and the light is reflected as blue from the posterior pigmented epithelium if the remainder of the stroma does not contain any pigment cells. More pigment cells in the anterior limiting layer result in a gray color, while a brown iris is due to the presence of many pigmented cells in that layer, as well as in the remainder of the stroma (Fig. 17–6).

The iris stroma consists of regularly arranged, arcuate bundles of collagen fibers that cross each other at wide angles at the periphery of the iris, where the bundles are arranged in an almost equatorial direction. Toward the pupillary margin, the crossing angles become more acute, and the fiber bundles have a more radial arrangement.

Each of the numerous blood vessels of the iris is surrounded by spiral collagen bundles that belong to several different ar-

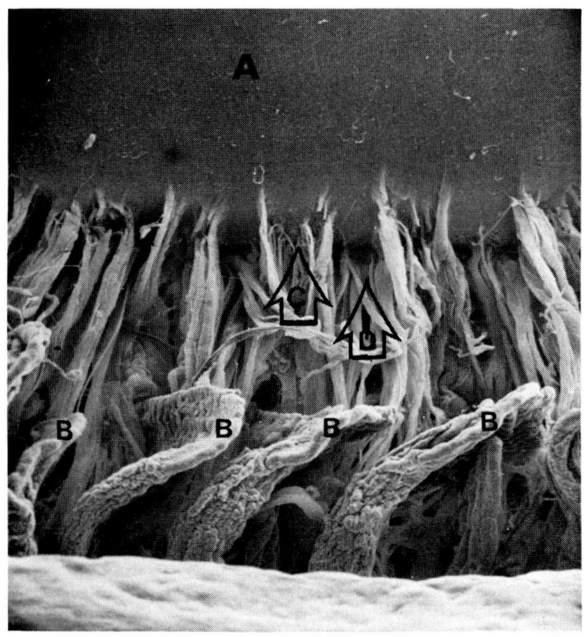

Fig. 17–5. *Scanning electron micrograph, ciliary processes and zonular attachments to the lens in a cat from a caudal view. A, Posterior lens; B, Ciliary process; C, Posterior zonular fibers; D, Anterior zonular fibers. Note the zonular fibers extending from the valleys and producing a clustering of fibers at their lenticular insertion with gaps between bundles. (From Gelatt, K.N.: Textbook of Veterinary Ophthalmology. Philadelphia, Lea & Febiger, 1981, Fig. 2–111.)*

cuate bundles. Consequently, the blood vessels change their position during contraction or dilatation of the iris in accordance with the collagen bundles that protect them against compression and kinking. Fibroblasts, mast cells, histiocytes, and melanocytes represent the majority of the cells in the iris stroma.

The arterial blood vessels originate from the *major arterial circle* (circulus arteriosus major) at the periphery of the iris and radiate, spirally wound, into the stroma, forming capillary loops in the vicinity of the pupillary margin. The veins have a straighter arrangement than the arteries and return to the base of the iris and the ciliary body.

Two muscles are present in the iris that regulate the size of the pupil. They are both of neuroepithelial (pigmented epithelium) origin. The *sphincter muscle* is composed of a network of smooth muscle cells,

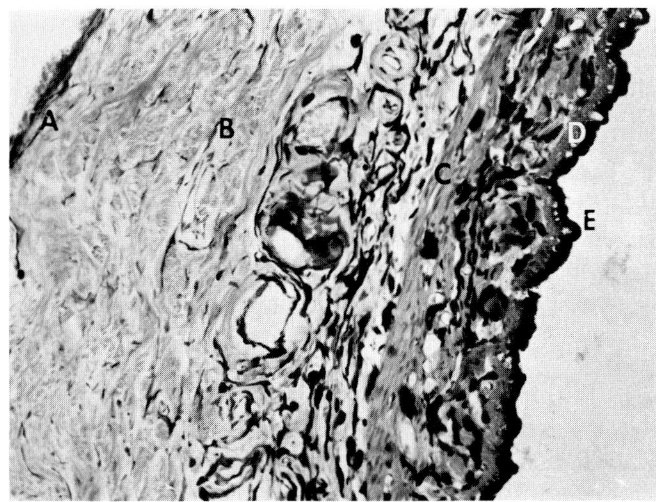

Fig. 17–6. *Iris, dog. Anterior limiting layer (A); stroma (B); sphincter muscle (C); dilator muscle (D); pigmented epithelial layer (E). The iris was sectioned near the pupillary opening, so that the fibers of the sphincter muscle were cut longitudinally. H & E. ×130.*

circularly arranged near the pupillary margin. The fibers cross each other at acute angles laterally and medially in animals with oval pupils, dorsally and ventrally in animals with slitlike pupils. The arches of the collagen bundles of the iris stroma loop through the muscle network, thus enabling the muscle fibers to act on them. The sphincter muscle receives parasympathetic innervation through the oculomotor nerve (nucleus of Edinger-Westphal; synapses in the ciliary ganglion).

The anterior epithelial layer, a continuation of the pigmented epithelial layer of the ciliary body, also forms the *dilator muscle.* The basal portions of the epithelial cells are elongated, branched, and infolded and possess the structural characteristics of smooth muscle cells; the apical portions have the structural features of typical pigmented epithelial cells (myopigmentocytes). The dilator muscle is innervated by sympathetic postganglionic neurons from the superior cervical ganglion.

The posterior pigmented epithelial layer (Fig. 17–6) of the iris is a continuation of the nonpigmented epithelial layer of the ciliary processes, which gradually becomes pigmented toward the base of the iris. Frequently, the epithelial cells are separated by wide intercellular spaces. On its posterior (inner) surface, the epithelium is covered by a basal lamina.

In ungulates, iris granules (granula iridica) are found at the ventral and dorsal pupillary margins. They represent highly vascularized proliferations of the stroma and the pigmented epithelium of the iris. They are cystic formations (small cysts in the horse; large cysts in the goat and sheep) lined by pigmented epithelial cells and associated with a complicated glomus-like capillary network. These granules may function in the production of aqueous humor.

Iris Angle

The periphery of the anterior chamber, at the level of the corneoscleral junction and the attachment of the ciliary body and the base of the iris, is extremely important functionally for the absorption of aqueous humor into the blood that maintains a continual circulation of aqueous humor. Structurally, it is a complicated meshwork, referred to as the iris angle (or iridocorneal, filtration, or drainage angle).

Toward the anterior chamber, bundles of collagen fibers, fibroblasts, and pigment cells, surrounded by flat cells (a continuation of the corneal endothelium), form the trabeculae of the *pectinate ligament* (ligamentum pectinatum), which attaches the base of the iris to the inner peripheral cornea (Fig. 17–7). Through the intertrabecular spaces, the anterior chamber communicates with the *spaces of Fontana,* which lie between endothelium-covered strands of collagen and occasional elastic fibers, fibroblasts, and melanocytes, which make up the uveal trabecular meshwork. The spaces of Fontana in turn are continuous with the *trabecular spaces* of the *corneoscleral trabecular meshwork* (trabeculae corneosclerales). This meshwork is formed by flat strands, or lamellae of fibroblasts, and by fibers, predominantly reticular fibers. Trabecular veins in this meshwork collect the aqueous humor, which then passes through the collecting veins into the *scleral venous plexus* (plexus venosus sclerae) located in the midsclera, posterior to the limbus. A canal of Schlemm, present in the human eye, is not found in domestic mammals.

RETINA

The retina is the sensory portion, also referred to as the pars optica retinae, of the neuroepithelial (optic cup origin) tunic. The nonsensory portion of this tunic, which begins at the ora serrata, covers the ciliary body and the iris as a double epithelial layer.

During embryonic development the optic vesicle, which originates as an outgrowth of the central nervous system (diencephalon), becomes indented to form the

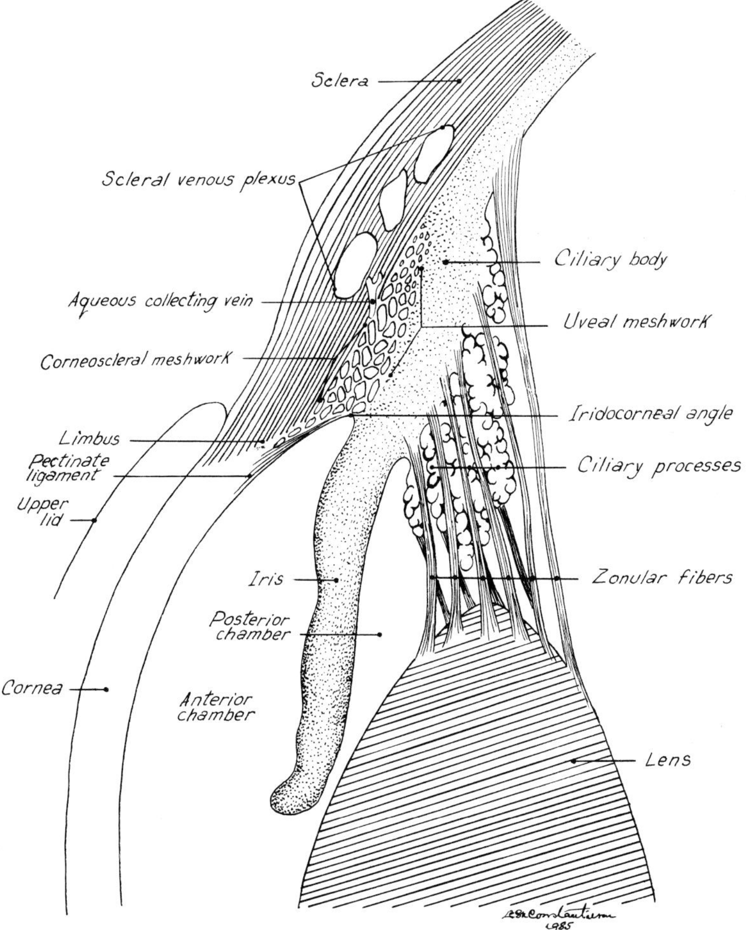

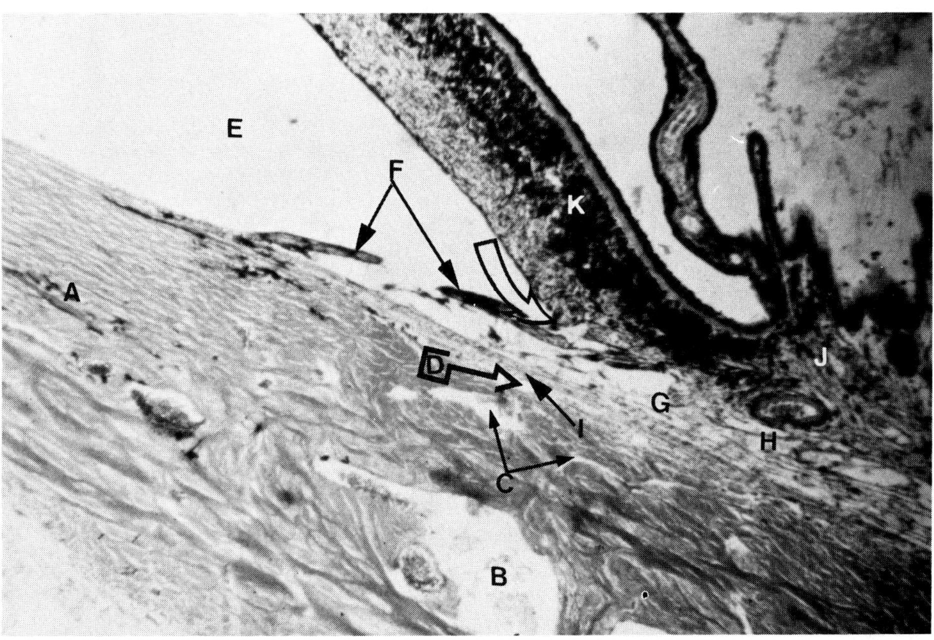

Fig. 17–7. *1, Schematic drawing, and 2, photomicrograph of the iridocorneal angle region of a dog. A, limbus with pigment; B, plexus venosus sclerae; C, collecting veins; D, trabecular veins; E, anterior chamber; F, accessory pectinate ligament (note the usual incomplete sectioning and relatively thin diameter); G, ciliary cleft (partially collapsed); H, uveal trabecular meshwork; I, corneoscleral trabecular meshwork (cribriform ligament); J, ciliary body; K, iris. Note: The pectinate ligament sectioned is part of the posterior row of accessory ligaments arising more posteriorly from the iris base. The primary ligament is not in this section but arises from the small protrusion on the iris (open arrow). (From Gelatt, K.N.: Textbook of Veterinary Ophthalmology. Philadelphia, Lea & Febiger, 1981, Fig. 2–80.)*

optic cup. The outer layer of the posterior part of this cup forms the retinal pigmented epithelium, while the inner layer differentiates into the remaining layers of the retina. The anterior part of the cup becomes the epithelium of the ciliary body and iris. In the normal eye, the cavity of the optic vesicle completely disappears by apposition of the two layers. However, under pathologic conditions and frequently as a consequence of histologic processing, it reappears.

Except at the transition toward the ora serrata and at the optic disk, the retina consists of the following layers (Fig. 17–8; see Fig. 17–11): (1) pigment epithelium, (2) layer of rods and cones, (3) external limiting membrane, (4) outer nuclear layer, (5) outer plexiform layer, (6) inner nuclear layer, (7) inner plexiform layer, (8) ganglion cell layer, (9) optic nerve fiber layer, and (10) internal limiting membrane.

The retinal *pigment epithelium* (RPE) is a simple squamous or cuboidal epithelium resting on a basal lamina (Figs. 17–9 and 17–10). Capillaries of the choriocapillaris frequently deeply indent the RPE cells. The base of the cell is characterized by deep infoldings of the plasma membrane and by the presence of numerous mitochondria. Laterally and apically, zonulae adherentes and occludentes are present. The cytoplasm contains extensive smooth and rough ER and numerous melanin granules. Melanin granules are lacking in the RPE overlying the tapetum lucidum. Tonguelike apical processes extend from the cells to surround the outer segments of the rods (Fig. 17–9). As many as five layers of flat, groovelike, nonpigmented processes surround (at least in the dog) the entire outer segments of the cones (Fig. 17–9).

The functions of the pigment epithelium are complex. They include transport of metabolites from the blood to the rods and cones, phagocytosis with lysosomal degradation and recycling of the shed outer segments of the photoreceptors, and absorption of light by the melanin.

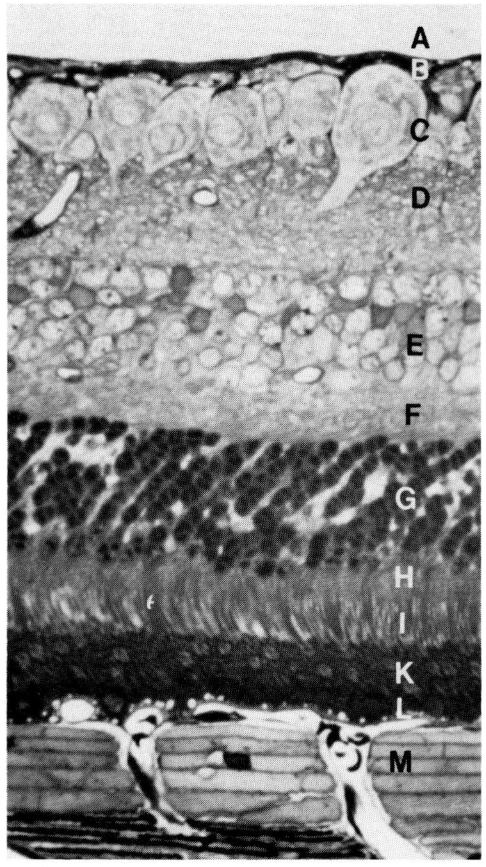

Fig. 17–8. *Semi-thin section through the retina and adjacent layers of the choroid at the level of the area centralis, dog. Vitreous body (A); optic nerve fiber layer (B); ganglion cells (C); inner plexiform layer (D); inner nuclear layer (E); outer plexiform layer (F); outer nuclear layer (G); external limiting membrane (H); inner segments of rods and cones (I); outer segments of rods and cones (K); pigment epithelium and choriocapillaris (L); cellular tapetum lucidum (M). Richardson's stain.* ×*800. (From Hebel, R.: Entwicklung und Struktur der Retina und des Tapetum lucidum des Hundes. In Ergebnisse der Anatomie und Entwicklungsgeschichte 45/2. Berlin, Springer-Verlag, 1971.)*

The outer segments of the photoreceptive *rods* and *cones* (first neuron) are readily distinguished with the light microscope as a layer adjacent to the pigment epithelium (Fig. 17–8). The outer segments consist of stacks of disks surrounded by the cell membrane. The disks are actually flattened membrane spheres, with molecules of visual pigment present in the membranes

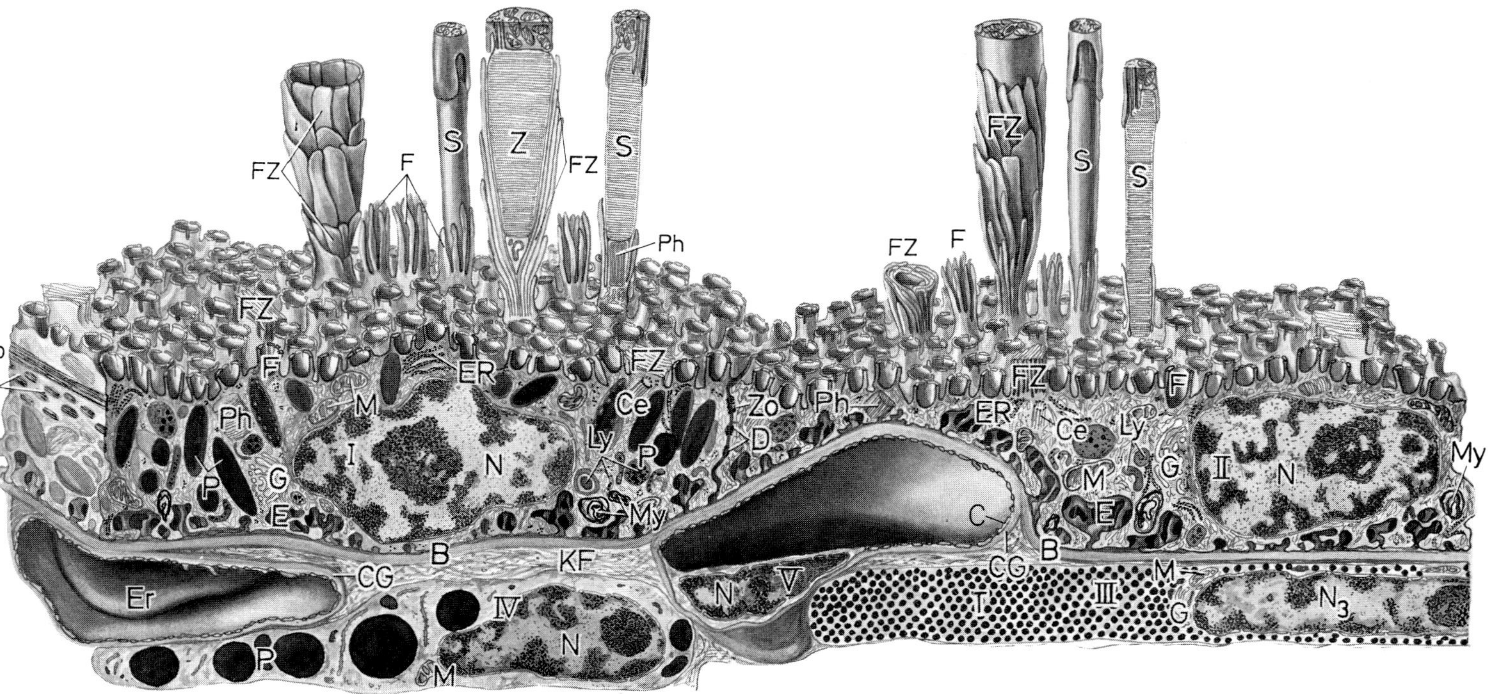

Fig. 17–9. *Three-dimensional schematic representation of the pigment epithelium and portions of adjacent layers. Pigment cell from the pigmented portion of the retina (I); pigment cell at the level of the tapetum (II); cell of the cellular tapetum (III); melanocyte in the choroid (IV); capillary endothelial cell (V); basal lamina of the pigment epithelium (B); fenestrated capillary endothelium (C); centriole (Ce); basal lamina of the capillary (CG); desmosome (D); basal cell invaginations (E); erythrocyte (Er); rough ER (ER); simple pigment cell processes surrounding rod (F); several layers of pigment cell processes surrounding cone (FZ); Golgi complex (G); collagen fibers (KF); lysosomes (Ly); mitochondria (M); myelin figures (dense bodies) (My); nucleus (N); nucleus of III (N_3); pigment granules (P); phagosomes (Ph); rod, outer segment (S); rodlike inclusions in III (T); cone, outer segment (Z); zonula occludens (Zo). (From Hebel, R.: Entwicklung und Struktur der Retina und des Tapetum lucidum des Hundes. In Ergebnisse der Anatomie und Entwicklungsgeschichte 45/2. Berlin, Springer-Verlag, 1971.)*

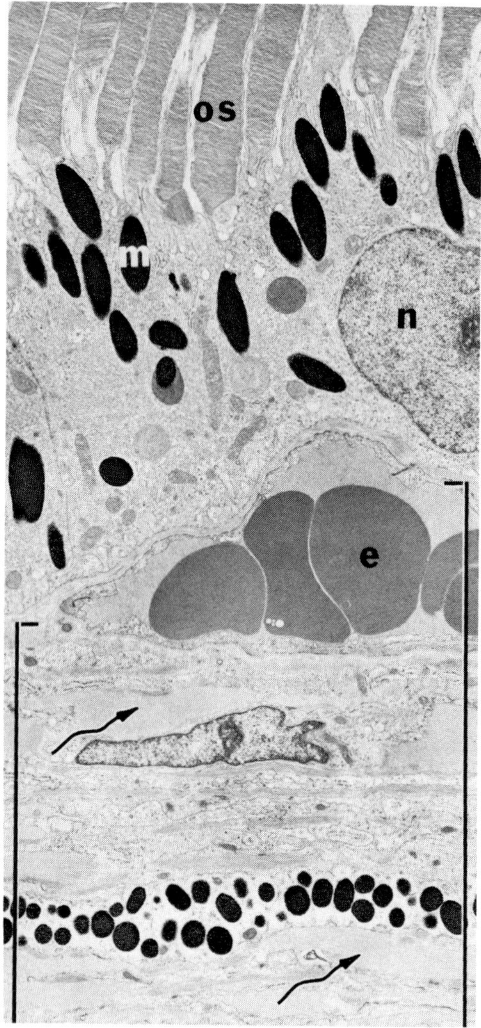

Fig. 17–10. *Electron micrograph, fundus, cat eye, illustrating the photoreceptor outer segments (os); a nucleus (n) and melanosomes (m) of the retinal pigmented epithelium. The inner choroid (brackets) contains a choriocapillary vessel with erythrocytes (e), part of a melanocyte with melanosomes, a fibroblast nucleus, and numerous collagen fibrils (arrows). ×4935. (Courtesy of E.J. King.)*

(Figs. 17–9 and 17–10). Each day, triggered by onset of morning light, short stacks of the oldest disks are shed from the distal ends of the photoreceptors and are subsequently phagocytized by, and degraded in, the RPE. New disks are continually added to the proximal ends of the outer segments, adjacent to the inner segments. Whereas the rods extend to the apical surface of the pigment epithelium, the cones terminate a certain distance from the epithelial surface. Apical processes from the pigment epithelium extend up around the outer segments of both rods and cones. Each outer segment is connected to its inner segment by a cilium. The inner segments contain the basal bodies of the cilia, as well as many mitochondria. The rod cells are responsible for vision in dim light, while the cone cells function in bright light and are responsible for color vision. Thus, animals who are mainly active at night have retinas with fewer cone cells than day-active animals.

The *external limiting membrane* histologically separates the layer of the rod and cone inner segments from the outer nuclear layer. It is not a true membrane, but rather the attachment sites (terminal bars, lacking zonula occludens) joining adjacent photoreceptor and radial glial (Müller's) cells. The radial glial cells' microvilli project peripherally between the inner segments of the rods and cones (Fig. 17–11). The *outer nuclear layer* contains the cell bodies and nuclei of the rods and cones (Fig. 17–8). The *outer plexiform layer* is composed of rod spherules and cone pedicles (the axonal terminations of the photoreceptor cells), the processes of the horizontal cells, and the dendrites of the bipolar cells (Fig. 17–11). The dendrites of rod bipolar cells and horizontal cell processes invaginate rod spherules and form synapses. The cone pedicles synapse with numerous horizontal cell processes and bipolar cells. The photoreceptor synapses contain synaptic vesicles and typical synaptic ribbons.

As many as four (in the dog) layers of nuclei make up the *inner nuclear layer* (Fig. 17–8). Most of the nuclei in the center of this layer belong to the bipolar cells (second neuron). Dendrites of the rod bipolar cell contact several rods, and the axon synapses with amacrine or ganglion cells (Fig. 17–11). The cone bipolar cells are either midget bipolar cells that contact a single cone or flat bipolar cells whose dendrites

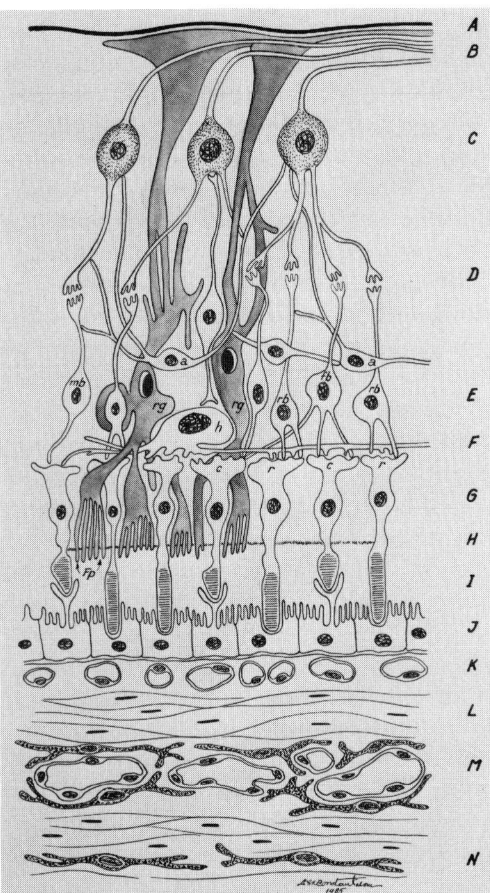

Fig. 17–11. *Schematic drawing of the organization of the retina and choroid. A through J represents retina and K through N represents choroid. Internal limiting membrane (A); nerve fiber layer (B); ganglion cell layer (C); inner plexiform layer (D); inner nuclear layer (E); outer plexiform layer (F); outer nuclear layer (G); level of the external limiting membrane (H); layer of rods and cones (I); pigment epithelium (J); choriocapillaris (K); connective tissue in lieu of the tapetum lucidum (L); vessel layer of the choroid (M); suprachoroid layer (N).*

The rod (r) spherules have synaptic contact with rod bipolar (rb) cells, which synapse with ganglion cells. The cone pedicles (c) have synaptic contacts with midget bipolar cells (mb) (which contact a single cone) and flat bipolar cells (fb), whose dendrites contact several cones, and whose axons then synapse with amacrine (a) and ganglion cells. Horizontal cells (h) contact rod spherules and cone pedicles. Amacrine cells (a) contact the axons of bipolar cells and dendrites of ganglion cells. Radial glial cells (rg) (dark cytoplasm) provide support to the retina, with their cytoplasmic processes extending between and around the other cells, and their foot processes (fp) expanded just under the internal limiting membrane.

contact several cones while their axons synapse with amacrine and ganglion cells. Those nuclei located in the outer portion of this layer belong to horizontal cells, and those located in the inner portion are amacrine cell nuclei. The amacrine cell nuclei are generally characterized by deep invaginations. Their cell processes extend into the inner plexiform layer and establish contact with the dendrites of ganglion cells and with the axons of bipolar cells. Amacrine cells also appear to be interconnected (Fig. 17–11). Between these lie the nuclei of the radial glial cells, readily recognizable because of the dark surrounding cytoplasm (Figs. 17–8 and 17–11). The radial glial cells are elongated, fibrous astrocytes extending between the inner and outer limiting membranes (Fig. 17–11). They provide mechanical support and nutrition to the retina. The *inner plexiform layer* contains cross and longitudinal sections of horizontally arranged fibers. This is the synaptic region between bipolar, amacrine, and ganglion cells. Radial glial cell processes are also present.

The *ganglion cell layer* (third neuron) is composed of large cell bodies. Their axons form a separate layer, the *optic nerve fiber layer* (Figs. 17–8 and 17–11). The axons converge and exit at the optic disk and course through the optic nerve. Dark processes of the radial glial cells cross these layers. Internal to the nerve fiber layer, they flare out and unite to form a continuous layer (Fig. 17–11). On their vitreal surface is a basement membrane that forms the *internal limiting membrane.* Occasional astrocytes, oligodendroglial cells, and microglial cells, identical to those found in other parts of the central nervous system, are present in the retina, especially in the ganglion cell and optic nerve fiber layers.

The retinal vasculature pattern varies greatly among species. In the holangiotic pattern (cat, dog, cow, pig, and sheep), blood vessels occur at the level of the optic nerve fiber layer. Wide capillaries are found at the periphery of the retina, and venules and arterioles are present toward the optic disk (papilla). Numerous capillaries are present in the inner zone of the outer plexiform layer. In the paurangiotic pattern (horse), the vessels are limited to the immediate peripapillary region.

The *area centralis retinae* is a small round or oval area of the retina located dorsally and laterally to the optic disk. It is characterized by an increased number of cones (the outer segments of these cones resemble those of rods), a thickening of the inner plexiform layer, an increased number of ganglion cells, thinning of the optic nerve fiber layer, and, finally, the absence of large blood vessels (Fig. 17–8). This is the area of most acute vision and corresponds to the area of the macula and fovea in primates.

LENS

The lens is a transparent, biconvex structure situated between the iris and the vitreous body and is suspended by the zonular fibers to the ciliary body (Fig. 17–7). It consists of the lens capsule, lens epithelium, and lens fibers.

The lens is entirely surrounded by the *lens capsule* (Fig. 17–12), which consists of several layers of lamellae of collagen fibrils alternating with basal lamina material. It is the basement membrane of the lens epithelium and is much thicker on the anterior lens surface than on the posterior surface.

Beneath the anterior lens capsule is the *lens epithelium* (Fig. 17–12), a layer of simple cuboidal epithelial cells. Their bases face the lens capsule and their apices face the lens fibers. The cells interdigitate heavily, especially at the equator, where they elongate and differentiate into *lens fibers* that make up the bulk of the lens. The elongated lens fibers extend toward the anterior and posterior poles, forming U-shaped cells. The lens grows throughout life by continual differentiation and addition of fibers. During elongation, the nuclei retain their central position within the cell and then move away from the surface of the lens. Fully differentiated lens fibers have lost their nuclei. They are long prismatic fibers, hexagonal in cross section (Fig. 17–12). They interdigitate extensively (especially when fibers from opposite sides of the equator meet to form lens sutures) and are connected through gap junctions and desmosomes. Mature lens fibers are practically devoid of organelles; with

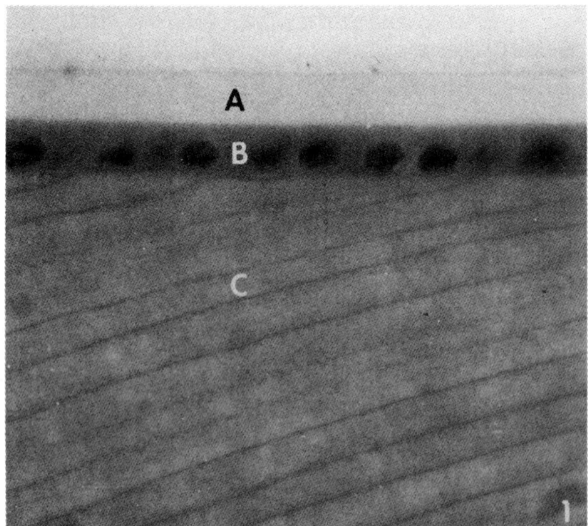

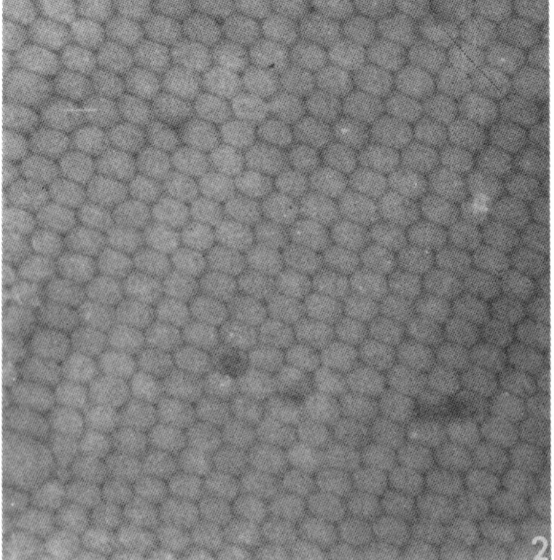

Fig. 17–12. *Lens, dog, 1, Rostral surface with capsule (A), epithelium (B) and fibers (C). 2, Cross section through lens fibers. H & E. ×615.*

the EM, their cytoplasm appears finely granular.

ZONULAR FIBERS

The zonular fibers originate from the ciliary inner limiting membrane, mainly between the ciliary processes and from the pars plana (Figs. 17–4 and 17–5). The fibers are composed of collagen fibrils and are attached to the lens capsule by fusion with its outermost layers anterior and posterior to the equator.

When the ciliary muscle contracts during accommodation, the choroid and the ciliary body are pulled forward with simultaneous relaxation of the zonular fibers and the lens. Consequently, the elastic lens capsule contracts and the lens assumes a more spherical shape, focusing the image on the retina. The ciliary muscle is less well developed in lower mammals than in primates and accommodation plays a lesser role.

VITREOUS BODY

The vitreous body occupies the posterior compartment, the space between the lens and the retina (Fig. 17–1). It is a hydrogel containing 98 to 99% water and adheres intensely to the optic papilla and the ora serrata from which it is separated by the internal limiting membrane. In most domestic mammals it is intimately attached to the posterior lens capsule as well. During cataract surgery (removal of the lens), the posterior lens capsule must remain intact to prevent the vitreous body from collapsing and prolapsing forward.

The vitreous body contains a network of sparse collagen fibrils that are concentrated at the retinal internal limiting membrane, forming the posterior hyaloid membrane, and are concentrated anteriorly, where the layer forms the anterior hyaloid membrane across the anterior face of the vitreous body. The vitreous body also contains hyaluronic acid and acid mucopolysaccharide.

LACRIMAL APPARATUS

The *lacrimal gland* is a compound tubuloacinar or tubuloalveolar gland, predominantly serous in ungulates with the exception of the pig, in which mucous cells predominate (Fig. 17–13). It is serous in the cat and seromucous in the dog. The acinar cells, which frequently contain lipid inclusions, are surrounded by numerous myoepithelial cells (Fig. 17–13). The interstitial connective tissue is composed predominantly of reticular fibers and some collagen fibers, and is rich in lymphocytes, plasma cells, and macrophages.

The intercalated and secretory ducts are lined with simple and stratified cuboidal epithelia, respectively (Fig. 17–13). The lacrimal ductules are lined with stratified cuboidal epithelium. In the pig, the initial portion of the ductules is surrounded by cartilage.

Excess tears accumulate in the *lacrimal lake* (lacus lacrimalis), a medially located widening of the conjunctiva lined by a stratified squamous and columnar epithelium. They enter the lacrimal canaliculi, which are lined with stratified squamous epithelium, through the puncta lacrimalia to reach the lacrimal sac and its continuation, the nasolacrimal duct.

The *nasolacrimal duct* is lined by a stratified columnar epithelium with goblet cells or by transitional epithelium (pig). It begins with an ampullar widening, the lacrimal sac, the propria of which contains a large amount of lymphoreticular tissue in the horse or a cavernous venous plexus. Toward the nasal end of the duct, simple branched tubuloacinar mucous (or seromucous in sheep and goat) glands are present.

SPECIES VARIATIONS

There are many variations in ocular anatomy and histology among species.

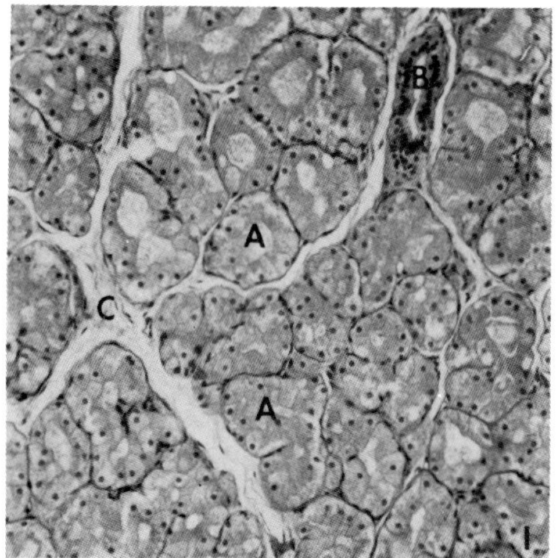

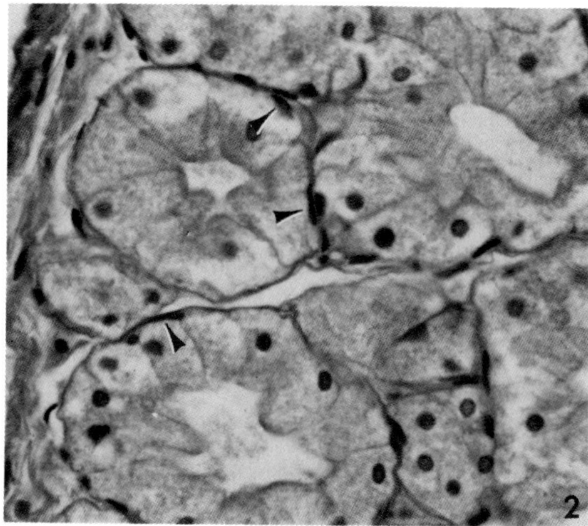

Fig. 17–13. *Lacrimal gland, pig. 1, Acini (A); small secretory duct (B); interlobular connective tissue (C). Trichrome. ×133. 2, The elongated flat nuclei (arrows) belong to myoepithelial cells. Trichrome. ×435.*

Among mammals, differences include size and shape of the globe, corneal size and shape, thickness of cornea and sclera, point of optic nerve exit, shape and orientation of the pupil, melanin granule shape and distribution, degree of development of the ciliary muscle, shape, relative size and color of lens, thickness of various retinal layers, retinal vascular patterns, absence of or location and type of tapetum lucidum, thickness of choroid, types of lacrimal glands, etc.

The differences between mammals and other vertebrates are much more striking. For example, bird eyes vary greatly in shape, and their scleras contain cartilage and, in many species, ossicles. In birds and some other vertebrates, such as snakes and lizards, a highly vascular structure called the pecten extends into the vitreous body from the optic disk region. There are a number of other differences between mammalian eyes and those of other vertebrates. For details of the structure of

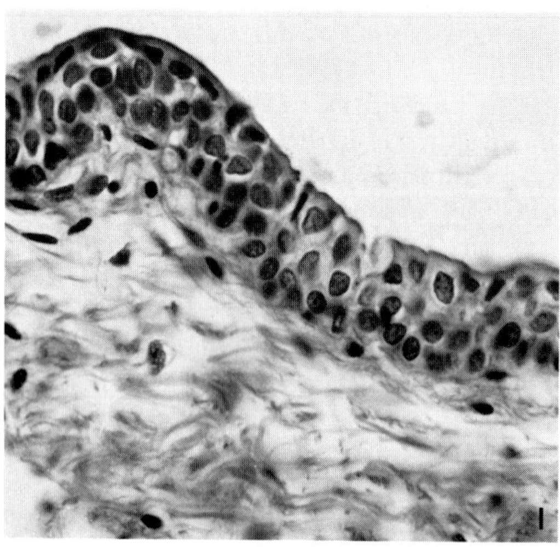

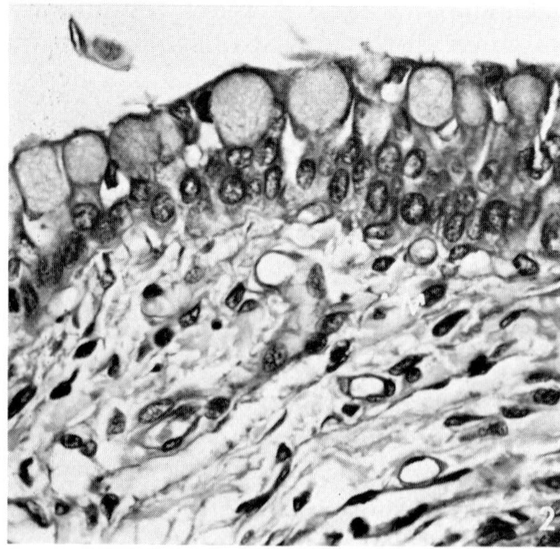

Fig. 17–14. *Conjunctiva. 1, Transitional epithelium, pig. H & E. ×435. 2, Pseudostratified columnar epithelium with many goblet cells. H & E. ×435.*

many nonmammalian eyes and of species differences among mammals, the student is referred to the listed references.

EYELIDS

The eyelids are movable folds of skin that protect the eyes. Their structure is discussed in Chapter 16.

THIRD EYELID

The third eyelid is a conjunctival fold fortified by hyaline (ruminants, dog) or elastic (horse, pig, cat) cartilage. The conjunctiva is a pseudostratified columnar (horse and carnivores) or transitional (pig, ruminants) epithelium with goblet cells (Fig. 17–14). It is based on a propria of highly vascularized loose connective tissue rich in fibrocytes, macrophages, mast cells, lymphocytes and plasma cells. It also may contain numerous lymphatic nodules. Superficial and deep glands are likewise present. The superficial gland of the third eyelid is serous in the horse and cat and seromucous in all other domestic mammals, with a predominantly mucous secretion in the pig. The deep gland of the third eyelid is present only in the pig and secretes a fatty product.

REFERENCES

Duke-Elder, S.: The Eye in Evolution. Vol. 1 of System of Ophthalmology. London, Henry Kimpton, 1958.

Fine, B.S., and Yanoff, M.: Ocular Histology, a Text and Atlas. 2nd Ed. Hagerstown, Maryland, Harper and Row, 1979.

Gelatt, K.N. (ed.): Veterinary Ophthalmology. Philadelphia, Lea & Febiger, 1981, pp. 3–121.

Prince, J.H., Diesem, C.D., Eglitis, I., and Ruskell, G.L.: Anatomy and Histology of the Eye and Orbit in Domestic Animals. Springfield, Illinois, Charles C Thomas, 1960.

Walls, G.L.: The Vertebrate Eye and Its Adaptive Radiation. Bloomfield Hills, Michigan, The Cranbrook Press, 1942.

18

Ear

ESTHER M. BROWN

The ear is composed of three divisions: the external ear, the middle ear, and the internal ear. The external ear, structured for sound collection, is composed of the auricle, or pinna, and the external auditory canal. The middle ear consists of the tympanic membrane, the tympanic cavity, and the three auditory ossicles and their associated muscles and ligaments. It is connected to the nasopharynx by the auditory tube. This air-filled cavity containing the ossicles is primarily for sound conduction. The inner ear, consisting of a membranous labyrinth enclosed within the petrous bone, is structured for both hearing and equilibrium.

EXTERNAL EAR

The microscopic description of the auricle and the external auditory canal is included in the chapter on the integument, p. 397.

MIDDLE EAR

The air-filled tympanic cavity, containing the three ossicles and their muscles and ligaments is lined with simple squamous or simple cuboidal epithelium resting on a thin layer of connective tissue. A few epithelial cells have cilia, particularly those on the floor of the cavity.

Tympanic Membrane

The thin tympanic membrane delimits the external auditory canal from the tympanic cavity (Fig. 18–1). It is covered externally by stratified squamous epithelium and internally by a layer of simple squamous epithelium continuous with that of the tympanic cavity. Between these two epithelial sheets is a connective tissue layer composed of inner circularly and outer radially oriented collagen fibers. Where the manubrium of the malleus attaches to the tympanic membrane the connective tissue is somewhat thicker and contains blood vessels and nerves that course along the manubrium and spread radially. The dorsal portion of the membrane, in which collagen fibers are sparse or even absent, is referred to as the *flaccid part.*

Ossicles

Three small bones, the *malleus, incus,* and *stapes,* traverse the middle ear connecting the tympanic membrane to the membrane of the vestibular (oval) window of the internal ear (Fig. 18–1). The manubrium of

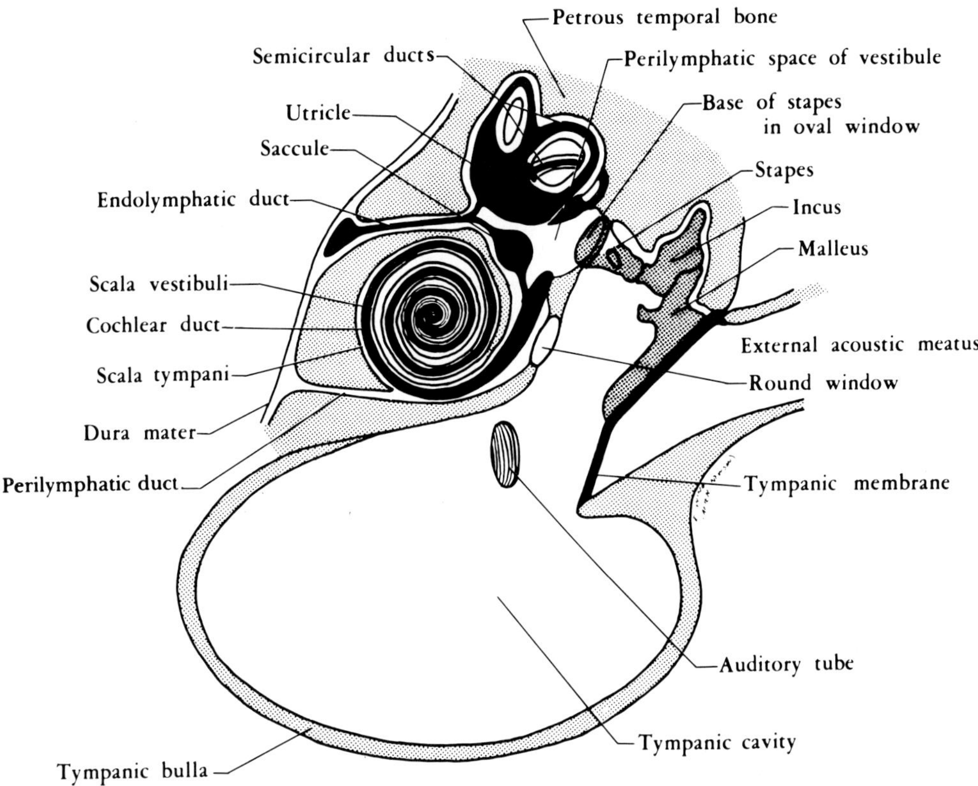

Fig. 18–1. *Diagram of the middle ear cavity (tympanum) and inner ear, dog. (From Jenkins, T.W.: Functional Mammalian Neuroanatomy. Philadelphia, Lea & Febiger, 1972; slightly modified from Getty, R., et al.: Am J Vet Res 17:364, 1956.)*

the malleus is firmly attached to the tympanic membrane, and a little hooklike process on the neck of the malleus serves as an attachment for the tensor tympani muscle tendon. Contraction of this muscle places tension on the tympanic membrane and tends to accentuate high frequencies. The head of the malleus articulates with both the petrous temporal bone and the incus, which, in turn, articulates with the stapes. Fibrous ligaments hold these synovial articulations in place. The footplate of the stapes is held to the vestibular membrane by an annular ligament. The stapedius muscle attaches to the head of the stapes, and contraction of the muscle relieves pressure on the vestibular window by moving the rostral end of the footplate caudolaterally, thus making low frequencies more audible.

Auditory Tube

The auditory tube connects the tympanic cavity to the nasopharynx. It is lined by ciliated pseudostratified columnar epithelium (with goblet cells) resting on loose connective tissue. The tube is surrounded by bone near the tympanum and by an incomplete cartilaginous tube toward the pharynx. The cartilage is hyaline near the bone and contains a gradually increasing number of elastic fibers toward the pharynx. The propria is thin and without glands in the osseous portion and becomes thicker and contains seromucous glands and lymphatic nodules in the cartilaginous part; at the pharyngeal extremity is a tubal tonsil. In the horse, the auditory tube expands ventrally to form the *guttural pouch,* which has the same histologic features as the pharyngeal portion of the tube but lacks a cartilaginous support.

INTERNAL EAR

Bony and Membranous Labyrinth

The inner ear is composed of the *bony labyrinth,* a system of bony canals and cavities within the petrous temporal bone, into which is fitted a similar series of membranous tubes and sacs, the *membranous labyrinth* (Fig. 18–2). Between the bony and membranous labyrinths and connected with the subarachnoid space via the perilymphatic duct is the *perilymphatic space* filled with fluid, *the perilymph* (Fig. 18–2). The membranous canals and sacs that fit into the bony labryinth are filled with *endolymph* and lined with mesothelium. The underlying loose connective tissue is continuous with the mesothelial-covered connective tissue trabeculae that span the perilymphatic space and anchor the membranous labyrinth to the bony wall (Fig. 18–3). The membranous labyrinth has two major divisions. The *vestibular* portion includes the organs of equilibrium, composed of the *semicircular canals,* the *saccule,* and the *utricle.* The *cochlear* portion contains the *spiral organ* of hearing (organ of Corti).

Vestibular Labyrinth

The vestibule is a small oval space adjacent to the medial wall of the tympanic cavity. It communicates rostrally with the cochlea and caudally with the semicircular canals. The medial wall has two depressions in which the membranous utricle (caudodorsal) and the saccule (rostroventral) are housed. These two structures are connected by the *utriculosaccular duct.* The three membranous semicircular canals, anterior, posterior, and lateral, lie at right angles to each other caudally and dorsally to the vestibule, and all communicate with the

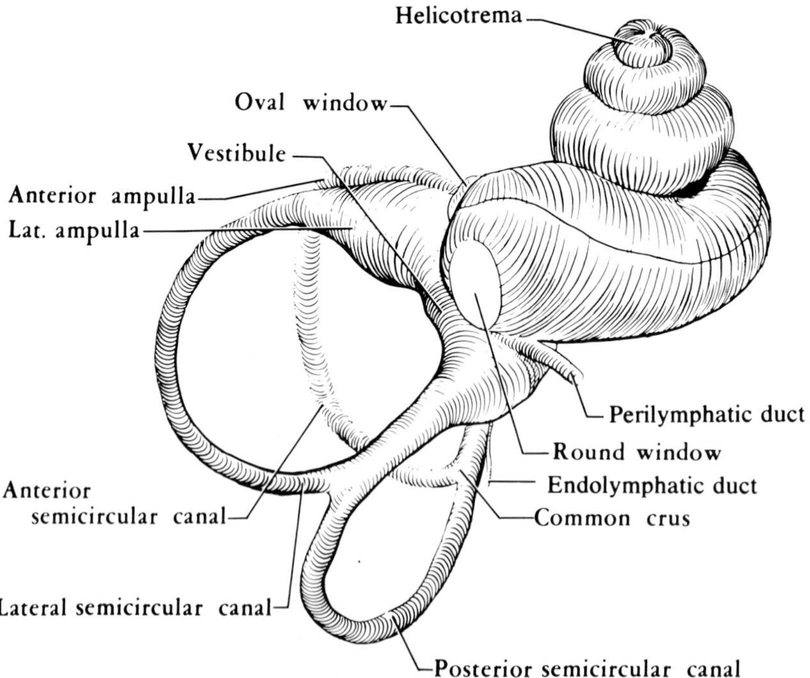

Fig. 18–2. *Ventroposteromedial view of the right osseous labyrinth, dog. (From Jenkins, T.W.: Functional Mammalian Neuroanatomy. Philadelphia, Lea & Febiger, 1972; after Getty, R., et al.: Am J Vet Res 17:364, 1956.)*

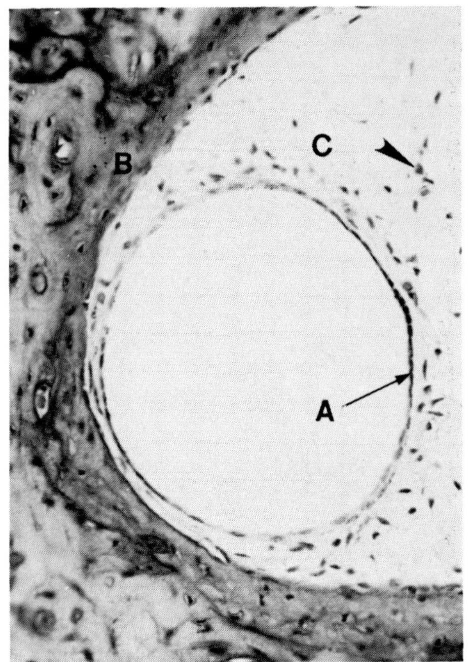

Fig. 18–3. *Semicircular canal, cat. The mesothelium-lined membranous tube (A) lies within the osseous labyrinth (B). The perilymphatic space (C) contains delicate mesothelium-lined connective tissue trabeculae (arrow) H & E. ×400.*

utricle. Each has an ampullated end; the ampullae of the anterior and lateral canals lie near each other and open into the superior end of the utricle, while the ampulla of the posterior canal opens into the inferior part. The opposite ends of the posterior and anterior canals are nonampullated and form a common crus, joining at the midportion of the utricle. The horizontal (lateral) duct also has a nonampullated end, and it, too, empties into the midportion of the utricle.

In certain areas within the vestibular membranous labyrinth, the squamous epithelial cells become tall columnar. These are the neuroepithelial areas of the utricle, saccule, and ampullae of the semicircular canals.

Semicircular Canals

The ampulla of each semicircular canal contains a sense organ sensitive to angular

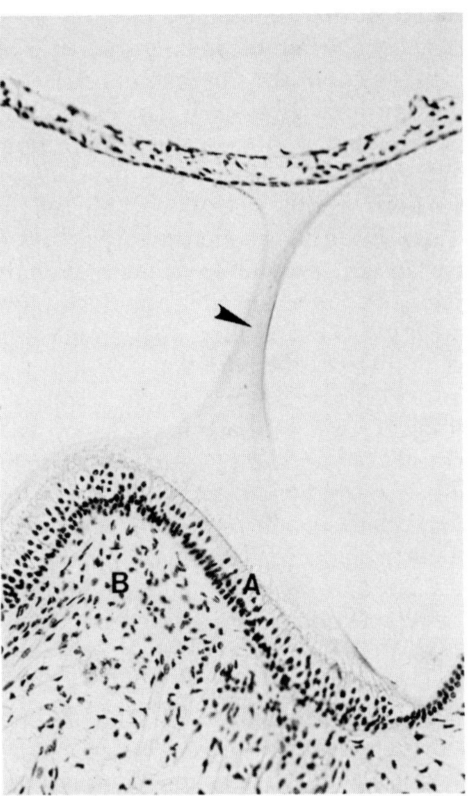

Fig. 18–4. *Crista ampullaris, guinea pig. The sensory and supportive cells (A) and the underlying connective tissue (B) form a crest within the ampulla. The gelatinous cupula (arrow) on top of the epithelium extends across to the opposite wall. H & E. ×400.*

acceleration, called the *crista ampullaris,* a ridge of neuroepithelium resting on a thickened connective tissue and projecting into the ampulla (Fig. 18–4). The neuroepithelium consists of *sensory hair cells* and sustentacular cells. Each hair cell has a cluster of 40 to 80 stereocilia, which are highly modified, long microvilli containing numerous actin filaments anchored in a complex terminal web of actin filaments called the *cuticular plate* located at the cell apex. The stereocilia increase in length progressively toward one pole of the cell. Adjacent to the longest stereocilium is a single *kinocilium* with an apical bulbous swelling and the typical 9 + 2 microtubule structure; however, it is incapable of independent motion. The stereocilia tilt toward the kinocilium so that the longest one touches it and the whole bundle is cone-shaped. This arrangement of the stereocilia and the single kinocilium gives each hair cell a functional polarization toward the kinocilium. Whenever the sensory hairs bend in the direction of the kinocilium, the cell increases its firing rate; conversely, movement in the opposite direction inhibits the excitation. Each hair cell bundle projects into a gel-like structure, the cupula, that extends across the ampulla. Two types of sensory cells are distinguishable ultrastructurally. Type I cells are flask-shaped with a constricted neck; the rounded portion fits into a cup-shaped afferent nerve terminal (nerve chalice), which is in contact with efferent fiber endings containing many vesicles that may have an inhibitory function. The type II cells are cylindric, and the base is innervated by afferent and efferent nerve fibers (Fig. 18–5).

The supporting cells are tall columnar with microvilli. Since they synthesize the matrix of the cupula, the cytoplasm contains numerous vesicles. The cupula is attached to the opposite wall of the ampulla and deflects in the direction of fluid movement, much like an elastic diaphragm. This deflection causes the hair bundles to bend. The motion of the cupula caused by the inertia of the endolymph controls movement of the eyeball, and thus the image of the visual field, by holding it stationary on the retina whenever the head is rotated (nystagmus reflex). Some nerve fibers from the crista give warnings about its position by the frequency of nerve impulses, while others detect changes in speed of rotation. The results of this neural activity help an animal maintain its normal posture during rotary acceleration.

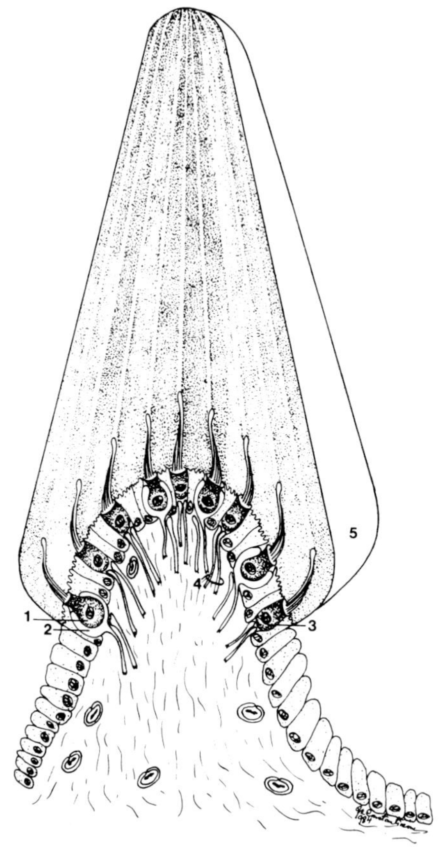

Fig. 18–5. *Crista ampullaris drawing illustrates the type I hair cells (1) surrounded by an afferent nerve chalice (2), type II hair cells (3) and their nerve fibers (4). The remaining cells are supportive. The stereocilia and kinocilium of each sensory cell project into the cupula (5).*

Utricle and Saccule

On the lateral wall of the utricle and on the medial wall of the saccule are regions where the simple squamous epithelium differentiated to form receptor organs, the *macula utricularis* and the *macula saccularis*. The macula saccularis is hook-shaped and is oriented vertically when the head is in the normal position. The macula utricularis is kidney-shaped and is oriented horizontally with the head in normal position. The sensory epithelium of both maculae rests on loose connective tissue containing blood vessels and nerves (Figs. 18–6 and 18–7).

The cells of these receptor organs are essentially the same as those of the crista. Type I and II cells are present along with the sustentacular cells. However, the gelatinous mass, into which the hair bundles penetrate, has calcium carbonate crystals called *statoconia* on the free surface. This

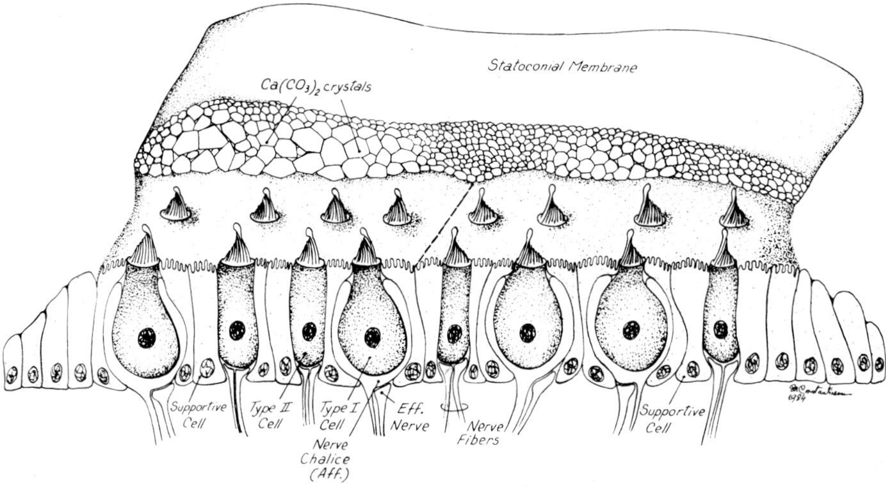

Fig. 18–6. *Macula utricularis drawing illustrates the type I sensory hair cells surrounded by a nerve chalice and the type II sensory cells. The numerous stereocilia (A) and the single kinocilium (B) of each cell form a conelike arrangement; each kinocilium faces the striola, represented here as a broken line. The statoconial membrane has been cut away to better illustrate the hair cells. (Modified and redrawn after H.H. Lindeman. Adv Otorhinolaryngol 20:405, 1973.)*

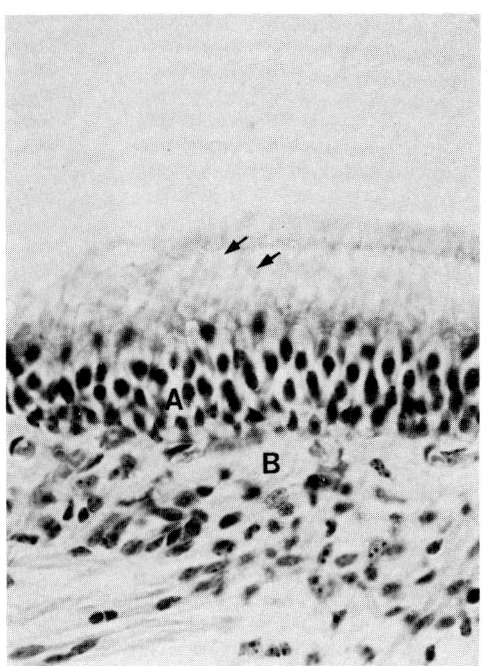

Fig. 18–7. *Macula utricularis, guinea pig. The sensory epithelium and support cells (A) rest on connective tissue (B). The $Ca(CO_3)_2$ crystals (arrows) are visible in the gelatinous membrane. H & E. ×600.*

gel-like mass with the overlying crystals is the *statoconial* (otolithic) *membrane.* Another morphologic difference is that the arrangement of the sensory cells of the macula utricularis is such that the kinocilium of each cell faces toward an arbitrary line, the *striola,* which divides the sensory cell population into two oppositely polarized groups (Fig. 18–6). In the macula saccularis, the hair cell polarization differs in that the kinocilium of each cell faces away from the striola.

Functionally, both maculae are receptors that detect the orientation of the head in a gravitational field and control posture, gait, and equilibrium. Linear acceleration or any change in head position causes a shear motion of the statoconic membrane relative to the hair cells that excites or inhibits the sensory cells, thus helping an animal to maintain a normal posture. Recent studies of the guinea pig inner ear indicate that the macula saccularis also probably functions partially as an acoustic organ. This acoustic activity is believed to be a function of the Type I sensory cells.

Cochlea

The bony cochlea is a rigid protective housing for the membranous cochlea (scala

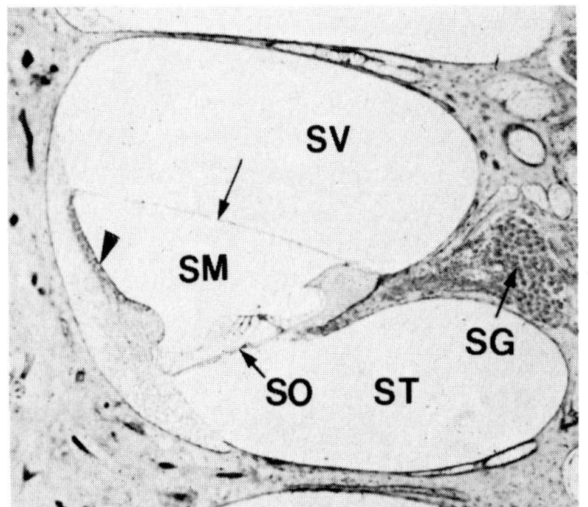

Fig. 18–8. *Cochlea, cat. Cross section through one turn of the cochlea illustrates the scala vestibuli (SV), the scala media (SM), and the scala tympani (ST). The SM is separated from the SV by the vestibular membrane (arrow) and from the ST by the spiral organ (SO) on the basilar membrane. The stria vascularis (arrow head) makes up the third wall of the scala media. The spiral ganglion (SG) is seen at the right in the osseous modiolus. H & E. ×66.*

media) containing the organ of hearing, the spiral organ. The canal of the osseous cochlea makes several turns around an axis of spongy bone, the *modiolus.* The number of coils is species-dependent, as follows: dog—3¼, cat—3, horse—2¼, pig—4, cow—3½, man—2½. The base of the modiolus forms the cranial part of the internal acoustic meatus where the cochlear nerve and blood vessels enter the cochlea. The bony canal is partially divided by a bony projection, the *spiral lamina,* which has two labia; the upper one is the vestibular lip, and the lower one, the tympanic lip.

The membranous cochlea extends into the bony cochlea from the saccule by a small duct and ends as a blind sac at the apex of the cochlea. The triangular-shaped scala media splits the osseous cochlea into two compartments above and below (Fig. 18–8). The dorsal compartment, or *scala vestibuli,* extends from the region of the vestibular window (oval) to the apex of the cochlea, where it becomes confluent with the ventral compartment, the *scala tympani,* in a structure called the *helicotrema.* The scala tympani ends at the *cochlear window* (round). Both the scalae vestibuli and tympani are filled with perilymph, whereas the scala media contains endolymph.

The scala media is separated from the scala vestibuli by the *vestibular membrane* (Reissner) and from the scala tympani by the *basilar membrane.* The basilar membrane is attached to the cochlea by the *spiral ligament* and extends to the other side, where it attaches to the spiral lamina. The vestibular membrane is covered on both sides with simple squamous epithelium interspersed with scant collagen fibers. The basilar membrane varies in width from the base coil, where it is narrowest, to the helicotrema, where it is widest. On the side facing the scala tympani it is lined with simple squamous epithelium and on the surface toward the scala media is the *spiral organ* of hearing. The *stria vascularis* makes up the third wall of the triangular-shaped scala media; it is lined with stratified cuboidal epithelium resting directly (with no basal lamina) on a layer of connective tissue containing numerous capillaries (Fig. 18–9). The epithelium has light-staining basal cells and darker-staining superficial or marginal cells containing many mitochondria. Electron microscopy has led to the identification of intermediate cells (basement cells), but their function is as yet obscure (see Fig. 18–11). The free surface of the marginal cells may have microvilli or may appear smooth, depending on species. Deep plasmalemma infoldings divide the basal cytoplasm into compartments containing numerous mitochondria. The basal cells have many processes that interdigitate with each other and with the marginal cells. These processes also partially surround and isolate each marginal cell from adjacent cells. Unlike in other epithelia, capillaries actually penetrate and course within the marginal cell layer (Fig. 18–9). Electron microscopy studies suggest the existence of an extremely narrow perivascular space between the capillaries and the epithelial cells. In all probability, the endolymph of the scala media is produced by the stria vascularis and regulates the ion

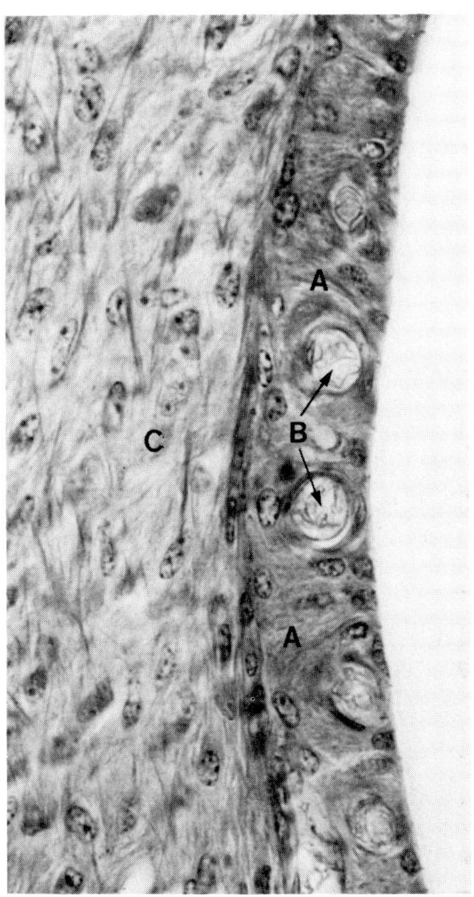

Fig. 18–9. *Stria vascularis, guinea pig. This stratified cuboidal epithelium (A) is traversed by numerous capillaries (B) and rests on loose connective tissue (C) Crossmon's trichrome ×600.*

content of the scala media endolymph, which has high potassium and low sodium levels. This concept is supported by the resemblance of the basal compartmentalization of the marginal cells to other cells involved in ion transport that have a similar basal structure. At the junction of the stria vascularis and the spiral organ, the stratified epithelium changes abruptly to simple cuboidal. This region is called the *spiral prominence* (see Fig. 18–11).

Spiral Organ

The sensory portion of the organ of hearing is a complex structure, most of which rests on the scala media side of the basilar membrane (Figs. 18–10 and 18–11). This receptor organ has three major components: (1) the sensory cells that transform mechanical energy into electrical energy, (2) a supportive structure for the sensory cells, and (3) the afferent and efferent nerve terminals (Fig. 18–11). The cells of the spiral organ, when viewed from the spiral limbus to the spiral ligament, include the border cells, inner and outer pillar cells, inner and outer hair cells (sensory), inner and outer phalangeal (Deiter) cells, outer limiting (Hensen) cells, and external supporting (Claudius) cells. With the exception of the sensory hair cells, all of the above-named cells have a supportive role. The hair cells are closely associated with the endings of the cochlear division of the vestibulocochlear nerve.

The columnar-shaped *border cells* rest on the tympanic lip of the spiral limbus, forming a single row on the inner side of the inner hair cells. Other than support, no particular function is known at this time.

The *inner and outer pillar cells* line a prominent triangular space, the *inner tunnel* (Corti). They have a broad base containing the nucleus and an elongated body packed with rigid tonofilaments that are attached to the cuticular plate on the free surface. The apex of the inner pillar cell is concave, whereas that of the outer pillar cell is convex; the two cells fit together much like a ball and socket (Fig. 8–11).

The sensory cells are in two groups: the inner hair cells form a single row adjacent to the inner pillar cells, and the outer hair cells lie in three to four rows just outside of the outer pillar cells.

The cylindric *outer hair cells* are slanted toward the inner tunnel (Fig. 18–12). From the apex of each cell is a bundle of approximately 100 stereocilia projecting from a prominent cuticular plate in a W pattern (V pattern in some mammals). The row of the longest stereocilia faces toward the stria vascularis; thus, these cells are morphologically polarized, much like the

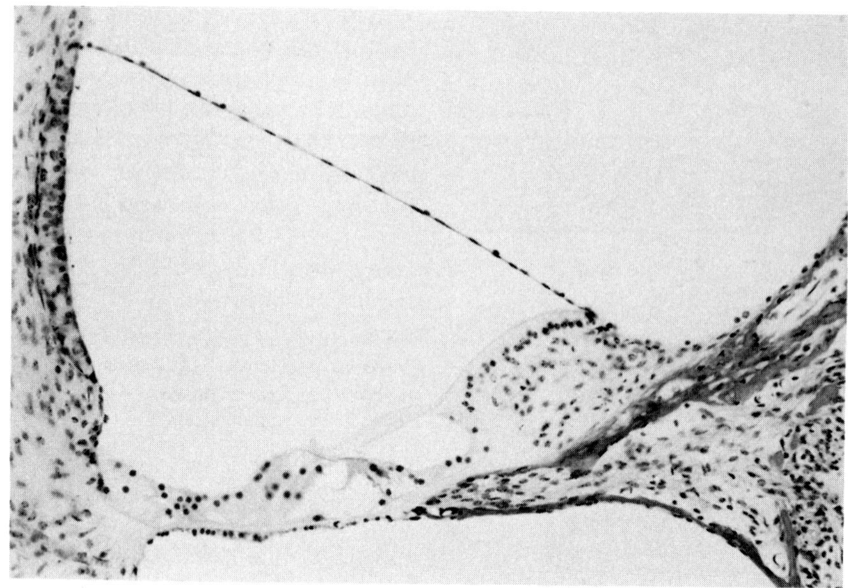

Fig. 18–10. *Scala media, guinea pig. The spiral organ rests on the basilar membrane. Compare this photograph with the drawing below for identification of cells and structure. H & E. ×165.*

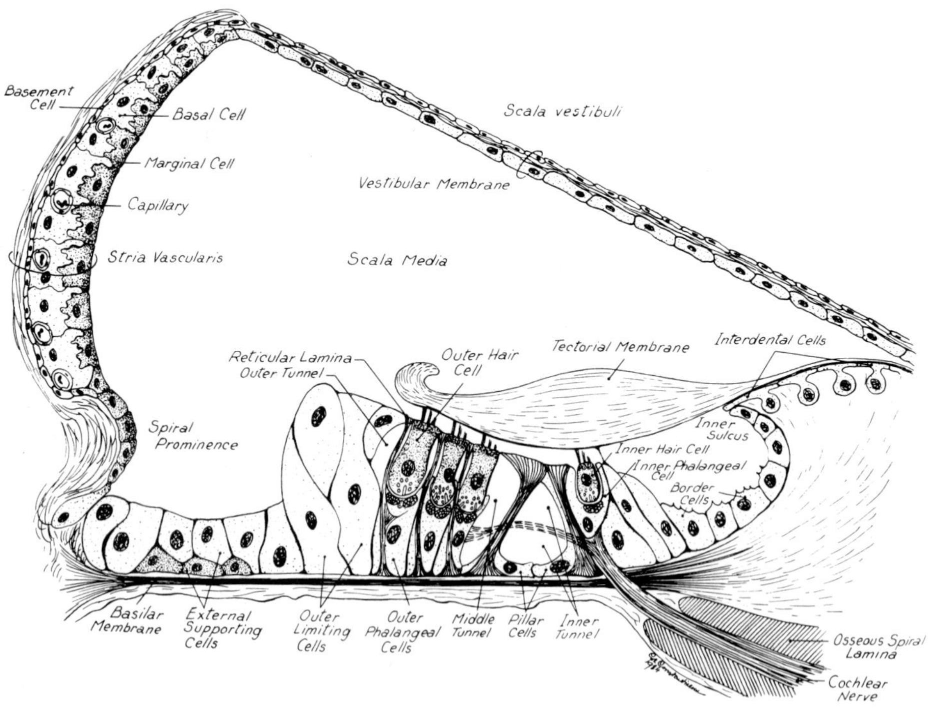

Fig. 18–11. *Spiral organ of hearing. (Modified and redrawn after P. Dallos: Handbook of Physiology. Am Soc Physiology section 1, Vol. 3, part 2, p. 601, 1984.)*

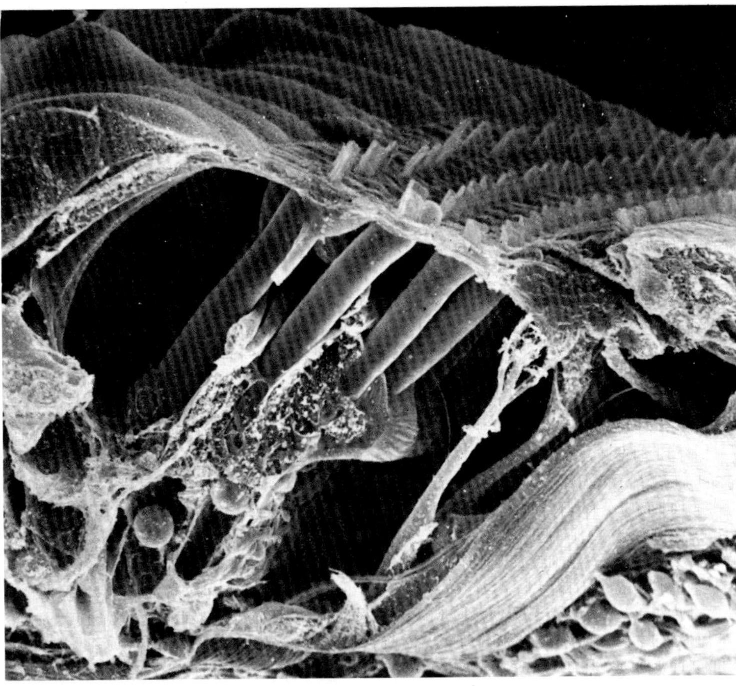

Fig. 18–12. *Scanning electron micrograph of the organ of Corti. (Reprinted by permission of the publisher from Weiss, L., Histology, Cell and Tissue Biology, 5th Ed., p. 1189. Copyright 1983 by Elsevier Science Publishing Co., Inc.)*

vestibular hair cells. At the base of the outer hair cells are a few afferent nerve endings and many efferent terminals containing vesicles. Both the inner and outer hair cells have synaptic ribbons identical to those seen in retinal cells where afferent synapses occur.

The *inner hair cells* are teardrop-shaped and their stereocilia form a straight row. At the base of these cells are many afferent nerve endings and a few efferent terminals. The inner hair cells are almost totally enveloped by *inner phalangeal cells,* and the outer hair cells are likewise enclosed by the *outer phalangeal cells.* These supportive cells rest on the basilar membrane and extend upward to cradle the base of the hair cell, then send long cytoplasmic processes toward the surface. The phalangeal cells have an elongated bundle of filaments originating from the basal cell membrane and extending to the apex. The phalangeal processes expand into a flat plate held to the hair cells by junctional complexes. The free surface of phalangeal cells and the hair cells, both of which have a massive terminal web, and the filamentous bundles in the phalangeal cells together make up a support structure, the *reticular lamina,* which holds the apical part of the hair cells rigid (Fig. 18–11).

The *outer limiting cells* and the *external supporting cells* complete the cellular component of the spiral organ. They are separated from the outer phalangeal cells by a space, *the middle tunnel* (space of Nuel).

Overlying the spiral organ is the *tectorial membrane,* a gelatinous structure extending from the spiral limbus over the hair cells. The lower surface of this membrane rests on the tips of the tallest stereocilia in each bundle. Where the tectorial membrane attaches to the spiral limbus are located the *interdental cells,* which apparently secrete the gel-like substance of the membrane.

Fibers from the spiral ganglion cells located in the osseous spiral lamina converge to form the cochlear division of the vestibulocochlear nerve. The peripheral processes of these ganglion bipolar cells course in bundles within the osseous spiral lamina, branch, and terminate in the spiral organ around the base of the hair cells.

MECHANISM OF HEARING

Sound vibrations impinge on the tympanic membrane, causing vibration at a given frequency. These vibrations are transmitted to the auditory ossicles and hence move the vestibular membrane. Because the perilymph is incompressible and lies in a bony chamber, the inward movement of the vestibular membrane produces pressure that is relieved by a compensating outward movement of the cochlear membrane. The transfer of such pressure changes are available by two routes: (1) sound waves transmitted as fluid pressure may travel the entire length of the scala vestibuli to join the scala tympani at the helicotrema and are then relieved by an outward bulging of the cochlear membrane, or (2) pressure waves may cross the vestibular membrane and transmit the energy to the endolymphatic fluid in the scala media, which in turn causes displacement of the basilar membrane. Embedded within the basilar membrane are stiff, reedlike fibers that are fixed at the basal but not at the distal end and hence vibrate at given frequencies. In general, low frequencies vibrate the basilar membrane near the apex, where the fibers are long and more limber, while high tones tend to move the membrane at the base, where the fibers are short and stiff. There is considerable overlap in this response to various frequencies along the basilar membrane so that the pitch and quality of a sound can be sorted out.

As stated previously, the hair cells are fixed in the reticular lamina, and the stereocilia of the outer hair cells are in contact with the tectorial membrane. Whenever the basilar membrane is deflected, the reticular lamina moves so that the hairs are moved by a shearing effect against the tectorial membrane. This is sufficient stimulus to translate mechanical energy into nerve impulses. Recent functional evidence suggests that the hairs of the inner sensory cells are embedded in the tectorial membrane and that they are probably velocity-sensitive. Moreover, the outer hair cells are thought to be concerned with the determination of sound intensity and the inner hair cells with pitch discrimination. Loudness of a sound is believed to be a function of the amount of basilar membrane in motion.

REFERENCES

Axelsson, A., and Vertes, D.: Vascular histology of the guinea pig cochlea. Acta Otolaryngol *85*:198, 1978.

Cazals, Y., Aran, J.-M., Erre, L.P., Guilhaume, A., and Aurousseau, C.: Vestibular acoustic reception in the guinea pig: A saccular function? Acta Otolaryngol *95*:211, 1983.

Dallos, P.: The Auditory Periphery. New York, Academic Press, Inc., 1973, pp. 196–211.

Flock, A.: Transduction in hair cells. *In* Handbook of Sensory Physiology. Edited by W.R. Loewenstein. Vol. 1, Principles of Receptor Physiology. Berlin, Springer-Verlag OHG, 1971, p. 396.

Hudspeth, A.J.: The hair cells of the inner ear. Sci Am *248*:154, 1983.

Johnson, W.H.: Experimental studies of otolithic function. Adv Otorhinolaryngol *20*:444, 1973.

Lindeman, H.H.: Anatomy of the otolith organs. Adv Otorhinolaryngol *20*:405, 1973.

Wilson, V.J., and Jones, G.M.: Mammalian Vestibular Physiology. New York, Plenum Press, 1979.

Index

Note: Numbers in *italics* indicate figures; numbers followed by a "t" indicate tables